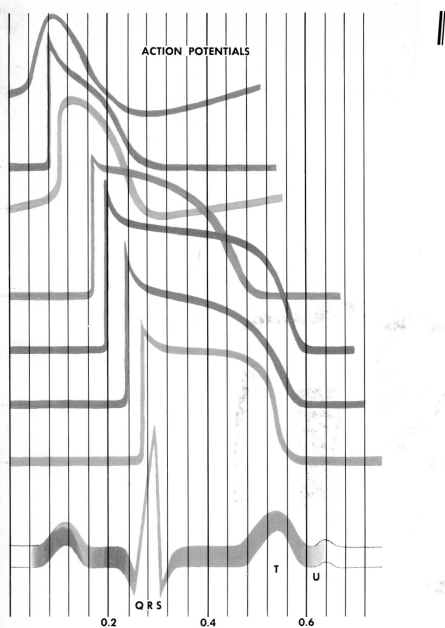

ACTION POTENTIALS

QRS

T

U

0.2   0.4   0.6

SECONDS

type of action potential to the normal electrocardiogram, and also the contribution of electrical activity in each type of cell to the ECG recorded from the body surface.

Activity of pacemaker fibres in the sinoatrial node precedes the first indication of activity in the electrocardiogram (the P wave) and cannot be demonstrated in the body-surface leads. Depolarization of atrial muscle fibres, in a sequence largely determined by the specialized atrial paths shown, causes the P wave. Repolarization of atrial fibres ordinarily is not seen in the ECG. Activity reaches the upper part of the A-V node early during the P wave. Propagation through the node is slow, and excitation of fibres in the His bundle does not occur until the middle of the P-R interval. The spread of activity through the common bundle, the bundle branches and parts of the Purkinje system precedes the earliest excitation of the ventricular muscle. There is no indication in the ECG of excitation of the fibres of the His-Purkinje system. The QRS complex results from activation of the muscle fibres of the ventricles. The isoelectric S-T segment corresponds to the plateau of the ventricular action potential, and the T wave results from repolarization of ventricular fibres. The U wave corresponds in time with repolarization of the specialized fibres of the bundle branches and Purkinje system, and it may reflect this event as recorded

at the body surface.

From these traces it is clear that, although the normal sequence of heart activation results from the anatomical distribution and unique electrical properties of specialized cardiac cells, there is no signal recorded in the electrocardiogram which corresponds to these events. Thus, the sequence of excitation of the specialized tissues can be determined only by implication when noting the temporal characteristics of the P and QRS complexes and their interrelationships. Finally, since excitation and the resulting depolarization cause contraction of the myocardial fibres, the coordinated mechanical activity of the heart depends on the anatomical distribution and the electrical properties of the specialized cardiac fibres.

This can now be further elucidated by recordings of His Bundle potentials at cardiac catheterization. NB Substances such as phosphate (see p. 54) affect conduction and the beating of the heart.

Resuscitation

Care of the Critically Ill

To Lesley

Dr David K. Brooks is an Editor of
Modern Emergency Department Practice.
(Edited by D. K. Brooks and A. J. Harrold).

Resuscitation

Care of the Critically Ill

Second Edition

David K. Brooks

MD (Lond.), PhD (Lond.), FRCPath, FACC, FACP
Consultant Physician, Accident and Emergency Department, St Mary's Hospital,
London and St Charles' Hospital, London.
Teacher in Emergency Medicine, University of London, St Mary's Hospital Medical School,
London.
Sub Dean, St Mary's Hospital Medical School, London.
Formerly Associate Professor of Medicine, Baylor College, Houston, Texas and University
of Texas in Houston.
Medical Director, Emergency Department and Cardiac Care Unit, Hermann Hospital,
Houston, Texas.

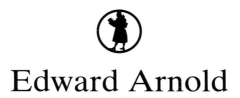

Edward Arnold

© David K. Brooks 1986

First published in Great Britain 1967 by
Edward Arnold (Publishers) Ltd,
41 Bedford Square,
London WC1B 3DQ

Second edition 1986

Edward Arnold (Australia) Pty Ltd,
80 Waverley Road,
Caulfield East,
Victoria 3145,
Australia

Edward Arnold,
3 East Read Street,
Baltimore,
Maryland 21202,
USA

British Library Cataloguing in Publication Data

Brooks, David K.
    Resuscitation.—2nd ed.
    1. Resuscitation
    I. Title
    615.8′043   RC86.7

ISBN 0-7131-4324-X

Whilst the advice and information in this book is
believed to be true and accurate at the date of going
to press, neither the authors nor the publisher can
accept any legal responsibility or liability for any
errors or omissions that may be made.

Text set in Times Roman Linotron 101
by Oxprint Ltd, Oxford
Printed in Great Britain by Butler & Tanner Ltd,
Frome, Somerset

Preface to the First Edition

The resuscitation of the seriously ill patient has three aspects of major importance and these are respiratory, cardiac and biochemical. Within the living organism the three are interdependent and a minor change in one may frequently produce a major change in the other two. When an endocrine disorder develops so that the water content of the body and the concentration of solutes is disturbed, cardiovascular function can become depressed and respiration impaired. Artificial ventilation of the lungs when performed incorrectly may so impair cardiac output and alter the body biochemistry that peripheral circulatory collapse is precipitated and death occurs. Many factors, therefore, must summate in order to improve the condition of the seriously ill patient and the neglect of any one of them may result in disaster.

Biochemical disturbances produce their own physical signs and what may appear to be relatively simple disorders, such as an excess or deficiency of water, may cause dramatic disturbances in the central nervous system, cardiovascular and respiratory systems. For example the violent convulsions and fits in a patient with water intoxication may, on their own, be indistinguishable from those of a patient with cerebral embolus or the more rare condition of magnesium deficiency, and in a similar manner it is possible to mistake the neurological signs in hepatic coma for cerebral thrombosis.

Doctors have become attuned to the concept that, in the presence of a metabolic acidosis, an increase in respiratory rate occurs and when there is a metabolic alkalosis the reverse process prevails. When this is examined in clinical practice we find that it is by no means true and this, perhaps somewhat heretical approach, is adopted in this book. The importance of changes in the osmolarity of body fluids is also stressed. Many of the numerous facets of acute disease processes are of importance in the after-care of patients who have suffered cardiac arrest or in preventing it from occurring and for this reason, this subject is dealt with fairly late in the book.

An understanding of physiological and pathophysiological processes is never of greater importance than in resuscitation and, wherever possible, an account of these factors is given before embarking upon treatment. An attempt is made to integrate the numerous aspects of practical resuscitation and scientific analysis so that treatment and investigation is more easily made. Repetition has not been excluded where the clarity has been considered to be necessary. On the other hand, only those aspects of a subject that are associated with the acute onset of a serious condition or its treatment have been covered and in this way much interesting material has been omitted.

London 1967   DKB

Acknowledgements to the First Edition

I am grateful to Professor W. T. Irvine of St Mary's Hospital who first suggested writing this monograph, the facilities he has given me and his continued encouragement. I am also grateful to Professor Roy Calne who independently suggested and encouraged the production of this work, and to Professor N. F. MacLagan and Mr Charles Drew for the facilities they have provided and their encouragement.

Permission to report the results from and the progress of patients which comprise case histories has kindly been given by Professor W. T. Irvine, Mr L. Lance Bromley and Mr J. R. Kenyon at St Mary's Hospital and Dr I. M. Anderson, Dr R. I. S. Bayliss, Mr R. Cox, Mr C. E. Drew, Mr E. H. Miles Foxen, Dr C. J. Gavey, Dr F. D. Hart, Mr P. H. Jones, Mr E. S. Lee, Dr R. D. Tonkin, and Mr G. Westbury. I am indebted to Mr G. Keen for the photographs of the patient with surgical emphysema and for the surgical details of the patient reported, and to Professor H. Ellis who gave access to his patients and assistance with some of the diagrams.

I am also grateful to Lt.-Col. S. H. Janikoun, R.A.M.C., for the early details of the patient with hydatid disease and for permission to report them, and to the Anaesthetic departments of both hospitals and particularly Professor G. S. W. Organe, Dr C. F. Scurr and Dr J. B. Wyman at Westminster and Dr C. A. Cheatle and Dr P. F. Knight at St Mary's.

I would like to thank Dr B. Strickland and his department for providing the X-rays, Dr P. Hansell and his photographic department for producing the illustrations and Dr D. C. O. James for his assistance with the chapter on Fibrinolysis.

I am particularly grateful to Miss Gillian Pentelow for the effort she has made in checking the references and successfully searching for obscure journals, Miss Ena Gallagher for her help and suggestions and Miss Margaret Wesson for the long hours she spent typing the manuscript.

The Welcome Historical Museum, *Anaesthesia*, the *Lancet* and the National Gallery kindly gave permission to reproduce some of the illustrations.

I would like to acknowledge the help and patient kindness I have had from the late Mr T. H. Clare, Miss B. Koster and Mr P. Bunyard of Messrs Edward Arnold.

Preface

During the time that has elapsed between publication of the 1st edition of this book and now, many changes have occurred in treatment and many advances have been made. In 1967 the routine use of beta-blockers, for example, had only just begun in Britain and their use in the USA was still restricted. Since that time of course practolol, although still used to treat acute arrhythmias when given intravenously, has been withdrawn from routine use, because of complications. Practolol was, however, used extensively for a considerable period of time and was found to be an extremely valuable anti-arrhythmic agent.

The hypoglycaemic agent phenformin has also been withdrawn, initially in the USA and later in Britain, although it is still used in other parts of the world. The treatment of lactacidosis, which results from phenformin administration, has therefore been included in this edition because visitors from abroad who are still taking this effective hypoglycaemic agent might be seen and because other preparations can have a similar effect.

Advances have been made in the field of cardiology, both in diagnosis and treatment, and the calcium blockers that are now available are a valuable adjunct in the treatment of hypertension, angina, acute cardiac arrhythmias and cardiomyopathies. Much more is now known about the pathophysiology of disease, and this has led to improved treatment. Similarly, the classification of anti-arrhythmic drugs by Vaughan Williams has allowed the clinician to have some knowledge of the action of some of the drugs he prescribes, although most are still given blindly based on clinical experience.

Advances have also been made in the understanding of the fluid compartments. The body fluid compartments have, quite correctly, been further subdivided. These subdivisions have, however, made the subject not only more difficult for the student to understand, but often confusing for the doctor who has to apply his knowledge to the seriously sick patient, frequently at speed with little warning. The volumes contained within the subdivisions are too small to influence therapy. I have therefore retained the basic subdivisions, popularized by Gamble, of intracellular, interstitial and vascular fluid compartments for the calculation of deficits of Na^+, H_2O and HCO_3^-, etc. and for explaining some of the pathophysiology of acute conditions.

The routine measurement of a number of biochemical parameters using automated analytical apparatus has alerted physicians to the consequences of changes of substances which were previously ignored, for example the plasma concentration of phosphate.

In critical care areas it is therefore important to have some knowledge of biochemistry, although a PhD in the subject is not necessary. It is important to have a knowledge of cardiology, although a precise study of all the congenital cardiac defects would normally be outside the scope of the attending physician in the critical care unit.

A study of the practical procedures, the effects and side-effects of drugs is, however, essential. The clinical management of the seriously ill patient is by no means a simple process and requires a breadth of knowledge that can only be obtained by taking an interest in the multiplicity of the problems that arise. Much work has been performed in this field, but there is scope for further research and clinical investigation. It is hoped that this book will encourage an interest in this field.

London 1986

DKB

Acknowledgements

In addition to those whom I acknowledged in the first edition, I am indebted to Mrs Margaret Ghilchik, BSc, MS, FRCS, at St Charles' Hospital, and Dr Barry Hulme, BSc, FRCP, for permission to publish details of their patients. Also to Dr Peter Cardew, MB BS from the Medical Illustration Department at St Mary's Hospital. I am also grateful to Dr John Kennedy, MD, for the photograph in the section on fat embolism.

I am indebted also for the earlier help in the preparation of this book that was given by Antoinette Jackson, BA, who searched the libraries to obtain original copies of early publications. Much help has been given to me in obtaining references for this book by the Chief Librarian at St Mary's Hospital, Mr Nigel Palmer, BA, ALA, and his assistants, Rachel C. Shipton, BA, ALA, and Sally E. Smith, BA, ALA, MLS. Julie Allum BA, ALA at St Charles' Hospital has also been of great assistance. I also have to thank Mrs Frances Daniels for spending long hours typing the manuscript, reading the proofs and checking the references.

I have to thank The *Lancet*, the CIBA Foundation, and the Year Book Medical Publishers for permission to reproduce some of the illustrations. I would also like to thank Mr John Atkinson for allowing me to publish the account, obtained from his family records, of surgery before anaesthesia.

London 1986   DKB

Contents

x   Contents

Chapter 1
Historical Outline to Resuscitation

The revival of the severely ill, the drowned, the dying and the dead has interested man since time began. The earliest account of the successful revival of the dead or dying was when Elisha breathed into the mouth of the son of the Shunammite woman and revived him (Fig. 1.1).[59]

Expired air ventilation has been used throughout history to expand the lungs of a subject who is not breathing and is the accepted practice in present-day methods of emergency treatment.

Until the work of Andreas Vesalius (1514–1564),[95] the teachings of Galen (AD 129–200) were accepted throughout the whole of Europe. This was with the encouragement of the Church which conferred the status of dogma upon his anatomical findings. Vesalius found these to be erroneous and that they applied mainly to animals. In 1543 he published De humani corporis fabrica libri septum and this aroused much heated dissent from the university physicians of Padua, who collectively denied the truth of his statements. Even his former teacher, Sylvius, joined forces against him and he left Padua for Madrid to become physician to the Emperor, Charles V, and on his death in 1556, to Philip II of Spain.

In the Fabrica he refuted Galenic teachings that when the thorax was opened, animals must necessarily die, and demonstrated that by artificial ventilation life could be maintained by insufflating air into the trachea.

William Harvey in 1628 observed that manual stimulation could restart the arrested heart of the pigeon.[43] These observations were made during his investigations into the anatomy of the vascular system. The resuscitation of the drowned person has been repeatedly attempted since the earliest times and the best method of doing so has been sought. In 1743 Heister's system of surgery[45] advocated the opening of the trachea with a scalpel to be followed by the blowing of air into the lungs either directly using the mouth or else via a tube. He noted that any delay was dangerous.

Dr Johnson reported that an Irish surgeon, called Glover, successfully resuscitated a tailor who had been hanged for street robbery in 1766.[56] He apparently incised both the temporal artery and

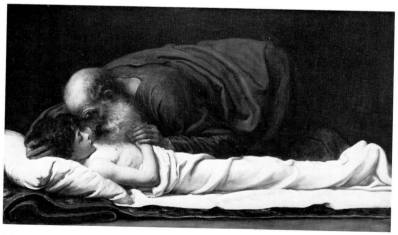

Fig. 1.1 'Elisha raising the son of the Shunammite.' Painting by Lord Leighton. (Reproduced by courtesy of the Royal Borough of Kensington and Chelsea Libraries and Arts Service, London.)

the external jugular vein. When blood failed to flow from both these incisions he proceeded to blow tobacco smoke into the rectum and to rub the body with spirits and with oil. When this treatment had been continued for 4 hours, he opened the trachea and blew vigorously into the lungs. After 20 minutes of this treatment the pulse became perceptible and a little later blood began to flow from the incised temporal artery. The tailor recovered sufficiently within 24 hours to walk a distance of 8 miles into the surrounding countryside and was thus able to elude the officers of the law who were searching for him.

James Boswell was an advocate but he was not always successful in his pleading. In 1773 some medical students from Edinburgh attempted to revive two of his clients called Brown and Wilson, who had been hanged for murder, by applying heat and by mouth-to-mouth ventilation.[9] This did not prove to be sufficiently effective. In the following year, Boswell approached Dr Munro in Edinburgh before the execution, to inquire the best way of setting about resuscitating John Reid who had been condemned to death for sheep stealing. Dr Munro advocated the application of heat, friction to start the blood flowing and blowing into the lungs. He suggested that preferably a hole should be cut into the trachea and air introduced by means of a pipe. Unfortunately, the resuscitative methods of Boswell on this occasion proved no more successful than his defence in court. However, in the same year Monsieur Janin of Paris successfully resuscitated two cases, one an infant who had suffocated in bed and the other a young man who had hanged himself in despair.[54] In both cases the method of resuscitation involved the application of artificial respiration, the blowing of tobacco smoke into the nostrils and the application of heat.

John Hunter also applied his fertile mind to the recovery of people who had been drowned and his recommendations were published in his monograph 'Proposals for the Recovery of Persons Apparently Drowned'.[52] He, quite correctly, believed that cardiac failure was caused by lack of ventilation and this was the cause of death. He described how he performed a tracheostomy on animals and introduced into the trachea a double action bellows which had a negative as well as a positive phase. He demonstrated that when he stopped the ventilation the heart went into arrest, but if he restarted the ventilation within a short period of time, then the heart would often beat again (Fig. 1.2). He also noted that electrical stimulation could restart the heart, but considered

A pair of double bellows were provided, conſtructed in ſuch a manner as by one action to throw freſh air into the lungs, and by another to ſuck out again the air which had been thrown in by the former, without mixing them together. The muzzle of theſe bellows was fixed into the trachea of a dog, and by working them he was kept perfectly alive. While this artificial breathing was going on, I took off the ſternum of the dog, and expoſed the lungs and heart; the heart continued to act as before, only the frequency of its action was conſiderably increaſed. When I ſtopped the motion of the bellows, the heart became gradually weaker and leſs frequent in its contractions, till it entirely ceaſed to move. By renewing the action of the bellows, the heart again began to move, at firſt very faintly, and with long intermiſſions; but by continuing the artificial breathing, its motion became as frequent and as ſtrong as at firſt. This proceſs I repeated upon the ſame dog ten times, ſometimes ſtopping for five, eight, or ten minutes, and obſerved that every time I left off working the bellows, the heart became extremely turgid with blood, the blood in the left ſide becoming as dark as that in the right; which was not the caſe when the bellows were working. Theſe ſituations of the animal appeared to me exactly ſimilar to drowning.

Fig. 1.2 Reproduced from the works of John Hunter.

it could only be applied as a last resort. He was critical of the use of tobacco smoke and of bleeding. In the same year he experimented with the induction of hypothermia, for it is to be noted that very often the person exposed to drowning was also very cold. He placed two carp in a glass vessel and froze them in winter. Both carp died, and he concluded that suspending animation in this way in man so that he could be revived many years later, was not possible.[53]

In 1764, in Wilkinson's Tutamen Nauticum, it was also concluded that death from drowning resulted from suffocation, even when no water was found in the lungs at post-mortem.[99] It was advocated that the patient should be stripped and a warm wrapping applied, that he should be held head downwards and shaken and the root of the tongue tickled with a feather so that he was stimulated to vomit and exhale any water contained in the stomach and air passages. Great stress was placed on ventilating the patient by blowing air through a variety of improvised tubes inserted into the mouth or nose. Here again tobacco smoke was employed as a means of stimulating circulation and respiration. Whitby, in his article 'Resuscitation in the North',[98] notes that in 1785 the doctors in Galloway Royal Infirmary purchased a resuscitation kit. This contained, amongst other things, an elastic leather blowpipe for inflating the lungs, an instrument for passing beyond the glottis and a blue leather tube for conveying fumes into the intestines. It also contained a bladder full of oxygen and a black leather tube for conveying medicines into the stomach.

In 1788 Kite presented a prize-winning essay on resuscitation to the Humane Society.[60] He discussed respiratory obstruction and pulmonary oedema in some detail and described an instrument for laryngeal intubation. Bellows could then be applied to the tube for ventilation, but he considered that those of the double acting type, described by Hunter, were no more effective than the simpler and cheaper ordinary forms. He stressed the importance of blowing air into the lungs for the reason of relieving congestion of the lungs and the work performed by the right side of the heart. Like John Hunter, Kite was critical of venesection and he believed that when no muscular response followed electrical stimulation, there was no possibility of recovery. It is interesting to observe that probably as a result of Kite's work the governors of the dispensary in Newcastle upon Tyne in 1789 issued pamphlets of instruction for the recovery of people apparently dead by drowning and suffocation or other causes. They circulated handbills containing short rules to be followed by any passer-by whose humanity might prompt him to give assistance. They also inserted an article on this subject in the Newcastle Advertiser. In addition, they established five receiving houses nearby the river at Newcastle and staffed them with medical assistants. They were equipped with a wooden pipe for expired air ventilation, a red leather tube with an ivory nozzle at one end for insertion into a nostril, a pair of bellows that could be attached to the other end of the tube and a black leather stomach tube. They also proposed to pay a premium of one shilling to any messenger who would bring the first surgeon to the drowned person and, as Whitby notes,[97] medical assistants were authorized to distribute a reward not exceeding 5 shillings to any person they employed to assist them, provided that they persevered by the means recommended for 4 hours or more. It was stressed that there were two essential factors in treatment, one was artificial respiration and the other the restoration of 'animal heat'. They also emphasized John Hunter's recommendation that by gently pressing the most prominent part of the windpipe backwards against the spine, the passage of air into the stomach, rather than the lungs, could be avoided. A silver catheter was also included in the resuscitation apparatus in the receiving houses and if artificial ventilation and friction were not effective, the removal of the patient to the receiving house was ordered so that the silver catheter could be inserted into the lungs and the bellows used. If necessary, a tracheotomy was to be performed, and while oxygen was preserved in bladders, it was considered to have little or no advantage over ordinary atmospheric air. If the patient was cold, rewarming was to take place slowly.

The success of these measures was first recorded in 1790, when a sailor fell into the Tyne, was taken from the water after 5 minutes and conveyed to the nearest receiving house. There the body was rubbed with warm flannels and had ether and volatile spirits applied to the temples. Hot bricks were applied to the feet. Whether artificial respiration was used is not noted, but the patient was observed to breathe after only 5 minutes and although he had various periods of apnoea and several convulsions, he made a complete recovery.

In the following year a child fell into the river and on being taken out of the water was quite lifeless. A surgeon in the village nearby inflated the lungs by mouth-to-mouth breathing, and signs of life soon appeared. He persisted, using the methods described in the Humane Society's pamphlet, and the child eventually recovered. As Whitby[97] notes, it is possible that the instructions of the Humane Society may not have had a wide public because of illiteracy, and successful resuscitation was infrequent, and by 1793 the 'preservation department' would only defray expenses that rescuers incurred if immersion of the subject in water had not been longer than 2 hours.

Although artificial respiration by means of blowing directly into the mouth or through a tube inserted into the nostril was described by Bell in his surgical textbook of 1785,[6] Ellis[30, 31] in Newcastle on Tyne, 83 years later, strongly advocated, on the grounds of simplicity, a method of artificial respiration described by Marshall Hall (Fig. 1.3).[41]

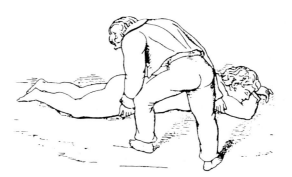

Fig. 1.3 The Marshall Hall method of artificial respiration. (Reproduced from the *Lancet*, 1856.)[41]

Herbert Williams, the Superintendent of the Hyde Park Receiving House, describes in a letter sent by Marshall Hall to the *Lancet* in February 1856,[42] how he attended St George's Hospital to watch a demonstration of the Marshall Hall method of artificial ventilation.

The mouth and one nostril were carefully closed by means of sticking-plaster to prevent the possibility of air finding its way through them. In the other nostril was inserted a caoutchouc tube about 3 feet long, at the end of which was fixed a bent glass tube of the same size, into which was poured a teaspoonful of water. The operator then took hold of the subject (who was lying in the prone position) by the left shoulder and hip and gently raised him until the whole body was resting on the 'right side'. This movement caused the air to enter the glass tube, creating bubbles in the water as it passed on into the lungs, and on the body being slowly replaced on the stomach, the air was freely expelled from the lungs and caused the same agitation in the water as it made its exit through the glass tube. Judging from the agitation, the quantity of air which passed into the lungs must have been considerable and quite sufficient for the purpose of artificial respiration. The great advantage of inflating the lungs by means of the rotatory movement or raising the body by the one shoulder and hip, is the readiness with which one person can perform the operation in the absence of any other assistance. This experiment appeared to be perfectly satisfactory.

The other method was then tried by raising the subject by the two shoulders, until the stomach was freed from any pressure, on a table, and then gently lowered down again. This movement produced precisely the same results as the rotatory, but required more strength to perform it.

By the early nineteenth century, the importance of ventilating the lungs with air was well established and resuscitation boxes were available containing endotracheal tubes and bellows very similar or identical to the fireside bellows that had been used by Paracelsus many years earlier. The annual report of the Royal Humane Society in 1824[86] illustrates the contents of such a box (Fig. 1.4) and the case in which it was stored (Fig. 1.5).

Another practice, that of rolling the patient to and fro on a barrel (Fig. 1.6a and b), was popular for many years and was practised from the seventeenth century to the early part of this century.[58] It was still used, even after it had been condemned by the Royal Humane Society in 1817, when it was considered to be ineffective and a waste of time.

Movement of the abdominal contents against the diaphragm was later advocated by Eve in 1932.[32] The patient was placed on a plank or door and rocked through an angle of 45°, head down, then head raised. The Eve method, or rocking bed, was still being used in the late 1950's in

APPARATUS FOR RESUSCITATION

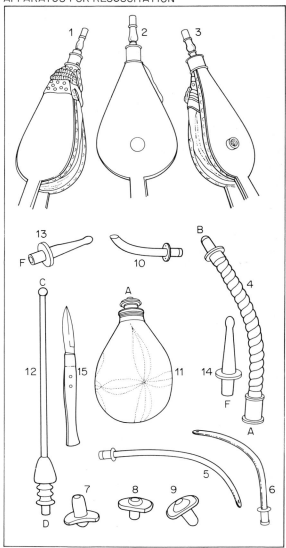

Fig. 1.4 Apparatus for resuscitation. **1**, **2** and **3** are different views of a pair of bellows, for inflating the lungs. **4**: a short flexible tube for conveying air into the lungs; **A**, the inferior extremity, to be attached to the nosel of the bellows; **B**, the other extremity, plugs into the silver tubes (**5** and **6**) and the nostril pipes (**7**, **8** and **9**) for inflating. **10**: a curved tube to be inserted into an artificial opening in the trachea, when it is thought proper to perform the operation of tracheotomy; and is to be connected with the bellows through the intervention of the flexible tube (**4**). **11**: an elastic bottle for injecting fluids into the stomach through the flexible tube (**12**); **A**, the mouth of the bottle, to be attached to the extremity of the flexible tube at **D**. **12**: a flexible tube (of the same composition as flexible catheters) to be introduced into the oesophagus for conveying spirits, etc. into the stomach, before the power of

swallowing be returned; **C**, the extremity, to be passed down the oesophagus; **D**, the other extremity, to be connected with the elastic bottle at **A**, containing the fluid to be injected. **13** and **14** are two clyster pipes for administering enemas: they fit at **F** into the elastic bottle at **A**. **15**: a scalpel for performing the operation of tracheotomy. (Reproduced by permission of the Royal Humane Society from their Report of 1824.) Instruments could be stored in a wooden box (see Fig. 1.5). The contents are clearly listed in the Royal Humane Society's Report.

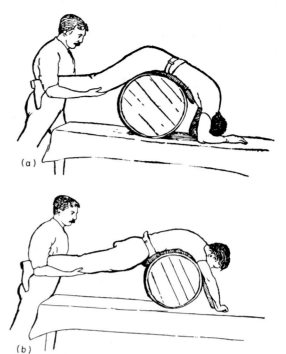

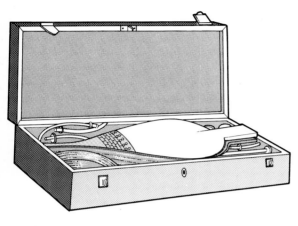

Fig. 1.5 The case in which the instruments listed in Fig. 1.4 could be stored and transported. (Reproduced by permission of the Royal Humane Society.)

Fig. 1.6 A barrel was used for many years and was popular during the eighteenth century. The expiratory phase is depicted in (a), and the inspiratory phase in (b). (Reproduced from the *Lancet*, 1909.)[58]

Britain to assist patients with respiratory insufficiency due to poliomyelitis.

The agony of surgery before anaesthesia is well illustrated by the records of the Higginbotham family, kindly loaned to the author by Mr John Atkinson.[3] Part of the account is reproduced in Fig. 1.7.

It may not be improper to state that William, son of the first-named Samuel Higginbotham, had been for some years sorely afflicted with stone in the bladder. Dr C. White of Manchester, having clearly ascertained its position and magnitude, repeatedly told him that there was no cure but by cutting. This operation he long resisted until worn out by the most excruciating pain and after having in vain the nostrums of every pretender who offered himself he at last consented to the truly dreaded operation in 1772. A number of relatives and friends came on the occasion. Dr White with his usual firmness, attended by two other surgeons, directed him to be placed on his back upon a strong table with his hands and feet fastened to each other to prevent him from offering any resis-

tance or obstruction during the operation. The gash was made between the privates and seat, this gave him but little pain compared with the extraction of the stone, which was literally torn from the part to which it was grown on the neck of the bladder (to which it was firmly cemented during its growth) by a strong clasp instrument. The first and second efforts failed and the instrument flew off the stone. This gave the sufferer the most indescribable pain and he begged with all the powers of persuasion and cries to be allowed to expire, and offered the doctor all his worldly property to allow it. To this the doctor answered 'I must go through my work'. He again placed his knee against the table and forcibly tore it out and also a smaller one which was forming but this dissolved. The other was much of the form of a hen's egg, but flatter. It measured 6½ inches round the long part and 3¾ round the middle, was a greyish or light brown colour and very rough resembling a moor stone. On being kept it reduced in size. The sufferer was put to bed with folded sheets under him which were frequently drawn from under the part. 8 pairs of sheets were constantly from the part to which it was grown on the neck of the bladder, (to which it was firmly cemented during its growth) by a strong clasp instrument. The first and second efforts failed and the instrument flew off the stone. This gave the sufferer the most indescribable pain, and he begged with all the powers of persuasion & cries to be allowed to expire, and offered the Dr all his worldly property, to allow it. To this the Dr answered "I must go through my work." he again placed his knee against the table and forcibly tore it out and also a smaller one, which was forming but was dissolved. The other was much of the form of a hen's egg, but flatter. It measured 6½ inches round the long part and 3¾ round the middle, was a greyish or light brown colour and very rough resembling a moor stone. On being kept it reduced in size.

Methodist New Connexion, and was the founder and liberal Supporter of several of their institutions. He was punctual

B.J.O.

Fig. 1.7 Part of the record of the Higginbotham family describing lithotomy before anaesthesia. (Reproduced with permission from J. Atkinson.)

in use and wash. The Dr left a young gentleman that was nearly loose from his apprenticeship for a whole fortnight and himself attended from Manchester 8 miles every day for 3 weeks and twice in one day on expecting him to die, and our relative Dr Lees frequently attended and gave great assistance throughout. His cries were heard by the family at nearly the bottom of the adjoining meadow to where they had been requested to withdraw. All his urine passed through the wound 8 weeks & 13 weeks in part. He, however, contrary to every expectation slowly recovered & survived 8 years without any repetition of the complaint. It was considered the first cure ever performed in this part of the country. Dr White said he never before had cut any of that complaint that was so far gone that recovered. Dr White's charge was 50 guineas and other expenses of the same amount, which, at that period was considered a large amount of money.

There is evidence that the chloroform anaesthesia was first used by Mr Holmes Coote at St Bartholomew's Hospital in the Spring of 1847[93] and was introduced into Edinburgh by Sir James Simpson in the latter part of that year. Its early use was associated with deaths and four deaths were reviewed by Simpson in 1848.[89] He believed that death was due to paralysis of the heart. One death that occurred was of a girl of 15 years of age called Hannah Greener who died when she had a toe-nail removed under chloroform anaesthesia. Murray[75] says that Simpson attributed the death to asphyxia because of the inhalation of brandy and water. This is probably the first case of cardiac arrest to occur as a result of general anaesthesia and was on 28 January 1848. Some deaths occurred when ether was introduced into general anaesthesia in America in 1846, and the Boston Society for Medical Improvement analysed, in 1860, 41 deaths that followed the use of this substance.

Deaths due to general anaesthesia, especially chloroform, encouraged Moritz Schiff to study the effects of cardiac arrest and how it might be treated.[87] He observed that when chloroform was used as an anaesthetic, cardiac arrest would often occur before the onset of respiratory failure and that respiratory depression, due to chloroform, was not reversible. This was unlike respiratory depression which occurred from using too high a concentration of ether. He also described the process of manual cardiac massage and noted that resuscitation could be produced even after several minutes and that the heart would undergo ventricular fibrillation before it returned to a normal beat. Cardiac massage in man, after death during anaesthesia, was attempted in 1889 by Niehaus in Berne[77] and in 1898 by Tuffier and Hallion in France[94] and in 1900 by Prus in Austria.[84] Probably the first successful case of resuscitation using internal cardiac massage was performed in Norway in 1901 when a woman died during an operation for carcinoma of the uterus.[57] In Britain the first patient to be resuscitated successfully after death during ether anaesthesia for appendicectomy, was a 65-year-old man reported by Starling in 1902.[92] Further successful accounts of resuscitation then followed and the probability of restoration of a normal heart beat became greater when Beck[5] electrically defibrillated a human heart after 75 minutes of cardiac massage. Since that time external cardiac massage and external electrical defibrillation have been developed (see p. 000). However, it is apparent that the value of an electric shock had been recorded very much earlier. John Currie,[19] in addition to investigating artificial ventilation of the lungs (he reported a successful case in his book in 1790), also advocated the use of electricity in resuscitation. In the annual report of the Royal Humane Society, London, he concluded:

This recommendation [for the use of electric current in cases of apparent death] does not depend upon mere theory but is drawn from instances of its success in real cases as well as in experiments made upon fowls and other small animals, which, after being completely deprived of sense and motion by a strong electrical shock passed through the heart or chest, were perfectly recovered by transmitting *slighter* shocks through the same parts: and in this way animation has been suspended and restored alternately, for a considerable number of times.

It is apparent that Galen was aware of the operation of tracheotomy and it is known that it was practised in the twelfth and thirteenth centuries. It was most commonly performed for resuscitation of people found drowned. Although the blowing of air into the open trachea by means of a tube inserted through the opening was practised from very early times, Paracelsus (1493–1541) is usually credited with the introduction of the common fireside bellows as a means of ventilation of the lungs. The opening of the windpipe and thus saving the life of a patient near to death because of an abscess which was obstructing the trachea, was described by Antonius Musa Brassabola (1500–1570).[13]

In the National Gallery in London hangs 'A Mythological Subject' (Catalogue No. 698) a painting by Piero di Cosimo, a Florentine artist who lived from about 1462 until 1521. He was a contemporary of Leonardo da Vinci (1452–1519) and doubtless had a good knowledge of anatomy. The painting (Figs. 1.8 and 1.9) portrays a Satyr kneeling at the head of a woman upon whom a tracheotomy had been performed. In Eastlake's Notebook (1858) it is referred to as 'The Death of Procris'. However, sitting at her feet is a retriever and in the background is a river. It would appear to be highly probable that the painting really depicts a successful attempt at resuscitation after drowning.[49] It is clear from the position of the hands and the rest of the body that the woman, although unconscious, is alive, but blood has been painted in such a way that it indicates that the opening in the throat was made while the subject was in an upright position. It is possible that this is the earliest pictorial record of a tracheotomy.

When an epidemic of diphtheria hit Naples, Marco Aurelio Severino (1580–1656) repeatedly performed tracheotomies to relieve obstruction. This operation had been recommended for the condition by Guidi (1500–1567) and Fabricius (1560–1654).[13] Since these early times tracheotomy has become a refined surgical procedure which has taken its place in medical practice for conditions such as acute respiratory failure and where positive pressure respiration has to be maintained for a prolonged period.

Because Britain was a seafaring nation and many of its sailors were exposed to cold when their ships came to grief, much interest was taken in this country in this aspect of resuscitation. In addition to experimenting with carp, John Hunter outlined in letters to Jenner in 1776, experiments that could be made on hedgehogs when hibernating.[53] The physiological effects of the immersion of man in cold water were studied by Currie,[20] who hoped that he could determine the cause of death from exposure following shipwreck. In 1803 Spallanzani investigated hypothermia in both non-hibernating and naturally hibernating animals, such as the porcupine, bat, dormouse and musk rat.[91] He observed that on cooling, the heart of the animals stopped, respiration ceased and, when they were placed in an oxygen-free atmosphere when cold, the bat especially was able to survive on rewarming. Walther[96] in 1862 observed that analgesia developed at approximately 25°C when rabbits were cooled and that at 20°C the rate of beating of the heart was reduced to 16–20/min. He also found that artificial respiration was necessary if the animals were to survive. Pembrey and Hale-White in 1896 showed that reduction in metabolism occurred at low temperatures and that less CO_2 was produced.[80] Simpson in 1902, cooled monkeys[90] which had been anaesthetized with ether to below 14°C and two of these survived. He observed that at 25°C the animal was insensitive to pain and that respiration ceased before the heart beat. Fay in 1940 cooled a patient with advanced cancer to a temperature in the region of 22–23°C for several days and was able to observe that the patient became free from pain and lethargic.[33] In 1950, after a series of experiments, Bigelow et al.[7] were the first to suggest that recovery from cooling to 28°C was relatively so safe that it could be used for open-heart surgery in man.

Because primitive man was unaware of the function of blood and the circulation itself and because loss of blood was so obviously associated with

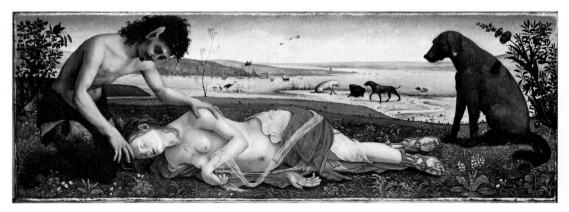

Fig. 1.8   Painting by Piero di Cosimo that hangs in the National Gallery in London, of what may be the first pictorial record of a tracheotomy. Piero di Cosimo was a contemporary of Leonardo da Vinci (1452–1519). (Reproduced by permission of the National Gallery.)

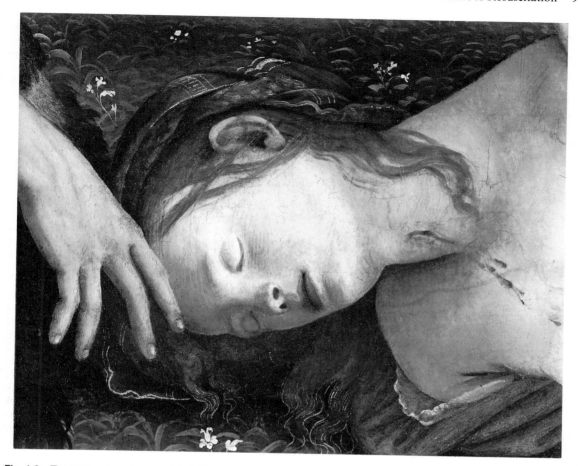

Fig. 1.9   The tracheotomy in more detail. (Reproduced by permission of the National Gallery.)

stupor, unconsciousness and death, it was invested from the earliest times with mystical qualities. Because it was considered that its character determined both the physical and mental characteristics of both man and animals, it played a great part in folklore, mythology and magic. It was common-place to prepare draughts of the blood from gladiators or animals slain in combat in order to acquire their strength and courage.

It is difficult to date accurately the time when the first blood transfusion was performed, but William Harvey[43] published his work on the circulation of blood in man in 1628, having described it at least 12 years earlier. It is probable that direct transfusion of blood into man had been attempted some 10 years previously. In 1628 Johannes Colle suggested blood transfusion as a means of resuscitation.[14] He was then a Professor at the University of Padua. In 1680 Francesco Folli,[34] a Florentine physician, published a work stating that he had been aware of William Harvey's treatise and was the originator of blood transfusion in man. Francis Potter, the Vicar of Kilmanton in Somerset, considered the concept of curing disease by blood transfusion in 1640, but when writing on the subject in 1652 had still achieved little success in the preparation of blood for transfusion.[4, 100]

In 1666 Pepys recorded in his diary his observations on blood transfusion:[81]

November 16th, 1666: "This noon I met with Mr. Hooke and he tells me the dog which was filled with another dog's blood is very well and likely to be so as ever, and doubts not its being of great use to men; and so do Dr. Whistler who dined with us at the taverne." (Dr Whistler was President of the Royal College of Physicians in 1683).

November 21st: "With Creed to a tavern

where dean Wilkins and others: and good discourse: among the rest of a man who is a little frantic, hath been a kind of minister now poor and debauched, hired for 20 shillings to have some of the blood of a sheep let into his body. They propose to let in about twelve ounces which they compute is what will be let in in a minute's time by a watch."

Another early account of an experimental blood transfusion that has been well recorded is that of Lower,[68] which was published in 1669. He describes the repeated bleeding of a small dog and repeated transfusion of this dog from the artery of two mastiffs used in turn. The artery of the mastiff was connected by a tube to a vein in the bled dog and after the repeated bleedings and re-transfusion and the vein having been repaired, the animal was able to get up and behave normally. Blood transfusions also appear to have been made 2 years earlier (1667) by Jean Denis,[26] Professor at Montpellier University and physician to Louis XIV. These workers were misguided in that the blood groups of the dog are of small consequence. Denis transfused the blood of a lamb into more than one human until the incompatibility of the two bloods caused one patient to die and for proceedings to be taken against him. In most of the experiments that were performed at this time a quill was used in order to transfer the blood from the donor animal to the recipient. Clotting usually occurred within the lumen, and venospasm, which resulted from the incompatibility, prevented too large a volume being transferred, so that in many cases a potentially dangerous situation was averted. Numerous accounts after this time include either descriptions or illustrations of transfusion of animal blood to man. This is probably because the procedure had gained notoriety and authors felt that it should be included. Even after the experience of Denis and the work of Blundell,[8] who showed at Guy's Hospital the incompatibility of blood transfused from one animal to another of a different species, accounts of the feasibility of using animal blood in man still appeared, and even as late as 1874, papers by Gesellius and Hasse were published advocating the use of lamb's blood.[35,44] In Britain, however, in 1857 Higginson produced his syringe for the purpose of blood transfusion from one person to another and this was used on numerous occasions.[48] The syringe is now used for other purposes and is better known to the nursing profession for the syringing of ears and sometimes still for the giving of enemas. With the advent of extracorporeal circulations becoming more widely used for purposes of resuscitation, the feasibility

of setting up such a Higginson syringe for left atrial to left femoral bypass of the heart and in so doing relieving the myocardium of its strain, the syringe, made of a plastic material, may return to its original function.

In August 1840, Mr Samuel Lane, a noted and respected surgeon at St George's Hospital Medical School in London, treated severe postoperative bleeding in an 11-year-old boy suffering from haemophilia by means of blood transfusion.[66] This inherited, sex-linked disorder of the coagulation of the blood, is now known to be a deficiency of Factor VIII. It has, however, been described throughout history, for example by Abulcasis (936–1013), in his treatise of medicine and surgery which was published in 1519.[1] The tendency to haemorrhage in the male members of certain families was reported in North America by Otto in 1803.[78] He concluded that it was probably transmitted by females. By 1820, the inheritance of the disease via the female was clearly established.[76] The clinical forms of the disease were, however, first described by Grandidier in 1855, and he gave it the name haemophilia.[36]

The boy named George Firmin was operated on by Samuel Lane 'to relieve the deformity of squinting'. He bled for 6 days and, as a last resort, Lane decided to transfuse blood from a 'stout, healthy young woman' who was bled by opening a vein in the arm with a lancet and the blood being allowed to fall into the funnel of Lane's transfusion syringe (depicted in Fig. 1.10). During the transfusion the pulse, which had previously been imperceptible, returned to the wrist and 'in the course of an hour or two, the boy sat up in bed and drank a glass of wine and water from his own hand'. There was no recurrence of bleeding. The account is not only interesting, it is also surprising because we know today that there would be, in all probability, an insufficient concentration of Factor VIII to have been effective, even if George Firmin had, what would appear to have been, one of the milder forms of haemophilia.

The presence of agglutinins and iso-agglutinins in the blood was detected by Landsteiner[65] in Vienna in 1901 and Shattock[88] in London in 1900 working independently. It required a further 6 years before Jansky[55] in Prague identified the four blood groups, O, A, B and AB. This work was repeated by Moss[73] in 1910. It appeared at that time that the major problems governing the transfusion of blood from one person to another had been solved and that blood replacement would immediately neutralize blood loss. However, apart from the difficulties of setting up blood

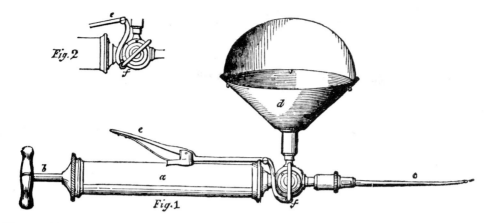

Fig. 1.—The syringe, with its pipe and funnel ready for use. *a,* the cylinder; *b,* the piston; *c,* the pipe, the extremity of which is introduced into the vein; *d,* the funnel; *e,* the lever which acting on *f,* the stop-cock opens or closes the communication of the syringe with the funnel or pipe as may be required.

Fig. 1.10 The syringe used by Mr Lane in his case of bleeding diathesis in 1840. *Fig. 2* in the diagram represents the stop-cock turned by the depression of the lever (*e* in *Fig. 1*). (Reproduced by permission of the *Lancet*.)[66]

banks and the organization of numerous suitable donors, a suitable anticoagulant had to be found. Sodium phosphate had been used by Braxton Hicks working at Guy's Hospital in 1863, but was too poisonous for use.[46,47] In 1891 Wright recommended the use of oxylated blood in man after experiments on dogs.[101] Sodium citrate was investigated just before the First World War and Agote gave his first transfusion of citrated human blood on 14 November 1914.[2] It was, however, not until 1917 that citrated blood was used in military hospitals in France and credit for this must be given to Oswald H. Robertson, a Canadian medical officer who produced the 'Robertson bottle'.[85] This was a large bottle of almost 2 pints capacity having a rubber bung pierced by three tubes. One of these tubes was connected by a short length of rubber tubing which ended in a wide-bore needle, through which blood flowed to be mixed with citrate inserted through one of the remaining two tubes in the bung. The remaining tube was connected to a Higginson's syringe, which could produce either positive or negative pressure in the bottle, so that it could be reversed for either taking or giving blood. It was soon found that not all forms of shock could be corrected by means of blood transfusion.

The work of Cannon in 1918 was a major step in those early days in elucidating some of the causes of the incompleteness of success.[10,11] As blood transfusions became more easily available, Cannon's work was forgotten, until in more recent times its importance has been recognized once more.

One of the earliest measurements of blood pressure, both venous and arterial, was performed by Stephen Hales (1677–1761). He also demonstrated the fall of blood pressure associated with haemorrhage.[40]

'6. Then laying bare the left carotid artery, I fixed to it towards the heart the brass pipe, and to that the wind-pipe of a goose; to the other end of which a glass tube was fixed, which was 12 feet 9 inches long. The design of using the wind-pipe was by its pliancy to prevent the inconveniences that might happen when the mare struggled, if the tube had been immediately fixed to the artery, without the intervention of this pliant pipe.

7. There had been lost before the tube was fixed to the artery, about 70 cubick inches of blood. The blood rose in the tube in the same manner, as in the case of the two former horses, til it reached 9 feet 6 inches height. I then took away the tube from the artery, and let out by measure 60 cubick inches of blood; and then immediately replaced the tube to see how high the blood would rise in it after each evacuation; this was repeated several times till the mare expired, as follows, viz.:

The Several Trials	Cubick Inches let out	Perpendicular Height after each Evacuation	
		Feet	Inches
1	70	9	6
2	130	7	10
3	190	7	6
4	250	7	3
5	310	6	5
6	370	4	9
7	430	3	9
8	490	3	$4\frac{1}{2}$
9	550	2	$9\frac{1}{2}$
10	610	3	$2\frac{1}{2}$
11	670	*4	5
		2	$9\frac{1}{2}$
12	730	3	6
13	790	3	5
14	820	2	0
15	833	2	5

*Deep Sighing raised the Blood. When the Force of the Blood was thus small, then faint Sweats came on.
Very faint.
Now expired.

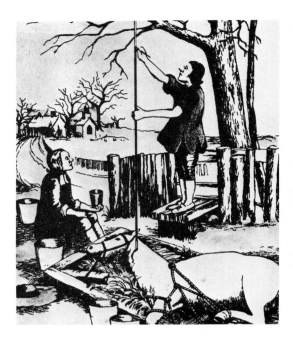

Fig. 1.11   The third experiment of Stephen Hales (1733), in which a glass tube was connected to the carotid artery of a horse that had been thrown and tied to a farm gate. (Reproduced by permission of the *Medical Times*, November 1944.)

8. We may observe that these three horses all expired, when the perpendicular height of the blood in the tube was about two feet.

9. These 833 cubick inches of blood weigh 31.82 pounds, and are equal to 14.4 wine quarts, the large veins in the body of the mare were full of blood, there was some also in the descending aorta, and in both ventricles and auricles.'

His own description is self-explanatory and is illustrated in Fig. 1.11. An indication of the blood pressure pulse wave was obtained by Landois (1872),[64] and it can be seen[69] that the pulse wave including the anacrotic notch was clearly demonstrated by this simple method (Fig. 1.12). Use of Korotkoff sounds is now universal. Shortly before the 'hemautogram' of Landois, but 100 years after the work of Stephen Hales, Poiseuille introduced his mercury manometer in 1828.[82] This was followed by the use of the kymograph by Ludwig in 1847.[70]

An inflatable cuff placed on the upper arm above the superficial part of the brachial artery, using the sounds described by Korotkoff[61,62] in Russia, has allowed the universal measurement of blood pressure by manometric means. Electrical transducers are today in common use in critical care units for the measurement of systemic arterial blood pressure, but the simple manometric method is still widely used for the measurement of central venous pressure in a manner similar to that of Stephen Hales. In his original description, he demonstrated that physical effort, which thereby raised the intrathoracic pressure, produced a marked rise in the venous pressure. Today, in clinical practice, a more accurate assessment from a constant baseline is required.

A further important step in medicine was the isolation of heparin. It was discovered by a medical student, Jay McLean, in 1916.[71]

I went one morning to the door of Dr. Howell's office, and standing there (he was seated at his desk), I said, 'Dr. Howell, I have discovered antithrombin'. He smiled and said, 'Antithrombin is a protein, and you are working with phosphatides. Are you sure that salt is not contaminating your substance?' . . . I told him that I was not sure of that, but it was a powerful anticoagulant. He was most skeptical. So I had the Diener, John Schweinhant, bleed a cat. Into a small beaker full of its blood I stirred all of the proven batch of heparphosphatides, and placed this on Dr. Howell's laboratory table

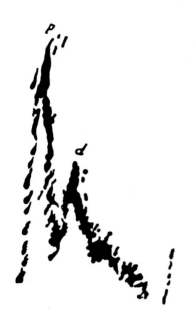

Fig. 1.12 The 'hemautogram', which established the presence of the dicrotic wave (d), was made by Landois by spraying blood from a needle placed in the tibial artery of a dog on to paper mounted on a rotating drum.

and asked him to tell me when it clotted. It never did clot.

McLean described his discovery of the anticoagulant in February 1916 in a talk to the Medical Society of Philadelphia and later in an article 'The Thromboplastic Action of Cephalin'.

Later, in 1918, Howell and Holt[50] published their classic paper on heparin. However, the value of heparin was not appreciated until 1936 when the pioneer vascular surgeon, Gordon Murray in Toronto, understood the immense benefit that it would have in clinical practice.[74]

Without heparin, extracorporeal circulation, such as the artificial kidney and the heart–lung machine, would not have been possible, although this substance may now be replaced by prostacyclin. Much vascular surgery would also not have been possible.

The concept of inserting sutures into blood vessels originated more than two centuries ago. Lambert suggested it to his surgeon colleague, Mr Hallowell, who repaired a damaged artery in the arm of one of his patients.[63] There appears to have been no further work in this field for more than 100 years until the use of the phenol spray by Lister to prevent sepsis. There then followed the repair of a damaged internal jugular vein,[21] the repair of a wound to the femoral artery,[83] and treatment of an aneurism of the brachial artery by Matas in 1888.[72]

The methods to be used for the suturing of blood vessels were advanced by Carrel,[12] and numerous other surgeons clearly demonstrated the feasibility of excising a segment of artery and restoring the continuity of blood flow following the end-to-end anastomosis of arterial grafts. In 1944, Craafoord and Nylin[18] in Sweden and Gross[37] in Boston reported the successful treatment of coarctation of aorta by end-to-end anastomosis. A short time later the use of homografts to replace the deficiency that resulted following excision of a coarctation was reported by Hufnagel[51] and by Gross and his co-workers.[38,39] Leriche identified the problems associated with occlusion of the abdominal aorta and suggested the possibility of surgical excision.[67] The first report of the treatment of occlusive disease of the lower abdominal aorta by excision and homograft replacement was that of Oudot in Paris (1951).[79] The following year, Dubost and his colleagues in Paris performed the first successful resection of an aneurysm of the abdominal aorta and its replacement with a homograft.[27]

Homografts, however, were found to have a number of serious disadvantages and this resulted in the development of a number of plastic substitutes, until the introduction of the woven Dacron graft in 1954,[22] which has proved to be satisfactory.[23–25]

Other forms of vascular surgery have developed.[15–17] The first carotid endarterectomy was performed by Mr H. H. G. Eastcott at St Mary's Hospital, London, in 1954[28] for the relief of stroke. Since then, vascular surgery has developed and expanded so that it can relieve many life-threatening and dangerous conditions. The patient reported by Eastcott *et al.* in 1954 remained well and free from all neurological symptoms until the time of her death in 1974, at the age of 84 from old age and heart disease.[29]

The various aspects of resuscitation have progressed more rapidly in recent times so that, as our knowledge of pathophysiology increases and new techniques develop, the probability of successfully reviving a severely ill person is very much greater. The scientific and humanitarian approach to this problem that was so outstanding in the efforts of the early clinicians and experimenters who had so little knowledge and equipment available to them, must be continued in our present time now that we have such improved facilities for research. Death itself in its early stages should be regarded only as an illness of penultimate severity.

References

1. Abulcasis (1519). *Liber theorucae*. S. Grimm and M. Vuirsung, Augsburg.
2. Agote, L. (1914–15). Nouveau procédé pour la transfusion du sang. *An. Inst. Clin. méd., B. Aires,* **1**, 25.
3. Atkinson, J. (1981). *Personal records of the Higginbotham family, 1772*. Private communication.
4. Aubrey, J. (1898). *Brief lives chiefly of contemporaries set down by J. Aubrey between 1669 and 1696*, Vol. **2**, p. 166. Oxford: Clarendon Press.
5. Beck, C. S. and Mautz, F. R. (1937). The control of heart beat by the surgeon; with special reference to ventricular fibrillation occurring during operation. *Ann. Surg.,* **106**, 525.
6. Bell, B. (1785). *A system of surgery*, 2nd edn, Vol. **2**, p. 414. Edinburgh: Elliot.
7. Bigelow, W. G., Lindsay, W. K. and Greenwood, W. F. (1950). Hypothermia, its possible role in cardiac surgery: an investigation of factors governing survival in dogs at low body temperatures. *Ann. Surg.,* **132**, 849.
8. Blundell, J. (1829).Successful case of transfusion. *Lancet,* **i**, 431.
9. *Boswell for the defence*, 1769–1774. (1960). Edited by W. K. Wimsatt and F. A . Pottle. London: Heinemann.
10. Cannon, W. B. (1918). A consideration of the nature of wound shock. *J. Amer. med. Ass.,* **70**, 611.
11. Cannon, W. B., Fraser, J. and Cowell, E. M. (1918). The preventive treatment of wound shock. *J. Amer. med. Ass.,* **70**, 618.
12. Carrel, A. (1907). The surgery of blood vessels. *Johns Hopkins Hosp. Bull.,* **18**, 18.
13. Castiglioni, A. (1947). *A history of medicine*. Translated by E. B. Krumbhaar. New York: Knopf.
14. Colle, J. (1628). *Methodus facile parandi tuta et nova medicamenta*, Chap. VII. Venetiis.
15. Cooley, D. A., Beall, A. C. Jr and Alexander, J. K. (1961). Acute massive pulmonary embolism: successful surgical treatment using temporary cardiopulmonary bypass. *J. Amer. med. Ass.,* **177**, 283.
16. Cooley, D. A., Beall, A. C. Jr and Grondin, P. (1962). Open-heart operations with disposable oxygenators, 5 per cent dextrose prime, and normothermia. *Surgery,* **52**, 713.
17. Cooley, D. A., Collins, H. A., Morris, G. C. and Chapman, D. W. (1958). Ventricular aneurism after myocardial infarction: surgical excision with use of temporary cardiopulmonary bypass. *J. Amer. med. Ass.,* **167**, 557.
18. Crafoord, C. and Nylin, G. (1945). Congenital coarctation of the aorta and its surgical treatment. *J. Thoracic. Surg.,* **14**, 347.
19. Currie, J. (1790). *Popular observations on apparent death from drowning, suffocation, etc.* London: Johnson.
20. Currie, J. (1798). *Medical reports on the effects of water, cold and warm, as a remedy in fever; appendix II.* Liverpool: Cadell & Davies.
21. Czerny, V. cited by Matas, R. (1909). Surgery of the vascular system. In *Surgery: Its principles and practices*, p. 171. Edited by W. W. Keen and J. C. DaCostal. Philadelphia: W. B. Saunders.
22. De-Bakey, M. E. Creech, O. Jr and Cooley, D. A. (1954). Occlusive disease of the aorta and its treatment by resection and homograft replacement. *Ann. Surg.,* **140**, 290.
23. De-Bakey, M. E., Cooley, D. A., Crawford, E. S. and Morris, G. C. Jr (1958). Clinical application of a new flexible knitted Dacron arterial substitute. *Arch. Surg.,* **77**, 713.
24. De-Bakey, M. E., Cooley, D. A., Crawford, E. S. and Morris, G. C. Jr (1958). Clinical application of a new flexible knitted Dacron arterial substitute. *Amer. J. Surg.,* **24**, 862.
25. De-Bakey, M. E. (1979). The development of vascular surgery. *Amer. J. Surg.,* **137**, 697.
26. Denis, J. (1667). A letter concerning a new way of curing sundry diseases by transfusion of blood, written to Monsieur de Montmor, counsellor to the French King, and Master of requests. *Phil. Trans.,* **2**, 489.
27. Dubost, C., Allary, M. and Oeconomos, N. (1952). Resection of an aneurysm of the abdominal aorta. Reestablishment of continuity by preserved human arterial graft, with result after five months. *Arch. Surg.,* **64**, 405.
28. Eastcott, H. H. G. (1981). Personal communication.
29. Eastcott, H. H. G., Pickering, G. W. and Rob, C. G. (1954). Reconstruction of internal carotid artery in a patient with intermittent attacks of hemiplegia. *Lancet,* **ii**, 994.
30. Ellis, R. (1868). On the Marshall Hall method of prone and postural respiration in drowning and other forms of apnoea and suspended respiration, with some suggestions for its more general adoption by the public. *Lancet,* **ii**, 538.
31. Ellis, R. (1868). The Marshall Hall method and memorial scholarship. *Lancet,* **ii**, 683.

32. Eve, F. C. (1932). Actuation of the inert diaphragm by a gravity method. *Lancet*, **ii**, 995.

33. Fay, T. (1940) Observations on prolonged human refrigeration. *N. Y. St. J. Med.*, **40**, 1351.

34. Folli, F. (1680). *Stadera medica nella quale altre la medicina infusoria, (ed altre novita, si bilanciano la regioni favore voli) e le contrario alla trasfusion der sangue*, p. 35. Florence.

35. Gesellius, F. (1874). *Zur Thierblut-Transfusion beim Menschen*, p. 1. St. Petersburg.

36. Grandidier, J. L. (1855). *Die Haemophilie Oder die Bluterkrankheit*. Wigand: Leipzig.

37. Gross, R. E. (1945). Surgical correction for coarctation of the aorta. *Surgery*, **18**, 673.

38. Gross, R. E. (1951). Treatment of certain aortic coarctations by homologous grafts; report of nineteen cases. *Ann. Surg.*, **134**, 753.

39. Gross, R. E., Bill, A. H. Jr and Peirce, E. C. (1949). Methods for preservation and transplantation of arterial grafts. Observations on arterial grafts in dogs. Report of transplantation of preserved arterial grafts in 9 human cases. *Surg. Gynecol. Obstet.*, **88**, 689.

40. Hales, S. (1733). *Statistical essays, containing haemastaticks*, Vol. **2**, London: W. Innys and R. Manby.

41. Hall, M. (1856). On a new mode of effecting artificial respiration. *Lancet*, **i**, 229.

42. Hall, M. (1856). Asphyxia, its rationale and its remedy. *Lancet*, **i**, 393.

43. Harvey, W. (1628). *The works of William Harvey*. Translated with a life of the author by Robert Willis, 1847, p. 28. London: Sydenham Society.

44. Hasse, O. (1874). *Die Lammblut-Transfusion beim Menschen*, p. 1. St. Petersburg.

45. Heister, L. (1743) *A general system of surgery*. Vol. **2**, Part 2, Sect. III, p. 4. London: Innys.

46. Hicks, J. B. (1863). Two cases of transfusion in childbed. *Lancet*, **i**, 265.

47. Hicks, J. B. (1869). Cases of transfusion, with some remarks on a new method of performing the operation. *Guy's Hosp. Rep.*, **14**, 1.

48. Higginson, A. (1857). Report of seven cases of transfusion of blood, with a description of the instrument invented by the author. *L'pool med.-chir, J.*, **1**, 102.

49. Holborow, C. A. (1959). A sixteenth century tracheostomy? *Bull. Hist. Med.*, **33**, 168.

50. Howell, W. H. and Holt, E. (1918). Two new factors in blood coagulation—heparin and pro-antithrombin. *Amer. J. Physiol.*, **47**, 328.

51. Hufnagel, C. A. (1947). Preserved homologous arterial transplants. *Bull. Amer. Coll. Surg.*, **32**, 231.

52. Hunter, J. (1776). Proposals for the recovery of persons apparently drowned. *Phil. Trans.*, **66**, 412.

53. Hunter, J. (1776). *The works of John Hunter, F.R.S., with notes*. Edited by J. F. Palmer, 1837, Vol. **1**, pp. 70; 284. London: Longman.

54. Janin, M. (1774). Abstract of a memoir published at Paris and the Hague, in 1773, on the causes of sudden and violent death; wherein it is proved, that persons who seemingly fall victims to it, may be recovered. *Scots Magazine*, **36**, 449.

55. Janský, J. (1906-7). Haematologické studie u psychotiků. *Sborn. Klinikhý*, **8**, 85.

56. Johnson, A. (1774). From Dr. Alex Johnson's Authentic Cases. *Scots Magazine*, **36**, 450.

57. Keen, W. W. (1904). A case of total laryngectomy (unsuccessful) and a case of abdominal hysterectomy (successful) in both of which massage of the heart for chloroform collapse was employed with notes of 25 other cases of cardiac massage. *Ther. Gaz.*, **28**, 217.

58. Keith, A. (1909). The mechanism underlying the various methods of artificial respiration practised since the foundation of the Royal Humane Society in 1774. *Lancet*, **i**, 825.

59. 2 Kings iv, 34, 35.

60. Kite, C. (1788). *An essay on the recovery of the apparently dead*. London: Dilly.

61. Korotkoff, N. S. (1905). On the subject of methods of determining blood pressure. *Bulletin of the Imperial Military Medical Academy of St Petersburgh*, **11**, 365.

62. Korotkoff, N. S. (1906). K voprosu o metodakh issledovaniya krovianogo davleniya. *Izv. Voen.-med. Akad.*, **12**, 254.

63. Lambert: cited by Rich, N. M. and Spencer, F. C. (1978). *Vascular trauma*, p. 6. Philadelphia: W. B. Saunders.

64. Landois. (1872). *Lehre vom Arterienpuls*. Berlin.

65. Landsteiner, K. (1901). Ueber agglutinationserscheinungen normalen menschlichen Blutes. *Wien. klin. Wschr.*, **14**, 1132.

66. Lane, S. (1840). Haemorrhagic diathesis: successful transfusion of blood. *Lancet*, **i**, 185.

67. Leriche, R. (1923). Des obliterations artérielles hautes (obliteration de la terminaison de l'aorte) comme causes des insuffisances circulatoires des membres inférieurs. *Bull. Mém. Soc. Chir. (Paris)*, **49**, 1404.

68. Lower, R. (1669). *Tractatus de corde*, p. 171. London: Redmayne.

69. Luciani, L. (1911). *Human Physiology*, Vol. 1, p. 592. Translated by F. A. Welby. London: Macmillan.

70. Ludwig, C. F. W. (1847). Beitrage zur Kenntniss des Enflusses der Respirationsbewegungen auf den Blutlauf im Aortensystem. *Arch. Anat. Physiol. wiss. Med.*, 242.

71. McLean, J. (1959). The discovery of heparin. *Circulation*, **19**, 75.

72. Matas, R. (1888). Traumatic aneurism of the left brachial artery. *Med. News*, **53**, 462.

73. Moss, W. L. (1910). Studies on isoagglutinins and isohemolysins. *Johns Hopkins Hosp. Bull.*, **21**, 63.

74. Murray, D. W. G., Jacques, L. B., Perrett, T. S. and Best, C. H. (1937). Heparin and the thrombosis of veins following injury. *Surgery*, **2**, 163.

75. Murray, E. W. (1848). *Chloroform in the practice of midwifery*, p. 25. London: Taylor & Walton.

76. Nasse, C. F. (1820). Von einer erblichen Neigung zu todtlichen Blutungen. *Archiv. fur medizinische*

Erfahring, **1**, 385.

77. Niehaus, (1889). Quoted by Zesas, D. G. (1903). Über Massage des freigelegten Herzens beim Chloroformkollaps. *Zbl. Chir.*, **30**, 588.

78. Otto, J. C. (1803). An account of an hemorrhagic disposition existing in certain families. *Medical Repository*, **6**, 1.

79. Oudot, J. (1951). La greffe vasculaire dans les thromboses du carrefour aortique. *Presse med.*, **59**, 234.

80. Pembrey, M. S. and White, W. H. (1896). The regulation of temperature in hibernating animals. *J. Physiol.*, **19**, 477.

81. Pepys on blood transfusion (1919). *Lancet*, **i**, 1098.

82. Poiseuille, J. L. M. (1828). Recherches sur la force du coeur aortique. Paris, *These* No. 166.

83. Postempski, P. (1886). La sutura dei vasi sanguini. Researche speramentali. *Arch. Soc. Ital. Chir, Roma*, **3**, 391.

84. Prus, J. (1900). Ueber die Wiederbelebung in Todesfällen in Folge von Erstickung, Chloroform-vergiftung und elektrischem Schlage. 3. Ueber die Wiederbelebung in den durch elektrischen Schlag bewirkten Todesfällen. *Wien. klin. Wschr.*, **13**, 482.

85. Robertson, O. H. (1918). A method of citrated blood transfusion. *Brit. med. J.*, **1**, 477.

86. Royal Humane Society (1824). *Annual Report.* London.

87. Schiff, M. (1874). Quoted by Zesas, D. G. (1903). Über Massage des freigelegten Herzens beim Chloroformkollaps. *Zbl. Chir.*, **30**, 588.

88. Shattock, S. G. (1900). Chromocyte clumping in acute pneumonia and certain other diseases, and the significance of the buffy coat in the shed blood. *J. Path. Bact.*, **6**, 303.

89. Simpson, J. Y. (1848). *The works of Sir James Y. Simpson, Bart.* Edited by Sir W. G. Simpson, Bart., 1871, Vol. **2**, p. 143. Edinburgh: A. & C. Black.

90. Simpson, S. (1902). Some observations on the temperature of the monkey. *J. Physiol.*, **28**, xxi.

91. Spallanzani, L. (1803). *Tracts on the natural history of animals and vegetables*, 2nd edn. Translated by J. G. Dalyell. Edinburgh: Creech & Constable.

92. Starling, E. A. (1902). Society of Anaesthetists report. Starling's paper entitled "Reflex inhibition of the heart during the administration of ether". *Lancet*, **ii**, 1397.

93. Sykes, W. S. (1961). *Essays on the first hundred years of anaesthesia*, Vol. **2**, p. 170. Edinburgh: E. & S. Livingstone.

94. Tuffier and Hallion (1898). De la compression rythmée du coeur dans la syncope cardiaque par embolie. *Bull. Soc. Chir.*, n.s. **24**, 937.

95. Vesalius, A. (1543). *De humani corporis fabrica libri septem.* Basileae: Oporini.

96. Walther, A. (1862). Beiträge zur Lehre von der thierischen Wärme. *Virchows Arch.*, **25**, 414.

97. Whitby, J. D. (1962). Some early manuals of resuscitation. *Anaesthesia*, **17**, 365.

98. Whitby, J. D. (1963). Resuscitation in the North. *Newc. med. J.*, **27**, 229.

99. Wilkinson (1764). Expedients for the recovery of persons supposed to be drowned. [Taken from Dr. Wilkinson's Tutamen Nauticum, or Seaman's Preservation just now published.] *Med. Mus.*, **3**, 316.

100. Wood, A. A. (1817). *Athenae oxonienses,* 3rd edn, Vol. **3**, p. 1155. London: Rivington.

101. Wright, A. E. (1891). A new method of blood transfusion. *Brit. med. J.*, **2**, 1203.

Chapter 2
Disturbances of Fluid and Electrolytes

The Composition of Body Fluids

Although an interest in transfusing blood from animals to man was present hundreds of years ago, the interest in the part played by water in maintaining normal metabolism is much more recent. Water depletion was most commonly manifest after infection with cholera. In 1831 O'Shaughnessy[232] analysed the blood of patients with cholera most carefully and laboriously and laid down the basis of present-day fluid therapy, although his work still went unrecognized 20 years later when cholera returned to Britain. The elegance of style and the scientific content of his letter to the *Lancet* (Fig. 2.1) might be the envy of all. He found haemoconcentration, sodium depletion and a gross metabolic acidosis, and that dehydration had led to uraemia. His observations were very soon applied clinically with good effect by Latta (1831)[178,179] in Leith, Scotland, so that a 50-year-old lady, very close to death, was resuscitated by injecting in the first instance 120 ounces (3300 ml) of Marcets Solution* and later maintained by the further injection of 330 ounces (9900 ml) of the same solution over 12 hours. He wrote.

> . . . I have already given an instance where deficiency in quantity was the cause of failure, which I will now contrast with one in which it was used freely. A female, aged 50, very destitute, but previously in good health, was on the 13th instant, at four a.m., seized with cholera in its most violent form, and by half-past nine was reduced to a most hopeless state. The pulse was quite gone, even in the axilla, and strength so much exhausted, that I had resolved not to try the effects of the injection, conceiving the poor woman's case to be hopeless, and that the failure of the experiment might affort the prejudiced and the illiberal an

opportunity to stigmatise the practice; however, I at length thought I would give her a chance, and in the presence of Drs. Lewins and Craigie, and Messrs. Sibson and Paterson, I injected one hundred and twenty ounces, when like the effects of magic, instead of the pallid aspect of one whom death had sealed as his own, the vital tide was restored, and life and vivacity returned: but diarrhoea recurred, and in three hours she again sunk. One hundred and twenty ounces more were injected with the same good effect. In this case 330 ounces were so used in twelve hours, when reaction was completely re-established; and in forty-eight hours she smokes her pipe free from distemper. She was then, for better accommodation, carried to the hospital, where probably, from contagion, slight typhoid symptoms were produced. She is now, however, convalescent.

One of the earliest analyses of tissue was performed by Berzelius (1840).[37] He noted that muscle ash contained sodium, magnesium, calcium phosphate, sodium and potassium chloride and lactate. Liebig (1847)[183] noted that blood contained much sodium and little potassium and that the reverse was true of muscle. Enderlin (1844)[87] found that the concentration of alkali phosphate in muscle exceeded that of alkali chloride. Bunge (1871 and 1873)[53,54] reported the influence of muscle extracts upon the heart rate and measured the urinary excretion of electrolytes in man. The inverse relationship between fat and tissue water content was investigated by Forster (1876)[109,110,111] and he observed that muscle and liver contained very little calcium and deduced that when eaten, these tissues alone would not assist in the deposition of bone. In 1896 Katz[164] demonstrated that muscle tissue contained twice to three times as much magnesium as calcium and that the mineral composition of individual tissues was constant. The classical views on cell permeability were published by Overton in 1902[233] and 1904.[234]

---

* Marcets Solution contained a mixture of saline and sodium bicarbonate. The solution used by Latta had an osmolarity just greater than 0.45% saline solution.

EXPERIMENTS ON THE BLOOD IN CHOLERA.

To the Editor of THE LANCET.

SIR,—Having been enabled to complete the experimental inquiries on which I have some time back been engaged in Newcastle upon-Tyne, I beg you will have the kindness to give insertion to the annexed outlines of the results I have obtained :—

1. The blood drawn in the worst cases of *the* cholera, is unchanged in its anatomical or globular structure.

2. It has *lost a large proportion of its water*, 1000 *parts of cholera serum having* but the average of 860 *parts of water*

3. *It has lost also a great proportion of its* NEUTRAL *saline ingredients.*

4. *Of the free alkali contained in healthy serum, not a particle is present in some cholera cases, and barely a trace in others.*

5. Urea exists in the cases where suppression of urine has been a marked symptom.

6. *All the salts deficient in the blood, especially the carbonate of soda, are present in large quantities in the peculiar white dejected matters.*

There are other results of minor consequence, to which I will not at present allude, neither shall I *on this occasion* offer any observation on the practical inference to which my experiments may lead. In a few days a detailed report shall be published, in which the mode of analysis, &c. will be minutely described. It will be found, I regret to say, in every essential particular, to contradict that recently given by Hermann. All my experiments, however, have been publicly performed, and can be authenticated by numerous witnesses, a precaution I thought it necessary to adopt, lest it might be supposed that I impugned, without sufficient foundation, the accuracy of the Moscow professor.

May I add, that until the publication of my report, I shall deem the suspension of discussion on the results now introduced as a matter of personal courtesy and obligation.   I am, Sir,
            Your obedient servant,
        W. B. O'SHAUGHNESSY, M.D.
London, 29 December, 1831.

Fig. 2.1   Reproduced by permission of the *Lancet*.[232]

Although Fagge (1874)[97] treated and first drew attention to the importance of dehydration in diabetic coma, credit for first appreciating the importance of the metabolism of water and electrolytes of the whole organism must be given to Claude Bernard (1859),[35] and for placing this subject on a precise, accurate, as well as scientific

foundation, we are indebted to the work of Peters and Van Slyke.[242] Van Slyke and Cullen produced their apparatus for measuring the CO_2 content of blood and the concept of alkali reserve in 1917[309] and laid down the concepts of acid–base balance in man.[308, 310–312] Benedict in 1915[31] examined the changes that occurred during starvation and these were examined further by Gamble, Ross and Tisdall (1923).[119] Loeb, Atchley and Palmer (1922) examined diabetic acidosis, and the equilibration of fluid between blood and serous cavities.[185]

The concept of tissue spaces had been laid down by Meigs (1912)[204] and Meigs and Ryan (1912)[205] and when Fenn *et al.*[100] (1934) calculated the volume of the chloride space and estimated the size and composition of the intracellular space, interest in the dynamic aspects of intracellular and extracellular electrolytes gathered force. When the flame photometer became available and isotopes could be detected with ease and their concentration measured with little difficulty, new doors were unlocked for research and clinical investigation. Isotopes especially, however, have produced difficulties related to their characteristics, partly because there is sometimes a limitation set to their usefulness, owing to the doubtful accuracy with which they can be measured for reliable results to be obtained. Also because the distribution of substances within the same anatomical 'space' differs. The same difficulties arise when measurements are made with substances other than radioactive isotopes, so that when we refer to the extracellular fluid compartment we sometimes use terms such as the inulin, thiocyanate, thiosulphate or chloride space, etc.

The measurement of blood volume by means of ^{51}Cr and albumin labelled with ^{131}I is probably of most value in every-day clinical practice and total exchangeable Na^+ and K^+ are the next most valuable measurements in detecting deficiencies in the body of these elements.

Body Water

The total volume of water within the body is represented by approximately 50–70% of the body weight. The amount is determined by the quantity of fat that is deposited subcutaneously. Adipose tissue contains relatively less fluid than other tissues. Thus in an obese person a figure of 50% of the body weight would more closely approximate to the total body water content, while 70% would be a more accurate determination in a lean person.

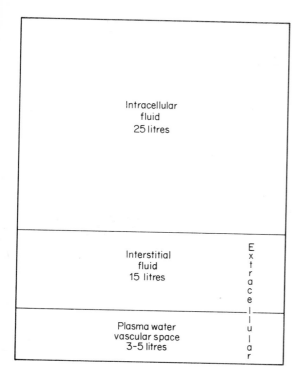

Fig. 2.2 The body water compartments in the average adult. The intracellular fluid space is approximately twice the volume of the extracellular fluid space. The latter is subdivided into interstitial fluid and plasma water. All three compartments are anatomically and functionally separate, discrete compartments. For example K⁺ is virtually excluded from the extra-cellular compartments but even this low concentration has to be maintained within narrow limits for the normal functioning of the myocardium. Na⁺ is virtually excluded from the intra-cellular compartment but moves rapidly into myocardial cells to initiate contraction. The interstitial fluid is protein free, but the semipermeable nature of the cell membranes and the 'gates' which allow individual ions to pass in a controlled manner enables equilibrium to be maintained with the plasma. (The figures in litres refer to the approximate volumes found in the adult.)

There is a fourth space which includes the cerebrospinal fluid, salivary glands and other organs (Richards and Truniger, 1983),[252] but this is quantitatively so small, even in the adult, that the author has excluded it from the diagram. The fourth space plays no significant part in the calculations for body water deficit and haemoconcentration.

The total body water content of a newborn pre-mature infant may be in the region of 80% of the body weight. Special problems are associated with water balance of the infant.

Both functionally and anatomically we can largely divide the body fluids into two main parts, the intracellular fluid (ICF) and extracellular fluid (ECF) (Fig. 2.2). Their volumes are approximately in the ratio of 2:1. Water which comprises roughly 40% of the body weight lies within the intracellular compartment and is referred to as intracellular fluid, and water comprising 20% of the body weight lies in the extracellular fluid compartment. The ECF can be further subdivided. That which comprises approximately one-quarter of the extra-cellular water (5% of the body weight) lies within the vascular compartment as plasma water. The remainder forms the interstitial fluid space, lymph, the cerebrospinal fluid and small pockets such as occur in bursae, intraoccular fluid, synovial cavities and that contained within relatively bio-chemically inert structures such as tendons and connective tissues. (There is some evidence that connective tissue may behave as one large deposit of 'ion exchange resin' and therefore is not as biochemically inert as is often supposed.)

The ICF is functionally even more greatly sub-divided than the ECF, for the contents of different cells vary with function, metabolic rate and oxygen consumption. Even within the cell, changes in mitochondrial and microsomal structure cause differences in ionic concentrations of elements such as magnesium and calcium.

The ECF and ICF are two completely separate entities both anatomically and chemically. Na⁺ and Cl⁻ are virtually excluded from the cell, while K⁺ and Mg⁺⁺ are almost entirely intracellular.

The major part of the body potassium is con-tained within the intracellular compartment, while sodium lies chiefly in the extracellular compart-ment. The mechanisms by which the gradients of potassium and sodium are maintained across the semipermeable membrane of the cell wall are not so far understood, but the process entails the expenditure of energy.[254]

Water is lost from the body by evaporation from the lungs with no loss of electrolyte; from the skin by insensible perspiration or by visible sweating, when it will contain variable quantities of sodium and potassium and is regulated in part by adreno-cortical function; from the gut via the faeces and by excretion through the kidneys by careful, dis-crete, incredibly accurate means under the control of endocrine and central nervous system functions. The approximate amounts of water lost from these sites in health, in a temperate climate, are as follows:

skin	300 ml
lungs	200 ml
faeces	200 ml
urine	1500 ml

In most living organisms, a very accurate balance between the amount of water taken in and the amount of water lost from the various pathways is maintained. In health, the balance is achieved by varying the water intake and the volume of water excreted in the urine.

In addition to being a universal solvent so that even 'insoluble' substances in fact dissolve to a very small degree, water has other physical characteristics that make it the ideal substance for the living organism. It has, for example, the greatest *specific heat* of any known solvent, and therefore the greatest heat capacity. It also has the highest *latent heat* of evaporation of any known solvent, allowing heat loss from the body to occur with relative ease.

Terminology of Expressing Concentration

When a salt is dissolved in water it dissociates into positive and negative ions. The positive ion migrates towards a negatively charged pole and is, therefore, referred to as a 'cation', while the negatively charged ion migrates towards a positively charged pole and is referred to as an 'anion'. Some ions possess more than one charge and if we are to understand the ionic composition of the body, it is necessary that we consider the different ions in terms of their chemical equivalents and electrical charge as well as their molar concentrations.

The milliequivalent (mEq)

The concentration of salts expressed as milligrams per cent has largely been discarded, although when thinking of total body composition it is also sometimes convenient to know the amount of a substance that is present in grams-weight, because the magnitude of an abnormal change is then more readily appreciated and oral replacement in tablet form using present methods of dispensing is made easier.

An equivalent is equal to the atomic weight or molecular weight expressed in grams divided by the valence. Thus:

(*a*)   1 Equivalent =

$$\frac{\text{Atomic weight or molecular weight (in grams)}}{\text{Valence}}$$

1 Milliequivalent = 1000th part of an equivalent, therefore

(*b*)   1 Milliequivalent =

$$\frac{\text{Atomic weight or molecular weight (in mg)}}{\text{Valence}}$$

Because sodium is univalent and has an atomic weight of 23, 1 mEq = 23 mg. Potassium is also univalent and has an atomic weight of 39 and, therefore, 1 mEq = 39 mg. 1 mEq of sodium chloride (NaCl) contains 1 mEq of Na^+ and 1 mEq of Cl^- which has an atomic weight of 35.5. Therefore 1 mEq of Na^+ is present in (23 + 35.5) = 58.5 mg of NaCl. 1 g of NaCl contains 17.1 mEq of Na^+, while 1 g of KCl contains 13.4 mEq of K^+.

The millimole (mmol) and solute concentration: the International System of Units (Systéme Internationale—SI units)

A 'molar solution' contains the molecular weight of a substance in grams (g-mol) per litre of solution. A millimole (mmol) is one thousandth part of a mole. This is the most accurate way of defining solute concentration. The 'concentration of' a substance is denoted by square brackets [ ].

A system of metric units has been introduced throughout the United Kingdom and Europe and many other parts of the world.[26,27] The USA has not adopted this system, although in some medical and other publications the SI unit (mmol) has been adopted. In this system, length is based on the metre (m), mass is based on the kilogram (kg), and the amount of substance is based on the mole (mol). The mole has now replaced the 'equivalent' and the millimole has replaced the milliequivalent in many international journals. However, a certain amount of controversy does exist in that some authors believe that where a particle has an electrical charge, as in the case of Na^+, K^+, HCO_3^-, etc., the term milliequivalent (mEq) should be retained. This is of some help in understanding the movement of the particles between the fluid compartments and eases the understanding of the significance of ionized and un-ionized substances with regard to osmotic pressure or osmolality. In traditional units, the plasma concentration of Ca^{++} was reported as having a normal value of 9–11 mg%. In milliequivalents per litre, the plasma $[Ca^{++}]$ is normally 4.6–5.6 mEq/l. However, in SI units (calcium being a divalent ion), the normal plasma $[Ca^{++}]$ is 2.3–2.8 mmol/l. The normal blood-urea concentration in traditional units is 20–40 mg% and in SI units it is 3.3–6.6 mmol/l. Similarly, the blood-glucose concentration, which was used by the author in the first edition of this publication in terms of millimoles and milliosmoles (mosmol), is now reported in mmol/l, 18mg% being equal to 1 mmol/l. When the blood-glucose concentration is high, the plasma $[Na^+]$ is misleadingly low. The plasma $[Na^+]$ does not then alert the clinician to the degree of dehydration present in the patient. The plasma $[Na^+]$, relative to the degree of dehydration and the water deficit, is assessed in a very simple manner when the blood sugar is reported in millimoles (SI units). Because glucose does not ionize, the figure reported in mmol/l (SI units) is merely halved and added to the reported plasma [Na^+] (see p. 422). However, when millimoles are used to report concentrations of drugs in the blood or plasma (the drug having been prescribed in milligrams), the clinician may not be alerted to the magnitude of an overdose, unless he is very familiar with the conversion of millimoles to milligrams, sometimes with serious consequences.[73,248,327] Pressure or partial pressure is now measured in pascals (Pa)* or kilopascals (kPa).

Osmotic pressure

If a solution of any solute, for example glucose or sodium, is separated from pure water by means of a membrane that is permeable to water, but not the solute, water tends to be drawn through the membrane in order to dilute the solution. The membrane, like the cell walls, is said to be 'semipermeable'. The movement of water can be prevented mechanically by exerting a pressure on the compartment containing the solution. The force that is required to prevent this movement is referred to as the 'osmotic pressure'.

We have seen how it is more convenient to work in milliequivalents and millimoles rather than milligrams. It is also more convenient in clinical practice to use the unit of osmotic force, the 'osmole', or rather, the one-thousandth part of this unit, the milliosmole (mosmol). This is because the osmotic pressure that a solution is capable of exerting is dependent upon the number of particles, molecules or ions present in the solution. Thus the same weight of a substance of high molecular weight, such as globulin, will exert a smaller osmotic force than the same weight of a substance of lower molecular weight, such as albumin. Substances of similar molecular weight, such as urea and sodium chloride, will exert widely different osmotic pressures, because the latter ionizes in solution and the former does not. The number of ions capable of exerting an osmotic force formed by the dissociation of the salt, is dependent upon valence, temperature and the presence of other ionizing solutes.

We can also refer to the osmotic pressure indirectly in terms of its osmotic activity, 'osmolar concentration' or 'osmolarity'.† In the case of a non-electrolyte, such as urea or glucose, 1 millimole = 1 milliosmole, but 1 millimole of NaCl = 2 milliosmoles when completely dissociated into Na^+ and Cl^-, and 1 millimole of $CaCl_2$ = 3 milliosmoles.

If we add up all the concentrations of all the cations in the plasma and multiply this figure by 2 and then add the figure for osmolality resulting from the blood or the plasma-glucose concentration, we obtain a figure of approximately 310 mosmol/l. When we measure plasma osmolality by other means (e.g. by freezing point depression), we reach a figure closer to 285 mosmol/l. It is generally accepted that the effective plasma osmolality is in the region of 300 mosmol/l.

A satisfactory calculation of the plasma osmolality can therefore be obtained from the formulae:

$$\text{osmolality} = 2 \times (Na^+ + K^+ \text{ in mmol/l}) + \frac{\text{glucose (mg/100 ml)}}{18}$$

$$\text{osmolality} = 2 \times (Na^+ + K^+ \text{ in mmol/l}) + \text{glucose (mmol/l)}$$

Plasma osmolality is measured for clinical purposes by freezing point depression or by vapour pressure determination, or more generally by estimating the sodium and potassium concentrations, doubling them and adding the osmolality resulting from the plasma-glucose concentration. The concentrations of other cations are so small that changes in these values will not materially alter the estimation of plasma osmolality as far as clinical purposes are concerned. Accurate estimations determined on healthy people show that there is little change in plasma osmolality from day to day; indeed, it appears to vary by less than 4 mosmol.[337] In practice, this is essential for it is often not recognized how enormous these forces are. The plasma osmolality of 300 mosmol/l represents a potential force of 7.7 atmospheres or 5800 mmHg; this is equivalent to a column of water the height of a twenty-storey building.[257] We can reflect on how insignificant a force a normal blood pressure of 120 mmHg appears to be in comparison to plasma osmolality, and yet how

---

*The pascal equals 1 newton per metre². The newton (N), the SI unit of force, equals that force needed to accelerate 1 kilogram by 1 metre per second² (or 1 N = 1 kg m s⁻²).

† The term 'osmolarity' is related to the solute concentration per unit volume of solution and the term 'osmolality' per unit weight. For dilute solutions the terms are virtually interchangeable. Plasma (not blood) concentrations of glucose, and indeed any solute, should be used, otherwise the concentration will be severely underestimated (Hilborne et al., 1984).[145] Urea does not need to be included because it can freely enter any cell.

comparatively minor deviations from normal values of blood pressure produce major alterations in function. When we have accumulated more information regarding the effects of changes in osmolality of body fluids, it may be found that these alterations may initiate as well as reflect disease processes. Evidence is accumulating that correcting the fall in the osmolality of the ECF during haemorrhagic shock (see p. 188) is important in protecting the kidney against tubular necrosis.

The regulation of the osmolality of body fluids is dependent upon the thirst mechanism, the availability of solute-free fluids and the control exerted by the kidneys upon water and solute excretion under the influence of endocrine secretions. The electrolyte content of the ECF is also dependent in turn upon these factors.

There is a further aspect, where osmotic forces may have an effect, which is of some importance in resuscitation. If, in addition to water depletion, there is also an excess of solute, that is to say electrolytes such as sodium in the ECF or glucose in the case of diabetic coma, then although the overall situation is largely identical to that of water depletion alone and contraction of the ECF is present, dehydration of the intracellular compartment is more marked than in dehydration alone. This is of great clinical significance if peripheral circulatory failure is to be avoided, for example during the treatment of diabetic ketosis (see page 416).

Renal Control of Water

The kidney is a complex organ and its anatomy and physiology are even now not completely understood. The account that follows, therefore, is a simplified version of what is thought to be largely true, although both in the anatomical and physiological sense only enough is covered for the purposes of resuscitation.

The glomeruli form the plasma filtrate and are situated in the cortex of the kidney. The glomerular filtrate traverses the proximal convoluted tubule while still within the cortex and then enters a hairpin-like loop known as the loop of Henlé. It then re-enters the cortex by passing through the distal convoluted tubule which in turn drains into the collecting tubule. This tubule begins in the cortex but passes straight through the medulla to open into the pelvis of the ureter. The loop of Henlé has a thin and a thick segment. The thin

segment extends along the descending limb and lower part of the ascending limb and the thick segment is confined to the upper part of the ascending limb. This minute structure allows the medulla to be divided into an inner and an outer zone. Some nephrons in man, however, especially those that originate from glomeruli placed less deeply in the cortex, have very short loops of Henlé which in fact never enter the medulla. These nephrons have extremely short thin segments. This makes the correlation of structure and function very difficult, but it is recognized that only those organisms that have loops of Henlé are able to concentrate glomerular filtrate, and the degree to which the concentration can be achieved is related to the relative lengths of the loops and how far they extend into the medulla.

Functionally, the system of tubules can be divided into three main parts: (*a*) an isotonic part, consisting of the proximal convoluted tubule in which 80–85% of the filtrated sodium is reabsorbed together with water so that there is no change in osmolality, (*b*) a diluting part in which sodium and other materials are selectively reabsorbed, this consists of the loop of Henlé and at least part of the distal convoluted tubule, and (*c*) a concentrating part, which consists of the collecting tubule and perhaps the distal part of the distal convoluted tubule (Fig. 2.3).

About 186 litres of fluid are filtered through the glomerulus every 24 hours; in other words the whole of the body water is turned over four and a half times every day. This is equivalent to 125 ml of filtrate every minute and is the same as the inulin clearance. Of the 186 litres, only 1–2 litres reach the bladder in each 24 hours, and in health this is dependent upon the fluid intake, diet and the environmental temperature.

In addition to reabsorption of 80–85% of the sodium filtered, all the glucose, all the potassium, some urea, by far the greater part of the protein, and most of the amino acid content* is reabsorbed in the proximal tubule, but no creatinine. Approximately 50 g of protein are filtered each day. If protein was not reabsorbed, it would represent a major loss to the body. In addition most of the bicarbonate ion is reabsorbed so that the pH falls. It can be seen, therefore, that although the reabsorption has taken place, iso-osmotically the tubular fluid has changed its character by the time it enters the loop of Henlé.

---

* Certain congenital conditions occur in which different amino acids fail to be reabsorbed, e.g. glycine in glycinuria, of neutral amino acids in Hartnup disease and of cystine, lysine, ornithine and arginine in 'cystinuria'.

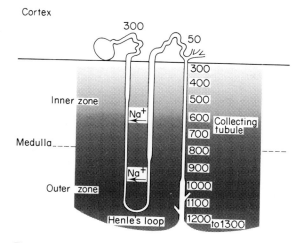

Fig. 2.3 A diagram showing the composition of a nephron. The transfer of Na⁺ from the ascending to the descending limb of the loop of Henlé leads to the production of zones of increasing osmolarity. The counter-current mechanism allows this to be achieved without large gradients of osmotic pressure between the two limbs. The figures refer to the osmolality of the tubular fluid in mosmol/l.

The loop of Henlé is considered to be anatomically designed in such a way that it could act as a counter-current multiplier system, so that the osmolality of the tissue adjacent to the loop increases the deeper the loop penetrates into the medulla, reaching a maximum at the bend of the loop, that is to say in man in the region of the papillae. All that would be necessary for this to occur would be the transfer of sodium ions from the ascending to the descending limb. We also know that the vasa-recta, which all arise from the juxtamedullary glomeruli, can act as a counter-current exchange system as the flow of blood within these vessels is in the opposite direction to that of the flow of tubular urine through the nephron. It has been observed that the erythrocytes in the vessels that are passing around the apex of the hairpin bend are crenated and there is cryoscopic evidence of hyperosmolality of the tissue in this area. Although the loop of Henlé is considered to function as the counter-current mechanism for producing hyperosmolality, it does so for the benefit of the collecting tubule so that water can be extracted from this segment of the nephron. In this way the active reabsorption of water in order to concentrate urine can be postulated without assuming that it is performed against an enormously powerful osmotic gradient. Although by its structure and function it is capable of producing the counter-current multiplier system

of hyperosmolality, the loop of Henlé produces dilution of the tubular fluid by the reabsorption of solutes, because as the tubular urine passes through the ascending limb it becomes diluted and is hypo-osmolar to plasma. The tubular urine in this region of the nephron may have an osmolality in the region of 50 mosmol/l as opposed to 300 mosmol/l when it left the glomerulus. The loop of Henlé, therefore, represents the second stage in the extraction of solute, especially sodium, from the tubular urine. It is influenced in this way by the secretion of hormones, especially aldosterone. We know that the kidney is capable of excreting a fluid which contains virtually no sodium at all, less in fact than tap water. Some substances are added to the urine by active tubular secretion, most if not all of the filtered K⁺, having been reabsorbed in the proximal tubule, appears in the tubular urine in exchange for the Na⁺ at this stage.

The last section of the nephron is the concentrating segment and is lined by cells which are made permeable to water by the influence of antidiuretic hormone (ADH). How this occurs is still largely unknown, but we do know that certain tissues are made more porous to water when ADH is injected into the animal. An example of this is the frog's skin. We can assume that in the absence of ADH the tubular urine passes on through the hypertonic medullary tissue largely unchanged because the collecting ducts are then impermeable to water.

When the antidiuretic activity is at its maximum, water is allowed to permeate readily and the osmolality of the tubular urine is raised from the region of 50 mosmol/l to 1200 mosmol/l and its volume is reduced.

Fluid Requirements and Therapy

Amount of fluid required

The insensible loss of water through the lungs, skin, faeces, etc. is often overestimated in patients living in a temperate climate. It may be as little as 400 ml in 24 hours, depending largely upon the nature of the disease, the presence of a pyrexia, sweating and the temperature and humidity of the environment.

If the patient has no fever and the room temperature is below 29°C (85°F), the insensible loss can be considered to be between 600 and 1000 ml in 24 hours. If the patient has a fever of greater than 38°C (101°F) and is sweating visibly but not excessively, or the temperature is above 29°C (85°F), then 1500 ml in 24 hours would be an expected loss of water.

In temperatures above 32°C (90°F) and pyrexias of greater than 39°C (102°F) associated with continuous visible sweating, then a water loss of 2 litres or more in 24 hours will be expected.

In the presence of continuous excessive sweating, 4 litres or more may be lost through the skin in 24 hours and only careful assessment by means of body weight, plasma electrolyte concentrations, packed cell volume (PCV), plasma protein estimations and urine specific gravity will permit accurate treatment (see p. 174). As much as 1 litre/hour may be lost as sweat when exposed in the desert.

Diarrhoea and hyperventilation will add to the degree of fluid loss and must be considered when estimates of water requirements are made. The volume of urine voided during the period of assessment must be added to the estimated fluid loss.

Except in the immediate postoperative period when blood transfusion and infusions of fluid may have been given in a volume sufficient to influence fluid balance significantly, the normal daily fluid requirements of the adult lie between 2% and 4% of the body weight. If a fluid deficit has occurred, 4–6% of the body weight may be given in electrolyte-containing or electroyte-free fluid.

When the water content of the body is less or greater than normal, abnormal concentrations of electrolytes appear in the body fluids.

Hyponatraemia

When the plasma sodium concentration falls below 130 mmol/l (mEq/l), hyponatraemia is said to be present. This is a purely arbitrary figure and it must be realized that abnormal responses may be seen when the plasma sodium is at a higher value. At levels well above 130 mmol/l (mEq/l) patients may have a feeling of lethargy and may even demonstrate muscle weakness. When Anderson et al. (1985)[14] performed a prospective study of 'in hospital' hyponatraemia, they found that the mortality was 60 times that of hospital patients who had a normal serum [Na+].

Hyponatraemia can occur in two ways, either by retention of water or by loss of electrolytes. It presents as three main syndromes.

(a) Simple sodium depletion or low salt syndrome.
(b) Water intoxication—primary retention of water.
(c) Symptomless hyponatraemia.

Symptomless hyponatraemia is a rare condition. The fall in the plasma sodium concentration implies that the osmolality of the plasma and other body fluids has fallen. Hyponatraemia is possibly more commonly seen today than hypernatraemia, especially since intravenous fluid can be given so easily and because there is a widespread regard for postoperative salt retention.

We have seen how sodium salts comprise the bulk of the electrolyte content of the ECF and how water diffuses freely into and out of the body cells. Gamble et al.[119] suggested that there was osmotic uniformity between the fluid compartments and this must be true for most of the body cells. This concept has one important consequence in the correction of electrolyte deficits. If we raise the osmolality of the ECF, for example by 10 mosmol/l, by the infusion of sodium salts, a redistribution of body water will result. The consequent withdrawal of water from the intracellular compartment will lower the tonicity of the ECF and raise the tonicity of the ICF. The final osmolality of both compartments will be related to the volumes of fluid that they contain.

The concept of osmotic uniformity has an important influence upon treatment. It implies that when corrections are made for abnormal electrolyte levels that are measured in the plasma, that is to say the ECF, they have to be calculated on the basis of total body water even though, in the case of Na+, there is quantitatively relatively little present in the ICF.

This is an important concept as it applies to all electrolytes. We shall see later that a similar concept, the isohydric principle (see p. 72), applies to changes in the acid–base state.

When we apply these principles in the process of treatment we find that the plasma concentrations do in fact follow the theoretically predictable values.

Sodium depletion

Many of the conditions that we are going to examine are also discussed in more detail.

Loss of Na+ occurs when renal conservation is poor, when there is extraneous loss from body cavities or the gut or when there is excessive sweating.

Renal salt loss

This is present in chronic nephritis (sometimes referred to as 'salt-losing nephritis'), during the osmotic pre-recovery phase of acute renal failure, and when severe sickness and fever of almost any aetiology are present. Renal salt loss occurs most commonly in the very old and the very young.

Adrenocortical insufficiency and Addison's disease result in a deficiency of salt-retaining hormones, especially aldosterone. This impairs the ability of kidneys to reabsorb Na^+, and salt depletion of a major degree can occur in the presence of a reduced potassium excretion.

Diuretic-induced hyponatraemia

Now that very potent diuretic agents are available, hyponatraemia is being observed with increasing frequency,[101,168,114] especially in advanced cases of congestive cardiac failure that have not been treated successfully by surgical means. When eight patients with severe congestive cardiac failure, who had developed hyponatraemia following prolonged diuretic therapy and demonstrated resistance to diuretics and continued to have oedema, were treated with magnesium sulphate infusions, marked improvement in the patients' condition occurred. The infusions resulted in a rising serum $[Na^+]$ and muscle biopsies showed a decrease in sodium and chloride content and increased muscle K^+. Dyckner and Wester[84] concluded that the improvement was probably mediated through the effect of Mg^{++} on membrane ATPase. It has been recognized that patients who have hyponatraemia and oedema appear to have an *increased* total body Na^+. While some of the changes in Na^+ metabolism can be explained by K^+ depletion, treatment with potassium salts alone usually does not improve the plasma $[Na^+]$.

Alimentary canal salt loss

The secretions from the gut often have a high Na^+ content of about 100–120 mmol/l (mEq/l), although frequently when fluid is lost because of vomiting, the concentrations are lower. When the losses are from an ileostomy or the result of gastroenteritis, a mixed depletion of both water and sodium results. Because these solutions are hypotonic to the ECF, hyponatraemia will result in a manner similar to that of excessive sweating.

Salt loss from paracentesis

The body can become depleted of Na^+ following repeated paracentesis of the thorax or the abdomen. The fluid removed contains an electrolyte content similar to that of the ECF and very often the amount of electrolyte removed is greater than that of a major diuresis of large proportions produced by diuretic therapy.

Case history. A child aged 10 years underwent a thoracic operation and fluid accumulated in both lung cavities following the operation. The pleural effusions were repeatedly tapped with marked relief of dyspnoea. Because she was unwell she ate little, and insufficient care was taken in making sure that blood analysis was repeated at frequent intervals. Eighteen days after the operation she began to hyperventilate at a fast rate and became disoriented, although there was very little fluid in the chest. Although acid–base measurements were not performed, it was considered erroneously that, because of the marked hyperventilation, a metabolic acidosis was present. She was therefore given sodium bicarbonate orally and showed some improvement. Acid–base analysis was performed the following day and she was found to have a moderate metabolic alkalosis, but the plasma revealed a Na^+ concentration of only 118 mmol/l (mEq/l). Paracentesis thoracis performed on the same day showed that the pleural effusion contained 120 mmol/l (mEq/l) of Na^+ and 3 mmol/l (mEq/l) of K^+. She was infused with 300 ml of 5% NaCl over a period of 9 hours, during which time a diuresis began. The hyperventilation ceased, the mental disorientation and bizarre behaviour disappeared. The patient made an uneventful recovery following careful oral treatment for the electrolyte disorder. Oral replacement kept pace with the removal of the substances from the thoracic cavity. In this case the treatment with sodium bicarbonate was of value because it replaced some of the sodium deficit and the bicarbonate ion was excreted in the urine. However, the use of alkali rather than sodium chloride would exacerbate the moderate potassium deficiency that was also present.

We must, therefore, take note that the sodium content of the urine, compared with that of the ECF, is low, especially during sodium depletion.

In all the conditions mentioned so far, hyponatraemia can only occur when a deficit in fluid volume is corrected with solutions which have either a low electrolyte content or are electrolyte free.

The sequence of events in sodium depletion when there is normal renal function and normal corticosteroid excretion and hypovolaemia is not present (i.e. in the otherwise normal person) takes the following pattern.*

When the plasma level of Na^+ falls, Na^+ retention by the kidneys follows. In order to restore the

---

* In order to make this account clear we are ignoring for the moment that some tissues, such as bone, contain relatively more Na^+ than other tissues. Most of this Na^+ is not, however, in dynamic equilibrium with the other compartments of body water.

balance of electrolyte to water and in this way correct the osmolality of the ECF, excretion of water occurs under the influence of the osmo-receptor of the hypothalamus. This leads to hypo-volaemia and generalized contraction of the body water, the packed cell volume (PCV) and plasma protein concentration becoming raised. Hypo-volaemia causes an increased secretion of ADH and results in oliguria which gives rise to a raised blood urea. It is at this stage that clinical interest is usually aroused in the patient who is not progressing favourably. Analysis of the serum or plasma then reveals a low [Na$^+$] (e.g. in the region of 125 mmol/l (mEq/l)), a low [Cl$^-$] of about 80 mmol/l (mEq/l) and a urea concentration which is above normal, 10–16.6 mmol/l (60–100 mg%). As the situation progresses, the blood urea rises and the plasma [Na$^+$] falls further; the plasma [K$^+$] and [HCO$_3^-$] may be high, normal or low depending upon numerous other factors.

If some of the lost fluid is replaced by drinking water only, a very low plasma sodium results, and if a large volume of water is infused or drunk, the volume of total body water will rise, but when the water intake is insufficient it is drawn into the cells from the ECF to level out the osmotic gradient that would otherwise be present.

Clinical features of sodium depletion

The patient has a sick, haggard, anxious appearance with sunken eyes. This is because of a reduced tissue turgor and reduced eyeball tension. With practice some people can detect an apparent 'translucent' appearance of the skin.

There is often a feeling of weakness and of nausea, and vomiting may occur. Muscle cramps are associated with this condition and mental disorientation producing bizarre behaviour and conversation is sometimes present. A man may, for example, relate the most intimate details of his life in a matter-of-fact manner. In extreme cases, the patient may have beads of perspiration on the forehead and elsewhere but, especially peripherally, the skin is cold because hypovolaemia has caused vasoconstriction. The blood pressure is low, the pulse pressure reduced and there is a tachycardia giving rise to a weak, rapid thready pulse which becomes impalpable if the condition progresses into frank peripheral circulatory failure.

Water intoxication

When a large volume of water is drunk it is rapidly absorbed from the gut, usually within 60 minutes, and dilutes the body fluids so that their osmolality falls a little. An attendant change of less than 1% of plasma osmolality stimulates the osmoreceptor and volume-receptor via the neurohypophysial-renin–angiotensin mechanisms, which in turn inhibits the excretion of ADH. This makes the distal part of the distal tubule and collecting ducts impermeable to water and a water diuresis ensues, so that within 3–4 hours, after drinking a litre of tap water, the water balance of the average adult returns to normal. There are circumstances in which water intake can exceed the diluting power of the normal kidney and water retention follows.

1. The mechanism of water excretion is impaired by specific disease processes such as renal or endocrine disorders and by generalized infective or traumatic processes.
2. Excessive intravenous infusion bypasses the thirst mechanism and can produce rapid changes in osmolality and consequently cause rapid alterations in the body solute concentration with attendant dramatic onset of symptoms. The giving of rectal water bypasses voluntary intake and the thirst mechanism. Tap water is virtually electrolyte-free and the method of administration often makes measurement or assessment of the volume given difficult or impossible.

We should now look at some of the clinical conditions dealing with each of these groups separately.

Impaired water excretion

(a) *Sickness and trauma.* A marked increase in ADH secretion is produced by severe infection which causes a generalized state of toxicity, trauma and haemorrhage. An increase in ADH secretion is maintained during the post-haemorrhagic period. Anxiety, fear, pain and discomfort have a similar effect. In clinical practice increased ADH secretion occurs most commonly following surgery, for during the postoperative period water-loading is not followed by a normal diuretic response and the 'escape mechanism' does not appear to operate in the same way. These effects can occur in the presence of a pre-existing hyponatraemia.[337]

(b) *Anoxia.* This produces a state of antidiuresis which is often overlooked when assessing fluid requirements. It is possible that the phenomenon can be explained in terms of inadequate cardiac output. For when the hypoxic patient is ventilated correctly with oxygen, not only does the systemic blood pressure rise, but also the urine output increases.

It is not uncommon, however, in the absence of any evidence of increased cardiac output, for severe oliguria to change to an adequate urine flow as the blood oxygen saturation rises. When an indwelling urethral cannula is *in situ*, it can be observed that the kidneys respond immediately following adequate oxygenation.

(*c*) *Cardiac failure*. When cardiac output begins to fall below pre-existing levels at rest, cardiac failure can be said to have occurred. It is important to define cardiac failure in this way because when there is shunting of blood from one side of the heart to the other, or from an artery to a vein, the cardiac output, even in failure, may be very much greater than normal. An arteriovenous aneurysm, possibly acquired during surgery, for example in the thigh, or following vascular or cardiac surgery, often presents as swelling of the ankles or sometimes jaundice of marked proportions, especially when associated with hepatomegaly. When pressure is applied to the site of the arteriovenous aneurysm, for example in the thigh, a slowing of the pulse rate will occur as the cause of the increased cardiac output is removed.

As the ability of the right side of the heart to pump blood falls, so an increase in the pressure on the venous side of the systemic circulation results consequent to redistribution of existing blood volume. The volume of blood in the high-pressure arterial system decreases and the mean blood pressure falls. There seems to be no doubt that under normal circumstances the veins are not filled to their capacity and an increase of some 10% in filling can occur before there is a detectable rise in venous pressure. This is the stage which we sometimes refer to as being a state of incipient cardiac failure, and oedema is not present. When the volume of blood in the arterial tree falls the secretion of aldosterone and ADH is stimulated and fluid and Na^+ are retained by the kidneys. As cardiac failure progresses further and the venous pressure rises, the balance between the volume of fluid filtered at the arterial end of the capillary network and the volume of fluid reabsorbed at the venule end is upset. In this way the volume of interstitial fluid increases and oedema is produced.

Another consequence of the reduced cardiac output and systemic blood pressure is a reduction in the glomerular filtration rate so that the passage of glomerular filtrate along the proximal tubule of the nephron is slow. Whereas, under normal conditions, 80–85% of the Na^+ content is reabsorbed isotonically with water, values of 90–95% reabsorption may be reached.

It can be seen that water and Na^+ excretion play an important part in the pathogenesis and treatment of cardiac failure and, conversely, minor

degrees of failure must be corrected in order to maintain a normal fluid balance. If the patient is placed on a low-salt or Na^+-free diet and a saluresis is induced by means of diuretics, the disproportionate sodium to water loss, because of the relatively low Na^+ content of urine compared with that of the ECF, will not apply if there is a negative sodium balance; that is to say, Na^+ excretion exceeds Na^+ intake. A rapid ingestion or infusion of electrolyte-free water can then produce water intoxication, especially if hyponatraemia is already marked. Diuretics of the chlorathiazide group that induce a potassium diuresis can, as described elsewhere (see p. 367) contribute to hyponatraemia in another manner.

(*d*) *Renal disease*. Any form of renal disease can give rise to water intoxication. Over-hydration can occur during the oliguria of acute nephritis, during the anuric phase of lower nephron nephrosis and during the terminal stages of chronic nephritis. It is necessary to appreciate that patients with only moderate azotaemia can develop severe and even lethal water intoxication and that the signs—mental disorientation, drowsiness, convulsions and coma— can be misinterpreted as being part of the primary disease. Water intoxication can sometimes occur before chronic nephritis has progressed to the stage of oliguria, and cases have been reported where it has occurred in patients with a 24-hour urine volume of more than 1000 ml following the drinking of a large volume of fluid (i.e. in preparation for a urea clearance test).[338] Similar cases have occurred when the water intake has been only moderately increased in order to produce a diuresis. Orthopnoea, a rise in body weight, oedema and increase in the volume of pleural effusion have accompanied this treatment.

(*e*) *Cirrhosis of the liver*. The marked retention of water in liver disease is largely a terminal event and is associated with gross oedema and ascites. Marked hyponatraemia occurs very often and this aspect is exacerbated by marked urinary potassium loss. Na^+ enters the cells to replace K^+ but hypokalaemia is frequently evident. It has long been recognized that cirrhosis of the liver gives rise to gynaecomastia, probably because the oestrogens produced are not metabolized. Increased oestrogens give rise to sodium and therefore water retention, and this may be one of the mechanisms by which body fluid volumes are expanded.

Water retention may be a complication of treatment of carcinoma of the prostate with stilboestrol. Repeated paracentesis abdominis—as repeated paracentesis thoracis (see p. 25)—gives rise to the hypoelectrolyteaemia, as the salt content of the fluid removed is almost identical with that of the ECF. It may also give rise to a major protein loss in the cirrhotic patient.

(f) *Self-induced water intoxication.* We have seen how water intoxication may be produced in patients who have chronic renal disease and drink too much water. It might be considered to be self-induced when an excess of electrolyte-free fluid is drunk by foundry workers and miners, producing the typical 'cramps'. However, it is also recognized that it may be associated with psychiatric disorders, especially schizophrenia[146] so that coma and convulsions develop. It must be borne in mind that a neurological lesion in these cases may be the primary cause.

(g) *Pitressin-induced intoxication.* When patients are undergoing a test for diabetes insipidus and are given injections of Pitressin, their subsequent water intake must be viewed with caution so that excessive dilution of the body fluids does not occur during the period of antidiuresis. People who are being treated with insufflation of posterior pituitary 'snuff' applied to the nasal mucosa sometimes produce the condition in themselves.

(h) *Oxytocin-induced intoxication.* Two cases of oxytocin-induced water intoxication have been reported by Mwambingu (1985).[218] These occurred during therapeutic abortion.

(i) *Inappropriate secretion of ADH.* This is most commonly seen following surgery and trauma. It is unrelated to the infusion of sodium-containing fluids. When water retention is a result of 'inappropriate ADH secretion' resulting from a neoplasm (e.g. carcinoma of the bronchus), then a gradual rise in body weight is observed and a small volume of urine of high osmolality (sp. gr. 1.018 or more) is excreted. The osmolality of urine is not reduced, nor is the volume of urine increased in response to a water load. As time progresses, the condition sometimes develops into one of partial adrenocortical insufficiency and a diuresis is produced when cortisone is administered.

Antidiuretic hormone is formed in the supra-optic nucleus of the hypothalamus and is transported along the supra-optico-hypophyseal tract and stored in the posterior lobe of the hypophysis or pituitary gland. The release of the hormone is determined by the plasma osmolality and ECF volume. At the distal tubule, the action of ADH is mediated by cyclic adenosine monophosphate (cyclic AMP), increasing the reabsorption of water in the collecting ducts. If the secretion of ADH is decreased (e.g. following head injury), the reabsorption of free water is reduced and the urine volume is increased.

Control of ADH secretion

Three factors appear to be associated with the control of ADH secretion and the supra-optico-hypophyseal system.[210] These appear to be:

(a) *osmoreceptors* located in the region of the median eminence which have receptor cells that can detect changes in plasma osmolality;

(b) *volume or stretch receptors* located in the left atrium: these are responsive to left atrial distension and are able to inhibit the release of ADH;

(c) *baroreceptors* which are located in the carotid sinuses and the aortic arch, and respond to a change in blood pressure.

A large number of stimuli can therefore be seen to initiate increased ADH secretion with retention of water. For example, haemorrhage, a fall in cardiac output, dehydration, hypoalbuminaemia, changes in body temperature, severe trauma and surgery. Some drugs also increase ADH release, including morphine, barbiturates and nicotine.

Factors which are known to decrease ADH secretion producing an increase in free-water excretion include concussion and brain damage, drugs and chemical preparations such as ethanol, diphenylhydantoin and possibly lithium. Total immersion of the body in water has produced suppression of ADH secretion.[93] Factors increasing and decreasing ADH secretion are listed in Table 2.1.

Table 2.1   Factors affecting ADH secretion

Factors which increase ADH secretion
  Increased plasma osmolarity and decreased blood volume
    Haemorrhage
    Decreased cardiac output
    Dehydration
    Hypoalbuminaemia
  Drugs and medications
    Nicotine
    Morphine
    Barbiturates
    General anaesthetics
    Beta-adrenergic agents
    Clofibrate (Atromid-S)
    Vincristine
    Cyclophosphamide (Cytoxan, Endoxana)
    Carbamazepine (Tegretol)
    Chlorpropamide
Factors which inhibit ADH secretion
  Ethanol
  Diphenylhydantoin
  Hypo-osmolarity
  Beta-adrenergic agents
  Morphine antagonists
  Total body immersion
  Hypervolaemia

Pathophysiology of inappropriate ADH secretion

The syndrome of inappropriate secretion of ADH causes an increase in total body water with subsequent dilution of body fluid compartments. The pathophysiology of the condition was first indicated by Schwartz *et al.* in 1957,[270] when they described its development in two patients suffering from bronchial carcinoma. Since that time, there have been a number of reports linking the condition with various disorders,[79, 268] including those of the chest and central nervous system. The continued reabsorption of body water, which would in the normal way be suppressed by the inhibition of ADH following stimulation of the volume, osmolar and other receptors, is allowed to proceed.

In 1967, Bartter and Schwartz[29] observed that when other causes of hyponatraemia were excluded (such as renal failure, salt depletion, corticoadrenal insufficiency), there remained a group of patients in whom inappropriate secretion of ADH appeared to be the aetiology of the condition. It was considered that the following factors should be present, although direct measurements of ADH were not made.

1. Hyponatraemia with consequent hyposmolality of the plasma.
2. Continued excretion of Na^+ in the urine.
3. Lack of clinical evidence of fluid loss and depletion.
4. Failure to dilute urine to a minimal degree and therefore assist concentration of plasma.
5. Normal renal function.
6. Normal corticoadrenal function.
7. The condition responded to water deprivation.[28,29]

While some tumours are known to produce ADH from amino acid precursors and to release the hormone quite independently from any control by the hypothalamus, other factors, such as aldosterone secretion, may be important. By far the greatest number of tumours associated with the inappropriate secretion of ADH are bronchogenic, especially the oat cell carcinoma, but tumours of many other organ systems have been implicated. Drugs such as vincristine are believed to act directly on the supra-optico-hypophyseal system. Chlorpropamide is considered to act directly on the renal tubules potentiating the action of ADH (see Table 2.1).

Some evidence of inappropriate ADH secretion is seen in patients who develop hyponatraemia following thoracotomy. It is also sometimes found in patients during artificial ventilation of the lungs. Here, the impairment of blood flow through the lungs (see p. 127) may result in decreased filling of the left atrium with subsequent suppression of the stretch receptors. There are a number of conditions, however, that are not necessarily due to inappropriate ADH secretion in which hyponatraemia occurs and water restriction produces an improvement in both the patient's condition and the plasma $[Na^+]$. Inappropriate ADH secretion, in some accounts, has been considered to be identical to water intoxication, although clinicians are aware that severe water intoxication can be iatrogenic (p. 30), or self-inflicted.[251]

It would appear, therefore, that when the term hyponatraemia is used, it should always be qualified indicating the aetiology of the condition, and not conveniently (and sometimes inaccurately) labelled inappropriate ADH secretion. This view is supported by Thomas *et al.*[299]

Symptoms and signs of water intoxication

The mode of onset of water intoxication depends largely on how it is produced. If it is the result of excessive intravenous infusions or the giving of large volumes of tap water rectally into patients of small size, then the first indications are dramatic and alarming and may presage a fatal outcome. At first they are mostly cerebral, the patient exhibiting anxiety, excitement or psychotic behaviour; delirium or coma and generalized convulsions may be present. Hyperventilation is often a marked feature and there may be nausea and repeated vomiting, profuse sweating and a flushed skin.

When the onset is more gradual the disorders of cerebral function are less acute. The patient is weak, drowsy and apathetic. There is often a severe headache and dimness or blurring of the vision. The tendon reflexes are hyperactive and exercise of muscles gives rise to cramping. As the condition progresses, drowsiness gives place to coma, hypertension is replaced by hypotension, tachycardia by bradycardia, and hyperventilation by a slow respiratory rate. Papilloedema may then be present.

The signs of water intoxication are the exact reverse of those of sodium depletion. Instead of loss of weight, weight is gained, the tissue turgor and skin elasticity are normal and the eyeball tension may be raised. The mucous membranes are moist, there may be excess salivation and fluid diarrhoea may occur.

In the early stages of water intoxication the kidneys may produce a large quantity of dilute urine, but as hyponatraemia develops this is replaced by oliguria which may become severe. The specific gravity of the urine is low.

Case history. An 18-year-old boy underwent an operation for subvalvar aortic stenosis under profound hypothermia. After the operation blood continued to drain from the thorax. In all he received 10 litres of blood from the beginning of the procedure. Although haemorrhage had ceased by the evening of the day of the operation and the pulse rate and blood pressure were maintained within normal values, in view of the experience of the preceding period two intravenous infusions were continued so that they would be available if rapid bleeding recurred. Both bottles contained dextrose 4.8% with saline 0.18%. The nursing staff were instructed, incorrectly, that the rate of infusion of one bottle should keep pace with the volume of urine excreted and that the other bottle should be infused at such a rate that the cannula was kept open. This regimen was maintained throughout the night and the following day and a large volume (greater than 3.5 litres) of dilute urine was passed. During this period the patient drank over a litre of water and fruit juice. The nursing staff, with admirable zeal, controlled the rate of infusion so that they had infused 500 ml in excess of the urine volume.

During the latter part of the afternoon following the operation the patient became drowsy and confused and a short while later had a generalized convulsion which recurred at irregular intervals, later interspersed with periods of a semicomatose state. These convulsions were considered to be the result of an air embolus which had been introduced during the surgical procedure and the fluid regimen was not suspected.

On examination the patient was warm with no sign of peripheral constriction. On the contrary the veins were full, the blood pressure and pulse were normal, but there was neck stiffness. The tendon reflexes were brisk and the plantar reflex was biphasic. The patient was passing urine at a rapid rate and the plasma sodium concentration was 124 mmol/l (mEq/l).

A careful assessment of the fluid balance from the time of operation demonstrated that a litre of glucose had been infused during the extracorporeal circulation in order to facilitate the giving of anaesthetic drugs. A further 540 ml of sodium bicarbonate solution (2.74%) had been infused to correct a metabolic acidosis. As each 540 ml (pint) of ACD blood infused represented a further 120 ml of fluid, the patient had also received 2400 ml of water from that source alone. In addition 300 ml of glucose had been infused via the arterial blood pressure cannula in order to keep it patent. By the time haemorrhage had ceased, therefore, the patient had acquired an excess of fluid of over 4 litres, although only a small proportion of this had been electrolyte free. In the ordinary way much of this would have been corrected by renal excretion, but because the infusion of fluid was keeping pace with urine output, this was prevented, and as the sodium content of the urine was lower than that of the ECF and because this water loss was being replaced by fluid of low-electrolyte concentration, the serum sodium fell. Furthermore, replacement exceeded urine output in two ways: (*a*) the thirst mechanism was not functioning normally and, although the volume was measured, the oral intake of fluid during the period of consciousness was not controlled; (*b*) a marked excess of fluid was infused because of wrong instructions given to the nursing staff as to the fluid requirement of the patient and also because a large volume of fluid was being infused in order to keep an intravenous drip functioning. As the nursing staff changed, the magnitude of this infusion was not realized.

The situation arose because it was not realized that patients who have received infusions of fluid and have, in addition, had a large volume of blood transfused because of haemorrhage, end the surgical procedure with a water load which requires time to be excreted. The second reason was the result of the nursing staff's zeal in performing their task correctly rather than neglecting any part of it. In the absence of a correctly arranged fluid regimen based on moderate water restriction, this situation can always arise.

On examination the clinical picture was predominantly that of water intoxication and a simple arithmetical assessment of water balance revealed a heavy water load. Fluid intake was reduced temporarily to 200 ml over the following 12 hours and 300 ml during the next 12 hours. Within 24 hours the patient had completely corrected his water balance and further recovery was uneventful.

Symptomless hyponatraemia

There is a group of people who demonstrate a low serum Na^+ level, but who are neither overhydrated nor dehydrated. There is never any evidence of abnormal renal function and while some subsequently demonstrate adrenocortical insufficiency, these particular patients respond normally to a water load and retain both water and salt when desoxycorticosterone acetate (DOCA) is administered. An increased Na^+ intake is followed by increased sodium excretion in the urine and, characteristically, when these patients are placed on a salt-free diet they are capable of passing Na+-free urine.

Although they may be a little lethargic and demonstrate slight muscle weakness, this is by no means marked and physical signs are virtually absent. There are, however, factors which are common to this group, for these patients rarely show marked improvement and the majority die within 2 years of diagnosis. They almost always suffer from malnutrition and while some suffer from chronic disease processes, such as carcinoma of the lung, advanced tuberculosis or cirrhosis of the liver, others have none of these disorders and the underlying condition is never discovered. Rarely, a tiny tumour of the pituitary gland has been found at autopsy.

The hyponatraemia is not associated with potassium retention and it must be assumed that a resetting of the osmoreceptor has occurred and is quite different, for example, from the chronic dilutional hyponatraemia of chronic cardiac failure.

Role of potassium depletion in hyponatraemia

When in chronic malnutrition K+ is lost from the body and when K+ depletion occurs from an abnormal K+ balance, then the Na+ replaces the K+ within the cells. This leads to a fall in the plasma Na+ level. It can be seen, therefore, that K+ depletion is one of the causes of hyponatraemia. When hyponatraemia is present in congestive cardiac failure there is a predisposition to digitalis intoxication resulting from K+ depletion. Also the severity of the condition, both in its action on the myocardium and its symptoms, is increased.

There are common clinical conditions in which the total body K+ is reduced. These are typically the metabolic response to surgery and trauma where Na+ and water are retained and K+ is lost via the urine, the serum Na+ level then falls. It is also seen when patients are treated with diuretics for congestive cardiac failure or for cirrhosis of the liver with ascites. When diuretics cease to work after a fall in the plasma Na+, K+ is still excreted in the urine in large quantities whenever they are used. K+ depletion is a cause of the onset of coma in hepatic insufficiency (see p. 427).

The treatment of hyponatraemia

(a) *Sodium loss.* Na+ depletion is associated with a reduction in body fluid. It is necessary, therefore, to restore both Na+ and water. This may be achieved by the infusion of isotonic NaCl either 0.85% (= 145 mmol/l) or 0·94% (= 153 mmol/l). In the first instance it is preferable to infuse a solution of NaCl, which has twice the

concentration of the isotonic solution; a 1.8% solution contains 300 mmol/l. The latter solution will restore the volume of the ECF without producing prolonged changes in plasma osmolality, and correction will be achieved by the renal excretion of water as renal function is improved. When difficult cases are being treated repeated estimation of the Na+ content of plasma and urine is necessary in order to control the body electrolyte and fluid content carefully.

The amount of Na+ required by the Na+-depleted patient may be calculated as follows:

Na+ deficit in mmol =
(140 − plasma [Na+]) × body weight in kg × 0.6

(b) *Water intoxication.* In this condition Na+ depletion is not of primary importance, although it may be present to a certain extent. The extracellular fluid space is already expanded above normal values, so that it is dangerous to infuse isotonic saline solution. This will merely expand the ECF still further without appreciably raising the Na+ concentration. This may exacerbate the cerebral oedema and may precipitate pulmonary oedema. The first step, therefore, is to stop all fluids immediately and sometimes this will be all that is necessary. Fluid restriction alone, however, will be of value only if a reasonably good renal function is still present, but severe serum hypotonicity is often associated with oliguria. Also, when convulsions continue, then treatment is essential because we know that in some cases there will be a fatal outcome. It is then advisable to infuse a 6% solution of NaCl (5.85% NaCl contains 1 mmol/ml). The solution should not be infused at a rate greater than 40 ml/hour unless the urine output improves markedly, when the rate of infusion may be increased to 50 or 60 ml/hour. When a water diuresis has been established it may be possible for the infusion to be terminated and, by continued water restriction, assisted by oral Na+ and renal function, the patient can correct the disorder spontaneously. Much stronger solutions containing 4 or 5 mmol/ml have been advocated.

The treatment of chronic water intoxication is difficult and rests largely upon the diagnosis. Basically, it might appear to depend upon which segment of the nephron is predominantly involved in the disease process.

When water retention is a result of excessive ADH secretion following trauma or surgery, time alone will reverse the situation if hypovolaemia is treated in the very early stages and if careful control is maintained over the water and electrolyte balance for a few days. The fact that there may be shifts of electrolyte into or out of the ICF must be taken into account. Other factors that require attention at this stage are pain and anxiety. Anaemia, hypoproteinaemia, inadequate vitamin intake and incipient cardiac failure need to be excluded. It is much more important to digitalize prophylactically patients who are severely ill and who may be moderately or severely anoxic from lung pathology, than to await the obvious signs of inadequate myocardial function. In adrenocortical insufficiency the delayed water excretion responds rapidly to injections of hydrocortisone either intravenously or intramuscularly. No harm will arise from the administration of a single 'test dose' of hydrocortisone (100–200 mg) intravenously. The treatment of inappropriate ADH secretion is water restriction and 9 α-fluorohydrocortisone. The condition is sometimes alleviated for a time by excision of the tumour and radiotherapy. When the disease process progresses, adrenocortical failure replaces inappropriate ADH secretion and fluid intake may have to be increased and cortisone (e.g. 25 mg b.d.) is usually effective.

A recurring problem is the hyponatraemia of chronic congestive cardiac failure. When the plasma [Na^+] falls to below 130 mmol/l, diuretics often fail to be effective and the prognosis of the patient becomes much worse. A salt-free diet exacerbates the condition and a sodium-restricted diet is often equally dangerous. Both diets contribute to the state of chronic malnutrition from which all these patients suffer. When the serum reaches very low levels, for example 120–127 mmol/l, water restriction is essential and 1 litre is an adequate intake over 24 hours in the adult. During this period the patient should be encouraged to take nourishing concentrated foods which are extra to the normal diet. For example, sweets, chocolate, biscuits, etc. should be encouraged and evaporated cows' milk, containing the concentrated easily absorbable homogenized fat globules, should be added liberally to puddings. The therapeutic dose of digitalis is often very close to the toxic dose and, while it is essential for the maximum therapeutic effect to be obtained, care must be taken under these circumstances that K^+ depletion does not occur, and K^+ supplements to the diet should be given, even when low doses of diuretics are employed. When hyponatraemia has been present for a considerable period, the plasma [Na^+] may have to reach 132 mmol/l before diuretics again produce an adequate urine output. Although osmotic diuretics such as mannitol and urea have been advocated, there is little evidence that they can be employed effectively in the majority of cases. K^+ salts may assist in the hyponatraemic patient by producing a K^+ diuresis.

Intravenous aminophylline (0.25–0.5 g) is sometimes effective when used in association with other diuretics because of its action in increasing renal blood flow and glomerular filtration rate (GFR). When Na^+ levels are returning to normal, spironolactone given daily may also be beneficial, and sometimes its effect is enhanced by cortisone (25 mg b.d.). Because of their low mineralocorticoid function, the use of triamcinolone 4–12 mg/day, prednisone or prednisolone 5–15 mg/day when given with diuretics is frequently effective.

Possibly the best preparation is triamcinolone acetonide which is a slow release 'depot' form of the corticosteroid. It is given in doses of 40 mg/ml by deep intramuscular injection. One or two millilitres at monthly intervals frequently assists in the control of this type of water retention and appears to be most effective in the elderly. In extremely resistant cases where the GFR is low, a combination of thiazide diuretic, e.g. chlorathiazide 1 or 2 g, or hydrochlorothiazide 50–100 mg given in two doses morning and noon with ethacrynic acid 25–75 mg i.v. or frusemide (Lasix) 50–400 mg i.v., may be effective. The diuretic bumetanide (Burinex) has been shown to be effective when the GFR is extremely low, for example 2.7–4.9 ml/minute in renal failure,[33] and, unlike frusemide, it has not caused ototoxicity when given in large doses.

Treatment of symptomless hyponatraemia
Except when it arises from an identifiable cause, such as inappropriate ADH secretion, and water restriction is effective, the treatment is difficult. Hypophysectomy and adrenalectomy do not offer much hope of success.

Hypernatraemia

The normal [Na^+] of the plasma or serum is between 135 mmol/l and 145 mmol/l. Hypernatraemia is usually said to be present when the plasma or serum [Na^+] is above 150 mmol/l, but it is advisable to consider any value above 145 mmol/l as a potentially serious condition. Hypernatraemia occurs whenever there is too little water within the body or when there is an excess of electrolyte, or when both factors are present.

Water loss from the body

When water is lost from the body and it is not replaced, the total body water is reduced and the concentration of the solutes in all the fluid compartments is increased. The volume of circulating blood falls because the plasma volume is reduced as a result of water loss. We are, therefore, able to detect a rise in the packed cell volume (PCV), the plasma protein concentration and the electrolytes. This condition is sometimes referred to as hyper-electrolytaemia and a raised serum Na^+ level is easily detected. It has already been pointed out that when a loss occurs from one of the fluid compartments a movement of water from the other compartments follows so that the fluid within most of the tissue cells maintains the same osmotic pressure as the ECF. Because of this, we are usually able to predict with a fair degree of accuracy the changes that occur within the human body. The usual example taken to illustrate this is a 70-kg man, although some of our adult patients will have body weights of 50 kg or less.

A 70-kg man will be expected to have approximately 40 litres of body water (60% of 70 = 42). His plasma $[Na^+]$ will be close to the normal value of 140 mmol/l (mEq/l). If he is allowed to lose 5 litres of body water without gain or loss of Na^+ from the body, then the rise in plasma Na^+ level can be calculated as follows:

$$140 \times \frac{40}{35} = 160 \text{ mmol/l (mEq/l)}.$$

This represents a rise in the plasma $[Na^+]$ of approximately 14%. Because equal concentration of all substances within the body follows a pure water loss, the normal PCV of 45% in the male patient will rise, so that it is just in excess of 51% when there is a deficit of water of 5 litres.

In practice, any PCV greater than 45% in the male and 40% in the female should be treated with suspicion when it has been established that there have been no recent blood transfusions, especially of packed cells, and that chronic lung pathology, congenital cardiac defects producing cyanosis and rare conditions such as polycythaemia vera are absent. The ratio:

$$\frac{\text{Normal PCV (haematocrit)}}{\text{Abnormal PCV (haematocrit)}}$$

can be used in a similar manner to the plasma $[Na^+]$ shown below.

The plasma protein concentration which may be expected to rise as haemoconcentration occurs may also reflect a disproportionate fluid loss. While PCV's and plasma protein concentration may be less reliable than serum sodium concentrations, especially in the presence of disease processes, serial estimations made over a number of days will reflect the changing fluid content of the extra-cellular space.

Estimation of fluid deficit

In order to estimate the volume of fluid required to correct the disproportionate water loss, these same principles may be applied. This is best illustrated by the following case.

Case history. A 58-year-old woman living alone developed a high fever. She was tended by an elderly neighbour and insisted that medical assistance should not be called. When 4 days had elapsed and she developed rigors, her neighbour, ignoring her wishes, sent for her medical practitioner who diagnosed pneumonia. On admission to hospital she had the physical signs of dehydration, fever and lung consolidation. The urine she passed was of low volume, had a specific gravity of 1.026 and contained less than 3 mmol/l (mEq/l) of Na^+. Her plasma $[Na^+]$ was 164 mmol/l (mEq/l). She weighed 62 kg and would, therefore, be expected to have a body content of approximately 37 litres, i.e.

$$62 \times \frac{60}{100} = 62 \times 0.6 = 37.2 \text{ litres}$$

We know that the plasma $[Na^+]$ is inversely proportional to the body water content. The volume of body water at the time of admission was, therefore, 31.6 litres, i.e.

$$\frac{140}{164} \times \text{body weight} \times 0.6$$

$$= \frac{\text{Normal } [Na^+]}{\text{Abnormal } [Na^+]} \times \text{body weight} \times 0.6$$

$$= \frac{140}{164} \times 37 = 31.6$$

As her normal body water content was 37 litres, her fluid deficit amounted to $37 - 31.6 = 5.4$ litres.

It should be noted that while Na^+ tends to be retained in the presence of pneumonic consolidation, any fever or severe illness impairs the kidneys' ability to concentrate, and hypernatraemia in the absence of a total body water deficit is well recognized. This patient was, however, able to achieve urine concentration to a satisfactory level. It should also be observed that even in the presence of a high fever and a very high plasma $[Na^+]$, the urine was relatively Na^+ free. A Na^+-free urine is commonly observed in the presence of hypernatraemia that has resulted from dehydration. It is sometimes suggested that this is a process evolved by the living organism to preserve the volume of circulating blood and in so doing other homoeostatic mechanisms are suppressed. Because in the early stage of her illness expert nursing care was absent, the patient had drunk an insufficient volume of water, and hyperventilation and high fever increased the amount of water lost through the skin and lungs.

The degree of dehydration or combined fluid and salt loss can be calculated from the haemoglobin. However, when this calculation is made in isolation, it gives no indication of the degree of electrolyte, particularly Na^+, change that has occurred. It is also of very little value where there is also blood loss.

Aetiology of hypernatraemia

We have seen how hypernatraemia is produced when the balance between water loss and water intake is upset, or when there is an excess of electrolytes within the body, or when both conditions prevail. We should now look at some of the clinical conditions in which it occurs and examine the mechanisms by which they develop.

Reduction of body water
Insufficient intake of water
We have seen how the thirst mechanism may not function when it is most needed, and the continued loss of water through the skin, lungs and kidneys makes fluid replacement essential. Even in the absence of diseases producing an excessive water loss, the requirements of the individual vary to such a degree, according, for example, to body size and the temperature of the environment, that attention to this factor must always be of concern to the medical and nursing staff.

Excessive water loss through the kidneys
Osmotic diuresis. The amount of fluid that is reabsorbed from the nephron is influenced by the nature and the quantity of solute in the filtrate produced by the glomerulus. When the filtrate contains a substance that is either not absorbed at all or is in such a high concentration that it can only be partially reabsorbed during its passage through the renal tubules, it exerts an osmotic force which counterbalances the mechanisms which are acting to withdraw water from the tubular urine. An increased urine flow then occurs even in the presence of dehydration. Any solute can produce an osmotic diuresis whether it is taken orally or whether it is infused intravenously. Glucose and urea are the most common examples but sodium salts, ammonium salts and potassium salts will have the same effects. The most convenient way of producing an osmotic diuresis is to infuse a non-reabsorbable solute such as mannitol. THAM (tris hydroxymethyl amino-methane) will also produce an osmotic diuresis as well as changing the acid–base balance. The infusion of concentrated sodium salts will have the same effect but with this difference: the urine during an osmotic diuresis will always contain less Na^+ than that contained in the plasma and usually contains between 5 and 100 mmol/l (mEq/l). It can thus be seen that an osmotic diuresis is an important process by which disproportion between water loss and body sodium content can occur. It is well recognized that infusions of hypertonic glucose and urea have this effect.

Osmotic diuresis occurring because of renal failure. This condition can be divided into its early and late stages. In the early stages the reduction in the number of nephrons in the kidney exposes the tubules to a high osmotic load so that a diuresis results from the excess solute. Some degree of polyuria is, therefore, one of the early signs of chronic renal insufficiency. Later, however, when the renal disease progresses towards its terminal stages, oliguria replaces polyuria for the kidneys become unable to excrete either solute or water.

Another form of osmotic diuresis occurs in the pre-recovery stage of acute renal failure, but this is also associated with renal insufficiency. Here the urine volumes may reach 10 litres or more in 24 hours. A very similar situation arises in patients who have suffered from obstructive anuria. It occurs most commonly after prostatectomy, the removal of renal calculi and the relief of congenital bladder neck obstructions in children. One interesting factor which is common to this group is the excretion of a large volume of very dilute urine, the osmolality being in the region of 200 mosmol/l. It will be seen that these conditions can lead rapidly to a hyperosmolar state reflected in raised plasma Na^+ levels.

Osmotic diuresis in the absence of renal failure. It can be seen that the kidney regulates the osmolality of the body fluids and that when the solute load exceeds the kidneys' ability to reabsorb the major part of it, then it is obligatory that water be excreted. Such a condition occurs in the uncontrolled diabetic. The presence of large quantities of ketone bodies and of glucose represents a vast increase in the osmotic load presented to the kidneys. Polyuria thus becomes a major symptom and dehydration of the body occurs rapidly. The flow of urine may increase to such an extent that the maximum reabsorbing 'capacity of the tubule for Na^+ may be exceeded and some Na^+ lost in the urine. However, an increase in plasma $[Na^+]$ is the general rule, and in extreme cases values of 175 mmol/l (mEq/l) or more may be reached. The treatment of this condition is dealt with on page 414.

Excessive ingestion of solute. It is a common practice during prolonged debilitating diseases and during prolonged unconsciousness, such as follows a head injury, to resort to feeding by means of an oesophageal or intragastric tube. This has many advantages. It is, however, possible to give nourishment in a concentrated form. Casilan, which is a form of concentrated protein, and Complan, which is a balanced diet manufactured by Glaxo, are popular preparations. These are excellent but it must be remembered that when a patient is sick the renal osmolar clearance is reduced and may be only 600 mosmol/l. If it is necessary, because of the high protein and electrolyte content of the diet, to excrete 1500–1800 mosmol/day, the patient will be obliged to pass 2.5–3 litres of urine every 24 hours. It can thus be seen that in this kind of patient excessive protein feeding can lead to rapid water depletion. Very clear and well documented accounts of this process occurring in patients and causing dehydration, azotaemia and hypernatraemia were reported by Gault *et al.*[123]

Diabetes insipidus. In this condition the action of ADH on the distal and collecting tubule of the kidney is absent. A large volume of dilute urine is passed by the patient who becomes water depleted unless an equally large volume of water is ingested. The treatment for this condition is to give 5–10 units of Pitressin subcutaneously in an aqueous solution each morning or evening. For more prolonged action, an intramuscular injection of 5–10 units (1–2 ml) of Pitressin tannate in oil can be given and will be effective for 48 hours. Another preparation is posterior pituitary extract snuff, which is insufflated into the nostrils. The daily requirements are in the region of 50–100 mg, but the precise dose and the frequency with which it has to be taken have to be determined in each individual case. A synthetic product, lysyl-8-vassopressin, in the form of a spray applied to the mucous membranes of the nose is effective in the mild case and is a useful adjunct to long-acting preparations.

Diabetes insipidus can be seen following trauma, especially when associated with concussion and fracture of the skull. The author has observed its development in children, for example a 3-year-old child (following fracture of the skull) and in adults. If correction of the fluid loss is not made, hypotension develops.

Case history. A 28-year-old man was struck by a car so that he received fractures of the right femur and skull and other minor injuries. He was unconscious and was ventilated artificially. Three days after the accident, at 6.30 p.m., he began to increase his urine output and between that time and 7.30 a.m. the following morning, he excreted approximately 8.5 litres of urine of low specific gravity. The increase in urine output was not reported to the medical staff and the prearranged intravenous fluid regimen was continued. The blood pressure fell from 150/90 mmHg to 80/40 mmHg. When the rate of fluid replacement was increased at 7.30 a.m. the following morning, the blood pressure began to rise and returned to its normal value. It was found that 5 units of Pitressin in water intramuscularly three times daily, or 10 units of Pitressin tannate in oil daily, maintained a normal fluid balance.

Nephrogenic diabetes insipidus. This is a congenital lesion which presents in a similar manner to that of ADH insufficiency, but is of renal origin. It can be differentiated from true diabetes insipidus by administering posterior pituitary gland extract. A very similar condition, in some ways indistinguishable from nephrogenic diabetes insipidus, except for the fact that it is rarely as severe, occurs in association with carcinomatosis.

Extrarenal water loss

(a) Sweating. Because water is the liquid with the greatest known latent heat it naturally forms an important means by which heat is dissipated from the body. It is not surprising, therefore, that it can play such an important part in electrolyte metabolism in relation to disease, industry and climatic conditions. The Na^+ content of sweat varies greatly and lies between 8 mmol/l (mEq/l) and 80 mmol/l (mEq/l). The K^+ content of sweat lies somewhere beween 3 mmol/l (mEq/l) and 10 mmol/l (mEq/l). Both the Na^+ content and the Na^+/K^+ ratio appear to be under the partial control of steroid secretion in a manner similar to that in which the electrolyte content of urine is controlled. It can be seen, however, that the Na^+ content of sweat and its osmolality are always well below those of plasma. Continued excessive sweating will thus lead rapidly to an imbalance between the water content of the body and sodium concentration of the ECF and thus to dehydration with hypernatraemia. The continuous unseen evaporation of water from the surface of the body is usually referred to as 'insensible fluid loss'. Insensible loss in a hot, dry atmosphere in a well-ventilated room may reach proportions similar to that of sweating in a humid atmosphere.

Excessive sweating is usually followed by the drinking of water which is electrolyte free. Thus if sweating causes a large fluid loss which contains a moderately high concentration of sodium, drinking tap water may lead to the reverse condition of hypernatraemia (i.e. hyponatraemia). This occurs in furnace or iron foundry workers and miners. It gives rise to the symptoms of acute water intoxication which in this case are usually manifested by muscle cramps and convulsions, and it has been known to cause death. Fortunately, the condition is now well recognized and care is taken that a sodium-free intake is avoided.

(b) *Losses from the gastro-intestinal tract.* Both the gastric juice and secretion of the small and large gut contain Na^+ so that both water and Na^+ depletion can occur as a result of vomiting and diarrhoea. In most cases, the intestinal juice is hypotonic to plasma so that hypernatraemia can develop. Infants, especially, can develop diarrhoea from almost any acute disease, for example, otitis media, and this can lead to marked hypernatraemia.

(c) *Hyperventilation.* This is an extremely important physical sign which is often neglected. As we have said elsewhere, it should always be regarded as a bad prognostic sign when it is an integral part of a disease process. It gives rise to a pure water loss and is commonly seen in conditions where water depletion has already occurred and hyperosmolality of the plasma is present. Its association with diabetic coma is discussed under that subject (see p. 413). It thus leads to an exacerbation of the abnormal state. In the later stages of dehydration, hyperventilation gives place to respiratory depression so that artificial ventilation may be necessary in addition to electrolyte-free fluid (i.e. 5% glucose or fructose). Positive pressure ventilation must be applied with care so that the hypotension and peripheral circulatory failure are not increased.

Many conditions produce hyperventilation. It occurs in the presence of hyponatraemia and in the absence of a metabolic acidosis so that the pathophysiology of the condition must in all cases be elucidated before special forms of therapy are instituted.

Reduction of body water absent (or of low significance)

Cerebral damage
In some cases of brain damage a resetting of the osmoreceptor centre in the hypothalamus occurs so that sodium is retained within the body and the plasma $[Na^+]$ is raised. Hypernatraemia sometimes appears in the newborn infant and is manifested by a failure to thrive and is associated with mental retardation. The plasma sodium level may be as high as a 170 mmol/l (mEq/l) in the presence of normal hydration. When a low-Na^+ diet is given the urine $[Na^+]$ falls.

It has been demonstrated that there is a reduction in the size and number of the cerebral gyri. It may be deduced in these circumstances that the osmoreceptors are 'set' at an abnormally high value. However, cerebral damage can also be caused by hypernatraemia following an excessive Na^+ intake, examples of which are given below.

Excessive electrolyte intake
This can occur in the following ways: (a) when too much electrolyte is prescribed by the medical attendant, (b) by voluntary over-ingestion, (c) by the administration of salt emetics, and (d) during infant feeding.

(a) Hypertonic electrolyte solutions are often infused during extracorporeal circulation for open-heart surgery, when a metabolic acidosis has to be corrected by adding sodium bicarbonate solution to the circulating blood. High plasma Na^+ levels are often encountered and values between 155 mmol/l(mEq/l) and 160 mmol/l(mEq/l) have been recorded. In the presence of a normal renal function the major part of the Na^+ is rapidly eliminated. Until recently it had been considered that the infusion of saline during surgery should be avoided as retention of Na^+, which is known to occur postoperatively, may lead to cardiac failure. There is growing evidence that this is not so. It is true that following trauma and surgery the urine contains very little Na^+ and this has usually been considered to be the result of altered renal function or of alterations in steroid secretion. We now know that if electrolyte infusions are given during surgery, the sodium concentration of the urine rises in the postoperative period and retention of Na^+ does not occur, even when further infusions of Na^+ are given in the postoperative period. During operative procedures it may be necessary to infuse hypertonic solution and this is the usual practice during extracorporeal circulations, such as the use of the heart–lung machines for heart–lung bypass, and profound hypothermia for open-heart surgery.

Long experience with the care of patients who have undergone open-heart surgery, some of whom have been in cardiac failure before surgical intervention, has confirmed that the hypernatraemia alone is not a contributory cause for cardiac failure. The volume of the water intake is, however, of major importance in this respect. When fluid intake is restricted cardiac failure arising from this cause may be avoided.

(*b*) Voluntary ingestion. Hyperelectrolytaemia arising from this cause almost invariably occurs when the patient is suffering from a peptic ulcer and is taking large quantities of sodium bicarbonate ($NaHCO_3$).

(*c*) Treatment of poisoning and drug overdose. Another source of serious hypernatraemia and hyperosmolality which may cause cerebral injury is the use of strong salt solutions as emetics. Numerous cases have been recorded.[22,49,60,104,132,266]

There is some controversy with regard to treatment because of the high incidence of convulsions developing during attempts to correct the abnormal plasma [Na^+]. The convulsions are said to be un-related to the severity of the hypernatraemia. Because it has been observed that rapid hydration with salt-free solutions may cause convulsions, the use of a glucose/saline solution has been advocated.[104]

(*d*) Hypernatraemia in infants has been associated with cot death. It is for this reason that the use of 'humanized cows' milk' has been attacked from some quarters. It has also been pointed out (Lucas, 1977)[187] that sterilizing the feeding bottle and the artificial teat in the sterilizing agent 'Milton', which contains sodium hypochlorite, can add significantly to the sodium concentration of the milk fed to infants. When 'Milton' is correctly diluted (1/80), the sodium concentration should be approximately 40 mmol/l (mEq/l) to which a small quantity of additional sodium from tap water must be added. Expressed human breast milk contains on average only 6.4 mmol/l(mEq/l).[78] Lucas also observed that when babies were fed humanized cows' milk, a third of the sodium in their diet originated from the sodium hypochlorite used to sterilize the bottles.

If the 'Milton' is diluted inaccurately, the average sodium content is found to be 79 mmol/l(mEq/l). It is apparent that, although the safety of using sodium hypochlorite as a sterilizing agent for infants' feeding bottles is well documented, a significant and possibly hazardous contribution to the dietary intake of sodium can be made and the implications are greater in babies of low birth weight if accurate dilution of the hypochlorite solution is not practised.

Potassium

We have already mentioned how K^+ is largely confined to the intracellular space, comprising the major cation in all cells in man including the erythrocytes. It plays a major part in maintaining the integrity of many specialized organ functions such as the beating of the heart, the conduction of impulses along nervous and other specialized tissues (such as the muscle end-plate) and renal function. The normal [K^+] within the ECF lies between 3.5 mmol/l(mEq/l) and 5.5 mmol/l (mEq/l). We refer to concentrations above this level as hyperkalaemia and those below this level as hypokalaemia.

Most evidence indicates that the renal control over K^+ is primarily one of tubular function.[34,216] The K^+ that is present in the urine appears to result from a process of secretion in which K^+ is exchanged for Na^+. Most, if not all, the K^+ that is present in the glomerular filtrate appears to be reabsorbed in the proximal tubule.[335] The normal dietary intake of K^+ is between 60 and 80 mmol/l (mEq/l) and the renal apparatus can cope with this quantity very readily. There is experimental evidence in animals that tolerance to continuous excessive K^+ loading may be acquired so that an increase in secretory rate that is 10–20 times greater than normal is achieved.[297]

Further work has indicated that potassium balance can be maintained in a markedly precise way during many forms of chronic progressive renal disease. Schultze *et al.*[269] maintained dogs on a constantly high dietary intake of potassium and then reduced the number of functioning nephrons by the surgical removal of one kidney. It was found that following the administration of a test dose of a potassium salt, the quantity of K^+ excreted in the first 5 hours by the remaining kidney alone was greater than that excreted pre-operatively by both kidneys together. Also, the 24-hour excretion of potassium by the remaining kidney averaged 92% of the administered load of potassium.

Part of the adaptation to an increased potassium load during chronic renal disease may be the increased excretion of potassium by the gut,[150] although the major adaptation would appear to be due to the increased excretion by the kidney. In this way, when the compensatory process has been developed to the full, a K^+ load which would normally be lethal can be well tolerated.

Two aspects with regard to K^+ excretion can be noted at this stage. The first is that K^+ excretion is largely independent of the GFR and, because of this, the retention of K^+ is not a feature of cardiac failure (that has not been treated with K^+-losing diuretics). Secondly, an excessively raised plasma [K^+] is a relatively late event in chronic nephritis, a disease in which there is a gradual reduction in the number of functioning nephrons. It is possible that an adaptive process such as that which occurs in K^+-loaded animals may develop in man[271] in order to excrete what might be considered to be a K^+ intake which is in excess of that with which a damaged kidney might be expected to cope.

Infusions of hypertonic glucose normally lower the serum $[K^+]$. This effect is mediated by insulin.[340] The distribution of $[K^+]$ between the fluid compartments is also influenced by aldosterone.[8] Some workers have found that, in the presence of aldosterone deficiency, the infusion of hypertonic glucose with insulin causes an *increase* in the serum $[K^+]$.[128,129] In addition, it has been demonstrated that patients suffering from diabetes mellitus who have normal aldosterone levels may also develop hyperkalaemia induced by glucose infusions.[12] Most of the patients who present in the emergency department suffering from severe diabetic ketosis have a high plasma $[K^+]$.

Acute gastric dilatation can occur in anorexia nervosa[48,95] and trauma. It is well recognized that perforation of the stomach can follow and that this is associated with a high mortality. Early treatment by means of gastric drainage and intravenous fluids is essential.

Because of the associated K^+ loss, a rough guide in therapy is the infusion of 40 mmol/l(mEq/l) of K^+ in the form of KCl for every litre of gastric fluid drainage.

The same regimen has been used successfully when prolonged paralytic ileus has occurred following surgery. The condition can arise after open-heart surgery, especially when respiratory failure develops and prolonged ventilation of the lungs is necessary. Careful K^+ replacement in these circumstances is essential.

Hyperkalaemia

Hyperkalaemia may occur in a number of clinical conditions and its reversal is frequently an important measure in resuscitation. It may occur acutely by the rapid infusion of K^+ salts or preparations such as triple-strength plasma, and in these circumstances may cause cardiac arrest. It occurs during acute renal failure and the rate of rise in concentration in the ECF is dependent upon the presence of tissue damage,[58] the amount of residual renal function and the time that has elapsed since the onset of the condition. A K^+-free intake must be maintained (see p. 108). A dangerous degree of K^+ intoxication may occur in patients with chronic renal disease when K^+ salts are given in association with diuretics or when there is an excessively high K^+ intake in food. The development of a gross metabolic acidosis contributes to hyperkalaemia. In this case, H^+ displace K^+ in the cells, and the

kidneys are then presented with an excessive load. These circumstances are exacerbated by dehydration and oliguria.

Hyperkalaemia due to K^+-sparing diuretics
Hyperkalaemia is a well-recognized risk associated with potassium-sparing diuretics. Spironolactone, one of the earliest products used for this purpose, has been the most frequently implicated agent. It has also been demonstrated to increase the degree of renal impairment in elderly patients.[155,219] Triamterene has also been found to have the same effect. Amiloride has been recognized to cause retention of K^+ and therefore hyperkalaemia, especially in the elderly.[20] Wan and Lye[320] found that amiloride induced both a metabolic acidosis and hyperkalaemia in an 80-year-old man, who returned to normal following the withdrawal of the diuretic agent. It required 10 days, however, for normality to be restored. It was noted that, in this particular case, the antiprostaglandin effect of indomethacin may have contributed to the condition. Nevertheless, patients of any age receiving potassium-retaining preparations during diuretic therapy need to be monitored carefully, so that severe hyperkalaemia is avoided.[117] Oral K^+ should never be prescribed in addition to a K^+-retaining agent.

Arginine-induced hyperkalaemia (cationic amino acid hyperkalaemia)
The amino acid arginine is usually administered in the form of the monohydrochloride, and it is regarded as a safe substance that can be given intravenously. It has been used, and indeed has gained acceptance, as a method of treating a severe metabolic alkalosis,[124] and to test the function of the pituitary gland.[206,207] It has been demonstrated that amino acid salts which, when ionized, have a cation in the form of an amino acid, can stimulate K^+ excretion in the urine.[4,80] Cationic amino acids, including arginine, have been demonstrated to cause a movement of K^+ from the cells into the ECF.[80,182]

In 1972, Hertz and Richardson[144] demonstrated that severe hyperkalaemia could be induced in patients who were being dialysed for terminal stage renal failure when arginine was administered therapeutically. The inability to excrete K^+ was considered to be a causative factor.

Two patients with alcoholic liver disease who received arginine monohydrochloride by intravenous infusion of the 10% solution in an attempt to reduce the persistent metabolic alkalosis that is associated with liver disease, developed severe hyperkalaemia.[56] In one patient the serum potassium rose to 7.5 mmol/l(mEq/l) 7 hours after the administration of arginine hydrochloride (600 ml of 10% solution; 285 mmol). The associated electro-cardiographic changes (see p. 92) developed. He was treated with calcium gluconate, glucose and insulin, and a potassium-binding resin. The plasma [K^+] fell and the patient survived. The second patient had a total CO_2 (TCO_2) of 59 mmol/l before the infusion of 40 g (190 mmol) of 10% arginine HCl. This patient died in spite of appro-priate treatment, and the plasma [K^+] rose from 4.0 mmol/l(mEq/l) to 7.1 mmol/l(mEq/l). These two patients, in a well-recorded report, illustrate the dangers of arginine and other cationic amino acids in the presence of an already abnormal meta-bolism even when renal disease is not present. The severity of the hyperkalaemia in these cases was probably due to the inability of the liver to meta-bolize the amino acid. The treatment of hyper-kalaemia, therefore, rests in maintaining a correct fluid balance, the withdrawal of a high oral or intravenous K^+ intake, the correction of the acid-osis with $NaHCO_3$ so that H^+ is displaced from the cells and replaced with K^+, and the facilitation of the excretion of K^+ by the renal tubules. The last is achieved by means of a K^+-losing diuretic such as hydrochlorothiazide. If these measures are ineffec-tive, the infusion of glucose and insulin (see p. 109) can be used for its temporary effect, even in conditions of chronic renal failure. When none of these measures is effective and ECG changes appear, then either blood (extracorporeal) or peritoneal dialysis may be performed. The giving of Ca^{++} salts may also be effective in reversing the effects of hyperkalaemia,[61] and when the meta-bolic acisosis is corrected in chronic renal failure with $NaHCO_3$ the addition of Ca^{++} to the diet or its injection intravenously may be necessary in order to avoid tetany.

Pseudohyperkalaemia and familial pseudo-hyperkalaemia

Familial pseudohyperkalaemia was reported by Stewart et al.[288] and refers to the leaching of K^+ from the red cells after blood has been withdrawn from a vessel and allowed to stand. In most people this process occurs relatively slowly. However, in people who have familial pseudohyperkalaemia, even if the red cells are separated almost immedi-ately by centrifugation, misleadingly high values of K^+ are found in the plasma. In the family that Stewart and his co-workers investigated, there appeared to be no identifiable disease; within 4 hours of withdrawing blood from a vein, however, the plasma [K^+] had risen from their normal value of 4 mmol/l (mEq/l) or less to 6 mmol/l (mEq/l) or more. The phenomenon of pseudohyperkalaemia had previously been recognized in leukaemia and thrombocythaemia.[30,46,65]

Hypokalaemia

Hypokalaemia commonly occurs in patients with cardiac failure who have been subject to prolonged diuretic therapy with inadequate replacement of KCl. [213,258] This can be exacerbated by chronic malnutrition which can often be seen prior to surgical correction of the cardiac defect. It is an important factor in determining the onset of arrhy-thmias following myocardial infarction (Solomon and Cole, 1981).[283] Gastro-intestinal disorders alone can give rise to hypokalaemia. Patients with chronic heart disease were found to have weight loss, nitrogen loss and potassium loss. The loss of weight, and therefore the loss of potassium and nitrogen, appears to be greater in men than in women.[298] Thomas et al. made their estimates using a total body counter after irradiation of the patient. It is well recognized that the total exchangeable potassium can underestimate the whole-body potassium in patients who have heart disease.[41] Gastric drainage can contain 40–60 mmol/l (mEq/l) of K^+. Plasma [K^+] can fall to as low as 1.8 mmol/l (mEq/l) in severe steatorrhea.[40] Vomiting and diarrhoea are associated with potas-sium loss, and chronic purgation can give rise to hypokalaemia.[286]

Hyperaldosteronism is characteristically asso-ciated with hypokalaemia and hyperkaluria. In primary hyperaldosteronism, resulting from tumours of the adrenal glands (aldosteronomas), changes in the plasma [Na^+] are not found consist-ently. The loss of potassium ions is often enor-mous,[64] and plasma values as low as 1.4 mmol/l (mEq/l) have been reported, with exchangeable K^+ levels of 30 mmol/kg body weight. These values can be increased 20 times by removal of the tumour. Hyperaldosteronism resulting from aldosteronomas is known as Conn's syndrome and the most consis-tent finding is muscle weakness which may be episodic and caused by the potassium deficiency. Tetany may occur as a result of the hypokalaemic alkalosis. Hypertension is not uncommon and, because of the muscle weakness, it can be mistaken for myasthenia gravis. Oedema is unusual. Condi-tions associated with hyponatraemia, such as cir-rhosis of the liver, nephrosis and renal artery stenosis, may produce secondary aldosteronism resulting in oedema. Chronic congestive cardiac failure may also occasionally give rise to similar changes. Both primary and secondary forms may respond to spironolactone.

In some patients adrenocorticoid therapy may give rise to hypokalaemia,[19] when large doses are used therapeutically. In most patients, however, an adequate oral intake compensates for any increased renal loss of K^+.

Liver disease sometimes gives rise to hypokalaemia and can be one of the precipitating causes of hepatic coma. Total body K^+ deficiency may be the cause of the metabolic alkalosis seen in cirrhosis of the liver. Hepatic coma can be induced when a K^+-losing diuretic is given without adequate oral replacement. Kwashiorkor, the disease seen in African children receiving a low-protein diet, is associated with a low total body K^+ and hypokalaemia.[122]

Hypothermia leads to a low plasma $[K^+]$, returning to normal on rewarming. Renal K^+ loss is usually only a feature of renal diseases in which the defect is primarily tubular, such as Fanconi's syndrome and renal tubular acidosis. In these conditions there is an inability to acidify the urine, amino aciduria and hypophosphataemia in the presence of a moderately raised blood urea. It is also seen in the pre-recovery phase of acute renal failure.

Hypokalaemia can develop after surgery. It is commonly seen following open-heart surgery when the heart–lung machine has been primed with 5% glucose solution. Postoperative hypokalaemia develops even when large volumes of blood have been transfused and much of the stored blood has a high plasma $[K^+]$.[47]

Liquorice hypokalaemia
Pseudo primary hyperaldosteronism is well recognized as a complication of ingestion of excessive amounts of liquorice. The mineralocorticoid activity of natural liquorice has been well documented.[71,136,291] Extracts of the root *Glycyrrhiza glabra* contains glycyrrhizinic acid and this substance has a marked aldosterone effect leading to hypokalaemia in those people who are addicted to foods or sweets containing the natural extract.[209] The synthetic form of liquorice used in the flavouring of many foods does not have this effect.

The biochemical picture seen in patients with mineralocorticoid excess is usually one of hypokalaemia, metabolic alkalosis, sodium retention, renal potassium wasting and depressed blood renin levels. Doses of glycyrrhizinic acid can range from 0.7 g to 4.0 g per day, and these have been observed to suppress both renin and aldosterone and lead to hypertension in addition to the metabolic effects.[92,186]

Chewing-tobacco hypokalaemia
Some chewing tobaccos contain large amounts of natural liquorice and therefore can produce pseudohyperaldosteronism. Most tobacco chewers expectorate, but one patient who did not, developed the classic symptoms of pseudohyperaldosteronism.[39]

Treatment of hypokalaemia
Hypokalaemia is treated by administering potassium salts. However, it has been shown by Aber *et al.*[2] that the chloride ion is essential. Some effervescent forms of medication contain potassium bicarbonate, and while this is better tolerated when given by mouth, this form of administration may lead to serious hypokalaemia, especially in the female receiving diuretic therapy. The oral route is the safest method of giving K^+ but there are many occasions when this is not possible or would be too slow. The plasma $[K^+]$ and not the total body K^+ is the most important factor in maintaining the normal rhythmic beating of the heart. When the plasma $[K^+]$ falls below 3.0 mmol/l (mEq/l), cardiac arrhythmias occur. Under certain circumstances, arrhythmias initiated by hypokalaemia can develop when the plasma $[K^+]$ is greater than 3.0 mmol/l (mEq/l).[83] This may be because of an associated decrease in $[Mg^{++}]$ (see p. 53). When an acute decrease in plasma $[K^+]$ occurs so that an arrhythmia has either developed or is threatened, then KCl must be given by intravenous infusion. It should not be infused at rates greater than 20 mmol/hour and should be administered in saline by means of a separate infusion so that its rate can be controlled and the danger of a massive infusion of K^+ is avoided, as this may result in cardiac arrest. It is rarely necessary to infuse at a faster rate because K^+ is confined initially to the extracellular space and the plasma $[K^+]$ begins to rise almost immediately following initiation of the KCl infusion. Intravenous infusion can be supplemented where possible with oral medication, for example, 600 mg every 4 hours. Care must be taken that an adequate urine output is being maintained; a rough guide to safety is 1 litre of urine in 24 hours. If this volume or more is being excreted, it is usually safe to administer K^+ by either route.

It must be borne in mind that the rate of equilibration of K^+ with tissue cells is highly variable and in some cases 24 hours is required before complete equilibration occurs. For this reason and the fact that K^+ depletion cannot be corrected properly for 24–28 hours, digitalis intoxication caused by body depletion of K^+ must be treated by the complete withdrawal of digitalis preparation for at least this period. Similarly, if operative mortality is to be reduced, a similar period is required for reparative measures to have effect before anaesthesia and surgery are begun.

Inherited disorders of potassium metabolism

There are three disorders that are generally recognized as distinct clinical entities at the present moment.

    (a) Familial periodic paralysis.
    (b) Adynamia episodica hereditaria.
    (c) Periodic paralysis caused by thyroid disease.

These conditions present clinically as a spontaneous flaccid paralysis of a transient nature. Although clinically they may appear to be very similar, the first condition (a) is associated with a reduced plasma [K+], the second (b) is associated with a raised plasma [K+], the third (c) occurs largely in people from the Far East who have thyrotoxicosis (see page 42).

    (a) *Familial periodic paralysis* usually begins in the second decade of life, the attacks coming on later in the day or at night. The muscles affected are those in the limbs and trunk. The muscles of the face, pharynx, larynx and diaphragm are not involved. During the attacks tendon reflexes are lost and the muscles fail to respond to electrical stimulus.

When the patient recovers from the condition the affected muscles regain their function in the reverse order to that in which the paralysis developed.

At the beginning of an attack, there appears to be a movement of K+ into the cells and the plasma [K+], which is normal or low before the attack, decreases. When the skeletal muscle K+ content is investigated it is found to be raised, while the Na+ content remains unchanged. The total exchangeable K+ of the body is found to be low and that of Na+ to be raised. The attacks are brought on by heavy exercise, over-eating, large positive changes in the Na+ balance, the administration of adrenocortical hormones and ACTH. The administration of glucose in large quantities or insulin may also precipitate an attack.

While the induction of paralysis has been related to a high-sodium diet or the retention of any Na+ by means of steroids, Conn *et al.*[67] and McDowell *et al.*[191] found that paralysis could be induced in the patient they reported only after restriction of sodium intake to 8 mmol/day. They postulated, therefore, that this form of periodic paralysis was different from that which generally benefited from sodium restriction. It is to be noted that Conn and

his co-workers provoked paralysis in two patients by giving a 208 mmol sodium-containing diet.

In 1971, Ishigami and his co-workers[153] found that, in addition to the constant fall in plasma [K+], there was a rise in plasma [Mg++] during an attack.

Familial periodic paralysis is said to be extremely rare amongst people with black skins. However, Corbett and Nuttall[69] reported two black brothers, aged 23 and 24 years, who had the typical characteristics associated with the condition.

One clinician will see only a small number of patients suffering from hypokalaemic periodic paralysis. Therefore, the reports from Johnsen[158] are of great value. The careful registration of 94 patients, in Denmark, from 12 affected families together with 12 additional patients who had no family history of this condition has provided encouraging results with regard to treatment and management.

There is one outstanding clinical effect that can be observed and that is that when the patients in this series were reviewed in 1959, a number of deaths had occurred in patients suffering from paralytic attacks between the ages of 14 and 31 years. When the subjects were reviewed again in 1978, only one additional patient had died during an attack and this followed the administration of digitalis. The life expectancy of people with this condition did not, therefore, differ from that of the normal Danish population.

The acute clinical picture had been clarified in this study. The development of total paralysis can appear gradually over a few hours and can last for up to 72 hours. There may also be short periods of weakness in one limb lasting an hour or more. The onset of paralysis tends to occur during rest following periods of vigorous exercise.

Because of the difficulty in measuring intracellular electrolytes, the aetiology of the condition still remains obscure, but the report by Johnsen[158] indicates that there is a shift of potassium and perhaps sodium together with water into the muscle cells. This can be associated with vacuolation.[91] The studies with regard to the electrical properties of skeletal muscle fibres and the membranes have yielded inconclusive and contradictory results.[158] The most common association with an attack appears to be a heavy carbohydrate intake. Oral or intravenous glucose combined with insulin appears to be the most consistent method of inducing an attack.[157]

    (b) *Adynamia episodica hereditaria* was the term used by Gamstorp[120] when she described 17 patients from two families who experienced periodic attacks of weakness and had normal or slightly raised serum [K+]. It begins in the first decade of life and logically, because the attacks are associated with a raised plasma [K+], can be caused by ingesting K+ when it is in high concentration either in natural foods or during medication. Unlike familial periodic paralysis, it is a condition of less clinical severity and is less likely to cause death. In this condition also, the exact aetiology is unknown and it may be similar to or identical with that of 'familial hyperkalaemic paralysis with myotonia' reported by Van der Meulen et al.[307] in which hydrochlorothiazide given intravenously was a successful form of treatment. In the absence of diuretic therapy, the urine [K+] is not raised during an attack of paralysis.

Treatment: A report of four patients[189] indicated that clinical improvement was obtained by giving glucose 20–40 g four times daily by mouth. An increased intake of NaCl may also be of assistance and *small* doses of 9-α flurohydrocortisone given intermittently (i.e. alternate days or every 3 or 4 days) so that Na+ balance is maintained but *excessive* Na+ retention is avoided, may also produce improvement. Calcium gluconate given intravenously may curtail an attack. Thiazide diuretics which produce a K+ diuresis may be used in the treatment of this condition.

(c) *Periodic paralysis caused by thyroid disease.* Periodic paralysis associated with thyrotoxicosis, although rare, is a recognizable syndrome. Most cases have been reported from Japan.

It is characterized by recurrent episodes of flaccid paralysis which commonly recover without any specific treatment and leave no residual weakness.[249] Norris et al.[225] investigated the condition and reported that there appeared to be a poor relationship between the serum potassium concentrations and the severity of the paralysis that was experienced by the patient.

The association of periodic paralysis with exophthalmic goitre was reported by Rosenfeld in 1902,[255] and this was probably the first account of the disorder, although it was also clearly reported by Kitamura in 1913.[170] A report from the Mayo Clinic by Dunlap and Kepler in 1931[81] also established the association. The condition is, however, largely confined to people from the Orient, and most of the subsequent reports have come from Japan. Okinaka et al.[230] studied 6333 patients suffering from thyrotoxicosis. They found that 8.2% of the males and 0.4% of the females had thyrotoxic periodic paralysis. This high incidence may have been due to confining the study to patients in hospital and thus excluding thyrotoxic ambulatory patients in the general population. Engel[88] noted that 90% of case reports of thyrotoxic periodic paralysis covering 228 patients originated from Japan. It is known, however, that the disease is seen in Korea,[169,180] in Chinese living in Hong Kong,[192] and in the Japanese population of Hawaii.[229] More recently, it has been reported in a Scotsman.[10]

An important difference between this condition and familial periodic paralysis is the response to thyroid medication. Administration of thyroid extract results in an increase in the severity of thyrotoxic periodic paralysis[279] but can cause improvement of the familial disorder.[334] Treatment of the thyrotoxicosis prevents the attacks.[153] Vacuolation can be seen in the muscles in both conditions.[89,90,224,263,264]

The author has seen only two cases. One was a young adult Chinese patient from Hong Kong resident in Britain who presented in the accident and emergency department with the sudden onset of generalized muscle weakness. On examination, his muscle strength was markedly diminished and his reflexes significantly reduced in sensitivity. He was admitted and found to have thyrotoxicosis and hypokalaemia. Investigations revealed, in a similar manner to those of Norris et al.,[225] that there was little or no correlation of the muscle weakness with either the plasma [K+] or carbohydrate metabolism.[175] The other case was a Japanese male who returned to Japan for treatment following oral KCl medication.

It appears that origin of the disease is related to the presence of two coincidental genetic abnormalities and these can be identified following investigation of the HLA antigens.[315,339]

The indication that the condition is primarily one of defective carbohydrate metabolism was first suggested by McArdle.[188] Other workers have suggested that insulin is the primary cause, and when pancreatic insulin release was blocked with the substance diazoxide, attacks of paralysis could not be provoked.[157] Other studies have suggested that there is an increased insulin secretion following intravenous glucose administration.[159]

Treatment: K+ salts, preferably KCl, should be given orally in doses of 6 g or more daily. Oral diazoxide would appear to be too toxic for long-term use and the most effective approach to both treatment and prophylaxis is with oral potassium salts. Careful monitoring of the serum potassium is, however, required, especially when potassium-retaining diuretics, such as spironolactone or amiloride, are given (see p. 38). Although limited, experience indicates that there may be some benefit from this form of treatment.[246,294] Because a fall in the [HCO_3^-] would appear to be of benefit, treatment with acetazolamide (Diamox) has been used, but the results have been inconclusive.[135,238] However, the current view held by Johnsen[158] is that a combination of acetazolamide and potassium appears to be indicated as the best prophylactic treatment available. There is some indication that the familial form of periodic paralysis may be improved, and attacks prevented by the administration of thyroid extract.[334] Three grains of dried thyroid, which contains 0.3 ml of L-thyroxine, were used. One patient developed factitious thyrotoxicosis because of excessive self-medication. Paralysis, however, returned in this patient when administration of thyroid was stopped. Similar findings were reported by Engel.[88]

Rules to be followed in K^+ replacement

1. The chloride ion is essential so that KCl must be used.
2. The female is much more prone to K^+ depletion than the male.
3. When a K^+-retaining hormone such as spironolactone, amiloride or triamterene is used, care must be taken that *hyperkalaemia* does not occur.
4. When a K^+-retaining hormone is used, K^+ supplementation in any form should *never* be given routinely, even to females.
5. When intravenous KCl is given, 20 mmol of K^+ hourly is a safe rate of administration and should not be exceeded except under serious circumstances (i.e. plasma [K^+] of 2 mmol/l (mEq/l) or less), and even then with careful ECG monitoring by a skilled clinician.
6. KCl should always be administered by a separate intravenous infusion so that, if for any reason the rate of intravenous fluid administration has to be increased, the rate of K^+ administration can be maintained at a constant rate. A convenient method of administration is adding 20 mmol of K^+ to the burette of a suitably designed infusion set.
7. When the urine output is 1 litre or more in 24 hours, the administration of K^+ preparations to the hypokalaemic patient is usually safe; however, if acute renal failure is suspected, K^+ should be administered cautiously and, if possible, withheld.

Calcium

The total amount of Ca^{++} within the body is approximately 1050 g, the major part of which lies within the skeletal system. The normal blood level of Ca^{++} is 2.3–2.8 mmol/l or approximately 5 mEq/l or 9–11 mg%. This element plays an important part in cellular function, the stability and the excitability of the cellular membrane, and the apposition of one cell to another by means of cement substance. When Ca^{++} metabolism becomes abnormal, it may have severe and fatal consequences, for example the hypercalcaemia that is a result of hyperparathyroidism.

It is well recognized that Ca^{++} plays an important part in all muscle contraction and we have been aware from the time of Ringer[253] of its importance in myocardial function.

Approximately 1 g of calcium is absorbed from the gut daily and the amount excreted into the urine by the average adult ranges between 100 and 400 mg (2.5 and 10 mmol) in 24 hours. Calcium exists in two forms: (a) that which is bound to protein, and (b) that which is in the ionized form. A number of different methods have been devised so that the concentration of ionized calcium can be expressed as a separate entity from the total calcium. Greenwald[134] proposed the following equation:

$$\text{ionized } Ca^{++} = \text{total calcium} - 0.87 \times \text{total protein}$$
$$\text{(mg\%)} \qquad \text{(mg\%)} \qquad \text{(g\%)}$$

However, some investigators in this field, Finlay *et al.* (1956)[102] concluded that only about one-third of the calcium in the plasma was in the ionized form as opposed to one-half of the total calcium. With this in mind, the following equation was derived:

$$\text{protein-bound calcium (\%)} =$$
$$7.6 \times \text{albumin} + 2.9 \times \text{globulin}$$
$$\text{(g\%)} \qquad \text{(g\%)}$$

Unfortunately, any equation is valid only when the plasma protein concentrations are normal and no other major metabolic change has occurred. It is, therefore, at the very time that it is desirable to the clinician to know the ionized calcium level that equations are of minimal value. It is readily apparent that when hypoproteinaemia in the form of a low plasma albumin is present, then the plasma [Ca^{++}] is low. Direct estimation of ionized calcium level is therefore difficult to obtain, but Ca^{++} specific electrodes are now available[281].

A correction factor for obtaining some estimation of the total plasma calcium in the presence of hypo- or hyperalbuminaemia is available. It can be estimated that for every gram per litre the plasma albumin is above or below normal, 0.02 mmol/l (0.08 mg%) should be subtracted from or added to the measured plasma calcium concentration. The following formulae can be used in the presence of hypoalbuminaemia:

Corrected plasma [Ca^{++}] (mmol/l) =
plasma [Ca^{++}] (mmol/l) ($\pm$)
normal plasma albumin (g/l) −
measured plasma albumin (g/l) $\times$ 0.02

Corrected plasma [Ca^{++}] (mg%) =
plasma [Ca^{++}] (mg%) ($\pm$)
normal plasma albumin (g/l) −
measured plasma albumin (g/l) $\times$ 0.08

The opposite sign (in brackets) has to be used in hyperalbuminaemia. Calcium-measuring electrodes have been available for more than 20 years. Major improvements in their design have been made, and have reached the stage of development that allows for their general use. The measurement of serum calcium has been reviewed by Kanis and Yates (1985).[163]

Ionized calcium is one of the factors involved in determining the degree of excitability of nerve and muscle tissues. A fall in the plasma [Ca^{++}] results in a reduction in the electrical resistance across the cell membrane and leads to an increase in the permeability of sodium and potassium ions.[222]

It is well recognized that the [Ca^{++}] is lower within the red cell than in the circulating plasma, and this gives rise to a number of physiological and buffering factors of great importance. A slight increase in the intracellular [Ca^{++}] leads to a marked increase in the K$^+$ permeability of the erythrocyte membrane. It is an important factor in the loss of K$^+$ from the metabolically depleted red cell in the presence of low plasma glucose concentrations. Very high intracellular [Ca^{++}] blocks the Na$^+$–K$^+$ pump mechanism within the red cell.[267]

Transmission of the impulses across the nerve synapse is reduced or inhibited by a lack of Ca^{++} because low calcium concentrations result in a fall in the availability of acetylcholine.

Conversely, a rise in plasma concentration results in a reduction in the excitability of the muscle membrane. The changes in the degree of excitability of tissues is also modified by the binding of calcium at various sites on cell membranes.[222] The activation of the contractile protein of striated muscle is considered to be due to the calcium ion,[321] as it is in cardiac muscle. Definitive changes in the Ca^{++} not only change the sensitivity of the contractile muscle, especially in the myocardium, but also the force of contraction.[330] Grossly abnormal electrocardiograms have been observed by the author in a doctor who had a parathyroid tumour; the electrocardiogram reverted to normal on removal of the gland (see p. 46).

Although it has never been established that low plasma calcium levels have been associated with an abnormality in blood-clotting mechanisms, Ca^{++} plays an important part in blood coagulation. The calcium ion has been found to act in combination with both Factor IX and Factor VII, especially when the latter forms a complex with serum thromboplastin.

Calcium excretion

Approximately two-thirds of the calcium ingested is normally excreted in the faeces.[222]

The average adult male, weighing approximately 75 kg, filters approximately 23 g of calcium through the glomeruli every 24 hours.[322] However, of this relatively large quantity of calcium, less than 400 mg (10 mmol) of the cation is actually concentrated in the urine in the male and less than 300 mg (7.5 mmol) in the female in 24 hours.[52] Most of the filtered calcium is reabsorbed at the proximal tubule.[177]

Renal excretion of calcium has a direct correlation with the excretion of other cations.[59] The relationship of sodium and magnesium and phosphate has an inverse correlation with calcium excretion. The urinary calcium concentration is virtually unaffected by the water content of the urine and the degree of hydration of the body. Infusion of chelating agents such as EDTA (ethylene-diamine-tetra-acetic acid) will increase the calcium diuresis by forming a chemical complex that is both more readily filtered at the glomerulus and also more actively secreted by the renal tubules.[50]

The reabsorption of calcium by the kidney is increased by the administration of parathormone. This hormone also affects the calcium and phosphorus levels in the blood by influencing the amount of calcium absorbed from the gut and bone. However, while the effects of parathormone have a relatively rapid influence on the kidneys, the effect on the gut and bone is slow.[322] In the normal person, there is an almost linear relationship between calcium excretion by the urine and gut and the calcium intake if ingestion of calcium does not exceed 600 mg/day.

Parathyroid hormone

Parathyroid hormone is secreted by the four para-thyroid glands that lie posterior to the thyroid gland. The main factor controlling parathyroid hormone secretion appears to be the concentration of calcium in the plasma. Reduction in $[Ca^{++}]$ stimulates secretion of the hormone and elevation of $[Ca^{++}]$ suppresses it. It is, however, apparent that magnesium may also play a role in parathyroid hormone secretion as, in long-term hypomag-nesaemia, impaired secretion of the hormone has been observed. The concentration of PO_4 appears to have no direct effect on secretion of the hormone, although recent studies suggest that some control may be mediated via the metabolites of vitamin D.

Mode of action

Parathyroid hormone appears to act primarily on the kidneys and on bone. Both these effects (as in the case of other hormones) appear to be mediated by the stimulation of adenylate cyclase.

Studies in man have shown that the phosphaturia that occurs after the administration of parathyroid hormone is preceded by the increase of urinary secretion of cyclic AMP. In addition to causing phosphaturia, parathyroid hormone increases the renal tubular reabsorption of calcium which, in association with the release of calcium from bone, results in elevation of the plasma $[Ca^{++}]$.

Recent work indicates that vitamin D (cholecal-ciferol), which is manufactured by the body when ultraviolet light acts on 7-dehydrocholesterol in the skin, or is absorbed by the body in the diet, is hydroxylated by the liver to 25-dihydroxy-cholecalciferol and by the kidney to 1,25-dihydroxy-cholecalciferol. Its production is influenced by parathyroid hormone. While parathyroid hormone is not the only factor regulating the metabolism of vitamin D, it is nonetheless an important influence. The function of 1,25-dihydroxycholecalciferol is not fully known but it has been established that it increases the proportion of calcium-binding pro-teins on the surface of the small intestine, thus increasing the absorption of calcium from the gut.

Calcitonin

The existence of a calcium-lowering hormone was first postulated by Copp et al. in 1962.[68] Until that time, the secretion of parathormone was considered to be the predominant method by which plasma calcium concentration was controlled.

Further investigations by Foster et al. in 1964[112] clearly demonstrated the presence of a calcium-lowering factor within the thyroid gland, released by cells, which are distinct from those that produce thyroxine and tri-iodothyronine, and which are referred to as 'C' cells. The presence of the plasma calcium-lowering agent, calcitonin, was demon-strated by Bussolati and Pearse in 1967[57] using an immunofluorescent technique. It is to be noted that, while in animals calcitonin is confined to the thyroid gland, in man the hormone has been found also in the parathyroid gland and thymic tissue.[118]

Calcitonin appears to lower the serum calcium concentration by acting principally on bone. This is achieved by inhibition of osteoplastic bone re-absorption so that calcium and phosphorus are prevented from leaving the bone but continue to be incorporated into bone.

Calcitonin has its greatest effect in producing a rapid fall in plasma $[Ca^{++}]$ when there is an in-creased exchange of calcium and phosphorus with the bone in such conditions as thyrotoxicosis and Paget's disease of the bone. It is to be noted that, as the osteoplastic activity is reduced, there is also a reduction in the breakdown of bone collagen, and as a consequence of this there is a diminution of the release of hydroxyproline and, therefore, a fall in the serum and urinary hydroxyproline con-centrations. One of the results of calcitonin, when given therapeutically, is to increase the excretion of calcium and phosphate in the urine, although this effect is not significant in lowering the plasma $[Ca^{++}]$.

Hypercalcaemia

Raised plasma calcium concentrations are being discovered with increasing frequency since the measurement of Ca^{++} has become a routine pro-cedure. A wide variety of conditions give rise to elevated plasma Ca^{++} levels (Table 2.2).

Table 2.2 The main causes of hypercalcaemia and hypo-calcaemia

Causes of hypercalcaemia	Causes of hypocalcaemia
Hyperparathyroidism	Hyperparathyroidism
Sarcoidosis	Rickets
Paget's disease of the bone	Osteoporosis
Metastatic carcinoma	Osteoplastic metastasis
Idiopathic hypercalcaemia	Cushing's syndrome
Milk-alkali syndrome	Acute pancreatitis
Hyperthyroidism	Acidotic states
Disuse atrophy	Acute hyperphosphataemia
Hypoadrenalism	
Hypervitaminosis D	
Tuberculosis	

Hyperparathyroidism

This condition is produced by an increase in circulating parathormone; it is one of the outstanding factors in the syndrome of hyperparathyroidism. This condition frequently presents with mental confusion and psychotic behaviour. The increased plasma $[Ca^{++}]$ results in various symptoms such as those of muscle weakness, fatigue, anorexia, constipation, bone pain, malaise and cardiac arrhythmias. Patients may die during a critical stage of this disease either from ventricular fibrillation, sometimes preceded by other arrhythmias,[317] or from respiratory failure induced by the neuromuscular disturbances. The plasma calcium concentration may reach levels of 5 mmol/l (20 mg%, 10 mEq/l) or more, so that immediate treatment with calcium-lowering agents is required.

Calcium is absorbed from the gut in excessive quantities in patients suffering from primary hyperparathyroidism; this ceases immediately following the surgical removal of the adenoma (Lafferty and Pearson, 1963).[174]

Patients suffering from hyperparathyroidism frequently develop nephrolithiasis.

Case history. A 59-year-old doctor who had been suffering from back pain for a considerable period of time which had not responded to self-administered prednisone during a period of 6 months, underwent a laminectomy and, immediately following the operation, became psychotic. Two previous estimations of his calcium concentration showed levels of 3 mmol/l (11 mg%, 6 mEq/l) and 2.25 mmol/l (9 mg%, 4.5 mEq/l). His chest X-ray showed marked hilar enlargement and the presence of enlarged lymphatic glands but did not have the typical appearance of sarcoid. When, however, a third estimation of his plasma calcium concentration once more demonstrated a level of 2.98 mmol/l (11.9 mg%, 6 mEq/l) which fell to 2.25 mmol/l (9 mg%, 4.5 mEq/l) when he was treated with 30 mg of prednisone daily, it was considered that the hypercalcaemia could be due to sarcoid. As the calcium fell, the patient's psychosis disappeared. He was, therefore, treated for 6 months with steroids at a dose similar to that which he had prescribed for himself. Sometimes the dose was reduced, being returned to the previous level of 30 mg% per day. It appeared that he benefited from this treatment which was accompanied by dietary restriction of calcium-containing foods.

However, the psychotic state returned and he developed muscle weakness. He was, therefore, unable to continue his medical practice and was admitted to hospital for further investi-gation. The ECG showed marked but non-specific ST–T change, first-degree A–V block, and intermittent tachyarrhythmias. An angiogram, performed bilaterally via the carotid arteries, revealed the probable enlargement of the left inferior parathyroid gland. Surgery was, therefore, performed and a parathyroid gland the size of a kidney bean was found and removed. An immediate fall in the serum calcium concentration occurred and 2–3 hours after the operation his systolic blood pressure fell to 90 mmHg. He also developed tetany in the limb muscles and a positive Chvostek sign. An infusion of calcium chloride was therefore given for 24 hours. The blood pressure and tetanic spasm were corrected immediately following the initiation of Ca^{++} therapy.

He made a relatively uneventful recovery from this surgery and began to improve markedly. His ECG returned to normal. Attempts to withdraw and reduce the steroid therapy resulted in a fall in blood pressure. It was, therefore, considered wise to continue administering steroids for a much longer period. He unfortunately developed a fistula between the stomach and the duodenum due to erosion through a gastric ulcer and he died some weeks later from toxic shock.

It would appear that the early medication with steroids for bone pain for an unknown and indefinite period which appeared to have given some relief obscured the diagnosis and made later management more difficult. It is also apparent that fluctuation in the serum calcium level gave the misguided impression that steroid therapy was beneficially affecting the serum calcium concentration

Paget's disease of the bone (osteitis deformans)

Paget's disease of the bone is a chronic, progressive disorder of unknown aetiology. It frequently gives rise to no symptoms and is found to be present when an X-ray is performed. Careful post-mortem studies have shown that it can be present in 3–4% of people of western European extraction who are over 55 years of age, and is probably present in 10% of the very old. The disease is frequently localized and cannot be detected by simple, clinical examination. In approximately 5% of patients, however, the disease is associated with symptoms of clinical importance.

Occasionally, the patient is aware of the thickening of the bone such as the tibia or clavicle but, in the pelvis, thickening can pass unnoticed. Sometimes, the overlying skin may be warmer because of the increased blood flow to the bone. When the disease becomes more widespread, the increased blood flow gives rise to a raised resting cardiac output and may induce cardiac failure. When the skull is affected, deafness can occur and, when there is vertebral disease, paraplegia can develop. Commonly, the diagnosis is made when a fracture develops in one of the affected bones, but bone pain on a weight-bearing bone is a common finding, especially if an incomplete fracture of the bone is present. However, bone pain which is persistent and lasting, unassociated with either deformity or fracture, and which is deep and dull in character, often develops.

In osteitis deformans, there is the osteoplastic resorption of normal bone and its replacement with a coarse trabeculated bone which is irregularly laminated. The normal architecture of the bone becomes distorted and the bone volume is increased. There is loss of collagen tissue and, because of the increased metabolism of both bone and collagen, there is a rise in plasma [Ca++].

Metastatic carcinoma
It has been recognized for some time that metastases to bone frequently result in hypercalcaemia.[260] Such metastases would, for example, be carcinoma of the breast and prostatic neoplasms. However, hypercalcaemia is also sometimes found in leukaemia and is considered to be the result of reabsorption of bone where the leukaemic cellular process[202] is most active and there is aggregation of leukaemic cells.

Raised serum calcium concentrations are, however, sometimes found where there is no direct skeletal involvement, such as in Hodgkin's disease, and surgical removal of the primary neoplasm is frequently associated with a fall in the serum calcium concentrations.[299]

Hypercalcaemia in all these conditions can produce muscle weakness and psychotic disturbances. Reduction of the raised serum calcium level in a patient with metastatic carcinoma of the breast has resulted in a complete disappearance of the psychotic state. In this patient in particular, the metastatic carcinoma was associated with a marked metabolic alkalosis.

Milk-alkali syndrome (Lightwood's Disease)
Patients treated with a high calcium intake and sodium bicarbonate frequently develop a raised serum calcium level. This can occur in adults being treated for peptic ulcer and also occurs in infants, as described by Lightwood.[184, 287]

Milk-alkali syndrome results in marked disturbances of the central nervous system and there is an associated increase in the protein concentration of the cerebrospinal fluid. In Milk-alkali syndrome, gross disturbance of muscle and other CNS symptoms occur. However, the explanation for this occurrence has not been fully elucidated.[173]

Hyperthyroidism
Thyrotoxicosis may lead to increased circulating calcium and increased calcium excretion in the urine and faeces.[18, 51] The hypercalcaemia is restored to normal when, as a result of therapy, the euthyroid state is once again restored.

Immobilization and disuse atrophy
When patients are immobilized, for example in a plaster cast, major loss of calcium from the body by renal excretion occurs. Raised serum calcium levels result and the urine concentration of calcium may be so high that it results in nephrolithiasis. Hypercalcaemia can also result from immobilization as a result of severe neurological impairment.[300] Hypercalcaemia also occurs in Paget's disease.

Disturbances of the adrenal gland
Patients suffering from Addison's disease sometimes develop hypercalcaemia and this may contribute to the associated psychological disturbances. Abnormal calcium deposits may sometimes occur. Conversely, the removal of the adrenal gland for such conditions as Cushing's disease or phaeochromocytoma results in hypercalcaemia in the postoperative phase. This condition is relieved by the administration of corticosteroids.

Hypervitaminosis D
It has long been established that vitamin D increases the absorption of calcium from the intestine, and this is particularly marked when vitamin D is given in conjunction with substances containing calcium salts. This method is used to relieve the decrease in calcium absorption which results in various conditions. It may also lead to a marked degree of hypercalcaemia[74,76,237] and should be avoided, for example, in conditions such as sarcoid and metastatic carcinomatosis. It is also considered that vitamin D can mobilize significant quantities of calcium from the bone.[148,300,301] For vitamin D to cause loss of calcium from the bone, the patient must be on a calcium-free diet. The role of the kidney in the metabolism of vitamin D has been emphasized by Peart, although the exact site of synthesis is still uncertain.[239]

It has ben reported that exposure to vitamin D in industry can give rise to prolonged hypercalcaemia (Jibani and Hodges, 1985).[156]

Tuberculosis

Abbasi et al.[1] found that patients with active tuberculosis developed hypercalcaemia following treatment. They observed that two factors were necessary: (a) the presence of tuberculosis, and (b) dietary supplementation with vitamin D. Patients suffering from chronic obstructive pulmonary disease who received the same dietary supplementation of vitamin D did not develop hypercalcaemia. Abbasi et al. defined hypercalcaemia as being 10.5 mg% (5.4 mEq/l; 2.6 mmol/l), and they were able to observe that when treatment for tuberculosis ceased, the serum calcium returned to normal levels within 4–16 weeks.[1]

Fulminating hypercalcaemia

In 1979 Notman et al.[226] reported a case of fulminating hypercalcaemia which developed suddenly in a patient who had had a radical cystectomy for an anaplastic transitional cell carcinoma of the bladder. Parathyroid hormone secretion was normal and renal function was not impaired. An increase in the content of nephrogenous cyclic AMP was, however, found in the urine.

Clinical manifestations of hypercalcaemia

1. *Cardiac arrhythmias*. It has long been recognized[167] that amongst the most life-threatening effects of hypercalcaemia is the action of Ca^{++} on the myocardium and His–Purkinje system. The most commonly described changes on the electrocardiogram are shortening of the Q–T interval,[21,168] prolongation of the P–R interval and changes in the configuration of the T–waves.[43,250] Bronsky et al.[45] found that the shortening of the Q–T interval was inversely proportional to the serum $[Ca^{++}]$ level in patients suffering from hyperthyroidism. They also found that when the $[Ca^{++}]$ was 16 mg% (4 mmol/l) there was also prolongation of the T–wave. They did not, however, find that the tachycardia present in patients with hyperparathyroidism was the result of the calcium concentration alone.

2. *Psychosis*. The onset of acute psychotic episodes, commonly transient in character, has been reported by a number of authors and is illustrated in the case history described on page 46. Unless a serum calcium estimation is performed, the origin of the psychosis is frequently overlooked.

3. *Muscle weakness*. The gradual onset of reduction in muscle power and tone can be insidious in patients with hypercalcaemia as a result of metastatic disease. The muscle weakness is often considered to be due to the primary disease rather than the secondary hypercalcaemia and treatment is therefore delayed. In some patients, the peripheral reflexes are suppressed as a result of the action of Ca^{++} on the peripheral nerves.

Treatment of hypercalcaemia

When hypercalcaemia presents as an acute and potentially lethal condition, treatment to lower the raised plasma $[Ca^{++}]$ must be instituted before the precise diagnosis of the disease is made and the aetiology of the hypercalcaemia established. This is because of the high mortality associated with the condition.[181] Treatment includes the following.

Increased fluid intake

The patient should be rehydrated after estimation of the plasma Na^+, K^+, urea, glucose and plasma protein concentrations. An estimate of the haemoglobin and PCV is also of value in assessing the degree of dehydration (see p. 33).

Saline infusions

Infusions of saline increase the urinary calcium excretion. There is some evidence that Na^+ inhibits reabsorption of Ca^{++} by the renal tubule.[318]

Thiazide diuretics

The treatment of both rehydration and saline infusions can be combined with the use of a 'loop' diuretic such as frusemide (Lasix). It can be given in doses of up to 100 mg i.v. every 1–2 hours.[290] When this method is used, careful monitoring of urine and plasma electrolyte concentration must be maintained and the appropriate volumes of fluid containing the cations that have been lost in the urine must be replaced. The effect of this treatment has been demonstrated not only by Suki and his colleagues, but also by Schweitzer et al.[272] In the absence of calcium replacement, severe hypokalaemia and hypomagnesaemia can develop. An infusion which is too rapid or too slow can also cause problems if cardiovascular insufficiency is present.

Sodium sulphate infusion

A calcium diuresis can be induced by the rapid infusion of sodium sulphate solution, which can be given at the rate of 1 litre every 3–6 hours. The solution is given as an isotonic solution containing 0.12 mol/l Na_2SO_4 with 0.002 mol/l $MgSO_4$ and 0.005 mol/l K_2SO_4. The sulphate anion inhibits tubular reabsorption of Ca^{++}, with a marked lowering of the serum $[Ca^{++}]$. Because there is an associated K^+ and Na^+ diuresis, it is the practice of some clinicians to add 20–60 mmol (mEq) of KCl to the sodium sulphate preparation when giving Na_2SO_4. In these circumstances, the infusion should be given with even greater caution and the rules for the infusion of K^+-containing compounds should be followed (see p. 43) and a separate infusion containing KCl may be necessary.

A further precaution is necessary with respect to the infusion of sodium sulphate because, as a consequence of the molecular weight of sodium sulphate, an isotonic solution provides a high concentration of Na^+ and in large doses hypernatraemia can develop.

It should also be noted that a sulphate diuresis is associated with an increased excretion of all divalent cations so that hypomagnesaemia is a possible complication. This increase in divalent cation excretion has a possible use in radiostrontium poisoning.[318]

Corticosteroids

The intravenous administration of very high doses of corticosteroids will frequently reduce the plasma $[Ca^{++}]$ depending upon its aetiology. Corticosteroids are highly effective in the presence of metastatic carcinoma, sarcoid and vitamin D intoxication, but are usually not effective in the presence of a parathyroid tumour. Corticosteroids are given in large doses, for example 500–1000 mg of hydrocortisone (Solu-Cortef) every 4–8 hours, or 240 mg of 6-methyl-prednisolone (Solu-Medrone) every 6 hours.

Mithramycin

This substance is a cytotoxic antibiotic which has been used in the treatment of some forms of neoplastic growth, especially those associated with hypercalcaemia. It is highly effective in lowering the serum $[Ca^{++}]$.[86] Mithramycin has toxic effects on normal tissues and may frequently give rise to renal insufficiency. It is, therefore, rarely indicated in the absence of associated malignant disease. It should be given in doses of 25 μg/kg body weight by intravenous infusion over a period of 3 hours. In very severe cases it can be given as a single intravenous injection, but the possibility of renal damage may be increased. It is considered by some to be the drug of choice[272] but, in addition to damage to the kidneys, mithramycin can also produce thrombocytopenia and liver damage. It acts by inhibiting bone reabsorption.

Phosphate infusions

A rapid lowering of the serum calcium in patients suffering from all forms of hypercalcaemia can be achieved by the infusion of the phosphate anion. The method of infusion that has been advocated[131] is a mixture of disodium phosphate and monopotassium phosphate. The disodium phosphate is in the form of a 0.1 mol/l solution and the monopotassium phosphate is given in the form that will provide 50 mmol of the salt or 1.5 g of phosphorus. The solution is infused over 6–8 hours and does not give rise to serious complications. The Boots company, Nottingham, England, produces a satisfactory solution of sodium phosphate 2.9%. This solution contains K^+ 19 mmol (mEq)/l, Na^+ 162 mmol (mEq)/l and phosphorus 100 mmol (mEq)/l.

Phosphates appear to act by depositing Ca^{++} in bone and, because their action is not dependent on renal excretion, they can be given to those patients who are suffering from renal insufficiency. It should be noted, however, that rapid infusion of very large quantities of phosphate may not only give rise to *hypo*calcaemia but may also induce hypotension and renal cortical necrosis. A rising blood urea or blood urea nitrogen, a significant elevation of the serum PO_4 which persists for more than 24 hours after treatment, oliguria and normal or low plasma $[Ca^{++}]$ are contraindications to the infusion of phosphate.

EDTA infusions and EDTA ethylene-diamine-tetra-acetic acid

This is given by intravenous infusion at an extremely slow rate in doses of 60 mg/kg body weight daily. EDTA is, however, as toxic to the kidneys as mithramycin and should be used only in the presence of severe cardiac arrhythmias when other methods have failed to act.

Calcitonin

There is much evidence that the injection of calcitonin reduces the plasma $[Ca^{++}]$ in a number of different conditions.[324] It is said to be highly effective in Paget's disease of the bone. It is given to adults in doses of 400 MRC Units 6–8-hourly. It is stated that doses in excess of 8 MRC Units/kg body weight, 6-hourly, have no additional benefit. The reabsorption of bone and the liberation of calcium are inhibited by calcitonin in a similar manner to that of mithramycin. The effectiveness of calcitonin may be lost after a few days so that little or no hypocalcaemic activity is produced. The activity of calcitonin may, however, be restored by adding steroids to the therapeutic regimen. Binstock and Mundy[38] found that a combination of calcitonin and glucocorticoids was the most effective form of therapy.

Frusemide (Lasix)

A comparison of the various treatments for hypercalcaemia, which included infusions of phosphates, sulphate and hydrocortisone, was made in 22 patients suffering from hypercalcaemia by Fulmer et al.[116] They found that, while hydrocortisone produced inconsistent changes in the serum [Ca^{++}], infusions of sulphate produced a maximum decrease of 1.87 mg% (0.94 mEq/l, 0.45 mmol/l). The greatest fall in serum [Ca^{++}] was produced by the infusion of phosphate. A mean maximum reduction in serum [Ca^{++}] of 6.01 mg% (3.0 mEq/l, 1.5 mmol/l) was obtained. This reduction in serum [Ca^{++}] was accompanied by a decrease in renal calcium excretion.

Dialysis

As can be expected, the calcium concentration can be reduced by dialysis, and dialysis can be used if all other forms of treatment are ineffective in a hypercalcaemic crisis. Hypercalcaemia, however, although uncommon, can occur during chronic dialysis as a result of increased circulating parathyroid hormone.[331] Parathyroidectomy has been advocated.[201] However, Lanier et al.[176] have reported the use of cimetidine (Tagamet) as an alternative treatment following the reduction of the severe hypercalcaemia in two patients who were receiving haemodialysis.

Cellulose phosphate

A relatively slow reduction of serum [Ca^{++}] can be obtained by the administration of 10 g of cellulose phosphate orally every day. Although cellulose phosphate was developed as a laboratory ion-exchange preparation, there have been a number of reports in which its effectiveness in treating hypercalcaemia and hypercalcuria has been demonstrated and during vitamin D intoxication.[77,235,236]

Hypocalcaemia

A number of metabolic conditions either induce or contribute to hypocalcaemia or a fall in the ionized [Ca^{++}]. It is well understood that the [Ca^{++}] as measured may be low but the ionized [Ca^{++}] may be normal when hypoproteinaemia is present. This will not give rise to tetany or to the physical signs associated with the condition. Nevertheless, tetany may occur in the presence of, for example, alkalaemia, when the plasma [Ca^{++}] is normal. Hypocalcaemia can occur in the following circumstances (see Table 2.2).

1. *Elevated serum phosphate:*
   (a) renal failure,
   (b) excessive treatment of hypercalcaemia with phosphate or other infusions,
   (c) hypoparathyroidism.
2. *Excessive renal Ca^{++} excretion:*
   (a) renal tubular acidosis.
3. *Post-parathyroidectomy.*
4. *Excessive loss of Ca^{++} from the alimentary tract:*
   (a) malabsorption syndrome,
   (b) vitamin D deficiency.
5. *Metabolic alkalosis:*
   (a) persistent vomiting,
   (b) excessive alkali intake.

Hypoparathyroidism and hypocalcitoninaemia

If, during thyroidectomy, the parathyroid glands are removed, a sudden, rapid fall in serum calcium occurs. This may result in a rapid onset of muscular irritability and tetany. A syndrome considered to be hypoparathyroidism was described by Albright et al. in 1942.[6] Hypocalcaemia associated with tetany has been observed as a complication of thyroidectomy and was indeed, described as early as 1879.[335] Wilkin et al.,[328] who studied 54 patients with Graves' disease, concluded that the fall in plasma [Ca^{++}] was due to a rise in the rate of release of the hormone thyrocalcitonin.[328]

Osteoporosis

This condition is rarely associated with a low plasma calcium level. It occurs in association with ageing, possibly due to an imbalance in calcium intake and metabolism.[223] Osteoporosis is commonly found in post-menopausal women and is exacerbated by steroid therapy. Therapy with oestrogen sometimes relieves the bone pain associated with osteoporosis but does not commonly alleviate its progress or increase the density of the bone.[142]

Studies of calcium balance indicate that a dietary deficiency of calcium-containing substances can be a factor in the aetiology of post-menopausal osteoporosis.[221] There is some indication that treatment with fluoride salts may be of benefit in the treatment of osteoporosis.[16]

Osteoblastic metastases

A fall in the serum calcium concentration is, only rarely, encountered when extensive osteoblastic metastases have occurred. In these conditions, a marked absorption of calcium into the bone following Ca^{++} infusions appears to occur.[223,259]

Acute pancreatitis

The low plasma calcium levels that are associated with this condition result mainly from a fall in the plasma albumin concentration in the circulating plasma.

Metabolic acidosis

It is well recognized that a metabolic acidosis is associated with osteoporosis. This can occur, for example, following transplantation of the ureters into the colon. Acidosis may then favour the renal excretion of calcium and in this way give rise to bone resorption.

Acute hyperphosphataemia

This can occur with the onset of marked renal insufficiency. It can develop acutely during the treatment of leukaemia and lymphomata.[162]

Drug therapy

Electrolyte imbalance including hypocalcaemia is recognized to occur following treatment of various conditions. The drugs causing hypocalcaemia include capreomycin, viomycin and gentamicin. Only the gentamicin has been associated with concomitant Mg^{++} and K^+ loss via the urine.[96,289,306] Hypocalcaemia occurring following antibiotic therapy has been documented by Bar *et al.*[23]

Symptoms and signs of hypocalcaemia

1. Paraesthesiae, which are frequently perioral and often in the extremities of the fingers and toes.
2. Cramping of individual muscles with production of carpopedal spasm. The following signs can be elicited.
   (a) Chvostek's sign can be elicited by tapping the facial nerve with one finger just anterior to the lower border of the external auditory meatus or lobe of the ear on either side of the face. This causes a contraction of the muscles supplied by the facial nerve, producing a 'twitch' which causes the angle of the mouth to rise and move backwards.
   (b) Trousseau's sign is elicited by a sphygmomanometer cuff on the upper arm as in blood pressure recording but maintaining a pressure midway between systolic and diastolic. This pressure is maintained for 3 minutes or until a response is obtained. When hypocalcaemic tetany is present, the procedure results in carpal spasm resulting in ulnar deviation of the hand. This is frequently referred to as 'main d'accoucheur', or the obstetrician's hand.

(c) Erb's sign is now rarely applied and is considered to be out of date, although it is still used by some anaesthetists. It is elicited by applying a direct galvanic current to the skin over a peripheral nerve such as the ulna or median nerve with increasing current up to 5 milliamperes. Contraction of the muscles is obtained with less than 5 milliamperes if the test is positive.
3. Grand mal convulsions.
4. Mental deterioration and dementia.
5. Laryngeal stridor, 'crowing inspiration'.
6. Abdominal pain, nausea, vomiting and sometimes severe constipation.

Treatment of hypocalcaemia

Treatment will depend upon the aetiology of the condition. If severe carpopedal spasm occurs, which can develop following parathyroidectomy, calcium gluconate can be given intravenously 10 ml of the 10% solution at a slow rate. In this condition, the elevation of the plasma alkaline phosphatase will be raised. Postoperatively, the patient should be placed on a high-calcium diet, for example one containing milk which has both Ca^{++} and PO_4 in large quantities. Additional vitamin D, 2000 i.u./day or, if tetanic symptoms appear, dihydrotachysterol (DHT) 2–8 mg/day, should be given and discontinued as soon as the tetany disappears.

In renal tubular acidosis, the patient may be treated with sodium and potassium citrate by mouth. With this form of therapy, an alternative cation is available for excretion. The reabsorption of phosphate from the tubular fluid is also corrected when the salts are given so that the osteomalacia is reversed without resort to vitamin D.

Uraemia

The presence of this condition usually requires a low-protein diet, and the diet will therefore be deficient in phosphate. Calcium infusions may repair the deficit of ionized calcium, and small doses of vitamin D may be necessary in chronic renal failure.

Malabsorption syndrome

This may lead to both rickets and osteomalacia and is corrected by large doses of vitamin D. In the acute stage, intravenous calcium preparations can be given because malabsorption of both calcium and vitamin D is associated with the disease.

Transplantation of ureters into colon

Because bone is used as a buffer, excess calcium

is excreted in the gut or, more precisely, in the urine which enters the gut. This may give rise to bone pain, due to osteomalacia, and a positive Chvostek's sign. Treatment with high doses of vitamin D and calcium corrects the condition.

Magnesium

We cannot leave the subject of water and electrolyte metabolism without at least being aware of the importance of Mg^{++} in some forms of resuscitation. Although its effects are usually produced in chronic conditions, Mg^{++} deficiency may appear as an acute emergency.

The normal serum $[Mg^{++}]$ lies between 1.5 and 2.8 mEq/l (0.7 and 1.4 mmol/l). The total body $[Mg^{++}]$ is in the region of 35 g.

Mg^{++} deficiency is well known in domestic farm animals, causing convulsions in suckling calves and 'grass staggers' in cows and horses. In man, it occurs predominantly during malabsorption syndromes, prolonged defects of water balance caused by vomiting, the pre-recovery diuretic phase of acute tubular necrosis, renal tubular acidosis, diuretic therapy, liver disease and chronic alcoholisms.[161,190] Parathyroid hypersecretion, hypercalcaemia and primary aldosteronism are also causes of this deficiency. A high calcium intake decreases Mg^{++} absorption and it has long been known that infusions of Ca^{++} into animals provoke an increased excretion of Mg^{++} in the urine.[198]

It is well recognized that a deficiency of Mg^{++} may give rise to hypocalcaemia.[13,63,66,85,94,98,107,130,203,217,231,277,289,304] Bar et al.[22] reported two patients who had developed hypocalcaemia associated with tetany, possibly because of increased renal magnesium excretion caused by gentamicin (Genticin, Garamycin). In both patients loss of renal potassium also occurred.

There is, under various physiological conditions,[94] an interrelationship between Mg^{++}, Ca^{++} and K^+, part of which is discussed below (see p. 53). In critical care medicine, abnormalities in Mg^{++} metabolism are of the greatest importance, but although this cation can now be measured with relative ease, these abnormalities are frequently overlooked.

The magnesium ion can have a profound effect on myocardial function.[149] Correction of the Mg^{++} deficit can be essential for maintaining a normal sinus rhythm and preventing the recurrence of ventricular fibrillation.

Severe hypermagnesaemia in which the plasma concentration has been in the region of 10–15 mEq/l (5–7.5 mmol/l) has been recognized to cause marked electrocardiogram changes.[149,282,316] Supression of the sinoatrial node and atrioventricular conduction leading to bradycardia and asystole have been observed. However, a moderate rise in plasma $[Mg^{++}]$ of 3.3–4.8 mEq/l (1.7–2.4 mmol/l) has been demonstrated to have caused severe bradycardia in a patient with chronic renal insufficiency.[36]

Severe hypotension and cardiovascular collapse can occur during marked hypermagnesaemia, and the hypotension is unresponsive to vasopressors.[211,212] Varying, but significant electrocardiogram changes, including heart block, develop;[211] these changes are reversible when the hypermagnesaemia is corrected. Even when hypermagnesaemia is acute, associated changes in plasma $[Ca^{++}]$ and $[PO_4]$ occur. Hypermagnesaemia has occurred following an enema of Epsom salt solution[99] and ingestion of magnesium sulphate.[121]

Hypomagnesaemia

In man hypomagnesaemia produces lethargy, muscle weakness, ataxia, vertigo and tremors. Bizarre behaviour, aggressiveness, mental instability and excitability also occur. The most dangerous effect of gross Mg^{++} deficiency is prolonged severe, potentially fatal, epileptiform attacks.

MacIntyre (1963)[195] described a case of steatorrhoea, in which serum Ca^{++} and K^+ levels had been returned to normal by treatment but during examination the patient complained of vertigo, suddenly vomited, developed epileptiform seizures and became unconscious. He appeared to be on the point of death. His serum $[Mg^{++}]$ was only 0.2 mEq/l (0.1 mmol/l). An infusion of 100 mEq (50 mmol) of $MgCl_2$ in 1 litre of 5% dextrose was given over 4 hours. During the next 24 hours he regained consciousness, but neurological signs persisted and then disappeared gradually during the following 5 days; 200 mEq (100 mmol) of $MgCl_2$ had to be administered by mouth to maintain a normal plasma Mg^{++} level.

Convulsions due to hypomagnesaemia occurring in an infant have been reported after severe diarrhoea.[265] Magnesium deficiency has occurred following massive intestinal resection[107] and coeliac disease.

Although it has been recognized that Mg^{++} depletion occurs in patients who have received diuretic therapy for long periods of time, and that this can induce digitalis intoxication,[314] it has also been demonstrated that digitalis-induced ventricular arrhythmias can be abolished by magnesium chloride, even when the plasma $[Mg^{++}]$ is normal.[125, 152] Because of this Holt and Goulding[147] have suggested that a far better method for demonstrating total body magnesium depletion is by the measurement of the intra-erythrocyte Mg^{++} level. Nevertheless, it was their view that measurement of the plasma digoxin level was of much greater value in determining digitalis intoxication, even in the presence of an abnormal blood $[Mg^{++}]$. This was because the administration of digitalis tended to raise the intra-erythrocyte concentration of Mg^{++}. Certainly, the administration of $MgSO_4$ intravenously appeared to improve the patient recorded on page 403 and others, and tended to confirm this observation. Magnesium deficiency associated with diuretic therapy was reviewed by Swales (1982),[292] and is one of the problems associated with treating the mildly hypertensive patient with diuretics.[240]

Relationship of magnesium and potassium

Although it is a divalent cation, magnesium would appear to have a close association with the monovalent cation potassium, especially in conditions of chronic illness. This has been reviewed by Wacker and Paresi,[316] MacIntyre,[196] and Walser.[319]

It has been demonstrated that, when animals are depleted of magnesium, a deficiency of K^+ within the muscles occurs and this is associated with a marked urinary potassium loss even when potassium supplements are given.[70, 193, 199, 243] However, neither hypokalaemia nor an increase in plasma HCO_3^- develops.

It has been demonstrated that, when animals are depleted of both cations, no increase in muscle potassium occurs when potassium alone is given to repair the one aspect of the deficit, but that a rise in muscle potassium occurs when magnesium is added to the diet. Thus, the concurrent depletion of both cations can rapidly lead to depletion of muscle K^+.

It is well recognized that infusions of glucose and insulin reduce the serum $[K^+]$. However, investigations in animals and in man indicated that the fall in plasma $[K^+]$ and shift of the monovalent cation K^+ into the cells are not accompanied by a similar shift of Mg^{++}.[3,325,326] Other clinical conditions in which there are coexisting changes in both potassium and magnesium are hyperaldosteronism,[197] acute renal failure (in which there is a rise in both cations)[139] and malabsorptive states (in which there is a decrease in both cations). It should be noted that, in addition to the rise in serum $[K^+]$ that is commonly demonstrated in patients suffering from diabetic ketoacidosis, even when total body depletion of the cation is present, hypermagnesaemia has also been demonstrated to coexist with the hyperkalaemia. In this condition, a fall in serum $[Mg^{++}]$ occurs in a similar manner to the fall of plasma $[K^+]$ following treatment with insulin.[316]

Relationship of magnesium and calcium

The close association between the body Ca^{++} and Mg^{++} has long been recognized. Major studies on the clinical aspects of Mg^{++} deficiency have been largely restricted to patients suffering from malabsorption syndrome or severe alcoholism.[203] Most of these studies have been incomplete because the dietary intake and faecal loss have been, in the main, unknown. Estimates of the size of the magnesium deficiency in hypomagnesaemic patients with malabsorption syndrome have varied greatly between 55 mmol and more than 200 mmol.[113,194,199] Dunn and Walser[82] studied two healthy patients in whom a reduction in Mg^{++} intake was achieved electively. They found that the major part of the external Mg^{++} loss was derived from bone and, unlike MacIntyre et al., no reduction in muscle magnesium was found. A fall in plasma $[Mg^{++}]$ occurred within one week of the onset of dietary deprivation of the cation. Shils (1964 and 1969)[276,277] found that, in two patients fed a liquid diet deficient in Mg^{++} but with added calcium and potassium, the patients became hypocalcaemic and hypokalaemic. Repletion of these cations only occurred following administration of Mg^{++}. Balance data, however, were not available from this study.

Because quantitatively moderate depletion of bone reserves of Mg^{++} would produce very little impact on total body Mg^{++}, it must be assumed that it would be unlikely to produce any marked clinical symptoms. A major loss of Mg^{++} from the body must occur before clinical manifestations can be observed. It would appear from these studies,[82,103] that the negative balance in magnesium-depleted patients is caused by faecal loss and that this is increased by a high oral intake of Ca^{++}.[140] While some investigators have found that, in man, a relatively minimal faecal loss of Mg^{++} occurs and falls almost to zero when the dietary intake of the cation is low,[24,25] these observations may have been the result of an accompanying relatively low intake of dietary Ca^{++}. It is possible that the reabsorption of Mg^{++} by the gut is decreased in the presence of high concentrations of Ca^{++} in the diet.

The conservation of Mg^{++} by the kidney was found to be high,[82] and the ingestion of large doses of alcohol did not increase urinary Mg^{++} loss, although other workers in this field have found that the prolonged ingestion of alcohol can induce excessive urinary Mg^{++} excretion.

It is quite apparent, therefore, that in the rapidly changing circumstances of a critical care unit, Mg^{++} cannot be viewed in isolation and the repletion of this and other cations is necessary.

Treatment of hypomagnesaemia

There are various oral preparations which can be given prophylactically in conditions where depletion of Mg^{++} is likely to occur, such as in diabetes, diuretic therapy, alcoholism and steatorrhoea.

In acute conditions, magnesium sulphate (1 g i.v.) can be given with safety, and repeated a short time later; this sometimes produces a dramatic improvement. Ampoules of $MgSO_4.7H_2O$, 50% w/v containing 1 g in 2 ml are available from Evans Medical, Liverpool, UK. Subsequent treatment can be given by adding $MgSO_4$ to the intravenous infusions if these are compatible, for example 0.9% NaCl infusion.

Zinc

It has long been known that zinc is an essential trace element which is required for the normal growth and development of animals.[241] Abnormalities in growth and sexual development associated with zinc deficiency have been reported in man.[247,262] The taste senses can also be affected.[141] This cation is also important in wound healing[261] and cell-mediated immunity.[241] Skin lesions are also an established factor in Zn^{++} deficiency.[295] An association between the inherited disorder of infants, *acrodermatitis enteropathica*, and Zn^{++} deficiency was observed by Moynahan and Barnes in 1973.[214,215,223] The characteristic features of the disease are an erythematous vesiculobullous dermatitis around the mouth and anus, alopecia and chronic diarrhoea. It can be cured by administering Zn^{++} salts orally.[138,284,285,305]

The normal plasma $[Zn^{++}]$ is approximately 90–100 µg% (12–17 µmol/l).

With the development of parenteral nutrition, skin eruptions similar to those of the inherited disorder have been noted.[228,323,334] These are related to the degree of Zn^{++} deficiency and they respond dramatically and rapidly to oral or parenteral Zn^{++} medication.[17] The fall in the body Zn^{++} during parenteral nutrition[165,166] is not surprising as many of these patients are in acute catabolic states, during which urinary Zn^{++} excretion is increased.[208] A prospective study by Fleming *et al.*[105] demonstrated that six patients receiving parenteral nutrition alone reduced their serum $[Zn^{++}]$ at a mean rate of 6.6 µg/ml per week.

The World Health Organisation's[336] recommended dietary intake of Zn^{++} for adult men is 5.5–22 mg/day, according to its source. Approximately one-third of the Zn^{++} taken orally is absorbed. Healthy adults on a normal daily oral Zn^{++} intake of 12.5 mg excrete approximately 500 µg daily in their urine, approximately 1000 µg through the skin as perspiration and 11 mg daily in their stool.[208,336]

There are no firm recommendations with regard to Zn^{++} requirements during complete parenteral nutrition. There is less Zn^{++} in synthetic crystalline amino acid solutions than in protein hydrolysates,[133] and the concentrations within these solutions vary between 7.2 µg/ml and 400 µg/ml. The skin eruptions and other manifestations of Zn^{++} deficiency have been reported to develop during alcoholic pancreatitis.[332] The skin rashes disappeared following medication with $ZnSO_4\,7H_2O$ in doses of 220 mg daily. This dose orally was recommended when this was possible. Alternatively, 10 mg of Zn^{++} in a soluble form (e.g. $ZnSO_4$) could be added to the infused fluid daily.

There are indications that burns heal more rapidly following administration of oral zinc.[44,143] Again, this may be due to increased catabolism leading to increased Zn^{++} excretion. When corticosteroids were administered to burn and surgical patients, a rapid and sustained fall in serum $[Zn^{++}]$ occurred.[108]

Phosphate

Acute hypophosphataemia (Table 2.3)

While inherited hypophosphataemia[127] has been recognized for many years, interest in the treatment of acute hypophosphataemia is of relatively recent origin. The most common cause of hypophosphataemia in recent years has been long-term parenteral nutrition[11,72] when the synthetic amino acid preparations have been used. When phosphate-

Table 2.3 Causes of hypophosphataemia

Malnutrition
Intravenous alimentation with:
   synthetic amino acid preparations
   glucose
   glucose with insulin
Liver disease
Alcoholism
Toxic shock (septicaemia)
Congenital inherited hypophosphataemia
Diabetes

containing casein hydrolysate preparations were used, the acute condition could not develop. With the development of chemically pure amino acid solutions with a pure carbohydrate solution such as sorbitol, phosphate-free infusions became possible. When the sole source of energy is derived from glucose, the prevention of hypophosphataemia is also an important factor in management.[137] There appears to be much evidence that the condition of hypophosphataemia will occur especially in those patients who are already nutritionally depleted and it is accentuated by the starvation that occurs quite frequently after major surgery.[256] The onset of hypophosphataemia may be particularly rapid when infusions of concentrated glucose are given in association with insulin.[293]

The normal plasma inorganic phosphate measured as PO_4 lies between 0.65 mmol/l and 1.4 mmol/l (2 and 4 mg%).

Hypophosphataemia has been associated with mental confusion (Table 2.4), intensive care unit (ICU) psychosis, hypoventilation, neuromuscular irritability[42] and acute haemolytic anaemia.[154,171] Acute respiratory failure has been reported in two alcoholics in whom the plasma phosphate level had fallen to less than 0.16 mmol/l (0.5 mg%). Ventilation improved following the intravenous infusion of phosphate. Phosphate depletion has been associated with hyperpara-thyroidism.[200]

Table 2.4 Clinical manifestations of hypophosphataemia

Cardiomyopathy (cardiac failure)
Convulsions
Respiratory failure
Mental confusion
Muscle weakness
Haemolytic anaemia
Manifestations of metabolic acidosis

As a result of their investigation into 19 patients following trauma, Sheldon and Grzyb[275] concluded that during the total parenteral nutrition it was

necessary to provide between 20 mmol and 25 mmol of potassium dihydrogen phosphate for each 1000 calories being given in the form of amino acids and carbohydrates.

When the content of 2,3-diphosphoglycerate within the red cell decreases, the oxygen dissociation curve moves to the left, so that the release of oxygen from oxyhaemoglobin to the tissues is impaired.[32,55,62,244,274,275,278,303] In the ordinary patient, this is not of great significance, but in those suffering from respiratory failure and who are not being artificially ventilated with high tensions of oxygen in the inspired gases, this small reduction in tissue oxygenation may be of clinical significance. The oxygen-carrying capacity of the circulation may be further reduced by the onset of haemolytic anaemia, which has also been reported in association with hypophosphataemia.

Hypophosphataemia has been observed in the presence of septicaemia in patients with faecal fistulae and in those patients who are undergoing dialysis for renal disease. As in other patients, a fatal fall in the plasma phosphate concentration may occur and pass totally unobserved unless special care is taken. In recent years, however, PO_4 has been measured routinely as part of a 'biochemical profile'.

In 1978, Darsee and Nutter[75] reported three cases of cardiomyopathy which appeared to result from hypophosphataemia. In all three cases there was a marked depression of the serum PO_4 concentration. Chest X-rays demonstrated cardiomegaly and interstitial pulmonary oedema. The electrocardiograms were typical of those seen in cardiomyopathy, as were the echocardiograms. The treatment of the patients included the use of diuretics, digitalis and oral phosphate supplements. The patients' serum phosphate levels returned to normal within 2–5 weeks, as did the cardiac function, electrocardiograms and echocardiograms.

Other workers have also shown that the serum phosphorus concentration can play an important part in myocardial function. O'Connor et al.[227] reported seven patients who were critically ill in whom the serum phosphorus concentration was less than 0.65 mmol/l (2.0 mg%) and, following an infusion of potassium phosphate salts and the return of the serum phosphate concentration to normal, the stroke work per beat increased. They concluded that the depression of myocardial contractility could result from the depletion of ATP, and that the reduced cardiac output observed in some hypophosphataemic patients could be corrected by phosphate repletion. Fuller et al.[115] made similar findings in phosphate-depleted dogs.

In view of these findings, hypophosphataemia must be considered in cases of cardiomyopathy.

In an extensive review of hypophosphataemia, Knochel[172] described several clinical conditions in which the serum phosphorus could be markedly reduced, for example to less than 0.323 mmol/l (1.0 mg%). These included diabetes mellitus, the recovery period following severe burns, intravenous nutrition,[217,280] alcoholism,[296] phosphate binding in the gut, and severe respiratory alkalosis. There are dangers when malnourished patients are fed a high-carbohydrate diet in which phosphorus-containing substances are absent. This can result in muscle weakness, haemolysis, platelet and leucocyte dysfunction and rhabdomyolysis and respiratory failure.[220]

In any patient who fails to improve postoperatively, or in the chronically sick patient, hypophosphataemia must be considered, especially when cardiac insufficiency is present.

Treatment of hypophosphataemia
Correction of hypophosphataemia is simple, and the solutions of potassium dihydrogen phosphate, to be given in doses of 20–25 mmol per 1000 kilocalories, are readily available for intravenous infusion.[15] Where possible, oral alimentation, with a liquid blended diet, is to be preferred. Alternatively, whole blood and plasma can be infused as a nutritive measure but expansion of the blood volume must be considered once myocardial insufficiency has developed.

Prepared solutions of sodium phosphate are available and described on page 49 in relation to the treatment of hypercalcaemia.

Hyperphosphataemia
Hyperphosphataemia occurs in chronic renal failure. The disturbances in calcium and phosphorus metabolism lead to the deposition of calcium–phosphorus aggregates in many tissues, particularly the blood vessels, myocardium, cornea and peri-articular membranes. Hyperphosphataemia occurs when the GFR falls below 20 ml/minute. It has been demonstrated experimentally by Ibels et al.[151] that restriction of phosphorus intake resulted in reduced plasma phosphate concentrations. Some control over the plasma $[PO_4]$ may be achieved by dietary phosphorus restriction combined with administration of phosphate-binding agents such as aluminium hydroxide, and this has been of value in chronic renal failure, hyperparathyroidism,[160] metastatic calcification,[313] excess parathyroid hormone,[200] and calciphylaxis.[126] However, some caution has to be used because, as demonstrated above, excessive PO_4 restriction may lead to osteomalacia, cardiomyopathy and congestive cardiac failure as well as acute respiratory failure. There is also increasing evidence that aluminium hydroxide, when given in excessive quantities, may be toxic in the uraemic patient.[9,106,245] It is possible that cimetidine (Tagamet) may be a preferable form of treatment in some cases.

References

1. Abbasi, A. A., Champlavil, J. K., Farah, S., Muller, B. F. and Arnstein, A. R. (1979). Hypercalcemia in active pulmonary tuberculosis. *Ann. Int. Med.*, **90**, 324.

2. Aber, G. M., Sampson, P. A., Whitehead, T. P. and Brooks, B. N. (1962). The role of chloride in the correction of alkalosis associated with potassium depletion. *Lancet*, **ii**, 1028.

3. Aikawa, J. K. (1960). Effect of glucose and insulin on magnesium metabolism in rabbits. *Proc. Soc. Exp. Biol. Med.*, **103**, 363.

4. Alberti, K. G. M. M., Johnston, H. H., Lauler, D. P. and Jagger, P. I. (1967). Effect of arginine on electrolyte metabolism in man (abstract). *Clin. Res.*, **15**, 476.

5. Albright, F. (1941). Case records of the Massachusetts General Hospital. Case 27461. *N. Engl. J. of Med.*, **225**, 789.

6. Albright, F., Burnett, C. H., Smith, P. H. and Parson, W. (1942). Pseudo-hypoparathyroidism. An example of 'Seabright-Bantom' syndrome. *Endocrinology*, **30**, 922.

7. Albright, F. and Reifenstein, E. C. (1948). *The Parathyroid Glands and Metabolic Bone Disease: Selected Studies*. Baltimore: The Williams and Wilkins Co.

8. Alexander, E. A. and Davinsky, N. G. (1968). An extrarenal mechanism of potassium adaption. *J. Clin. Invest.*, **47**, 740.

9. Alfrey, A. C., Le Grendrere, G. R. and Kaehny, W. P. (1976). The dialysis encephalopathy syndrome. Possible aluminium intoxication. *N. Engl. J. of Med.*, **294**, 184.

10. Ali, K. (1975). Hypokalaemic periodic paralysis complicating thyrotoxicosis. *Brit. Med. J.*, **4**, 503.

11. Allen, T. R., Ruberg, R. L., Dudrick, S. J., Long,

J. M. and Steiger, E. (1971). Hypophosphataemia occurring in patients receiving total parenteral hyper-alimentation. *Fedn. Proc.*, **30**, 580.

12. Ammon, R. A., May, W. S. and Nightingale, S. D. (1978). Glucose-induced hyperkalaemia with normal aldosterone levels: Studies in a patient with diabetes mellitus. *Ann. Int. Med.*, **89**, 349.

13. Anast, C. S., Mohs, J. M. and Kaplan, S. L. (1972). Evidence of parathyroid failure in magnesium deficiency. *Science*, **177**, 606.

14. Anderson, R. J., Chung, H. M., Kluge, R. and Schrier, R. W. (1985). Hyponatraemia: A prospective analysis of its epidemiology and the pathogenic role of vaso-pressin. *Ann. Int. Med.*, **102**, 164.

15. Anonymous (1981). Treatment of severe hypophos-phataemia. *Lancet*, **ii**, 734.

16. Anonymous (1984). Fluoride and treatment of osteo-porosis. *Lancet*, **i**, 547.

17. Arakawa, T., Tamura, T., Igarashi, Y., Suzuki, H. and Sanstead, H. H. (1976). Zinc deficiency in two infants during total parenteral alimentation for diarrhea. *Am. J. Clin. Nutr.*, **29**, 197.

18. Aub, J. C., Bauer, W., Heath, C. and Ropes, M. (1929). Studies of calcium and phosphorus meta-bolism. Part III. The effects of the thyroid hormone and thyroid disease. *J. Clin. Invest.*, **7**, 97.

19. Bagshawe, K. D., Curtiss, J. R. and Garnett, E. S. (1965). Effective prolonged hydrocortisone adminis-tration on potassium metabolism. *Lancet*, **i**, 18.

20. Bailey, R. R. (1978). Diuretics in the elderly. *Brit. Med. J.*, **i**, 1618.

21. Ballins, M. (1932). Parathyroidism. *Ann. Surg.*, **96**, 649.

22. Banister, A., Matin-Siddiqi, S. A. and Hatcher, G. W. (1975). Treatment of hypernatraemic dehydra-tion in infancy. *Arch. Dis. Child.*, **50**, 179.

23. Bar, R. S., Wilson, H. E., Mazzaferri, E. L. (1975). Hypomagnesemic hypocalcaemia secondary to renal magnesium wasting. A possible consequence of high dose gentamicin therapy. *Ann. Int. Med.*, **82**, 646.

24. Barnes, B. A., Cope, O. and Gordon, E. B. (1960). Magnesium requirements and deficits. An evaluation in two surgical patients. *Ann. Surg.*, **152**, 518.

25. Barnes, B. A., Cope, O. and Harrison, T. (1958). Magnesium conservation in the human being on a low Mg diet. *J. Clin. Invest.*, **37**, 430.

26. Baron, D. N. (1974). S. I. Units. *Brit. Med. J.*, **4**, 509.

27. Baron, D. N., Broughton, P. M. and Cohen, M. (1974). The use of S. I. Units in reporting results obtained in hospital laboratories. *J. Clin. Path.*, **27**, 590.

28. Bartter, F. C. (1977). *Acid-Base and Electrolyte Balance. Normal Regulation and Clinical Disorders.* Edited by A. B. Schwartz and H. Lyons, New York. Grune & Stratton.

29. Bartter, F. C. and Schwartz, W. B. (1967). The syn-drome of inappropriate secretion of anti-diuretic hormone. *Amer. J. Med.*, **42**, 790.

30. Bellevue, R., Dosik, H., Spergel, G. and Gussoff, B. D. (1975). Pseudohyperkalaemia in extreme leuko-cytosis. *J. Lab. Clin. Med.*, **85**, 660.

31. Benedict, F. G. (1915). *A study of prolonged fasting.* Carnegie Institute Publication No. 203, Washington: Carnegie Institute.

32. Benesch, R. and Benesch, R. E. (1967). The effect of organic phosphates from the human erythrocyte on the oxygen equilibration of human erythrocytes. *Biochem. Biophys. Res. Commun.*, **26**, 162.

33. Berg, K. J., Tromsdal, A. and Widerøe, T. (1975). Bumetanide in severe chronic renal insufficiency. (Abstract) *Postgrad. Med. J.*, **51** (Suppl. 6), 50.

34. Berliner, R. W., Kennedy, T. J. and Hilton, J. G. (1950). Renal mechanisms for excretion of potassium. *Amer. J. Physiol.*, **162**, 348.

35. Bernard, C. (1859). *Leçons sur les propriétés physio-logiques et les alterations pathologiques des liquides de l'organisme*, Vol. **1**, Paris: Balliere.

36. Berns, A. S. and Killmeyer, K. R. (1976). Magnesium induced bradycardia. *Ann. Int. Med.*, **85**, 760.

37. Berzelius, J. J. (1840). *Lehrb. de. Chemic. deutsch. v. Wohler*, **9**, 567.

38. Binstock, M. L. and Mundy, G. R. (1980). Effect of calcitonin and glucocorticoids in combination on the hypercalcemia of malignancy. *Ann. Int. Med.*, **93**, 269.

39. Blachley, J. D. and Knochel, J. P. (1980). Tobacco chewer's hypokalemia: licorice revisited. *N. Engl. J. of Med.*, **302**, 784.

40. Blainey, J. D., Cooke, W. T., Quinton, A. and Scott, K. W. (1954). The measurement of total exchange-able potassium in man, with particular reference to patients with steatorrhoea. *Clin. Sci.*, **13**, 165.

41. Boddy, K., Davies, D. L., Howie, A. D., Madkour, M. M., Mahaffy, M. E. and Pack, A. I. (1978). Total body and exchangeable potassium in chronic airways obstruction: a controversial area? *Thorax*, **33**, 62.

42. Boelens, P. A. (1970). Hypophosphataemia with muscle weakness due to antacids and hemodialysis. *Amer. J. Dis. Child.*, **120**, 350.

43. Bradlow, B. A. and Segel, N. (1956). Acute hyper-parathyroidism with electrocardiographic changes. *Brit. Med. J.*, **2**, 197.

44. Brodribb, A. J. M. and Ricketts, C. R. (1971). The effect of zinc in the healing of burns. *Injury*, **3**, 25.

45. Bronsky, D., Dubin, A., Waldstein, S. S. and Kushner, D. S. (1961). Calcium and the electrocardio-gram. II. The electrocardiographic manifestations of hyperparathyroidism and of marked hypercalcaemia from various other etiologies. *Amer. J. Cardiol.*, **7**, 833.

46. Bronson, W. R., DeVita, V. T., Carbone, P. P. and Cotlove, E. (1966). Pseudohyperkalaemia due to release of potassium from white blood cells during clotting. *N. Engl. J. of Med.*, **274**, 369.

47. Brooks, D. K. (1972). Organ failure following surgery. *Advances in Surgery*, p. 289. Chicago: Year Book Medical Publishers.

48. Brook, G. D. (1977). Acute gastric dilatation in anorexia nervosa. *Brit. Med. J.*, **2**, 499.

49. Bruck, E., Abal, G. and Aceto, T. (1968). Therapy of infants with dehydration due to diarrhoea. *Amer. J. Dis. Child.*, **115**, 281.

50. Brull, L. and Barac, G. (1961). Sur l'excretion urinaire du calcium chez le chien. *Arch. Int. Pharmacodyn.*, **135**, 482.

51. Buckle, R. M., Mason, A. M. S., Middleton, J. E. (1969). Thyrotoxic hypercalcaemia treated with porcine calcitonin. *Lancet*, **i**, 1128.

52. Bulusu, L., Hodgkinson, A., Nordin, B. E. C. and Peacock, M. (1970). Urinary excretion of calcium and creatinine in relation to age and body weight in normal subjects and patients with renal calculus. *Clin. Sci.*, **38**, 601.

53. Bunge, G. (1871). Ueber die physiologische Wirking der Fleischbrühe und der Kalisalze. *Pflüg. Arch. ges Physiol.*, **4**, 270.

54. Bunge, G. (1873). Ueber die Bedeutung des Kochsalzes und das Verhalten der Kalisalze im menschlichen Organismus. *Z. Biol.*, **9**, 104.

55. Bunn, H. F. and Jandl, J. H. (1970). Control of hemoglobin function within the red cells. *N. Engl. J. Med.*, **282**, 1414.

56. Bushinsky, D. A. and Gennari, F. J. (1978). Life-threatening hyperkalemia induced by Arginine. *Ann. Int. Med.*, **89**, 632.

57. Bussolati, G. and Pearse, A. G. E. (1967). Immuno fluorescent localization of calcitonin in the 'C' cells of pig and dog thyroid. *J. Endocrinol.*, **37**, 205.

58. Bywaters, E. G. L. (1944). Ischemic muscle necrosis; crushing injury, traumatic edema, the crush syndrome, traumatic anuria, compression syndrome; a type of injury seen in air raid casualties following burial beneath debris. *J. Amer. med. Assoc.*, **124**, 1103.

59. Caniggia, A., Gennari, C. and Cesari, L. (1965). Intestinal absorption of Ca in stone-forming patients. *Brit. Med. J.*, **i**, 427.

60. Capper, J. (1975). Salt and water to induce vomiting? *St. Bartholomew's Hospital Journal*, **79**, 365.

61. Chamberlain, M. J. (1964). Emergency treatment of hyperkalaemia. *Lancet*, **i**, 464.

62. Chanutin, A. and Curnish, R. R. (1967). Effect of organic phosphates from the human erythrocyte on the oxygen equilibration of human erythrocytes. *Biochem. Biophys. Res. Commun.*, **26**, 162.

63. Chase, L. R. and Slatopolsky, E. (1974). Secretion and metabolic and metabolic efficacy of parathyroid hormone in patients with severe hypomagnesemia. *J. Clin. Endocrinol. Metab.*, **38**, 363.

64. Chobanian, A. V., Burrows, B. A. and Hollander, W. J. (1961). Body fluid and electrolyte composition in arterial hypertension. (2) Studies in mineralocorticoid hypertension. *J. Clin. Invest.*, **40**, 416.

65. Chumbley, L. C. (1970). Pseudohyperkalaemia in acute myelocytic leukaemia. *J. Amer. med. Assoc.*, **211**, 1007.

66. Cockburn, F., Brown, J. K. and Belton, N. R. (1973). Neonatal convulsions associated with primary disturbance of calcium, phosphorus and magnesium metabolism. *Archives of Disease in Childhood*, **48**, 99.

67. Conn, J. W., Louis, L. H., Fajans, S. S., Streeten, D. H. P. and Johnson, R. D. (1957). Intermittent aldosteronism in periodic paralysis. *Lancet*, **i**, 802.

68. Copp, D. H., Cameron, E. C., Cheney, B. A., Davidson, A. G. F. and Henze, K. G. (1962). Evidence of calcitonin—a new hormone from the parathyroid that lowers blood calcium. *Endocrinology*, **70**, 638.

69. Corbett, V. A. and Nuttall, F. Q. (1975). Familial hypokalemic periodic paralysis in blacks. *Ann. Int. Med.*, **83**, 63.

70. Cotlove, E., Holliday, M. A., Schwartz, R. A. and Wallace, W. M. (1951). Effects of electrolyte depletion and acid-base disturbance on muscle cations. *Amer. J. Physiol.*, **167**, 665.

71. Cotterill, J. A. and Cunliffe, W. J. (1973). Self-medication with liquorice in a patient with Addison's disease. *Lancet*, **i**, 294.

72. Craddock, P. R., Yawata, Y., Van Santen, L., Gilberstadt, S., Silvis, S. and Jacob, H. S. (1974). Acquired phagocyte dysfunction. A complication of the hypophosphatemia of parenteral hyperalimentation. *N. Engl. J. of Med.*, **290**, 1403.

73. Crome, P., Widdop, B., Volans, G. N. and Goulding, R. (1978). SI, moles and drugs. *Brit. Med. J.*, **1**, 1277.

74. Cruickshank, E. M. and Kadicek, E. (1958). The antagonism between cortisone and vitamin D: experiments on hypervitaminosis D in rats. *J. Endocrin.*, **17**, 35.

75. Darsee, J. R. and Nutter, D. O. (1978). Reversible severe congestive cardiomyopathy in three cases of hypophosphatemia. *Ann. Int. Med.*, **89**, 867.

76. De Luca, H. F. (1976). Recent advances in our understanding of the vitamin D endocrine system. *J. Lab. Clin. Med.*, **87**, 7.

77. Dent, C. E., Harper, M. and Parfitt, A. M (1964). The effect of cellulose phosphate on calcium metabolism in patients with hypercalciuria. *Clin. Sci.*, **27**, 417.

78. Department of Health and Social Security (1977). *The Composition of Human Milk*. London: H. M. Stationary Office.

79. De Rubertis, F. R. and Michelis, M. F. (1970). Complications of severe alkalosis and syndrome resembling inappropriate secretion of antidiuretic hormone. *Metabolism*, **19**, 709.

80. Dickerman, H.W. and Walker, W. G. (1964). Effect of cationic amino acid infusion on potassium metabolism *in vivo*. *Amer. J. Physiol.*, **206**, 403.

81. Dunlap, H. F. and Kepler, E. J. (1931). Occurrence of periodic paralysis in course of exophthalmic goiter. *Proc. Mayo Clin.*, **6**, 272.

82. Dunn, M. J. and Walser, M. (1966). Magnesium depletion in normal man. *Metabolism*, **15**, 884.

83. Dyckner, T. and Wester, P. O. (1978). Ventricular

extrasystoles and intracellular electrolytes in hypo-kalemic patients before and after correction of the hypokalemia. *Acta. Med. Scand.*, **204**, 375.

84. Dyckner, T. and Wester, P. O. (1981). Effects of magnesium infusions in diuretic induced hyponatrae-mia. *Lancet*, **i**, 585.

85. Editorial (1974). Neonatal calcium magnesium and phosphorus homoeostasis. *Lancet*, **i**, 155.

86. Edwards, C. R. W. and Besser, P. G. M. (1968). Mithramycin treatment of malignant hypercalcaemia. *Brit. med. J.*, **iii**, 167.

87. Enderlin, C. (1844). Physiologisch-chemische Unter-suchungen. *Ann. Chem. u. Pharm.*, **50**, 53.

88. Engel, A. G. (1961). Thyroid function and periodic paralysis. *Amer. J. Med.*, **30**, 327.

89. Engel, A. G. (1966). Electron microscopic observations in thyrotoxic and corticosteroid induced myopathies. *Mayo Clin. Proc.*, **41**, 785.

90. Engel, A. G. (1966). Electron microscopic observa-tions in primary hypokalaemic and thyrotoxic periodic paralysis. *Mayo Clin. Proc.*, **41**, 797.

91. Engel, A. G., Lambert, E. H., Rosevear, J. W. and Tauxe, W. N. (1965). Clinical and electromyographic studies in a patient with primary hypokalemia periodic paralysis. *Amer. J. Med.*, **38**, 626.

92. Epstein, M. T., Esouberm, E. A., Donald, R. A. and Hughes, H. (1977). Effect of eating liquorice on the renin–angiotensin aldosterone axis in normal subjects. *Brit. Med. J.*, **1**, 488.

93. Epstein, M., Pins, D. S. and Millar, M. (1975). Suppression of ADH during water immersion in normal man. *J. Appl. Physiol.*, **38**, 1038.

94. Estep, H., Shaw, W. A. and Watlington, C. (1969). Hypocalcemia due to hypomagnesemia and reversible parathyroid hormone unresponsiveness. *J. Clin. Endocrinol. Metab.*, **29**, 842.

95. Evans, D. S. (1968). Acute dilatation spontaneous rupture of the stomach. *Brit. J. Surg.*, **55**, 940.

96. Evans, R. A. and Watson, L. (1966). Urinary excretion of magnesium in man. *Lancet*, **i**, 522.

97. Fagge, C. H. (1874). A case of diabetic coma treated with partial success by the injection of a saline solution into the blood. *Guy's Hosp. Rep.*, **19**, 173.

98. Fankushen, D., Raskin, D. and Dimich, A. (1964). The significance of hypomagnesemia in alcoholic patients. *Amer. J. Med.*, **37**, 802.

99. Fawcett, D. and Gens, J. P. (1943). Magnesium poisoning following an enema of epsom salt solution. *J. Amer. med. Assoc.*, **123**, 1028.

100. Fenn, W. O., Cobb, D. M. and Marsh, B. S. (1934). Sodium and chloride in frog muscle. *Amer. J. Physiol.*, **110**, 261.

101. Fichman, M. P., Vorherr, H., Kleeman, C. R. and Telfer, N. (1971). Diuretic-induced hyponatremia. *Ann Int. Med.*, **75**, 853.

102. Finlay, J. M., Nordin, B. E. C. and Fraser, R. (1956). A calcium infusion test. "Four-hr Skeletal retention": Data for recognition of osteoporosis. *Lancet*, **i**, 826.

103. Fitzgerald, M. G. and Fourman, P. (1956). An experi-mental study of magnesium deficiency in man. *Clin. Sci.*, **15**, 635.

104. Fitzpatrick, C. (1975). Salt overdosage. *Brit. Med. J.*, **2**, 517.

105. Fleming, C. R., Hodges, R. E. and Hurley, L. S. (1976). A prospective study of serum copper and zinc levels in patients receiving total parenteral nutrition. *Am J. Clin. Nutr.*, **29**, 70.

106. Flendrig, J. A., Krus, H. and Das, D. A. (1976). Aluminium intoxication: the causes of dialysis dementia? *Proc. Eur. Dial. Transplant Ass.*, **13**, 355.

107. Fletcher, R. F., Henly, A. A. and Sammons, H. G. (1960). Case of magnesium deficiency following massive intestinal resection. *Lancet*, **i**, 522.

108. Flynn, A., Pories, W. J., Strain, W. H., Hill, O. A. Jr. and Fratianne, R. B. (1971). Rapid serum-zinc depletion associated with corticosteroid therapy. *Lancet*, **ii**, 1169.

109. Forster, J. (1876). Ueber den Ort des Fettansatzes im Tiere bei verschiedener Fütterungsweise. *Z. Biol.*, **12**, 448.

110. Forster, J. (1876). Ueber die Verarmung des Körpers, speziell der Knochen, an Kalk bei ungenügender Kalkzufuhr. *Z. Biol.*, **12**, 464.

111. Forster, J. (1876). Valentine's meat-juice und Fleischbrühe. *Z. Biol.*, **12**, 475.

112. Foster, G. V., Baghdiantz, A., Kumar, M. A., Slack, E., Soliman, H. A. and MacIntyre, I. (1964). Thyroid origin of calcification. *Nature*, **202**, 1303.

114. Fuisz, R. E., Lauler, D. P. and Cohen, P. (1962). Diuretic-induced hyponatremia and sustained anti-diuresis. *Amer. J. Med.*, **33**, 783.

115. Fuller, T. J., Nichols, W. W., Brenner, B. J. and Peterson, J. C. (1978). Reversible depression in myo-cardial contractility in the dog with experimental phosphorous deficiency, *Clin. Res.*, **26**, 32A (Abstract).

116. Fulmer, D. H., Dimich, A. B., Rothschild, E. O. and Laird Myers, W. P. (1972). Phosphate infusion effec-tively reduces serum calcium. *Modern Medicine*, **17**, 73.

117. Gabow, P. A., Moore, S. and Schrier, R. W. (1979). Spironolactone-induced hyperchloremic acidosis in cirrhosis. *Ann. Int. Med.*, **90**, 338.

118. Galante, L. (1968). Thymic and parathyroid origin of calcitonin in man. *Lancet*, **ii**, 537.

119. Gamble, J. L., Ross, G. S. and Tisdall, F. F. (1923). The metabolism of fixed base during fasting. *J. biol. Chem.*, **57**, 633.

120. Gamstorp, I. (1956). Adynamic episodica hereditaria. *Acta paediat. (Uppsala)*, **45**, **Suppl.**, 108.

121. Garcia-Webb, P. and Bhagat, C. (1984). Hyper-magnesaemia and hypophosphataemia after ingestion of magnesium sulphate. *Brit. med. J.*, **288**, 759.

122. Garrow, J. S. (1965). Total body potassium in kwashiorkor and marasmus. *Lancet*, **ii**, 455.

123. Gault, M. H., Dixon, M. E., Doyle, M. and Cohen, W. M. (1968). Hypernatremia, Azotemia, and

dehydration due to high-protein tube feeding. *Ann. Int. Med.*, **4**, 778.

124. Gennari, F. J. (1977). Differential diagnosis and treatment of metabolic alkalosis *Acid-Base and Electrolyte Balance*, p. 74. Edited by A. B. Schwartz and H. Lyons. New York: Grune and Stratton.

125. Ghani, M. F. and Smith, J. R. (1974). The effectiveness of magnesium chloride in the treatment of ventricular tachyarrhythmias due to digitalis intoxication. *Amer. Heart J.*, **88**, 621.

126. Gipstein, R. M., Coburn, J. W., Adams, D. A., Lee, D. B. N., Khosrow, P., Sellers, A., Suki, W. N. and Massry, S. G. (1976). Calciphylaxis in man. A syndrome of tissue necrosis and vascular calcification in 11 patients with chronic renal failure. *Arch. Int. Med.*, **136**, 1273.

127. Glorieux, F. H., Scriver, C. R., Reade, T. M., Goldman, H., Roseborough, A. (1972). Use of phosphate and vitamin D to prevent dwarfism and rickets in x-linked hypophosphatemia. *N. Engl. J. of Med.*, **287**, 481.

128. Goldfarb, S., Cox, M., Singer, I. and Goldberg, M. (1976). Acute hyperkalaemia induced by hyperglycemia: hormonal mechanisms. *Amer. Int. Med.*, **59**, 744.

129. Goldfarb, S., Strunk, L. and Goldberg, M. (1975). Paradoxical glucose induced hyperkalaemia: combined aldosterone and insulin deficiencies. *Amer. J. Med.*, **59**, 744.

130. Goldman, A. S., Van Fossan, D. D. and Baird, E. E. (1962). Magnesium deficiency in celiac disease. *Pediatrics*, **29**, 948.

131. Goldsmith, R. S. and Ingbar, S. H. (1966). Inorganic treatment of hypercalcaemia of diverse etiologies. *N. Engl. J. of Med.*, **274**, 1.

132. Goodbody, R. A., Middleton, J. E. and Gamlen, T. R. (1975). Saline emetics and hypernatraemia. Report on two fatalities. *Medicine, Science and the Law*, **15**, 261.

133. Greene, H. L. (1977). Trace metals in parenteral nutrition. *Zinc Metabolism: Current Aspects in Health and Disease*, p. 87. Edited by G. J. Brewer and A. S. Prasad. New York: Alan R. Liss.

134. Greenwald, I. (1931). Relation of concentration of calcium to that of protein and inorganic phosphate in serum. *J. Biol. Chem.*, **93**, 551.

135. Griggs, R. C., Engel, W. K. and Resnick, J. S. (1970). Acetazolamide treatment of hypokalemic periodic paralysis. *Ann. Int. Med.*, **73**, 39.

136. Gross, E. G., Dexter, J. D. and Roth, R. G. (1966). Hypokalemic myopathy with myoglobinuria associated with licorice ingestion. *N. Engl. J. of Med.*, **274**, 602.

137. Guillou, P. J., Morgan, D. B. and Hill, G. L. (1976). Hypophosphatemia: a complication of "innocuous dextrose-saline". *Lancet*, **ii**, 710.

138. Hambridge, K. M., Walravens, P. A. and Nelder, K. H. (1977). The role of zinc in the pathogenesis and treatment of acrodermatitis enteropathica. In *Zinc Metabolism: Current Aspects in Health and Disease*, p. 329. Edited by G. J. Brewer and A. S. Prasad. New York: Alan R. Liss.

139. Hamburger, J. (1957). Electrolyte disturbances in acute uremia. *Clin. Chem.*, **3**, 319.

140. Heaton, F. W., Hodgkinson, H. and Rose, G. A. (1964). Observations on relation between calcium and magnesium metabolism in man. *Clin. Sci.*, **27**, 31.

141. Henkin, R. I. and Bradley, D. F. (1970). Hypogeusia corrected by Ni^{++} and Zn^{++}. *Life Sci.*, **9**, 701.

142. Henneman, P. H. and Wallack, S. (1957). The use of androgens and estrogens and their metabolic effects. A review of the prolonged use of estrogens and androgens in post-menopausal and senile osteoporosis. *Arch. Int. Med.*, **100**, 715.

143. Henzel, J. F., DeWeese, M. S. and Lichti, E. L. (1970). Zinc concentrations within healing wounds. *Archs. Surg., Chicago*, **100**, 349.

144. Hertz, P. and Richardson, J. A. (1972). Arginine-induced hyperkalemia in renal failure patients. *Arch. Int. Med.*, 130, 778.

145. Hilborne, L. H., Howanitz, P. J. and Howanitz, J. H. (1984). Serum osmolality. *N. Engl. J. of Med.*, **310**, 1608.

146. Hobson, J. A. and English, J. T. (1963). Self-induced water intoxication; case study of a chronically schizophrenic patient with physiological evidence of water retention due to inappropriate release of antidiuretic hormone. *Ann. Int. Med.*, **58**, 324.

147. Holt, D. W. and Goulding, R. (1975). Magnesium depletion and digoxin toxicity. *Brit. Med. J.*, **I**, 627.

148. Howard, J. E. and Connor, T. B. (1954). Some experiences with the use of vitamin D in the treatment of hypoparathyroidism. *Trans. Assoc. Amer. Physicians*, **67**, 199.

149. Hurst, J. W., Logue, B. R. and Schlant, R. C. (1974). *The Heart*, 3rd ed. p. 1500. New York: McGraw-Hill.

150. Hyes, C. P., McLeod, M. E. and Robinson, R. (1967). An extrarenal mechanism for the maintenance of potassium balance in severe chronic renal failure. *Trans. Ass. Amer. Physicians, Philadelphia*, **50**, 207.

151. Ibels, L. S., Alfrey, A. C., Haut, L. and Huffer, W. (1978). Preservation of function in experimental renal disease by dietary restriction of phosphate. *N. Engl. J. of Med.*, **298**, 122.

152. Iseri, L. T., Freed, J. and Bures, A. R. (1975). Magnesium deficiency and cardiac disorders. *Amer. J. Med.*, **58**, 837.

153. Ishigami, R., Shiotani, S., Yoshida, A., Kawaya, T., Ohmoto, J., Akiyama, Y., Osawa, K., Kawaguchi, Y., Kadota, I. and Shinobe, N. (1971). Changes in serum magnesium levels in periodic paralysis (Jap.). *Arch. intern. Med.*, **18**, 17.

154. Jacob, H. S. and Amsden, T. (1971). Acute hemolytic anemia with rigid red cells in hypophosphatemia. *N. Engl. J. of Med.*, **285**, 1446.

155. Jaffey, L. and Martin, A. (1981). Malignant hyperkalaemia after amiloride/hydrochlorothiazide treat-

ment. *Lancet*, **i**, 1272 (c).

156. Jibani, M. and Hodges, N. H. (1985). Prolonged hypercalcaemia after industrial exposure to Vitamin D3. *Brit. Med. J.*, **290**, 748.

157. Johnsen, T. (1977). Endogenous insulin fluctuations during glucose-induced paralysis in patients with familial periodic hypokalaemia. *Metabolism*, **26**, 1185.

158. Johnsen, T. (1981). Familial periodic paralysis with hypokalaemia. *Dan. Med. Bull*, **28**, 1.

159. Johnsen, T. and Beck-Nielsen, H. (1979). Insulin receptors, insulin secretion and glucose disappearance rate in patients with periodic hypokalaemic paralysis. *Acta Endocrinol.*, **90**, 272.

160. Johnson, W. J., Goldsmith, R. S., Beabout, J. W., Kelly, P. J. and Arnaud, C. D. (1974). Prevention and reversal of progressive secondary hyperparathyroidism in patients maintained by hemodialysis. *Amer. J. Med.*, **56**, 827.

161. Kalbfleisch, J. M., Lindemann, R. D., Ginn, H. E. and Smith, W. O. (1963). Effects of ethanol administration on urinary excretion of magnesium and other electrolytes in alcoholic and normal subjects. *J. Clin. Invest.*, **42**, 1471.

162. Kanfer, A., Richet, G., Roland, J. and Chatelet, F. (1979). Extreme hyperphosphataemia causing acute anuric nephrocalcinosis in lymphosarcoma. *Brit. med. J.*, **1**, 1321.

163. Kanis, J. A. and Yates, A. J. P. (1985). Measuring serum calcium. *Brit. med. J.*, **290**, 728.

164. Katz, J. (1896). Die mineralischen Bestandteile des Muskelfleisches. *Pflüg. Arch. ges. Physiol.*, **63**, 1.

165. Kay, R. G., Tasman-Jones, C., Pybus, J., Whiting, R. and Black, H. (1976). A syndrome of acute zinc deficiency during total parenteral alimentation in man. *Ann. Surg.*, **183**, 331.

166. Kay, R. G. and Tasman-Jones, C. (1975). Acute zinc deficiency in man during intravenous alimentation. *Aust. NZJ Surg.*, **45**, 325.

167. Kellogg, F. and Ker, W. J. (1936). Electrocardiographic changes in hyperparathyroidism. *Amer. Heart J.*, **12**, 346.

168. Kennedy, P. G. E., Mitchell, D. M. and Hoffbrand, B. I. (1978). Severe hyponatremia in hospital in-patients. *Brit. Med. J.*, **ii**, 1251.

169. Kim, Y. T. and Cha, Y. M. (1975). *Kor. J. intern. Med.*, **8**, 237. Quoted by McFadzean and Yeung, 1967.

170. Kitamura, K. (1913). On periodic paralysis (In Japanese). *J. Jap. Soc. Int. M.*, **1**, 22.

171. Klock, J. C., Williams, H. E. and Mentzen, W. C. (1974). Hemolytic anemia and somatic cell dysfunction in severe hypophosphatemia. *Arch. Int. Med.*, **134**, 360.

172. Knochel, J. P. (1977). The pathophysiology and clinical characteristics of severe hypophosphatemia. *Arch. Int. Med.*, **137**, 203.

173. Krawitt, E. L. and Bloomer, H. A. (1965). Increased cerebrospinal fluid protein secondary to hypercalcaemia of the milk alkali syndrome. *N. Eng. J. of Med.*, **273**, 154.

174. Lafferty, F. W. and Pearson, O. H. (1963). Skeletal, intestinal and renal calcium dynamics in hyperparathyroidism. *J. Clin. Endocrin.*, **23**, 891.

175. Lancaster, R. (1981). Personal communication.

176. Lanier, D., Favre, H., Allan, I., Jacob, and Bourgoignie, J. J. (1980). Cimetidine therapy for severe hypercalcemia in two chronic hemodialysis patients. *Ann. Int. Med.*, **93**, 574.

177. Lassiter, W. E., Gottschalk, C. W. and Mylle, M. (1963). Micropuncture study of renal tubular re-absorption of calcium in normal rodents. *Amer. J. Physiol.*, **204**, 771.

178. Latta, T. (1831–2). Malignant cholera . . . relative to the treatment of cholera by the copious injection of aqueous and saline fluids into the veins. *Lancet*, **ii**, 274.

179. Latta, T. (1831–2). Reply to some objections offered to the practice of venous injections in cholera. *Lancet*, **ii**, 428.

180. Lee, T. S., Kim, J. Y., Lee, J. K. and Lee, M. (1964). *J. Kor. med. Ass.*, **7**, 247. Quoted by McFadzean and Yeung 1967.

181. Lehmann, J. and Donatolli, A. A. (1964). Calcium intoxication due to primary hyperparathyroidism. *Ann. Int. Med.*, **60**, 447.

182. Levinsky, N. G., Tyson, I., Miller, R. B. and Relman, A. S. (1962). The relation between amino acids and potassium in isolated rat muscle. *J. Clin. Invest,.* **41**, 480.

183. Liebig, J. (1847). Ueber die Bestandtheile der Flüssigkeiten des Fleisches. *Ann. Chem. u. Pharm.*, **62**, 257.

184. Lightwood, R. and Stapleton, T. (1953). Idiopathic hypercalcaemia in infants. *Lancet*, **ii**, 255.

185. Loeb, R. F., Atchley, D. W. and Palmer, W. W. (1922). On the equilibrium condition between blood serum and serous cavity fluids. *J. gen. Physiol.*, **4**, 591.

186. Louis, L. H. and Conn, J. W. (1956). Preparation of glycyrrhizinic acid, the electrolyte-active principle of licorice: its effects upon metabolism and upon pituitary-adrenal function in man. *J. Lab. Clin. Med.*, **47**, 20.

187. Lucas, A. (1977). Hypochlorite sterilising fluid as source of dietary sodium in gavage fed infants. *Lancet*, **ii**, 144.

188. McArdle, B. (1956). Familial periodic paralysis. *Brit. Med. Bull.*, **12**, 226.

189. McArdle, B. (1962). Adynamia episodica hereditaria and its treatment. *Brain*, **85**, 121.

190. McCollister, R. J., Flink, E. B., Lewis, M. D. (1963). Urinary excretion of magnesium in man following the ingestion of ethanol. *Amer. J. Clin. Nutr.*, **12**, 415.

191. McDowell, M. K., Herman, R. H. and Davis, T. E. (1963). The effect of a high and low sodium diet in a patient with familial periodic paralysis. *Metabolism*, **5**, 388.

192. McFadzean, A. J. S. and Yeung, R. (1967). Periodic

paralysis complicating thyrotoxicosis in Chinese. *Brit. Med. J.*, **1**, 451.

193. MacIntyre, I. and Davidson, D. (1958). The production of secondary potassium depletion, sodium retention, nephrocalcinosis and hypercalcemia by magnesium deficiency. *Biochem. J.*, **70**, 456.

194. MacIntyre, I., Hanna, S., Booth, C. C. and Read, A. E. (1961). Intracellular magnesium deficiency in man. *Clin. Sci.*, **20**, 297.

195. MacIntyre, I. (1963). Magnesium metabolism. *Sci. Basis Med. Ann. Revs.*, [**10**], 216.

196. MacIntyre, I. (1967). Magnesium metabolism. *Adv. Intern. Med.*, **13**, 143.

197. Mader, I. J. and Iseri, L. T. (1955). Spontaneous hypopotassemia, hypomagnesemia, alkalosis, and tetany due to hypersecretion of corticosterone-like mineralocorticoid. *Am. J. Med.*, **19**, 976.

198. Mandel, L. B. and Benedict, S. R. (1909). The paths of excretion for inorganic compounds. V. The excretion of calcium. *Amer. J. Physiol.*, **25**, 23.

199. Manitus, A. and Epstein, F. H. (1963). Some observations on the influence of a magnesium-deficient diet on rats, with special reference to renal concentrating ability. *J. Clin. Invest.*, **42**, 208.

200. Massry, S. G. (1977). Metabolic acidosis in hyperparathyroidism. Role of phosphate depletion and other factors. In *Phosphate Metabolism*, p. 301. Edited by S. G. Massry and E. Ritz. New York: Plenum Press.

201. Massry, S. G. and Coburn, J. W. (1976). Divalent ion metabolism and renal osteodyotrophy. In: *Clinical Aspects of Uraemia and Dialysis*, p. 304. Edited by S. G. Massry and A. L. Sellers. Springfield, Illinois: Charles C. Thomas.

202. Mawdsley, C. and Holman, R. L. (1957). Hypercalcaemia in acute leukaemia. *Lancet*, **i**, 78.

203. Medalle, R. and Waterhouse, C. (1973). A magnesium-deficient patient presenting with hypocalcemia and hyperphosphatemia. *Ann. Int. Med.*, **79**, 76.

204. Meigs, E. B. (1912). Contributions to the general physiology of smooth and striated muscle. *J. exp. Zool.* **13**, 497.

205. Meigs, E. B. and Ryan, L. A. (1912). The chemical analysis of the ash of smooth muscle. *J. biol. Chem.*, **11**, 401.

206. Merimee, T. J., Rabinowitz, D., Riggs, L., Burgess, J. A., Rimoin, D. L. and McKusick, V. A. (1967). Plasma growth hormone after arginine infusion. *N. Engl. J. of Med.*, **276**, 434.

207. Merimee, T. J., Lillicrap, D. A. and Rabinowitz, D. (1965). Effect of arginine on serum-levels of human growth-hormone. *Lancet*, **ii**, 668.

208. Mills, C. F., Quarterman, J., Chester, J. K., Williams, R. B. and Dalgarno, A. C. (1969). Metabolic role of zinc. *Am. J. Clin. Futr.*, **22**, 1240.

209. Molhuysen, J. A., Gerbrandy, J., de Vries, L. A., de Jong, J. C., Lenstra, K. B., Turner, K. P. and Borst, J. G. G. (1950). A liquorice extract with desoxycortone-like action. *Lancet*, **ii**, 381.

210. Moran, W. H. (1971). CPPB and vasopressin secretion. *Anaesthesiology,* **34**, 501.

211. Mordes, J. P., Swartz, R. and Arky, R. A. (1975). Extreme hypermagnesemia as a cause of refractory hypotension. *Ann. Int. Med.*, **83**, 657.

212. Mordes, J. P. and Wacker, W. E. C. (1977). Excess magnesium. *Pharmacol. Rev.*, **29**, 273.

213. Morgan, D. B. and Davidson, C. (1980). Hypokalaemia and diuretics: an analysis of publications. *Brit. med. J.*, **280**, 905.

214. Moynahan, E. J. (1974). Acrodermatitis enteropathica. A lethal inherited human zinc-deficiency disorder. *Lancet*, **ii**, 399.

215. Moynahan, E. J. and Barnes, P. M. (1973). Zinc deficiency and a synthetic diet for lactose intolerance. *Lancet*, **i**, 676.

216. Mudge, G. H., Foulks, J. and Gilman, A. (1948). The renal excretion of potassium. *Proc. Soc. exp. Biol. (N.Y.)*, **67**, 545.

217. Muldowney, F. P., McKenna, T. J. and Kyle, L. H. (1970). Parathormone-like effect of magnesium replenishment in steatorrhea. *N. Engl. J. of Med.*, **281**, 61.

218. Mwambingu, F. T. (1985). Water intoxication and oxytocin. *Brit. med. J.*, **290**, 113.

219. Neale, T. J., Lynn, K. L. and Bailey, R. R. (1976). Spironolactone-associated aggravation of renal function impairment. *N.Z. Medical Journal*, **83**, 147.

220. Newman, J. H., Neff, T. A. and Ziporin, P. (1977). Acute respiratory failure associated with hypophosphatemia. *N. Engl. J. of Med.*, **296**, 1101.

221. Nordin, B. E. C. (1960). Osteoporosis and calcium deficiency. In *Bone as a tissue.* p. 46. Edited by K. Rodahl, J. T. Nicholson and E. M. Brown. New York: McGraw-Hill.

222. Nordin, B. E. C. (1962). Calcium balance and calcium requirement in spinal osteoporosis. *Amer. J. Clin. Nutr.*, **10**, 384.

223. Nordin, B. E. C. and Fraser, R. (1956). A calcium-infusion test. 1. Urinary excretion data for recognition of osteomalacia. *Lancet*, **i**, 823.

224. Norris, F. H., Panner, B. J. and Stormont, B. M. (1968). Thyrotoxic periodic paralysis. Metabolic and ultrastructural studies. *Arch. Neurol. (Chic).*, **19**, 88.

225. Norris, F. H., Clarke, E. C. and Biglieri, E. (1971). Studies in thyrotoxic periodic paralysis. *J. of the Neurological Sci.*, **13**, 431.

226. Notman, D. D., Krauss, D. J. and Moses, A. M. (1979). Fulminating hypercalcemia and markedly increased nephrogenous cyclic AMP in a patient with transitional cell carcinoma of the bladder. *Amer. J. of Med.*, **66**, 870.

227. O'Connor, L. R., Wheeler, W. S. and Bethune, J. E. (1977). Effect of hypophosphatemia on myocardial performance in man. *N. Engl. J. of Med.*, **297**, 901.

228. Okada, A., Takagi, Y., Itakura, T., Satani, M., Manabe, H., Iida, Y., Tanigaki, T., Iwasaki, M. and

Kesahara, N. (1976). Skin lesions during intravenous hyperalimentation. *Surgery*, **80**, 629.

229. Okihiro, M. M. and Beddow, R. M. (1965). Thyrotoxic periodic paralysis in Hawaii: its predilection for the Japanese race. *Neurol. (Minneap.).*, **15**, 253.

230. Okinaka, S., Shizume, K., Iino, S., Watanabe, I., Irie, M., Noguchi, A., Kuma, S., Kuma, K. and Ito, T. (1957). The association of periodic paralysis and hyperthyroidism in Japan. *J. of Clin. Endoc.*, **17**, 1454.

231. Opie, L. H., Hunt, B. G. and Findlay, J. M. (1964). Massive small bowel resection with malabsorption and negative magnesium balance. *Gastroenterology*, **47**, 415.

232. O'Shaughnessy, W. B. (1831–2). Proposal of a new method of treating the blue epidemic cholera by the injection of highly oxygenised salts into the venous sytem. *Lancet*, **i**, 115.

233. Overton, E. (1902). Beiträge zur allgemeinen Muskel- und Nervenphysiologie. *Pflüg. Arch. ges. Physiol.*, **92**, 115.

234. Overton, E. (1904). Beiträge zur allgemeinen Muskel- und Nervenphysiologie. III. Mittheilung. Studien über die Wirkung der Alkali– und Erdkalisalze auf Skelettmuskeln und Nerven. *Pflüg. Arch. ges. Physiol.*, **105**, 179.

235. Pak, C. Y. C., Wortsman, J., Bennett, J. E., Delea, C. S. and Bartter, F. C. (1968). Control of hypercalcemia with cellulose phosphate. *J. Clin. Endocrinol. Metab.*, **28**, 1929.

236. Pak, C. Y. C., Williams, H. E. and Ruskin, B. (1971). Physicochemical basis for the formation of Ca-containing renal stones. *Clin. Res*,. **19**, 482.

237. Paterson, C. R. (1980). Vitamin-D poisoning: survey of causes in 21 patients with hypercalcaemia, *Lancet*, **i**, 1164.

238. Pearson, C. M. and Kalyanaraman, K. (1972). Periodic paralysis. In *The Metabolic Basis of Inherited Diseases*. 3rd edn, p. 1181. Edited by J. B. Stanbury, J. B. Wyngaarden and D. S. Fredrickson. New York: McGraw-Hill.

239. Peart, W. S. (1977). The kidney as an endocrine organ. *Lancet*, **ii**, 543.

240. Peart, W. S. (1981). The problem of treatment in mild hypertension. *Clin. Sci.*, **61**, 403.

241. Pekarek, R. S., Hoagland, A. M. and Powanda, M. C. (1977). Humoral and cellular immune responses in zinc deficient rats. *Nutr. Rep. Int.*, **16**, 267.

242. Peters, J. P. and Van Slyke, D. D. (1931). *Quantitative Clinical Chemistry*. Vols. 1 and 2. London: Bailliere, Tindall and Cox.

243. Peterson, V. P. (1963). Metabolic studies in clinical magnesium deficiency. *Acta med. Scand.*, **173**, 285.

244. Pizak, L. R., Watkins, G. and Sheldon, G. F. (1972). Hyperalimentation and the oxy-hemoglobin dissociation curve. In *Intravenous Hyperalimentation*, p. 197. Edited by G. S. M. Cowan and W. L. Scheetz. Philadelphia: Lea and Febiger.

245. Platts, M. M., Goode, G. C. and Hislop, J. S. (1977). Composition of the domestic water supply and the incidence of fractures and encephalopathy in patients on home dialysis. *Brit. Med. J.*, **ii**, 657.

246. Poskanzer, D. C. and Kerr, D. N. S. (1961). Periodic paralysis with response to spironolactone. *Lancet*, **ii**, 511.

247. Prasad, A. S., Miale, A., Farid, Z., Sanstead, H. H. and Schulert, A. R. (1963). Zinc metabolism in patients with the syndrome of iron deficiency anemia, hepatosplenomegaly, dwarfism, and hypogonadism. *J. Lab. Clin. Med.*, **61**, 537.

248. Prescott, L. F., Stewart, M. J. and Proudfoot, A. T. (1978). SI moles and drugs, *Br. Med. J.*, **1**, 1620.

249. Ramsay, I. (1974). *Thyroid Disease and Muscle Dysfunction*. London: Heinemann Medical Books.

250. Rapoport, A., Sepp, A. H. and Brown, W. H. (1960). Carcinoma of the parathyroid gland with pulmonary metastases and cardiac death. *Amer. J. Med.*, **28**, 443.

251. Resnick, M. E. and Patterson, C. (1969). Coma and convulsions due to compulsive water drinking. *Neurology, Minneapolis*, **19**, 1125.

252. Richards, P. and Truniger, B. (1983). *Understanding Water, Electrolyte and Acid-Base Balance*. London: William Heinemann.

253. Ringer, S. (1880–2). Regarding the action of hydrate of soda, hydrate of ammonia, and hydrate of potash on the ventricle of the frog's heart. *J. Physiol.*, **3**, 195.

254. Robinson, J. R. (1960). Metabolism of intracellular water. *Physiol. Rev.*, **40**, 112.

255. Rosenfeld, M. (1902). Acute Aufsteigende Lähmung bei Morbus Basedow. *Berl. klin. Wschnschr.*, **39**, 538.

256. Rowlands, B. J. and Giddings, A. E. (1976). Postoperative hypophosphataemia. *Lancet*, **ii**, 1077.

257. Rushmer, R. F. (1961). *Cardiovascular Dynamics*. 2nd edn. Philadelphia: W. B. Saunders.

258. Ryan, M. P., Ryan, M. F. and Counihan, T. B. (1981). The effect of diuretics on lymphocyte magnesium and potassium. *Acta. Med. Scand.*, **S647**, 153.

259. Sackner, M. A., Spivack, A. D. and Balian, L. J. (1960). Hypocalcemia in the presence of osteoblastic metastases. *N. Engl. J. of Med.*, **262**, 173.

260. Sanderson, P. H. (1959). Hypercalcaemia and renal failure in multiple secondary carcinoma of bone; report of a case. *Brit. med. J.*, **2**, 275.

261. Sandstead, H. H., Lanier, V. C., Shepard, G. H. and Gillespie, D. D. (1970). Zinc and wound healing. *Am. J. Clin. Nutr.*, **23**, 514.

262. Sandstead, H. H., Harold, H., Prasad, A. S., Schulert, A. R., Farid, Z., Miale, A., Bassilly, S. and Darby, W. J.. (1967). Human zinc deficiency, endocrine manifestations, and response to treatment. *Am. J. Clin. Nutr.*, **20**, 422.

263. Satoyoshi, E., Murakami, K., Kowa, H., Kinoshita, M. and Nishiyama, Y. (1963). Periodic paralysis in hyperthyroidism. *Neurology (Minneap.)*, **13**, 746.

264. Satoyoshi, E., Suzuki, Y. and Abe, T. (1963). Periodic paralysis. A study of carbohydrate and thiamine

metabolism. *Neurology (Minneap.)*, **13**, 24.

265. Savage, D. C. L. and McAdam, W. A. F. (1967). Convulsions due to hypomagnesaemia in an infant recovering from diarrhoea. *Lancet*, **ii**, 234.

266. Schatz, W. J. (1937). Treatment based on physical principles followed by recovery in sodium chloride poisoning. *Medical Record*, **145**, 487.

267. Schatzmann, H. J. and Buergin, H. (1978). Calcium in human red blood cells. *New York Acad. Sci.*, **307**, 125.

268. Scheiner, E. (1975). The relationship of ADH to the control of volume and tonicity in humans. *Adv. Clin. Chem.*, **17**, 1.

269. Schultze, R. G., Taggart, D. D., Shapiro, H., Pennell, J. P., Caglar, S. and Bricker, N. S. (1971). On the adaptation in potassium excretion associated with nephron reduction in the dog. *J. of Clin. Invest.*, **50**, 1061.

270. Schwartz, W. B., Bennett, W., Curelop, S. and Bartter, F. (1957). A syndrome of renal sodium loss of hyponatraemia probably resulting from inappropriate secretion of ADH. *Amer. J. Med.*, **23**, 529.

271. Schwartz, W. B. and Polak, A. (1960). Electrolyte disorders in chronic renal disease. *J. chron. Dis.*, **11**, 319.

272. Schweitzer, V. G., Thompson, N. W., Harness, J. K. and Kishiyama, R. H. (1978). Management of severe hypercalcemia caused by primary hyperparathyroidism. *Archs. Surg.*, **113**, 373.

273. Sheldon, G. F. (1973). Hyperphosphatemia, hypophosphatemia and the oxyhemoglobin dissociation curve. *J. Surg. Res.*, **14**, 367.

274. Sheldon, G. F., Jelinek, C. and Fuchs, R. (1974). The role of inorganic phosphate in recovery from transfusion. *Surg. Forum*, **25**, 430.

275. Sheldon, G. F. and Grzyb, S. (1975). Phosphate depletion and repletion: relation to parenteral nutrition and oxygen transport. *Ann. Surg.*, **182**, 683.

276. Shils, M. E. (1964). Experimental human magnesium depletion. I Clinical observations and blood chemistry alterations. *Amer. J. Clin. Nutr.*, **15**, 133.

277. Shils, M. E. (1969). Experimental human magnesium depletion. *Medicine (Baltimore)*, **48**, 61.

278. Shils, M., Wright, W. and Turnbull, A. (1970). Long-term parenteral nutrition through an external arteriovenous shunt. *N. Engl. J. of med.*, **283**, 341.

279. Shinosaki, T. (1926). Klinische Studien über die periodische Extremitätenlahmung. *Z. ges. Neurol. Psychiat.*, **100**, 564.

280. Silvis, E. S. and Paragas, P. D. (1972). Parasthesias, weakness, seizures and hypophosphatemia in patients receiving hyperalimentation. *Gastroenterology*, **62**, 513.

281. Simon, W., Ammann, D., Oehme, M. and Morf, W. E. (1978). Calcium-selective electrodes. *Ann. New York Acad. Sci.*, **307**, 52.

282. Smith, P. K., Winkler, A. W. and Hoff, H. E. (1939). Electrocardiographic changes and concentrations of

magnesium salts. *Amer. J. Physiol.*, **126**, 720.

283. Solomon, R. J. and Cole, A. G. (1981). Importance of potassium in patients with acute myocardial infarction. *Acta. med. Scand.*, **S647.**, 87.

284. Spencer, H., Vankinscott, V., Lewin, F. and Samachson, J. (1965). Zinc metabolism during low and high calcium intake in man. *J. Nutr.*, **86**, 169.

285. Spencer, H., Osis, D., Kramer, L. and Norris, C. (1976). Intake, excretion, and retention of zinc in man. *Trace Elements in Human Health and Disease*, p. 345. Vol. 1. Edited by A. S. Prasad and D. Oberleas. New York: Academic Press.

286. Staffurth, J. S. (1964). The total exchangeable potassium in patients with hypokalaemia. *Postgraduate Med. J.*, **40**, 4.

287. Stapleton, T., Macdonald, W. B. and Lightwood, R. (1956). Management of idiopathic hypercalcaemia in infancy. *Lancet*, **i**, 932.

288. Stewart, G. W., Corrall, R. J. M., Fyffe, J. A., Stockdill, G. and Strong, J. A. (1979). Familial pseudohyperkalaemia—a new syndrome. *Lancet*, **ii**, 175.

289. Suh, S. M., Tashjian, A. H. and Matsuo, N. (1973). Pathogenesis of hypocalcemia in primary hypomagnesemia. Normal end-organ responsiveness to parathyroid hormone, impaired parathyroid gland function. *J. Clin. Invest.*, **52**, 153.

290. Suki, W. N., Yium, J. J., Von Minden, M., Saller-Herbert, C., Eknoyan, G. and Martinez-Malonado, M. (1970). Acute treatment of hypercalcemia with Furosemide. *N. Engl. J. of Med.*, **283**, 836.

291. Sundaram, M. B. M. and Swaminathan, R. (1981). Total body potassium depletion and severe myopathy due to chronic liquorice ingestion. *Postgraduate Medical Journal*, **57**, 48.

292. Swales, J. D. (1982). Magnesium deficiency and diuretics. *Brit. med. J.*, **285**, 1377.

293. Swaminathan, R., Morgan, D. B., Inonescu, M. and Hill, G. L. (1978). Hypophosphataemia and its consequences in patients following open heart surgery. *Anaesthesia*, **33**, 601.

294. Talso, P. J., Glynn, M. F., Oester, Y. T. and Fudema, J. (1963). Body composition in hypokalemic familial periodic paralysis. *Ann. New York Acad. Sci.*, **110**, 993.

295. Tasman-Jones, C. and Kay, R. L. (1975). Zinc deficiency and skin lesions. *N. Engl. J. of Med.*, **293**, 830.

296. Territo, M. C. and Tanaka, K. R. (1974). Hypophosphataemia in chronic alcoholism. *Archs. Int. Med.*, **134**, 445.

297. Thatcher, J. S. and Radike, A. W. (1947). Tolerance to potassium intoxication in the albino rat. *Amer. J. Physiol.*, **151**, 138.

298. Thomas, R. D., Silverton, N. P., Burkinshaw, L. and Morgan, D. B. (1979). Potassium depletion and tissue loss in chronic heart-disease. *Lancet*, **ii**, 9.

299. Thomas, T. H., Morgan, D. B., Swaminathan, R.,

Ball, S. G. and Lee, M. R. (1978). Severe hyponatraemia: A study of 17 patients. *Lancet*, **i**, 621.

300. Thomas, W. C. and Howard, J. E. (1964). In *Comar and Bronner's Minimal Metabolism*, Vol. **II**, Part A. New York: Academic Press.

301. Thomas, W. C. and Morden, H. G. (1958). The effect of cortisone experimental hypervitaminosis D. *Endocrinology*, **63**, 57.

302. Tomlinson, S., Hendy, G. N. and O'Riordan, J. L. H. (1976). Simplified assessment of response to parathyroid hormone in hypoparathyroid patients. *Lancet*, **i**, 62.

303. Travis, S. F., Sugerman, H. J., Ruberg, R. L., Dudrick, S. J., Delivoria-Papadopoulos, M., Millier, L. D. and Oski, F. A. (1971). Alterations of red-cell glycolytic intermediates and oxygen transport as a consequence of hypophosphatemia in patients receiving intravenous hyperalimentation. *N. Engl. J. of Med.*, **285**, 763.

304. Tsang, R. C., Kleinman, L. I. and Sutherland, J. M. (1972). Hypocalcaemia in infants of diabetic mothers. *J. Pediatr.*, **80**, 384.

305. Tucker, S. B., Schroeter, A. L., Brown, P. W. and McCall, J. T. (1976). Acquired zinc deficiency. *J. Amer. med. Assoc.*, **235**, 2399.

306. Vanasin, B., Colmer, M. and Davis, P. J. (1972). Hypocalcemia, hypomagnesemia and hypokalemia during chemotherapy of pulmonary tuberculosis. *Chest*, **61**, 496.

307. Van der Meulen, J. P., Gilbert, G. J. and Kane, C. A. (1961). Familial hyperkalemic paralysis with myotonia. *N. Engl. J. of Med.*, **264**, 1.

308. Van Slyke, D. D. (1923). The determination of chlorides in blood and tissues. *J. biol. Chem.*, **58**, 523.

309. Van Slyke, D. D. and Cullen, G. E. (1917). Studies of acidosis. 1. The bicarbonate concentration of the blood plasma; its significance and its determination as a measure of acidosis. *J. biol. Chem.*, **30**, 289.

310. Van Slyke, D. D., Hastings, A. B., Hiller, A. and Sendroy, J. (1928). Studies of gas and electrolyte equilibria in Blood. XIV. The amounts of alkali bound by serum albumin and globulin. *J. biol. Chem.*, **79**, 769.

311. Van Slyke, D. D. and Neill, J. M. (1924). The determination of gases in blood and other solutions by vacuum extraction and manometric measurement. *J. biol. Chem.*, **61**, 523.

312. Van Slyke, D. D., Wu, H. and McLean, F. C. (1923). Studies of gas and electrolyte equilibria in the blood. V. Factors controlling the electrolyte and water distribution in the blood. *J. biol. Chem.*, **56**, 765.

313. Verbeckmoes, R., Bouillon, R. and Krempien, B. (1975). Disappearance of vascular calcifications during treatment of renal osteodystrophy. Two patients treated with high doses of Vitamin D and aluminium hydroxide. *Ann. Int. Med.*, **82**, 529.

314. Vitale, J. J., Hellerstein, E. E., Nakamura, M. and Lown, B. (1961). Effects of magnesium-deficient diet upon puppies. *Circulation Research*, **9**, 387.

315. Volpé, R. (1981). Hypokalaemic thyrotoxic periodic paralysis. *J. of Roy. Soc. Med.*, **74**, 170C.

316. Wacker, W. E. and Parisi, A. F. (1968). Magnesium metabolism. *N. Engl. J. of Med.*, **278**, 712.

317. Waife, S. O. (1947). Hyperparathyroidism and partial heart block. *J. Lab. and Clin. Med.*, **32**, 185.

318. Walser, M. (1961). Calcium clearance as a function of sodium clearance in the dog. *Amer. J. Physiol.*, **200**, 1099.

319. Walser, M. (1967). Magnesium metabolism. In *Rev. Physiol. Bichem. Exp. Parmac.*, p. 189. New York: Springer.

320. Wan, H. H. and Lye, M. D. W. (1980). Moduretic-induced metabolic acidosis and hyperkalaemia. *Postgraduate Med. J.*, **56**, 348.

321. Weber, A., Hertz, R. and Reiss, I. (1963). On the mechanism of the relaxing effect of fragmented sarcoplasmic reticulum. *J. Gen. Physiol.*, **46**, 679.

322. Weisberg, H. F. (1962). *Water Electrolyte and Acid-Base Balance*. Baltimore: Williams and Wilkins.

323. Weismann, H., Hjorth, N. and Fischer, A. (1976). Zinc depletion syndrome with acrodermatitis during long term intravenous feeding. *Clin. Exp. Dermatol.*, **1**, 237.

324. West, T. E. T., Joffe, M., Sinclair, L. and O'Riordan, J. L. H. (1971). Treatment of hypercalcaemia with calcitonin. *Lancet*, **i**, 675.

325. Whang, R. and Brandfonbrener, M. (1966). The effect of hemorrhagic shock on serum electrolytes. *Clin. Res.*, **14**, 157.

326. Whang, R. and Reyes, R. (1967). The influence of alkalinization on the hyperkalaemia and hypermagnesemia in uremic rats. *Metabolism*, **16**, 941.

327. Widdop, B. (1980). Molar concentrations in toxicology. *Lancet*, **ii**, 87.

328. Wilkin, T. J., Isles, T. E., Paterson, C. R., Crooks, J. and Swanson Beck, J. (1977). Post-thyroidectomy hypocalcaemia; a feature of the operation or the thyroid disorder? *Lancet*, **1**, 621.

329. Wilkinson, R. (1984). Treatment of hypercalcaemia associated with malignancy. *Brit. med. J.*, **288**, 812.

330. Winegrad, S. and McClellan, G. B. (1978). Regulation of the calcium sensitivity of the contractile system of heart muscle by the sarcolemma. *New York Acad. Sci.*, **307**, 477.

331. Wing, A. J., Curtis, J. R., Eastwood, J. B., Smith, E. K. M. and De Wardener, H. E. (1968). Transient and persistent hypercalcemia in patients treated by maintenance hemodialysis. *Brit. med. J.*, **2**, 150.

332. Williams, R. B., Russell, R. M., Dutta, S. K. and Giovetti, A. C. (1979). Alcoholic pancreatitis: patients at high risk of acute zinc deficiency. *Amer. J. Med.*, **66**, 889.

333. Wirz, H. and Bott, P. A. (1954). Potassium and reducing substances in proximal tubule fluid of the rat kidney. *Proc. Soc. exp. Biol. (N. Y.)*, **87**, 405.

334. Wolf, A. (1943). Effective use of thyroid in periodic paralysis. *N. Y. St. J. Med.*, **43**, 1951.

335. Wolfler, A. (1879). Weitere Beitrage zur Chirurgischen Behandlung des Kropfes. *Wien. med. Wshr.*, **29**, 758.
336. World Health Organisation (1973). *Trace Elements in Human Nutrition*. World Health Organisation Technical Report Series No. 532, Geneva, WHO, p. 9.
337. Wynn, V. and Houghton, B. J. (1957). Observations in man upon the osmotic behaviour of the body cells after trauma. *Quart. J. Med.*, **26**, 375.
338. Wynn, V. and Rob, C. G. (1954). Water intoxication: differential diagnosis of the hypotonic syndromes. *Lancet*, **i**, 587.
339. Yeo, P. P. B., Chan, S. H., Lui, K. F., Wee, G. B., Lim, P. and Cheah, J. S. (1978). HLA and thyrotoxic periodic paralysis. *Brit. Med. J.*, **2**, 930.
340. Zierler, K. L. (1960). Effect of insulin on potassium efflux from rat muscle in the presence and absence of glucose. *Amer. J. Physiol.*, **198**, 1066.

Further Reading

Ayus, J. C., Olivero, J. J., Frommer, J. P. (1982). Rapid correction of severe hyponatremia with intravenous hypertonic saline solution. *Amer. J. Med.*, **72**, 43.
Dandona, P., Fonseca, V. and Buron, D. N. (1985). Hyponatremia and hypovolemia. *N. Engl. J. of Med.*, **313**, 387.
Editorial (1985). Treatment of refractory ascites. *Lancet*, **ii**, 1164.
Ferrier, I. N. (1985). Water intoxication in patients with psychiatric illness. *Brit. Med. J.*, **291**, 1594.
Finberg, L., Harper, P. A., Harrison, H. E. and Sack, R. B. (1982). Oral rehydration for diarrhea. *J. of Paed.*, **101**, 497.
Fonseca, V. and Havard, C. W. H. (1985). Electrolyte disturbances and cardiac failure with hypomagnesaemia in anorexia nervosa. *Brit. Med. J.*, **291**, 1680.
Schuman, C. A. and Jones III, H. W. (1985). The 'milk-alkali' syndrome: two case reports with discussion of pathogenesis. *Quart. J. Med.*, **55**, 119.
Worthley, L. I. G. and Thomas, P. D. (1986). Treatment of hyponatraemia seizures with intravenous 29.2% saline. *Brit. Med. J.*, **292**, 168.

Chapter 3
Acid–Base Equilibrium
(hydrogen ion regulation)

Hydrogen Ion Concentration

In health, the hydrogen ion concentration of the body is stricly controlled and kept within narrow limits. The pH of arterial blood normally lies between 7.38 and 7.43. The extremes of pH compatible with life are about 6.8 and 7.8. The constancy of the blood pH is maintained by a complex arrangement of biophysical reactions and physiological changes, the two main physiological processes being the gas exchange processes that occur in the lungs and the ability of the kidneys to control the H^+ content of the body by excretion in the urine. In man the kidney is normally unable to produce urine which has a pH lower than 4.5 or greater than 7.9, but this latter figure is raised when a subject is unnecessarily loaded with sodium bicarbonate which is excreted in the urine. The normal plasma concentration of HCO_3^- is 24 or 25 mmol/l (mEq/l).

Because the ability of the kidney to excrete acid is limited, a strong anion must be accompanied by an equivalent cation other than H^+. This can be achieved by the renal tubular apparatus, either by the excretion of a cation, such as Na^+, K^+, Ca^{++} or Mg^{++}, or by the excretion of monobasic phosphate in place of the more alkaline dibasic form, or by the production of ammonia. In all cases, however, the kidney responds slowly to changes from a normal acid–base state and normally the urine contains only 40–50 mmol (mEq) of titratable acid every 24 hours. On the other hand, the rate at which the lungs are able to remove CO_2 is great, and approximately 13 000 mmol (mEq) of titratable acid are removed every day. The diffusing capacity of CO_2 across the alveolar membrane is 20 times that of O_2. The retention of CO_2 under normal circumstances, is therefore impossible. The CO_2 tension of arterial blood (PCO_2) in the normal person at sea level is 40 mmHg (5.3 kPa).* Simultaneous measurement of the gas tension in arterial

---

*1 mmHg = 133.3 pascals (Pa)
 1 kilopascal (kPa) = 7.5 mmHg

blood and alveolar air show that, for practical purposes, the two are identical in the absence of major lung pathology. The rapid carriage of carbon dioxide by the haemoglobin of the erythrocytes involving the chloride shift mechanism is an important factor in the maintenance of a constant blood pH. Although this can be looked upon as a transport mechanism, it is also an important buffering mechanism. When rapid changes in $[H^+]$ of the body occur, the body buffers represent the first stage in the involved and complicated processes by which these changes and the resulting functional effects are minimized.

Buffer Solutions

In physiological solutions a buffer almost invariably consists of a mixture of a weak acid which is *poorly* ionized and the salt of the weak acid which, in contrast, is almost *completely* ionized. There is, therefore, a common ion and when the salt of a weak acid is added to a solution of the weak acid, the dissociation of the acid is decreased. The $[H^+]$ of the acid solution is then lower and the pH value is higher than when the salt is absent. The change in the $[H^+]$ is proportional to the ratio of the salt to the acid in solution. This effect is very clearly seen when sodium acetate is added to 0.2 mol/l solution of acetic acid:

(1) $CH_3COOH \rightleftharpoons CH_3COO^- + H^+$

(2) $CH_3COONa \rightleftharpoons CH_3COO^- + Na^+$

It can be seen from equations (1) and (2) that there is a common ion (CH_3COO^-).

The pH of the 0.2 mol/l solution of acetic acid at 25°C is 2.7, but when sodium acetate is added to the solution, so that the ratio of salt to acid is unity, then the pH is raised to 4.7. As more sodium acetate is added the pH of the solution rises further.

This can easily be demonstrated in the laboratory.

If a strong acid such as HCl is added to the mixture of acetic acid and sodium acetate, more CH_3COOH is formed so that the $[H^+]$ does not rise to the same degree as it would if these substances were not present.

When a strong alkali such as NaOH is added to the solution, more CH_3COO^- is formed because the OH^- joins with the H^+ of CH_3COOH to form water. The ratio of acetate ions to acid increases and the $[H^+]$ falls, but not to the same extent as would occur if the buffer pair were not in solution.

Acids and Bases

The older terminology which considered an acid to be a substance that ionizes in solution giving $[H^+]$ and a base to be a substance which ionizes giving $[OH^-]$ has been replaced and the concepts formulated by Brönsted (1923)[24] and Lowry (1923)[85] are now generally accepted. Van Slyke termed sodium (Na^+) 'fixed base'.[120–122]

In the Brönsted and Lowry classifications, an acid is considered to be any substance capable of donating H^+ or protons; these classifications are therefore similar to the older classification. This is readily understood when considering the primary dissociation of monobasic acids. (Monobasic means the possession of one ionizable hydrogen atom, while polybasic signifies the ability to ionize, giving rise to more than one hydrogen atom, as in the case of phosphoric acid, H_3PO_4.)

In this terminology a base is any substance that can combine with protons (hydrogen ions) and, therefore, the term has a much broader implication. For example, when carbonic acid dissociates it does so into a hydrogen ion or proton and a bicarbonate ion or base:

(3) $\underset{\text{Acid}}{H_2CO_3} \rightleftharpoons \underset{\text{Proton}}{H^+} + \underset{\text{Base}}{HCO_3^-}$

In a similar way water dissociates into a proton and a hydroxyl ion:

(4) $\underset{\text{Proton}}{H^+} + \underset{\text{Base}}{OH^-} \rightleftharpoons \underset{\text{Acid}}{H_2O}$

The OH^- (or base) combines with a proton (or H^+) and the water molecule formed is an acid.

Sodium ions (Na^+) are now, therefore, referred to correctly, as cations, as are all positively charged ions, and the old Van Slyke terminology of 'fixed base' is avoided, so that confusion does not occur.

If HA represents the general formula for a monobasic acid, then it dissociates into a proton H^+ and a base A^-:

(5) $HA \rightleftharpoons H^+ + A^-$

It is conventional to depict the 'molar concentration' of a substance or ion by placing it within square brackets, such as [ ]. The extent to which a substance ionizes in solution at any given temperature depends upon the intrinsic characteristics of the substance itself. This is termed 'dissociation constant', K. According to the Law of Mass Action, which states that the velocity of a reaction is proportional to the product of the molecular concentrations of the reacting substances, the rate at which HA dissociates (R_1), is proportional to the molar concentration of HA ($[HA]$) and to the intrinsic ability of HA to dissociate (k_1). In this way the rate at which reaction (5) moves to the right is depicted by:

(6) $R_1 = k_1 [HA]$

The rate at which reaction (5) moves to the left (R_2) will then be dependent upon the molar concentrations of H ($[H]$) and A ($[A]$) and to the intrinsic affinity of H and A for each other when in collision (k_2). In this way:

(7) $R_2 = k_2 [H^+][A^-]$

When equilibrium is attained R_1 must equal R_2 so that:

(8) $k_1[HA] = k_2 [H^+][A^-]$

(9) $\dfrac{k_1}{k_2} = \dfrac{[H^+][A^-]}{[HA]}$

and

(10) $K = \dfrac{[H^+][A^-]}{[HA]}$

where K = the equilibrium constant for the reaction. Equation (10) is fundamental to the understanding of acid–base balance as K denotes the 'strength' of acids and alkalies. When equation (10) is rearranged:

(11) $[H^+] = K\dfrac{[HA]}{[A^-]}$ and $[H^+] = K\dfrac{[Acid]}{[Base]}$

It can, therefore, be seen that the hydrogen ion concentration of a solution containing a weak acid is equal to the dissociation constant multiplied by the ratio of the molecular concentrations of undissociated acid to its base. When a solution contains a weak acid (HA) and the salt of the weak acid (BA), it can be assumed that because of the almost complete ionization of the salt, the concentration of base is derived from the salt itself. We can write the equation as follows:

$$(12) \quad [H^+] = K\frac{[HA]}{[BA]}$$

This is the Henderson[66-68] approximation equation for dilute buffer solutions. K is usually written K' to indicate that it is not the true dissociation constant because it is realized that the presence of other salts and solutes in solution alter this factor. The equation can also be written:

$$(13) \quad [H^+] = K'\frac{[Acid]}{[Base]} = \frac{[Proton\ donor]}{[Proton\ acceptor]}$$

Sørensen[112] introduced the logarithmic notation for the hydrogen ion concentration and Hasselbalch[63-65] converted the Henderson equation into the negative logarithmic form, where:

$$(14) \quad -\log[H^+] = -\log K' - \log\frac{[HA]}{[BA]}$$

or

$$(15) \quad pH = pK' + \log\frac{[BA]}{[HA]}$$

or

$$(16) \quad pH = pK' + \log\frac{[A^-]}{[HA]}$$

This equation is called the Henderson–Hasselbalch equation and when the buffer pair consists of CO_2 and $NaHCO_3$ it may be written:

$$(17) \quad pH = pK' + \log\frac{[NaHCO_3]}{[H_2CO_3]}$$

pK'

We have seen how pK' is the logarithmic notation for the dissociation constant K. Substances which dissociate readily will have numerically large K values and, therefore, numerically small values for pK'. The 'stronger' the acid, therefore, the smaller its pK', while the weaker the acid the greater its pK. This is readily seen in the case of phosphoric acid which is an important body buffer and dissociates in stages becoming weaker each time.

$$H_3PO_4 \rightleftharpoons H^+ + H_2PO_4^- \quad pK = 1.96$$

Phosphoric acid — Proton — Primary phosphate anion

$$H_2PO_4^- \rightleftharpoons H^+ + HPO_4^{--} \quad pK = 6.8$$

Primary phosphate anion — Proton — Secondary phosphate anion

$$HPO_4^{--} \rightleftharpoons H^+ + PO_4^{---} \quad pK = 12.4$$

Secondary phosphate anion — Proton — Tertiary phosphate anion

It can be seen from the Henderson–Hasselbalch equation that when the molar concentration of base equals the molar concentration of acid, then the ratio of base to acid is 1, the log of which = 0. Therefore, pH = pK. In other words, pH = pK, when the gram molecular concentrations of a buffer pair in solution are equal. This is of great physiological importance.

The buffering capacity of any buffer system is maximum in the region of pK, for carbonic acid this is 6.1, which is well below the physiological range of the pH of blood and extracellular fluid (ECF). If we look at Fig 3.1, we can see that we are not using the bicarbonate–carbonic acid buffer system to its best advantage, and that small changes in either the $[CO_2]$ or $[HCO_3^-]$ produce major changes in blood pH. It must be realized, therefore, that this system is a poor buffer system and that if we are going to maintain a constant pH of the ECF and plasma, we must do so by the changes of renal and respiratory function, rather than by pure biochemical means. It is important to grasp this point when investigating and treating patients, because the Henderson–Hasselbalch equation is often regarded as being similar to a reversible reaction of chemicals undergoing changes in a test tube. Scant attention is paid to the fact that the Henderson–Hasselbalch equation can largely apply only *in vivo* in the presence of active biological function. Because a normally functioning ventilatory, renal and central nervous system are necessary, it is not surprising that the body often responds to alterations of the acid–base state in a manner which is not mathematically predictable.

The Body Buffers

We have seen how the buffer systems consist of an acid together with its common anion or conjugate base. These are regarded as a buffer pair, and the body fluids contain numerous buffer pairs. Within the cells or intracellular fluid (ICF) space, the main buffers, placed in order of quantitative importance, are:

Acid	Base
Protein	Protein anion
Organic phosphate	Organic phosphate anion
Carbonic acid	Bicarbonate anion

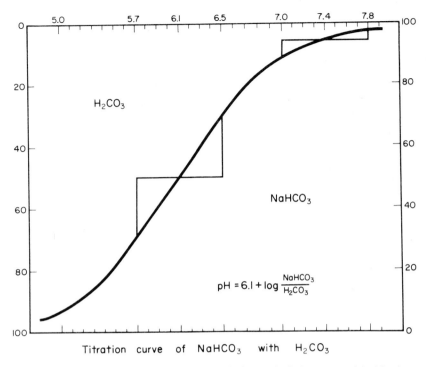

$$pH = 6.1 + \log \frac{NaHCO_3}{H_2CO_3}$$

Titration curve of NaHCO₃ with H₂CO₃

Fig. 3.1 Titration curve of NaHCO₃ with H₂CO₃ showing the relatively poor buffering power of the bicarbonate–carbonic acid buffer system within the physiological range of pH (after Peters and Van Slyke).[102]

In the ECF compartment the main buffers are, in order of quantitative importance:

Acid	Base
Carbonic acid	Bicarbonate anion
Plasma protein	Protein anion
Di-hydrogen phosphate	Mono-hydrogen phosphate

The pH within the cells varies with each particular tissue and is in the region of 6.8, while the pH of the ECF is about 7.4. This represents a marked gradient of [H⁺]. If we were to regard the buffer systems as being divided between the intracellular and extracellular fluid compartments this would still be an over-simplification of the true circumstances. The buffering capacity within the different compartments is dissimilar because of the protein-rich ICF and the relatively protein-free interstitial fluid. Further buffering compartments are also easily recognizable. In the plasma the bicarbonate–carbonic acid buffer system, together with the plasma proteins, is predominant, but by far the most important buffer system within the vascular space is that formed by the erythrocytes containing large quantities of amphoteric protein (haemoglobin) together with the bicarbonate ion. Further subdivisions of buffer compartments can be considered. For example, lymph and cerebrospinal fluid (CSF) behave in a similar way to plasma, except for their varying protein content, but the CSF may take many hours to equilibrate with the rest of the ECF when rapid changes in the acid–base state occur.

In theory it should be possible to summate all the anions of the body capable of accepting hydrogen ions, that is to say, the total amount of base that is available. Included in this estimate would be contributions from connective tissue as well as all the weak acids with their respective bases and materials such as the myoglobin of muscles. In practice this is not possible and reliable figures are not available, however between 600 and 900 mmol (mEq) of acid can be added to the adult body without causing the pH to reach such low values that irreversible changes are produced and death occurs.

If we consider all the buffer anions available in whole blood, including bicarbonate, phosphate and proteins of the plasma and the haemoglobin, phosphate and bicarbonate of the erythrocytes, it is reasonable to infer that a similar state prevails in the rest of the body. If conditions are not changing rapidly, this must be largely true. Singer and Hastings[111] produced a nomogram for the assessment of the acid–base state in terms of 'buffer-base' (Fig. 3.2). They used the old terminology of Van Slyke in which cation was referred to as 'fixed base'. They designated 'buffer-base' as the fraction of the blood cations that was electrically equivalent to the buffer anions, these being protein and bicarbonate ions (Fig. 3.2). To make an assessment of buffer-base, it is necessary to know the pH, the plasma bicarbonate ion concentration and the haemoglobin concentration or packed cell volume (PCV). The normal value for buffer-base lies between 46 and 52 mmol/l (mEq/l).

The predominant buffer system in the ECF space is the carbonic acid-bicarbonate system. The

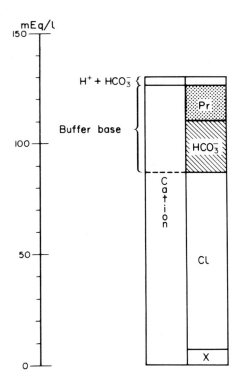

Fig. 3.2 The concept of 'buffer base' of Singer and Hastings.[111] They used the older terminology of Van Slyke in which sodium is referred to as 'fixed base'. It consists of the number of milliequivalents of cation that give electrical neutrality to the buffer anions (protein and bicarbonate anions). The protein is very largely haemoglobin.

Henderson–Hasselbalch equation, as we have seen, is written:

$$(17) \quad pH = pK' + \log \frac{[NaHCO_3]}{[H_2CO_3]}$$

The H_2CO_3 concentration is related to the partial pressure (tension) of CO_2 (PCO_2 in mmHg) multiplied by its solubility factor for plasma converted to STP. The equation, therefore, can be written:

$$pH = pK' + \log \frac{[HCO_3^-]}{PCO_2 \times 0.0301} = 6.1 + \log \frac{24.0 \text{ mmol/l*}}{1.2 \text{ mmol/l}}$$

The bicarbonate ion concentration of the plasma is largely controlled by the kidneys, while the tension of carbon dioxide depends upon respiratory function. The equation is sometimes written:

$$pH = pK' + \log \frac{\text{Kidney function}}{\text{Lung function}}$$

We see, therefore, that when we investigate the acid–base state of the ECF there is a 'respiratory' or 'gaseous' component and a 'metabolic' component. These two components determine the pH of the blood and plasma.

The *total* amount of CO_2 present in a sample of plasma (TCO$_2$) can be estimated manometrically by the method of Van Slyke and Neill.[122] This quantity expressed either in volumes per cent (vols %) or, more usually in mmol/l, is the amount of CO_2 present both as $NaHCO_3$ and H_2CO_3; in other words, the metabolic and respiratory components of acid–base balance.†

The Henderson–Hasselbalch equation can be rearranged so that the PCO_2 can be calculated from a knowledge of the pH and plasma TCO$_2$.

$$(18) \quad PCO_2 \text{ mmHg} = \frac{TCO_2 \text{ mmol/l}}{(1 + \text{antilog} (pH - 6.1) \times 0.0301)}$$

When plasma is equilibrated with 5.6% CO_2 in oxygen saturated with water vapour ($PCO_2 = 40$ mmHg), the TCO$_2$ represents the 'alkali reserve'.

A measurement of acid–base state can be made by equilibrating a sample of blood or plasma with two gas mixtures of known CO_2 tension and plotting the pH of the samples on a log PCO_2–pH graph.[22] This method gave rise to the 'standard bicarbonate' of Astrup[12,13] and also the concept of 'base excess' of Siggaard–Andersen.[5] These estimations are measurements of the 'metabolic

*Normal values for human plasma.

†In clinical practice today, is most parts of the world, these measurements are made indirectly using pH and PCO_2 electrodes. TCO$_2$ is then calculated.

component' of acid–base balance and can be applied to blood or plasma alone.[5,110]

Response to an Altered Acid–Base Balance: acidaemia, acidosis, alkalaemia, alkalosis

We have seen how the pH of a solution is dependent upon the ratio of base to acid and, for plasma and the ECF, this is related to the ratio of bicarbonate ion to carbonic acid: HCO_3^-/H_2CO_3.

When the pH of the blood is lowered (pH equals 7.35 or less), we refer to the condition as *acidaemia*. As we shall see, *acidaemia* can occur in the presence of either a low or a high plasma $[HCO_3^-]$. When the pH of the blood is raised (pH equals 7.45 or more), we refer to the condition as an *alkalaemia*. Within certain limits, alkalaemia can occur in the presence of both a reduced and a raised PCO_2.

The term *acidosis* is used to describe a quantitative decrease in plasma $[HCO_3^-]$, referred to as a *metabolic acidosis*, or a quantitative increase in blood PCO_2, referred to as a *respiratory acidosis*.

The term *alkalosis* is used to describe a quantitative increase in plasma $[HCO_3^-]$, referred to as a *metabolic alkalosis*, or a quantitative decrease in PCO_2, referred to as a *respiratory alkalosis*.

The terms acidosis and alkalosis therefore have to be qualified whenever they are used if they are to have any meaning. It is clear that a *metabolic acidosis* can occur in the presence of *alkalaemia*, for example in salicylate poisoning (see p. 431), and that *metabolic alkalosis* can occur in the presence of *acidaemia* when there is an associated rise in PCO_2.

The Isohydric Principle

When we measure changes in blood pH we must remember that these changes are occurring in the ECF as a whole, although the time taken for equilibration with its subdivisions, such as the CSF, may take many hours. Furthermore, it may take a considerable time for intracellular metabolic changes which alter the intracellular pH to equilibrate with the ECF. In a common solution, however, all weak acids must be at the same pH and adjustments in the ratio of base to acid must be made in order for this to be achieved, so that:

$$(19) \quad pH = pK_1 + \log \frac{Base_1}{Acid_1}$$
$$= pK_2 + \log \frac{Base_2}{Acid_2}$$
$$= pK_3 + \log \frac{Base_3}{Acid_3}$$

A solution of different buffers, such as shown in equation (19), is known as a buffer system and, while equilibrium is attained within such a system, it must also be attained within similar but separate systems contained in other fluid compartments. This must be so even though the pH of ICF is 6.8 and that of ECF 7.4. The concept of the isohydric principle is of great importance when correcting a metabolic acidosis with infusions of sodium bicarbonate because it is necessary to calculate a base deficit in terms of total body water in a similar way to that of changes in sodium concentration (see p. 33).*

This becomes significant in clinical practice only in conditions such as phenformin acidosis, diabetic ketosis and toxic shock when almost all the buffering capacity of the body (approximately 900 mmol in the adult) has been utilized.

Effects of a Changing PCO_2

The PCO_2 or carbon dioxide tension of the arterial† blood and alveolar air is calculated from the percentage concentration of the gas. The alveolar air is at 38°C and is fully saturated with water vapour. It is, therefore, composed of H_2O, N_2, O_2 and CO_2. The concentration of CO_2 is 5.6%. To find the partial pressure of CO_2 in the mixture we have to subtract the partial pressure resulting from water vapour, which at 38°C is 50 mmHg, from the

---

*Formulae for correcting a base deficit (low $[HCO_3^-]$) have been published calculating the deficit within the ECF alone. These, for example, correct the deficit in one third of the total body water. By ignoring the isohydric principle, the quantity required to correct the deficit is grossly underestimated. This is not important when the deficit is small and spontaneous correction takes place, but when the acidosis is due to bypass of the ileum, phenformin or diabetic acidosis (ketosis), this may have serious consequences.

†Venous blood taken from the back of the hand after warming the hand and arm with electric pads is arterialized and may be used for acid–base estimations in the absence of shock.[29]

atmospheric pressure and calculate 5.6% of the remainder thus:

$$(760 - 50) \times \frac{5.6}{100} = 40 \text{ mmHg}$$

When pathological changes in the lungs impair the removal of CO_2, the PCO_2 rises and the pH of the blood therefore falls. This is inevitable in the first instance because of the poor buffering capacity of the carbon dioxide–bicarbonate buffer system (Fig. 3.1). The fall of pH is diminished a little because of the presence of protein, especially haemoglobin, and phosphate within the body. To restore the pH of the body fluids to normal, a process of compensation begins. The kidneys retain bicarbonate ion and excrete an acid urine, thus the concentration of bicarbonate ion in the plasma and ECF increases and the chloride ion concentration falls. Retention of carbon dioxide is not possible without hypoxia in a patient breathing air, because the rate of diffusion of CO_2 through

the lungs is 20 times greater than that of oxygen. When a low tension of oxygen is present over a considerable period of time, it leads to a rise in the PCV and, therefore, of haemoglobin, thereby adding to the increased buffering capacity of the blood. In practice the process of compensation, which is dependent upon a healthy and intact renal apparatus, is slow; it takes 48 hours or more. Complete compensation is rare and a respiratory acidosis is generally associated with low blood pH values.

If for any reason hyperventilation occurs, the CO_2 tension of the alveoli decreases and the pH rises above normal values; this is referred to as a 'respiratory alkalosis'. It occurs in a variety of conditions such as cerebral tumour, hepatic coma and salicylate poisoning, but it is most commonly seen during prolonged controlled artificial ventilation. In some conditions, as the PCO_2 falls, compensation of the respiratory alkalosis takes place and bicarbonate ion is excreted in the urine. The

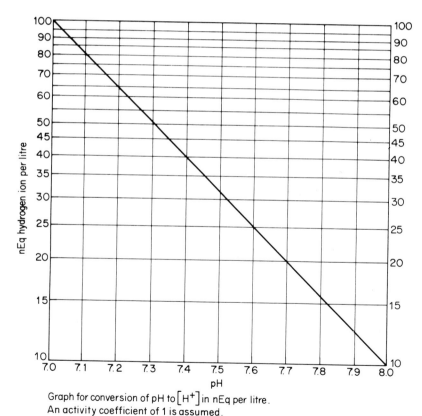

Graph for conversion of pH to $\left[H^+\right]$ in nEq per litre.
An activity coefficient of 1 is assumed.

Fig. 3.3 Graph for conversion of pH to $[H^+]$ in nEq/l. An activity coefficient of 1 is assumed. (Reproduced with permission from the *Lancet* and Professor Whitehead.)[126]

pH of the urine may be alkaline in reaction. Reduction of the bicarbonate ion concentration of the plasma occurs during excessive hyperventilation under anaesthesia; this is not, however, because of the loss of bicarbonate into the urine, but it is largely due to metabolic acidosis caused by a reduction in cardiac output.[50]

Effects of a Change in the Bicarbonate Ion Concentration

It follows from the previous section that when the bicarbonate ion concentration of the ECF is raised, an increase in respiration should occur so that the pH is reduced from its raised level. Here again, full compensation is rarely produced in practice and the condition is referred to as a metabolic alkalosis. In clinical medicine a metabolic *acidosis* is the more commonly observed acid–base defect, and often increased alveolar gas exchange reduces the PCO_2 below its normal value and the pH of the blood sometimes approximates closely to 7.4. This is most commonly seen in conditions in which a chronic metabolic acidosis is present for a long period of time (e.g. following uretrocolic transplant).

pH and H⁺ Concentration in Nanomoles per Litre

A number of workers prefer to work in nanomoles of H^+ per litre rather than in the terms of pH. This is a logical step and is an extension of the use of SI units and moles per litre. A graph (see Fig. 3.3) and a conversion table (Table 3.1) for pH and the equivalent in $[H^+]$ are given here. In this publication, the author has retained the pH terminology throughout. The equivalent value in kPa for PCO_2 can be obtained from the alignment nomogram (Fig. 3.4) opposite.

Measurement of Acid–Base Components

The measurement of pH by means of a glass electrode containing HCl, a platinum wire connected to a millivolt meter via a KCl bridge, and a

Table 3.1 pH–H⁺ concentration conversion table

pH		H⁺ nEq/l	pH		H⁺ nEq/l
7.00	=	100.0	7.41	=	38.9
7.01	=	97.7	7.42	=	38.0
7.02	=	95.5	7.43	=	37.2
7.03	=	93.3	7.44	=	36.3
7.04	=	91.2	7.45	=	35.5
7.05	=	89.1	7.46	=	34.7
7.06	=	87.1	7.47	=	33.9
7.07	=	85.1	7.48	=	33.1
7.08	=	83.2	7.49	=	32.4
7.09	=	81.3	7.50	=	31.6
7.10	=	79.4	7.51	=	30.9
7.11	=	77.6	7.52	=	30.2
7.12	=	75.9	7.53	=	29.5
7.13	=	74.1	7.54	=	28.8
7.14	=	72.4	7.55	=	28.1
7.15	=	70.8	7.56	=	27.5
7.16	=	69.2	7.57	=	26.9
7.17	=	67.6	7.58	=	26.3
7.18	=	66.1	7.59	=	25.7
7.19	=	64.6	7.60	=	25.1
7.20	=	63.1	7.61	=	24.5
7.21	=	61.7	7.62	=	24.0
7.22	=	60.3	7.63	=	23.4
7.23	=	58.9	7.64	=	22.9
7.24	=	57.5	7.65	=	22.4
7.25	=	56.2	7.66	=	21.9
7.26	=	55.0	7.67	=	21.4
7.27	=	53.7	7.68	=	20.9
7.28	=	52.5	7.69	=	20.4
7.29	=	51.3	7.70	=	20.0
7.30	=	50.1	7.71	=	19.5
7.31	=	49.0	7.72	=	19.1
7.32	=	47.9	7.73	=	18.6
7.33	=	46.8	7.74	=	18.2
7.34	=	45.7	7.75	=	17.8
7.35	=	44.7	7.76	=	17.4
7.36	=	43.7	7.77	=	17.0
7.37	=	42.7	7.78	=	16.6
7.38	=	41.7	7.79	=	16.2
7.39	=	40.7	7.80	=	15.8
7.40	=	39.8			

standard Ag/AgCl electrode has been possible for many years and many types of apparatus for this purpose have been available since the late 1950s. The HCO_3^- component was measured manometrically by the Van Slyke apparatus.[120-122] This gave the value for the total CO_2 (TCO_2) which included both the HCO_3^- component and dissolved CO_2 in the plasma. Recent advances in technology have allowed the almost automated measurement of blood gases and the acid–base state, including measurement of the blood oxygen tension, PO_2. The invention by Clarke (1956)[35] of an oxygen-measuring PO_2 electrode allowed the direct

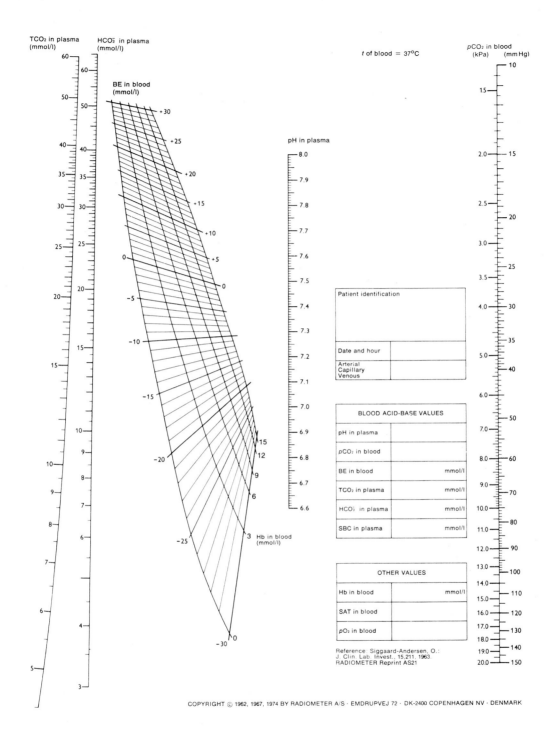

Fig. 3.4 Siggaard-Andersen alignment nomogram. Reproduced from Siggaard-Andersen (1974)[110] by kind permission of Radiometer Ltd.

measurement of the oxygen tension in the blood for the first time.

As long ago as 1916 Hasselbalch[64,65] argued that the buffering capacity of blood could be measured by equilibrating blood with CO_2 at a tension of 40 mmHg. In 1918, Henderson and Haggard[68] suggested measuring the TCO_2 of whole blood, equilibrated in a similar manner. It was not until 1957 when Jørgensen and Astrup[79] demonstrated that the measurement of the bicarbonate ion concentration of whole blood at a PCO_2 of 40 mmHg was not only a valid clinical measurement but was technically easy to obtain at 37°C, that rapid progress was made towards using the components of buffer-base in clinical medicine. Jørgensen and Astrup called this concept (i.e. whole blood containing 15 g haemoglobin/100 ml equilibrated at 37°C with CO_2 at 40 mmHg) *standard bicarbonate*.

Standard Bicarbonate and Base Excess

We have seen how the buffering capacity of the blood is influenced by the concentration of bicarbonate, plasma proteins and haemoglobin; this is reflected in the concept of buffer-base.

It had been realized that, if the log of the PCO_2 was plotted against the pH, the curve for oxygenated blood was virtually linear.[11,102,120] Brewin et al.,[22] while investigating the acid–base state of the living organism at low temperatures, demonstrated that the slope of this curve increased with the haemoglobin concentration. They also advocated that the shift to the left of the curve, that occurs as the bicarbonate concentration falls, should be used to estimate the degree of metabolic acidosis that develops when the body is cooled. If, therefore, specimens of blood and plasma containing the same $[HCO_3^-]$ were equilibrated with gas mixtures containing two known tensions of CO_2 and the pH was measured, the lines intersected when the results were plotted on the log PCO_2/pH graph. This was used by Siggaard-Andersen who observed that, by joining up the points of intersection of the curves made by whole blood and plasma, the buffering capacity of the blood could be measured. Once established, the components of the curve could be calculated mathematically, Siggaard-Andersen called this concept *base excess*. He called values above the normal base excess *positive base excess* and they indicated a metabolic alkalosis, and values below normal were called *negative base excess* and they indicated a metabolic acidosis. It is to be noted that these measurements are made on whole blood and indicate, in a similar manner to buffer–base (see p. 71), changes in all the buffer components of the blood such as haemoglobin, plasma protein, etc., in addition to the H_2CO_3 : HCO_3^- ratio. Base excess does not follow either buffer base or standard bicarbonate in a linear fashion. When the haemoglobin concentration is normal (and does not change between measurements) base excess can be calculated from the standard bicarbonate,[110] but these stable conditions rarely prevail in clinical practice.

The PCO_2 Electrode

The technical measurement of the acid–base state of whole blood was greatly simplified when Severinghaus developed his PCO_2 electrode. It consisted of a glass pH electrode covered by a layer of filter paper soaked in $NaHCO_3$. The whole electrode was covered with a plastic membrane through which CO_2 could diffuse. Thus, when the filter paper was moist, changes in PCO_2 initiated changes in the HCO_3^- : H_2CO_3 ratio (i.e. the Henderson–Hasselbalch equation) on the surface of the pH electrode. These changes in pH could be calibrated on the pH meter in terms of PCO_2, using humidified gases of known CO_2 content.

Causes of Metabolic Alkalosis

1. Blood transfusion. This is probably the most common cause of a raised blood $[HCO_3^-]$ seen by the clinician, as the citrate in the anticoagulant, either acid citrate dextrose (ACD) or citrate phosphate dextrose (CPD) is converted into bicarbonate. It is usually not observed until 24 hours after the transfusion.

2. Infusions of $NaHCO_3$.

3. Vomiting. As HCl is lost from the stomach and the plasma $[Cl^-]$ falls, the plasma $[HCO_3^-]$ rises. The loss of K^+ from the body in gastric secretions is also a contributory cause, and patients suffering from pyloric stenosis commonly require treatment with NaCl and KCl before surgery.

4. Potassium depletion can occur following inadequate intake, excessive diuretic therapy, excessive renal loss, vomiting etc., and because of the competition between K^+ and H^+. As K^+ is lost from the cells, the cation is replaced by H^+. There is therefore an intracellular acidosis in the presence of an extracellular alkalosis.

5. Cirrhosis of the liver. A raised plasma bicarbonate is commonly found in chronic liver disease. It may be the result of or exacerbated by K^+ depletion. During hepatic coma, hyperventilation and the resulting decrease in PCO_2 increase the degree of alkalaemia.

6. Cushing's syndrome and ectopic ACTH (adreno-cortico-tropic hormone) secretion. Adrenocortical hyperfunction leads to urinary K^+ loss and sometimes to a rise in plasma $[HCO_3^-]$. Both pituitary- and adrenal-induced Cushing's syndrome have a similar effect.

Causes of Metabolic Acidosis

Metabolic acidosis may develop as a consequence of: (1) an increase in acid load or intake, (2) increased acid production, (3) decreased acid excretion by the kidneys, or (4) increased loss of alkali from the gut or kidneys.

1. Increased acid load or intake.
    (a) NH_4Cl (given orally or intravenously).
    (b) Poisoning:
        (i) methanol producing formic acid,
        (ii) ethylene glycol causing hepatic failure,
        (iii) paraldehyde producing acetic acid,
        (iv) salicylic acid (see p. 431).*
2. Increased acid production.
    (a) Diabetic ketoacidosis producing beta-hydroxybutyric acid, aceto-acetic acid and acetone.
    (b) Lactic acidosis, seen with:
        (i) hypoperfusion syndrome, cardiogenic shock, haemorrhagic shock etc.,
        (ii) 'washout acidosis' which follows the release of lactic acid and other products of anaerobic metabolism when the clamp on a major vessel (e.g. the aorta) is released during surgery,
        (iii) phenethylbiguanide (phenformin) acidosis, also produced by metformin and dithiazanine,
        (iv) hyperventilation and positive end-expiratory pressure (PEEP), especially when causing a marked fall in cardiac output,
        (v) impaired metabolism seen in diabetic ketosis, acute hepatic dysfunction,

tricyclic antidepressant overdose, hypothermia, starvation.
3. Decreased renal acid excretion.
    (a) Acute renal failure.
    (b) Chronic renal failure, decreased excretion of buffers resulting from decreased filtration, and decreased ammonia production because of loss of functioning nephrons.
    (c) Renal tubular acidosis, defect in H^+ secretion.
4. Increased loss of alkali.
    (a) Gastro-intestinal loss:
        (i) gastroenteritis, cholera,
        (ii) drainage of pancreatic juice.
    (b) Renal tubular acidosis, 'proximal type' associated with loss of HCO_3^- in the urine.

Causes of Respiratory Alkalosis

1. Cerebrovascular accident causing hyperventilation.
2. Hepatic coma.
3. Aspirin (salicylate) poisoning.
4. Early stages of pulmonary oedema.
5. Fibrotic changes in the lungs causing anoxia, with compensatory hyperventilation.
6. Diabetic ketosis.
7. Non-ketotic diabetic crisis ('hyperosmotic non-ketotic diabetic coma').
8. Raised $[Ca^{++}]$ as a result of hyperparathyroidism, sarcoid, metastatic carcinoma.
9. Cerebral metastasis.

Causes of Respiratory Acidosis

1. Chronic obstructive lung disease.
2. Rebreathing CO_2.
3. Ventilation blood flow disturbances.
4. Respiratory distress syndrome, especially in the infant.
5. Increase in the physiological dead space.
6. Increase in the dead space by means of endotracheal tubes and tubes attached to respiratory apparatus.
7. Disturbances of diffusion such as pulmonary oedema and bilateral bronchograms performed simultaneously on both lungs.
8. Respiratory depression, for example drug induced, narcotics, barbiturates etc.

---

*This can occur when therapeutic doses of salicylates are given but are combined with acetazolamide (Cowen et al., 1984).[43]

Renal Control of the Acid–Base State

Bicarbonate resorption by renal tubules

The resorption of bicarbonate is accomplished by both proximal and distal tubular mechanisms. Most of the HCO_3^- resorption is achieved, as with other substances, at the proximal tubule (see p. 22), but the mechanism in this region of the nephron is characterized by a high capacity to reabsorb and a low pH gradient between the plasma and tubular fluid. Approximately 80–90% of the bicarbonate is reabsorbed in this region, and the method by which this is achieved is demonstrated in Fig. 3.5. Sodium moves from the tubular fluid into the cell against an electrochemical gradient. Hydrogen ions are secreted actively from the cell into the tubular fluid where they react with HCO_3^- to form H_2CO_3 which, under the action of carbonic anhydrase, dissociates into CO_2 and water. The CO_2 thus formed diffuses into the cell where it is rehydrated under the catalytic action of carbonic anhydrase to form H_2CO_3. The

H_2CO_3 thus formed dissociates into H^+ and HCO_3^-, the H^+ becoming available for secretion and the HCO_3^- for resorption into the renal vein. It can be seen that this mechanism depends upon the catalyst, carbonic anhydrase, so that when an inhibitor of this substance such as acetazolamide (Diamox) is given, increased excretion of bicarbonate occurs in the urine.

The distal tubular mechanism for the resorption of bicarbonate is very similar to that of the proximal tubule except for two factors. The first is that, quantitatively, it accounts for only approximately 10% of the total bicarbonate resorption. Nevertheless, it is a sensitive mechanism which is capable of conserving virtually all the remaining bicarbonate in the tubular fluid in response to an appropriate stimulus. The second major difference is that, in order to accomplish the resorption of the remaining bicarbonate, it is necessary for the distal tubular cells to secrete H^+ against a steep $[H^+]$ gradient which, in the collecting ducts, is in the region of 1000 to 1, in other words, when the blood pH is 7.4 and the urine pH 4.4.

Resorption of bicarbonate from the tubular fluid is influenced by a number of different factors

1. Probably the most important factor influencing resorption of bicarbonate is the arterial PCO_2. This mechanism responds appropriately both in respiratory acidosis (when it causes bicarbonate resorption) and in respiratory alkalosis (when resorption is inhibited).

2. Bicarbonate resorption is also influenced by the total body K^+ balance. The intracellular $[K^+]$ rather than the plasma $[K^+]$ alone is probably the most important influence. Loading with potassium salts results in the movement of K^+ into the cells in exchange for H^+. The hydrogen ions liberated from the cells are buffered by the extracellular bicarbonate, and the reduced intracellular $[H^+]$ in the tubular cells results in less bicarbonate being reabsorbed. The potential consequence of loading a patient with potassium salts is therefore the induction of an intracellular alkalosis and an extracellular acidosis associated with the excretion of an alkaline urine containing potassium bicarbonate. In contrast, it is well recognized that depletion of intracellular potassium from whatever cause increases the renal tubular resorption of bicarbonate, resulting in an increase in plasma bicarbonate concentration. The reduced concentration of intracellular potassium is accompanied by an increase in the $[H^+]$ within the cell. It is assumed that a similar circumstance exists within the renal tubular cells, resulting in an increase in H^+ excretion and bicarbonate resorption.

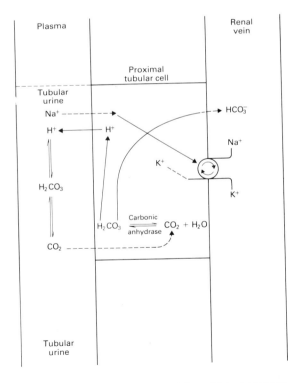

Fig. 3.5 Diagrammatic representation of bicarbonate reabsorption in a proximal tubular cell. Solid lines indicate active transport. Interrupted lines represent passive diffusion assisted by electrochemical gradients.

Hypokalaemia, therefore, is associated with an intracellular acidosis and an extracellular alkalosis and the excretion of urine with a low pH as its acid content is increased.

3. Bicarbonate resorption is also influenced by the plasma and the ECF [Cl⁻]. When total body depletion of Cl⁻ and hypochloraemia occur, plasma bicarbonate is increased. Conversely, an increase in the total body chloride leading to hyperchloraemia depresses bicarbonate resorption and this results in a fall in the plasma bicarbonate concentration. The mechanism of this reciprocal relationship between bicarbonate and chloride is not yet fully elucidated, although in some circumstances the presence of hyperchloraemia (see p. 91) is partially understood.

4. There is one further factor that is important in influencing bicarbonate resorption from the tubular urine. This is the variation that occurs in the secretion of adrenocortical hormone. Increased exogenous or endogenous levels of mineralocorticosteroids or 17 0H-glucocorticosteroids increase the propensity for renal tubular HCO_3^- resorption. It is not clear whether this effect is secondary to the primary stimulation of sodium resorption, H^+ secretion from the cells, or merely a consequence of the increased K^+ excretion observed in these circumstances.

Generation of bicarbonate by renal tubules

In maintaining the acid–base state of the body, the renal tubules, in addition to reabsorbing bicarbonate filtered at the glomerulus, also have the capacity to regenerate HCO_3^- and therefore to replenish the bicarbonate stores which are depleted during the buffering of strong acids. While the neutralization of acids occurs by the formation of a neutral salt, the production of H_2CO_3, as we have seen dissociates into H_2O and CO_2; the CO_2 is excreted by the lungs.

$$H_3PO_4 + 2NaHCO_3 \rightleftharpoons Na_2PO_4 + 2H_2O + 2CO_2$$

The renal tubules regenerate the bicarbonate lost as CO_2 and H_2O by converting the disodium phosphate to the monosodium phosphate, as shown in Fig. 3.6.

Sodium ions are reabsorbed from the glomerular filtrate and returned to the body water accompanied by a bicarbonate ion that is generated within the distal renal tubular cell. In these circumstances, when a H^+ is excreted from the body and a new HCO_3^- is added to the body fluids, a net loss of acid occurs and a replenishment of the body buffers is achieved. At the pH of body fluids, phosphate is present, four-fifths as the mono-

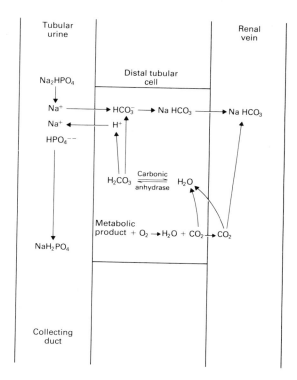

Fig. 3.6 Generation of bicarbonate anion (HCO_3^-) and thus replenishment of the body buffer occurs under the influence of carbonic anhydrase within the tubular cell. It is accomplished by converting Na_2HPO_4 into the monosodium form, NaH_2PO_4. A hydrogen ion is excreted and a 'new' bicarbonate ion is added to the circulating blood. This mechanism forms the 'titratable acid'.

hydrogen anion, HPO_4^{--}, and one-fifth as the dihydrogen anion, $H_2PO_4^-$. In the Henderson–Hasselbalch equation the formula is defined as follows:

$$7.4 = 6.8 + \log \frac{[HPO_4^-]}{[H_2PO_4^-]}$$

It can be seen from the Henderson–Hasselbalch equation that, as the urine is made more acid, the concentration of H_2PO_4 increases so that, when the pH of the urine is at its lower limit (pH = 4.5), virtually all the HPO_4^{--} has been converted to the acid form, H_2PO_4. Other weak acids present in the urine become increasingly important quantitatively as the pH of the urine falls.

The concentration of buffer anions in the urine determines and limits the quantity of hydrogen ions that can be excreted as 'titratable acids'. Furthermore, there seems to be a lower limit to the pH of the urine because of the enormous gradient which exists at the lower limit between the plasma pH and the urine pH. Nevertheless, even more hydrogen ions can be excreted by a highly efficient mechanism, which is a further prodigious phenomenon achieved by the renal apparatus.

The process consists of the deamination of amino acids, principally glutamic acid, thus producing ammonia (NH_3). This small molecule, which has no electrical charge, can pass quite freely across the cell membrane. Having done so, it joins with a H^+ to form NH_4^+ and when it has received a charge, it can no longer pass through the cell membrane and is trapped within the fluid in the tubular compartment (Fig. 3.7). The conversion of the H^+ to NH_4^+ which, in regard to pH values, is neutral, results in a decreased $[H^+]$ in the *urine* and an increased excretion of H^+ from the *body*. This has to be performed within the physiological limits set by the gradient of pH that is possible between plasma and human urine.

When the urine pH is 4.5* the concentration of free H^+ is less than 0.1 mmol/l (mEq/l).† By means of the excretion of 'titratable acids' and ammonium formation, the net removal of H^+ per litre of urine can greatly exceed its content of free H^+.

The term 'titratable acids' was produced a long time ago to describe a measurement which can be made in terms of millimoles (milliequivalents) of sodium hydroxide which must be added to a litre of urine to return its pH to that of plasma, (i.e. 7.4). This value, plus the NH_4 content of the urine, minus the bicarbonate content of the urine, is a quantitative measurement of the net acid excretion from the body (Fig. 3.8).

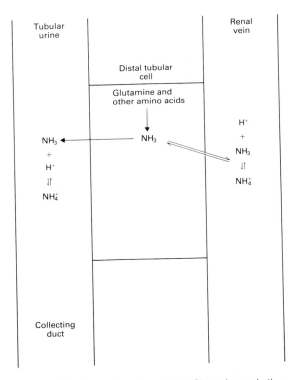

Fig. 3.7   Renal excretion of ammonia. Glutamine and other amino acids give rise to the free base NH_3 which can diffuse readily (but passively) through the cell wall. When combined with a hydrogen ion to form ammonium (NH_4), it becomes relatively non-diffusable.

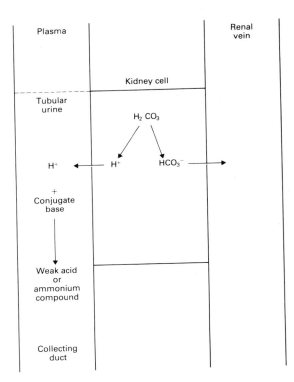

Fig. 3.8   Summary of the changes taking place in the tubular urine in which HCO_3^- is regenerated and excretion of acid is achieved in the presence of a low hydrogen ion concentration.

*This is close to the lower limit of urinary pH.

†pH	8.00	7.00	6.00	5.00	4.00
Free $[H^+]$ in mmol/l (mEq/l)	0.00001	0.0001	0.001	0.01	0.1

Thus if 2 litres of urine were passed at a pH of 4.0, only 0.2 mmol (mEq) of the approximately 50–70 mmol (mEq) which need to be excreted in 24 hours can be in the form of free H^+.

Because any bicarbonate in the urine indicates a loss of alkali or a gain of acid by the body, any bicarbonate excreted in the urine must be subtracted from the sum of 'titratable acids', plus ammonia to obtain the value of the net excretion of acid in the urine. At a pH of 4.5, the quantity of bicarbonate present in the urine is negligible.

It is, however, necessary to estimate the bicarbonate in the urine almost immediately after it is voided if an accurate assessment is to be made before bacterial action converts urea into ammonium carbonate.

The average diet in Britain results in the excretion of approximately 70 mmol of H^+ per day. Of this, the excretion of 'titratable acids' may be expected to account for approximately 40 mmol of acid excretion. The excretion of ammonia accounts for most of the remainder.

The excretion of ammonia, however, may attain levels of 200–300 mmol/day or more in conditions of chronic acidosis, such as diabetic ketoacidosis, or following prolonged administration of acidifying salts, such as ammonium chloride (Table 3.2). As with most factors in the kidney, the adaptation of the tubules to the raised acid load is relatively slow and 4–6 days are required before the formation of NH_3 is such that NH_4^+ excretion achieves its maximum.

Through the years, the site of acidification of the tubular urine within the nephron has been the subject of much speculation. Recent and direct measurement by micropuncture techniques and the inhibition of carbonic anhydrase by increasing quantities of acetazolamide have indicated that bicarbonate resorption occurs largely by means of H^+ excretion. While it is possible that some of the bicarbonate filtered at the glomerulus is reabsorbed directly as the anion, it is well established that, at the proximal tubule, resorption of bicarbonate is achieved with little or no change in the pH of the tubular fluid. A relatively small addition of H^+ is, therefore, required when the tubular urine reaches the distal tubule in order to lower the pH of the urine which is finally excreted.

Acidosis of renal origin

It can be seen that in chronic renal failure, acidosis (which is a consequence of the failure to remove H^+ from the plasma in adequate quantities) develops. The degree of acid excretion by the kidney is reduced for the following reasons:

1. The number of functioning nephrons are reduced; this leads to decreased filtration of phosphate buffers, thus limiting the quantity of acid excreted as H_2PO_4.
2. There is a decrease in NH_3 formation by the renal tubules, thereby reducing the amount of H^+ that can be excreted as NH_4^+.

Decreased acid excretion results in the buffering of H^+ by the body fluids and by the tissue buffers. Bone is probably one of the tissues involved in buffering excess acid, and it is the buffering by bone with resultant loss of Ca^{++} that may contribute to the development of renal osteodystrophy.

Renal tubular acidosis
Renal tubular acidosis[130] (RTA) is the result of either a deficiency in the excretion of H^+ by the tubules or an inability to reabsorb HCO_3^-, or it may be the result of the coexistence of both deficiencies. Unlike the acidosis which occurs in chronic renal failure, there is no impairment of glomerular filtration rate (GFR).

There are therefore two forms of RTA. One form is characterized by impairment of HCO_3^- resorption at the proximal tubules; this form is the result of the excretion of bicarbonate and is

Table 3.2 Excretion of acid by man

	Acid excreted per day (mmol)	Ratio NH_3 : titratable acid
Normal man		
Acid combined with ammonia	30–50	
Titratable acid	10–40	1–2.5
Diabetic ketosis		
Acid combined with ammonia	300–500	
Titratable acid	75–250	1–2.5
Chronic renal failure (Bright's disease)		
Acid combined with ammonia	0.5–15	
Titratable acid	2.0–20	0.2–1.5

therefore associated with a change in the pH of the urine. The other form occurs because of the inability of the distal tubules to excrete H^+ and establish a gradient of pH between the plasma and the urine. An alkaline urine is excreted even when acidaemia is present, because the acidaemia is the result of the inadequate excretion of 'titrable acids' and NH_4^+ resulting in a positive acid balance within the body.

RTA can be diagnosed in two ways: (a) by determining the response of the patient to an HCO_3^- load and determining the renal threshold for HCO_3^-, and (b) by determining the response of the patient to an acid load and measuring the capacity of the distal tubular mechanism to secrete H^+ against a gradient.

In *proximal RTA*, the patient has a reduced HCO_3^- threshold but can maximally acidify the urine in response to an acid load.

In *distal RTA*, the HCO_3^- threshold is normal but patients are unable to acidify their urine to a maximal degree when given an acid load.

Undetermined anion or anion gap

When attempting to analyse and identify the cause of a metabolic acidosis, some light is sometimes shed by the size of the 'anion gap'. In the normal person, the anion gap refers to anions such as SO_4^{--} or PO_4^{--}, lactate or pyruvate, which are not usually measured in the routine biochemistry department.

The anion gap can be calculated by subtracting the sum of the plasma chloride and bicarbonate concentrations from the plasma sodium concentration.

$$\text{Anion gap} = [Na^+] - ([Cl^-] + [HCO_3^-])*$$

In the healthy, normal adult the anion gap is approximately 12 mmol/l. A normal anion gap in the presence of a low bicarbonate ion concentration indicates the presence of a hyperchloraemic metabolic acidosis. An increase in the anion gap indicates that the retention of anions other than chloride, for example ketoacids, lactic acid or, in acute renal failure, PO_4^{--} and SO_4^{--}, has occurred. Those conditions which give rise to a metabolic acidosis with an increase in the anion gap are typical of those found in Table 3.3A. Patients that are found to have a low HCO_3^- associated with no

*The 'anion gap' has been defined as the difference between the sum of *both* major plasma cations ($Na^+ + K^+$) and the major anions ($Cl^- + HCO_3^-$). It is usual to omit not only K^+ from the calculations but also Ca^{++} and Mg^{++} because of the quantitatively very small fluctuations that can occur in these cations. This view has been confirmed by Emmett and Narins.[53]

Table 3.3 Metabolic acidosis associated with an increased (A) or unchanged (B) undetermined anion (anion gap)

A With increase in unmeasured anions	B Without increase in unmeasured anions
Diabetic ketoacidosis	Diarrhoea
Renal failure	Renal tubular acidosis
Lactic acidosis	Ammonium chloride
Salicylate poisoning	administration
Methyl alcohol poisoning	Carbonic anhydrase inhibitors
Ethylene glycol poisoning	Ureterosigmoidostomy
Paraldehyde (rarely)	Drainage of pancreatic
	secretions

increase in unmeasured anions have conditions that are listed in Table 3.3B.

In patients in whom diabetic ketosis has developed but who are mainly suffering from an increase in concentration of the 3-hydroxy-butyrate component rather than the aceto-acetate, the raised anion gap may be the only method by which the acidosis can be diagnosed. This is because it is only the aceto-acetate reaction with the nitroprusside reagent that gives the accepted colour change in the conventional 'Acetest'.

Decreased anion gap (Table 3.4)

The significance of a low anion gap has been emphasized by Murray *et al.*,[95] who reported a significant decrease in the anion gap in 50 patients suffering from a multiple myeloma. In these patients, the anion gap was approximately 9 mmol/l and was related to the retention of chloride or bicarbonate. In 1977, Schnur *et al.*[106] described a reduced anion gap in patients with plasma cell dyscrasias who were asymptomatic. These patients demonstrated an anion gap of 6 mmol/l or less.

Table 3.4 Conditions which give rise to a reduced concentration of unmeasured anions (anion gaps)

Multiple myeloma
Plasma cell dyscrasias
Bromism
Hypernatraemia
Hypercalcaemia
Hypermagnesaemia
Hypoalbuminaemia

Other causes of reported decreased, undetermined anion concentrations have included the ingestion of bromide,[19] severe hypernatraemia,[95] hypoalbuminaemia, hypercalcaemia and hypermagnesaemia.[52] In some conditions, however, the decrease is artificial because the abnormal serum biochemistry disturbs the measurements made when these are performed on an Auto Analyser.

Limitations and errors in the anion gap

It is well recognized that the anion gap may have certain limitations; a normal value may be obtained when bicarbonate loss is the result of diarrhoea and when the acidosis is the result of renal tubular acidosis or uteroenterostomy.

Also, the anion gap may be raised, in the absence of a metabolic acidosis, in dehydration and during treatment with sodium salts of acids, such as lactate and acetate, especially when these salts are metabolized slowly. Treatment with large doses of antibiotics intravenously, for example sodium carbenicillin, also gives rise to an increase in the undetermined anion value.

A low anion gap may also be deceptive when the plasma is diluted as in water intoxication and hypoalbuminaemia. It can also be seen that the anion gap which would normally be raised may be returned to normal by hypoalbuminaemia.

There are certain technical considerations which would also alter the anion gap when values are obtained from the routine laboratory. For example, the flame-photometer may be non-linear when high values of $[Na^+]$ such as 170 mmol/l (mEq/l) are present. The Na^+ may therefore be underestimated, thus reducing the anion gap. The paraproteinaemias have such a high viscosity that the dilution may be incomplete in the Auto Analyser circuit and inaccuracies may therefore result; a very low or even negative anion gap can be reported, for example, in myeloma.[92] The paraproteins themselves have a net *positive* charge and may be found to have produced a lowered anion gap, in addition to the problems caused by the viscosity of the plasma.

Bromism is a further example where the measured results may be misleading. In the circulating blood, some bromide ions replace chloride ions *in vivo*; this is, however, inaccurately reflected when measurements are made by Auto Analysers. This is because the apparatus is unable to distinguish precisely between the two halides. In addition, Auto Analysers are more sensitive to bromide than to chloride. The result obtained can therefore be such that the 'observed' plasma $[Cl^-]$ is greater than that of the total concentration of halide actually present, thus reducing the observed anion gap.

Lactic acidosis

The measurement of blood lactate has been performed for many years.[41,49,60,87] The author's first measurements were made in the 1950s in order to explain the acidosis associated with extracorporeal circulations using the heart–lung machine especially during hypothermia. Clausen, in 1925,[36] reported the presence of lactic acidosis in children who had developed dehydration and severe hypovolaemia as a result of diarrhoea. Friedemann *et al.* (1945)[55] reported the presence of pyruvic and lactic acids in the blood of man in relation to anoxia at high altitude and to muscular activity. Litwin *et al.* (1959)[83] reported the presence of lactacidaemia during extracorporeal circulation.

Numerous workers in this field have instituted infusions of sodium bicarbonate with marked therapeutic effect. It is of some interest, therefore, that the infusion of bicarbonate itself, or oral intake of bicarbonate, can produce an increase in the blood lactate concentration. This is considered by some workers to be the result of a modification of the glycolytic pathway and the stimulation of anaerobic glycolysis.[59] Tris hydroxymethyl aminomethane (THAM) (see p. 97) has a similar effect,[118] indicating that the sudden change in the acid–base state, rather than the HCO_3^- itself, is the cause. However, the increase in blood lactate is insignificant and does not quantitatively decrease the metabolic *alkalosis* produced by the bicarbonate infusion.

Classification of lactic acidosis (lactacidosis)

Attempts have been made to classify the types of lactic acidosis occurring in patients. Huckabee[72] differentiated the types of lactacidosis on the basis of the blood lactate:pyruvate ratio and devised the term 'excess lactate'. This approach has been questioned by several authors including Cohen and Woods[39] who divided the patients into two groups: type A, in whom the blood lactic acid concentration rose due to poor tissue perfusion resulting from hypoxaemia; and type B, in whom the lactic acidosis was associated with other disorders in which hypotension and poor tissue perfusion were not initiating factors or of any major importance. It must be noted that the pyruvate concentration in the blood seldom makes a major impact on the degree of metabolic acidosis, while the concentration of lactate can be more than equal to the normal plasma $[HCO_3^-]$. A sudden increase in the number of patients with type B lactacidosis has been observed because of the use of the hypoglycaemic agent phenformin hydrochloride, and the bypass gut operation for gross obesity.[45]

Attempts have also been made in numerous reports, some of which are quoted in this chapter, to define lactacidosis arbitrarily by the concentration of lactate in the blood, for example concentrations above 5 mmol/l. In the author's opinion, this is an unsatisfactory method of defining the condition because for example in diabetic ketosis, the addition of just 2 mmol of lactate to the already severe metabolic acidosis can be of enormous clinical significance. The contribution of 5 mmol of lactate, far from being the level at which we consider lactic acidosis to be present, can, in some circumstances, be lethal. Cohen and Woods' classification[39] would, therefore, appear to be preferable for clinicians engaged in the resuscitation of the severely ill patient. However, as described below, opinion with regard to the conditions to be included in each division could be modified with clinical practice.

Lactic acidosis can, therefore, be said to occur in two separate groups of conditions. The first type (A) is that associated with reduced perfusion of tissues—hypoperfusion lactacidosis. The second type (B) is one in which there is no impairment of the circulation or of the maintenance of the blood pressure. In rare cases, lactic acidosis is an inherited metabolic disturbance—metabolic lactacidaemia. Type B lactacidosis can be induced by drugs, or the infusion of substances used in intravenous nutrition; it can be one of the manifestations of acute or chronic disease.

Causes of anoxic tissue lactacidosis (Type A) (hypoperfusion lactacidosis)

1. Hypotension:
   (a) haemorrhagic
   (b) cardiogenic
   (c) toxic
   (d) neurogenic
   (e) dehydration
   (f) plasma loss
   (g) drug induced
   (h) diabetes.
2. Arterial blood desaturation:
   (a) intrinsic lung disease
   (b) respiratory depression caused by drugs
   (c) pulmonary oedema
   (d) respiratory distress syndrome.
3. Specific localized tissue anoxia:
   (a) embolic occlusion of major vessels
   (b) clamping of major vessels during surgery
   (c) impaired perfusion due to trauma, tourniquet, atheroma, etc.

Causes of lactacidosis not precipitated by a primary defect in the cardiovascular system (Type B)

1. Drugs:
   (a) phenformin
   (b) metformin
   (c) dithiazanine iodide
   (d) anthelmintics
   (e) sodium nitroprusside
   (f) tricyclic antidepressants.
2. Poisoning:
   (a) methanol
   (b) salicylate
   (c) paraldehyde
   (d) ethanol.
3. Energy substrates (intravenous alimentation):
   (a) sorbitol
   (b) ethyl alcohol
   (c) fructose.
4. Common diseases:
   (a) diabetes mellitus
   (b) liver disease
   (c) renal failure
   (d) infection
   (e) leukaemia and reticuloses
   (f) pancreatitis.
5. Inherited metabolic disorders:
   (a) glycogen storage disease Type 1
   (b) hepatic fructose 1.6 diphosphatase deficiency
   (c) methylmalonic aciduria
   (d) Leigh's encephalomyelopathy.
6. Other causes:
   (a) fasting
   (b) gut bypass operation.

Lactacidosis; clinical conditions

Hypoxia
Hypoxia causes a progressive rise in the blood lactate concentration in animals which is proportional to the degree of anoxia;[30,105] this correlation is not, however, usually seen in man.

A rise in blood lactate concentration does not appear to be produced by anoxia alone in the presence of, for example, pulmonary disease.[73] This observation was confirmed by Eldridge and Salzer,[51] and was in agreement with the author's own observations at that time that, in the absence of circulatory insufficiency, blood lactate concentrations (e.g. in Pickwickian syndrome) were not significantly higher than normal. The cause of the rise in blood lactate and pyruvate is sometimes difficult to identify.[4,15]

Acute hypoxia, however, has been found to produce marked lactacidaemia. In 1958, Huckabee[71] found that breathing gases of low oxygen tension produced a rise in the arterial blood lactate concentration. A rise in the lactate concentration was found to be between 3 and 4 mmol/l when the arterial PO_2 was between 26 and 32 mmHg. Exercise in patients suffering from chronic obstructive lung disease can elicit a fall in HCO_3^- and a rise in blood lactate.

As already noted, severe metabolic acidosis develops during acute attacks of severe bronchial asthma. The author has found that this is due to lactic acidosis; this is in agreement with the findings of Mitheofer et al.[93] and Strauss et al.[114]

Hypotension (shock)

The observations of Cannon[32] have been mentioned and must have resulted from the accumulation of lactate. Cournand et al.[42] and Cruz et al.[44] found a correlation between the degree of acidosis and the severity of shock. Cruz et al. were able to demonstrate a direct correlation between the rate of survival and the arterial blood lactate concentration in dogs suffering from anaphylactic shock. Tranquada et al.,[119] in a series of 46 cases of lactic acidosis, most of whom were hypotensive, found that lactacidosis was present. This is in keeping with the findings of Oliva.[98] However, lactic acidosis occurs in patients suffering from cardiogenic and septic shock as well as from shock produced by haemorrhage.[70,86,100]

Haemorrhagic shock

As explained in Chapter 6, the degree of lactate accumulation within the body is related to the fall in bicarbonate ion concentrtion. We know that the fall in bicarbonate concentration is due to the degree of haemorrhagic shock and the length of time that this has existed (see Fig. 6.5). There does, however, appear to be a limitation with regard to the concentration of lactate in the blood, and the mechanism of this limitation is unclear.

Endotoxin shock

In 1965, Hopkins et al.[70] examined patients suffering from endotoxin shock and compared the concentrations of lactate in the blood with those in the blood of patients suffering from haemorrhagic shock. They found that the mean value in the patients suffering from endotoxin shock was 6.6 mmol/l, while in patients suffering from haemorrhagic shock the mean value was 7.2 mmol/l. The patients with haemorrhagic shock had a low blood pressure; in patients with endotoxin shock, however, the blood pressure varied greatly. This indicated that impaired tissue perfusion could occur in patients with endotoxin shock even though no major fall in blood pressure occurred. The series reported by Tranquada et al. in 1966[119] indicated that the raised blood lactate could be seen in numerous patients suffering from endotoxin shock.

Cardiogenic shock

The development of left ventricular failure results in the induction of pulmonary oedema. Both metabolic and respiratory acidosis have been described in patients in whom pulmonary oedema has developed.[1,3,14,56]

Pulmonary oedema

It was found by Fulop et al.[56] that 18 patients with acute pulmonary oedema had an arterial blood pH of less than 7.36. The blood lactate concentration was also raised and reverted to normal following treatment of the pulmonary oedema and improvement in the degree of left ventricular failure. No sodium bicarbonate was given and it was concluded that the fall in lactate was due to a return of adequate tissue perfusion.

Beri-beri (alcohol-induced)

Alcohol-induced beri-beri can also give rise to lactacidosis. Majoor[88] has reported a severely acidotic patient with a serum lactate concentration of 24.5 mmol/l caused by a fulminating form of 'cardiac beri-beri'. One patient had rapid respiration without impairment of pulmonary function, was cold and cyanotic peripherally, had distended jugular veins and severe abdominal pain which was associated with an extremely tender and swollen liver. Infusions of sodium bicarbonate improved the degree of acidosis but increased the central venous pressure (CVP). Injections of thiamine produced recovery with dissipation of the lactacidosis and the abnormal acid–base state.

Fasting and gut bypass surgery

A rise in blood lactate occurs during fasting.[45] The treatment of obesity by anastomosing the gut, so that a large section of it is bypassed, may give rise to severe and sometimes lethal lactacidosis.

Diabetes and lactic acidosis

The blood lactate concentration is not raised in diabetic patients unless the control of the diabetes is lost.[6,72,75,119] However, raised blood lactate levels have been found in patients who have developed diabetic ketosis with hyperglycaemia.[8,62,69,90,103,124,125,132]

While Cohen and Woods[39] consider this type of lactic acidosis to be contained in the type B group, the author's opinion is that there is much evidence (see p. 417) that cases of diabetic ketosis should be included in group A because of the reduction in blood volume and reduced tissue perfusion exacerbated, in many cases, by hypothermia.

The presence of a raised blood lactate is not necessarily a consequence of the ketosis itself. It occurs in non-ketotic, hyperosmolar diabetic crisis and, in the author's own experience and that of others,[8,124,125] the presence of lactate in the blood is a common finding in the severely ill diabetic patient who has become hypotensive.

Extracorporeal circulation

A lactic acidosis was found during the experiments performed when dogs were cooled to low temperatures so that a circulatory and respiratory arrest was possible for 45 minutes.[80] It was noticed that in the untreated dog, a syndrome of hypotension (refractory to vasopressor agents and Ca^{++} infusions), respiratory arrest and complete central nervous system depression (associated with areflexia) developed. This was corrected by infusions of isotonic (1.4%) bicarbonate. The development of a similar syndrome was later observed in man (see p. 137).

The lactic acidosis which developed during extracorporeal circulations[83] was found to occur during profound hypothermia in man when the lungs were perfused. It was noted that lactic acidosis was present in addition to marked changes in the anion gap (Fig. 3.9).

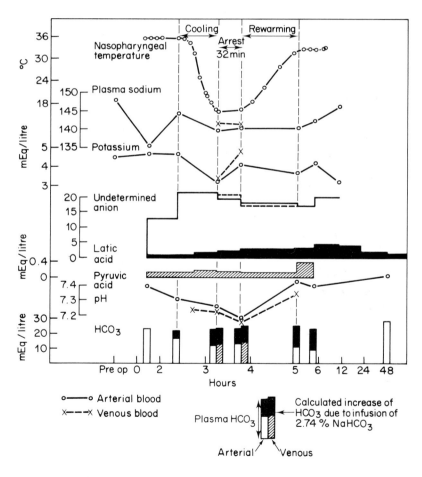

Fig. 3.9   Nasopharyngeal temperature, plasma [Na+], undetermined anion, lactic acid concentration, pyruvic acid concentration, arterial and venous pH and [HCO3] in a patient cooled to low temperatures for open-heart surgery using the Drew technique. Note that no correction for temperature or pH was made and 2.74% NaHCO3 was infused throughout the procedure.

Treatment of lactacidosis

It is apparent that treatment of lactacidosis must be directed towards the underlying cause, but this in itself is not always a simple task. The patients reported by Tranquada et al.,[119] frequently had more than one pathological condition and, indeed, the development of hypotension produces a number of physiological changes which themselves potentiate the condition, for example as found by Brooks and Feldman in 1962.[27] Relatively low concentrations of lactate, as little as 2 mmol/l,[23] in patients have been associated with a very high mortality. Studies by Seligman et al. (1947)[109] and Beatty (1945)[17] supported the conclusion that low values of blood lactate indicated, in many cases, a poor prognosis. It would seem, however, that the low values of lactate were merely an indication of the stage reached in the progress of the disease, just as a moderately reduced oxygen tension may, in some cases, represent an early state of hypoxia which progresses later to severe respiratory failure. Although this can often be reversed, at other times it frequently leads to death. Nevertheless, blood lactate metabolism is so complex, involving a fully functioning liver, actively metabolizing peripheral tissues, an adequate cardiac output, the absence of hypoxia and a normal total body tissue perfusion, that the isolated estimation of the lactate concentration in the blood is of only limited value. Peretz et al.,[100,101] showed that, in 52 patients suffering from shock of various aetiologies, the concentration of blood lactate correlated well with the survival rate. The mortality rate rose to over 90% of the patients when the lactate concentration was above 8.9 mmol/l. In the author's experience the lactate concentration alone is not an absolute indicator to the prognosis of the patient, but the response of the patient to infusions of bicarbonate is a clear and almost absolute indicator as to whether the patient will survive or not. Those patients whose acid–base state is improved by bicarbonate infusions tend to survive, while those in whom an immediate improvement in the acid–base state does not occur when adequate quantities of sodium bicarbonate are infused, rarely survive.

A formula for the calculation of the volume of bicarbonate solution required is given on p. 96.

Intracellular pH

It would not be surprising if the cells of different tissues had different values for intracellular pH. It is well recognized that, because of the difference in concentration of salts and hydrogen ions, a negative potential amounting to approximately 90 mV exists across the membrane of skeletal and cardiac muscle. With a membrane potential within that region, the intracellular pH could be as low as 5.9.

Numerous techniques have been used to estimate intracellular pH; these include: (a) use of dyes as pH indicators, (b) application of the Henderson–Hasselbalch equation to estimate the concentration of intracellular bicarbonate and plasma PCO_2, (c) distribution of weak organic acids, particularly DMO (5.5–dimethyl-2, 4-oxazolidinevione), between the extracellular and intracellular fluids, and (d) direct measurements with small, glass electrodes into individual muscle cells. There appears, however, to be little uniformity in the findings; most reports agree that intracellular pH is lower than that of plasma, although opinions differ as to whether the intracellular pH is nearer to 6.0 or to 7.0.

Acid–Base in Clinical Practice

Phenformin-associated lactic acidosis*

Because of its importance and high mortality, this aspect of lactacidosis should be regarded as a separate entity requiring special treatment. Although phenformin has been withdrawn from general use in many countries, it is still being used in many parts of the world.

Since the introduction of the hypoglycaemic agent, phenformin, more than 550 cases of lactic acidosis have been reported, although, of course, many more cases have occurred. A number of cases have been very well documented; the pathogenesis of lactic acidosis in these diabetic patients is, however, still poorly understood. The knowledge that we do have is derived from animal experiments, from the study of patients who have taken overdoses, and from the study of patients who have developed lactic acidosis when receiving only therapeutic quantities of the substance. A small rise in blood lactate is observed in all patients treated with phenformin.[123] It seems that, while lactate oxidation is increased by phenformin, the increase in rate is not sufficient to keep pace with lactate production.[108] It would also appear that, with regard to lactate production, some patients are abnormally sensitive and may have an inborn error of metabolism which is only revealed during phenformin therapy.[108,113,115]

---

*Phenformin has been withdrawn from general use in the USA and United Kingdom, but it is still being prescribed in some countries, and metformin and similar preparations are still being used.

Both animal experiments and observations in man have indicated that diabetes itself predisposes towards a raised blood lactate level. It is also well recognized (for reasons discussed elsewhere, pp. 83 & 416) that patients who develop ketoacidosis also develop an elevated blood lactate concentration in the absence of any treatment with phenformin or other hypoglycaemic agents.[125,129] Pyruvate levels are also raised in healthy diabetic patients, indicating an abnormality in lactate metabolism.[94]

There is no direct evidence that lactic acidosis in patients receiving phenformin results from alterations in lactate metabolism which can be directly attributed to the oral hypoglycaemic agent itself. Elevated concentrations of ketone bodies are found in most diabetic patients suffering from phenformin-associated lactic acidosis. This indicates that one contributory factor is a deficiency of insulin.

Further evidence of the part played by insulin in the production of phenformin lactacidosis is based on the observations of Loubatieres et al.,[84] who found that the expected rise in blood lactate in dogs, given a large single dose of phenformin, was reduced when pretreatment with insulin was given.

There is evidence that diabetes alone predisposes towards lactic acidosis.[128] The presence of raised levels of lactate during diabetic coma in three patients who had not received phenformin was reported by Daughaday et al.;[47] other cases have been reported by Watkins et al.[125] and Wise et al.[129]

Case history. A 70-year-old male who had suffered from maturity onset diabetes for some years came to visit his son from another city in America. The family was of Oriental extraction and the patient was taken to see an osteopath because he was feeling tired. The osteopath prescribed an injection of vitamin B_{12} and a tablet of frusemide (Lasix), probably of 40 mg. The following day, the patient felt worse and somewhat weak and was, therefore, taken once more to visit the osteopath, who prescribed on this occasion another injection of vitamin B_{12} and also, this time, frusemide (Lasix) 80 mg i.m.

Twelve hours later, the patient presented at the Emergency Center by ambulance. His blood pressure on admission was 75/50 mmHg. The patient was of short stature, thin, weighing approximately 55 kg, and underweight but not cachectic. There were signs of dehydration and there was moderate cyanosis of the peripheries. The respiratory rate varied (was not Cheyne–Stokes) but was in the region of 28 breaths per minute. The pulse was of poor volume. The patient appeared to be mentally well orientated, aware of his surroundings and able to answer questions, but was so weak that he had some difficulty in talking because he tired so quickly. The history was, therefore, obtained from the son and, in addition to the above, it transpired that the patient had been receiving phenformin hydrochloride (DBI, Meltrol, Dibotin, Dipar) 150 mg daily from his medical practitioner in another city. The patient had, however, noted from time to time that his urine contained glucose, so that he had either not been properly controlled or had not been taking his medication at regular intervals.

Examination revealed no marked intrinsic abnormality of the heart. There was no increased jugular venous pressure, the heart was of normal size and the heart sounds were normal and regular with no gallops audible. There was a grade II/6 ejection systolic murmur which decreased on inspiration. It did not radiate into the axilla or towards the sternum and was audible predominantly at the apex. The electrocardiogram demonstrated a regular sinus rhythm at a rate of 95 per minute. No acute changes were present and there were minimal non-specific S–T changes which could be accounted for by the heart rate. On examination of the blood, it was revealed that the blood sugar was 185 mg% (10.3 mmol/l), no plasma acetone was present, the blood urea nitrogen was 45 mg%. The serum electrolytes demonstrated Na^+ 128 mmol/l (mEq/l), K^+ 5.0 mmol/l (mEq/l), Cl^- 96 mmol/l (mEq/l), TCO_2 6 mmol/l. The blood lactate concentration was found to be 26 mmol/l. The blood pyruvate was not estimated. Arterial blood-gas estimation demonstrated a pH of 6.80, HCO_3^- 5.9 mmol/l (mEq/l) and PCO_2 36 mmHg. An intravenous infusion of 0.9% saline was instituted immediately in order to rehydrate the patient and replace some of the sodium that may have been lost in the urine. The urinalysis revealed only a trace of ketones, no glucose, no proteins, and no blood. The pH of the urine was 5.0. An injection of 50 ml of 8.4% $NaHCO_3$ was given intravenously and this resulted in an immediate, but temporary, rise in blood pressure to 110/60 mmHg. The patient was transferred to the intensive care unit and, because of the enormity of the acidosis, an infusion of 500 ml of 8.4% $NaHCO_3$ was started. By the evening of the same day, the blood pressure was being maintained at 100/60 mmHg and blood analysis revealed that the pH of the blood was 7.22, the standard bicarbonate 10.6 mmol/l and the PCO_2 28 mmHg.

Although the patient had taken his phenformin on the day of admission and on the previous day, no other hypoglycaemic therapy had been given. The blood sugar at this time was 160 mg% (8.9 mmol/l) and the blood lactate concentration was 24 mmol/l. When the second blood sample was taken, approximately 250 mmol of sodium bicarbonate had been infused. Because of the apparent clinical improvement in the patient's condition, it was decided to continue the infusion of bicarbonate during the night until a further 500 mmol had been given. In the early hours of the following morning, the patient's blood pressure fell so that it became temporarily unrecordable. Hyperventilation was visible and the patient became comatose and able to speak only with difficulty, his words were not comprehensible. A blood sample taken at that time showed that, in spite of the infusions of bicarbonate, the plasma bicarbonate concentration had fallen to a standard bicarbonate of less than 4 mmol/l, the pH was 6.8 and the PCO_2, measured by the PCO_2 electrode, was 25 mmHg.

A rapid infusion of sodium bicarbonate of 8.4% was instituted so that a further 300 mmol were given over a period of 3 hours. Virtually no improvement in the acid–base state occurred as approximately 3.5 hours later the pH values were 6.84, the standard bicarbonate measurement was 5.3 mmol/l and the PCO_2 was 33 mmHg. The bicarbonate infusion was continued and, because of the apparent lack of response to bicarbonate infusions and the absence of hyperglycaemia, it was decided to institute blood dialysis in a vain attempt to improve the patient's metabolic condition. The patient, however, died while the catheters were being inserted for the dialysis procedure. No glucose-insulin infusions had been given.

Precipitation of phenformin lactacidosis by diuretics has been observed in published reports. The use of mercaptomerin sodium (Thiomerin) as an initiating cause has been questioned.[103] In one of the patients reported by Johnson and Waterhouse,[78] aldactazide was given three times daily in addition to phenformin. The lactic acidosis developed only when the patient changed from tolbutamide to phenformin. It would, therefore, seem that it is possible that one of the precipitating factors may be hypovolaemia induced by a diuretic, or perhaps a direct action of the diuretic itself upon the metabolism of lactic acid in the liver or peripheral tissues. If other published reports are examined, it is possible to note that diuretic therapy in association with phenformin has been used, although this has not necessarily appeared to be a precipitating factor in the development of lactic

acidosis. Assan et al.[9,10] published reports in which all four of their patients given frusemide (Lasix) after the development of phenformin lactic acidosis survived, but it is evident from their graphs that the diuretic was not given until after the acidosis had been corrected with $NaHCO_3$. The following case history, in which there was a successful outcome and a glucose–insulin mixture was infused, illustrates some of these factors. The glucose–insulin mixture is considered to enhance lactate metabolism.

Case history. A 46-year-old woman was admitted through the Emergency Center because she complained of feeling very unwell, dizzy and disorientated. She had also had a feeling of nausea for approximately 3–4 hours. A history was obtained which demonstrated that she had been given hydrochlorothiazide (Direma, Esidrex, Hydrosaluric, Hydrolevril) 50 mg twice daily for hypertension. Some weeks after the initiation of the treatment, it was noted that she was also suffering from diabetes. Treatment with tolbutamide (Tolanase, Orinase, Rastinon, Pramidex) 500 mg was given twice daily. She felt extremely unwell when taking the tolbutamide and this was exacerbated when she drank alcohol, from which she was reluctant to abstain. One week before her admission to hospital, her treatment had been changed to phenformin hydrochloride (DBI, Meltrol, Dibotin, Dipar) 50 mg twice a day. After phenformin therapy, glycosuria ceased.

She presented at the Emergency Center having felt unwell and nauseated for 24 hours. She was unable to stand because she felt weak. Her temperature was 37.0°C. Her blood pressure was 100/60 mmHg, respiration 28 breaths per minute with an observable large tidal volume. A venous blood sample revealed the following: Na^+ 128 mmol/l (mEq/l), K^+ 5.4 mmol/l (mEq/l), Cl^- 98 mmol/l (mEq/l), TCO_2 4.0 mmol/l, anion gap 26 mmol, blood glucose 62 mg% (3.4 mmol/l), Hb 14.2 g%, WBC 8200/mm³.

An infusion of sodium bicabonate was instituted immediately and an arterial blood sample was taken when only a few millilitres had been given. This revealed the following: Na^+ 131 mmol/l (mEq/l), K^+ 5.1 mmol/l (mEq/l), Cl^- 96 mmol/l (mEq/l), pH 7.1, PCO_2 25 mmHg, base excess −21.6 mmol/l, standard bicarbonate 7.2 mmol/l, anion gap 28 mmol, lactate 17.6 mmol/l, blood glucose 73 mg% (4.0 mmol/l).

Shortly after this blood sample was taken, and before the blood values were known, the blood pressure fell to 65/45 mmHg; the rate of infusion of $NaHCO_3$ was increased and 10 ml of $CaCl_2$ 10% was given. Blood pressure increased only slightly, to 80/65 mmHg and, over the next 3 hours, 340 mmol/l of $NaHCO_3$ were infused. An arterial blood sample revealed only a marginal improvement in the acid–base state, pH 7.24, PCO_2 27 mmHg, standard bicarbonate 11.6 mmol/l, base excess −14.7 mmol/l, lactate 31 mmol/l, Na^+ 134 mmol/l (mEq/l), K^+ 5.4 mmol/l (mEq/l), blood glucose 68 mg% (3.8 mmol/l).

An infusion of 500 ml of glucose 20% with insulin 45 units was begun and given at the rate of 15 drops per minute, and the infusion of $NaHCO_3$ was continued overnight until, by the following morning, a further 520 mmol had been given. The patient's condition had improved, by 2 a.m. the following day her blood pressure had risen to 110/70 mmHg, her heart rate had fallen to 85 beats/min, and, although tidal volume had increased, respiratory rate had fallen to 26/min. This improvement was maintained and a blood sample taken at 8 a.m. revealed the following: Na^+ 138 mmol/l (mEq/l), K^+ 4.8 mmol/l (mEq/l), Cl^- 96 mmol/l (mEq/l), pH 7.39, PCO_2 35 mmHg, HCO_3^- 20.4 mmol/l, anion gap 24 mmol/l, blood sugar 98 mmol/l. A second infusion of glucose with insulin was given at the same rate, being completed over a period of approximately 6 hours, and a slow infusion of $NaHCO_3$ was continued. By midday, the patient was able to take a little water by mouth and could move unassisted in bed but was still very weak. A total of 1220 mmol of $NaHCO_3$ had then been given since her admission.

A blood sample taken at 2 p.m. demonstrated that continued improvement with a fall in the anion gap and lactate concentration occurred: Na^+ 142 mmol/l (mEq/l), K^+ 4.6 mmol/l (mEq/l), Cl^- 98 mmol/l (mEq/l), pH 7.41, PCO_2 37 mmHg, HCO_3^- 22.8 mmol/l, blood sugar 125 mg% (6.9 mmol/l), lactate 4.6 mmol/l. During the evening of the same day, the patient was sitting up in bed, still feeling very tired and weak but drinking bland fluids such as milk in small quantities. The blood pressure was maintained at 125/70 mmHg and the heart rate had fallen to 72 beats/minute. Respirations were no longer laboured and arterial blood sample revealed Na^+ 142 mmol/l (mEq/l), K^+ 3.5 mmol/l (mEq/l), Cl^- 100 mmol/l (mEq/l), pH 7.43, PCO_2 38 mmHg, HCO_3^- 24 mmol/l, blood sugar 135 mg% (7.5 mmol/l).

The next day, both infusions of bicarbonate and 20% glucose/insulin were discontinued, and the patient felt much stronger and was thirsty; she took water and other fluids by mouth.

At no time was acetone found in the urine or in the blood, and urine output continued in adequate quantities. Blood analysis on that day gave the following results: Na^+ 148 mmol/l (mEq/l), K^+ 4.0 mmol/l (mEq/l), Cl^- 105 mmol (mEq/l), pH 7.48, PCO_2 39 mmHg, HCO_3^- 28.4 mmol/l, lactate 1.2 mmol/l, glucose 165% (9.2 mmol/l), urine glucose 25 mg%.

An uneventful recovery from this episode occurred; phenformin was discontinued and treatment with insulin was begun.

Treatment of phenformin lactic acidosis

The primary treatment should be directed towards correcting the precipitating cause, when this is known (e.g. toxaemia from infection, dehydration etc.), and *hypo*glycaemia, when this is found to be present[48] with insulin-glucose.

However, no precipitating cause may be evident and the aetiology of phenformin lactic acidosis has yet to be correctly identified.[10,38,40,57,129] A number of authors have attempted to review the possible causes. It would appear that myocardial insufficiency, hypotention, infection, alcohol ingestion[81] and shock of various forms are frequent causes of lactic acidosis in the patients receiving phenformin therapy. The author's own experience has been confined to sepsis, haemorrhage and the apparently mistaken prescription of thiazide diuretics (see case histories), and one case in which there was no known cause. In almost all cases, a decreased fluid intake or abnormal fluid balance has been present on admission to hospital. It would appear that renal insufficiency where the serum creatinine is greater than 133 μmol/l (1.5 mg%) should be an absolute contraindication to phenformin therapy. This is notwithstanding the fact that pre-renal azotaemia may be present prior to therapy because of dehydration resulting from the osmotic diuresis produced by glycosuria.

Therapy

In view of the above, treatment of lactic acidosis produced by phenformin should be directed in the following way.

1. Correction of the deficiency of insulin by infusing a glucose/insulin mixture (e.g. glucose 20% with insulin 45 units per 500 ml).
2. Correction of the metabolic acidosis by means of sodium bicarbonate (e.g. 4.2 or 8.4%). In the first instance 500–800 mmol will be required. As much as 1200 mmol has been given.
3. Rehydration and correction of blood volume.
4. Haemodialysis.

Spontaneous Ventilation and Acid–Base Changes

The application of mathematical reasoning to alterations in acid–base equilibrium, together with the observation of 'air hunger' by Kussmaul (1874)[82] occurring in diabetic coma, has led to the belief that clinically detectable hyperventilation occurs in all cases of metabolic acidosis. A closer examination of the response of patients to acid–base disorders reveals that a reappraisal of these concepts, and the conditions in which changes in alveolar ventilation and respiratory rate occur, may be necessary.

Hyperventilation

Hyperventilation infers an increase in the volume of air breathed per minute with the consequent slight rise of oxygen tension (PO_2) and decrease of carbon dioxide tension (PCO_2) in the alveoli. The only routine measurement made is that of respiratory rate, and it is upon this that the clinical assessment usually depends, although true evaluation is possible only by knowing the volume of air breathed per minute (minute volume) and the respiratory dead space. We can see from Chapter 5 that increased alveolar ventilation can be produced by an increase in the tidal volume and respiratory rate which is imperceptible by ordinary clinical observation.

We should at this point, therefore, examine some common clinical conditions in which hyperventilation might be expected to occur because of a metabolic acidosis.

Acute renal failure

An account of the condition of acute renal failure is given in Chapter 4 and the acid–base changes are briefly mentioned there. It would be expected that the accumulation of fixed acids resulting in a marked metabolic acidosis would result in obvious and easily recognizable hyperventilation. Table 3.5 shows the values obtained from five patients. The acid–base data of the first three patients demonstrate a marked reduction of base, but not one was considered by clinical observation to be acidotic. No increase in respiratory rate was detectable and observations on numerous other patients with this condition confirm these findings.

Hyperventilation is, in fact, rarely seen unless there is some complicating factor such as cardiac failure, severe pyrexia or gross overhydration. Cardiac failure is commonly produced by a raised serum potassium concentration or overhydration.

The results taken from patient No. 4 in Table 3.5 show a rise in respiratory rate associated with a raised plasma PCO_2. The metabolic acidosis was only of moderate severity. The patient was 35 years of age and had oedema extending well above the thighs into the lower abdomen. Overhydration was the prime cause of the increased respiratory rate. Patients given a large volume of fluid and who developed dyspnoea due to overhydration were said, in the past, to be suffering from 'uraemic lung'.

Table 3.5 Blood pH, TCO_2, PCO_2, $[HCO_3^-]$, respiratory rate and $[K^+]$ in five patients with acute renal failure

	pH	TCO_2	PCO_2	$[HCO_3^-]$	Respiratory rate	$[K^+]$
1	7.20	12.9	32	11.6	20	5.6
2	7.11	11.4	35	10.4	19	5.2
3	7.24	14.8	35	13.8	22	5.6
4	7.17	18.5	48	17.1	30	4.8
5	7.26	14.5	31	15.6	37	7.9

TCO_2 = Plasma total CO_2 content (mmol/l).
PCO_2 = Plasma CO_2 tension (mmHg).
$[HCO_3^-]$ = Plasma bicarbonate ion concentration (mmol/l)
$\qquad = (TCO_2 - 0.0301 \times PCO_2)$.
$[K^+]$ = Plasma potassium concentration in mmol/l (mEq/l).
Respiratory rate is in breaths/minute.

Patient No. 5 in Table 3.5 was an elderly woman with carcinoma obstructing both ureters. Excessive hydration was not present, but she had a raised venous pressure and her plasma potassium concentration was increased to a cardiotoxic level. The electrocardiogram (Fig. 3.10) showed the absence of a P wave, slurring of a widened QRS complex and a high peaked T wave. These are the typical electrocardiogram changes that occur in this condition and they precede the onset of ventricular tachycardia and fibrillation. Hyperventilation can be explained in this patient by cardiac failure.

It has been repeatedly observed that, in the well-controlled patient, when the plasma potassium is low and excessive hydration is absent, hyperventilation is not to be expected even in the presence of a major metabolic acidosis.

Ureteric transplant

Another condition which gives rise to a gross metabolic acidosis, when there is a reduced plasma bicarbonate and raised plasma chloride concentration, is that which follows transplant of the ureters into the lower colon. This is performed to prevent

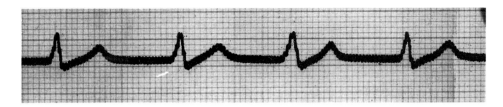

Fig. 3.10 The electrocardiogram taken from the patient with cardiotoxic levels of K^+ in the plasma, whose acid–base data are reported in Table 3.5. Note the absent P wave, the widened QRS complex and the tall T wave which is not as 'spiked' as usual. Cardiac failure in this case caused hyperventilation.

obstruction as a result of pelvic carcinoma, usually of the bladder. Changes in electrolytes were first demonstrated by Boyd,[21] who showed that metabolic acidosis was present in a 10-year-old boy who, 3 years earlier, had undergone uretero-colic anastomosis for bladder exstrophy. Jewett[76,77] also observed the production of a metabolic acidosis in dogs after he had transplanted ureters into the rectum. Ferris and Odel[54] clearly demonstrated the main biochemical disorders that follow the operation when they reported their investigations in 141 cases that underwent uretero-colostomy at the Mayo Clinic. Although many patients remained well, some developed a syndrome of malaise, excessive thirst, a salty taste in the mouth and marked loss of weight. Similar findings have since been reported from numerous sources. A marked reduction of PCO_2 is not always present.

One of the fundamental problems in the clinical management and treatment of this condition was in deciding whether relative emphasis should be placed upon impaired renal function or upon the reabsorption of electrolytes from the urine. Most evidence indicates that the cause of the metabolic acidosis is the migration of ions across the gut wall.[54] This aspect was been reviewed by Irvine *et al.*[74]

In the complicated condition of ureteric transplant in which a large number of major metabolic disturbances occur, changes in respiratory function might well be expected.

Table 3.6 gives the acid–base data and respiratory rates of a patient examined at 2-monthly intervals over a period of 6 months. He was treated with sulphaguanidine, to reduce the gut flora, and cachets of sodium bicarbonate. On no occasion was a tachypnoea detected even though a gross metabolic acidosis was present. Investigation of a series of patients has demonstrated that tachypnoea need not occur even when the $[HCO_3^-]$ is as low as 6 mmol/l (mEq/l). A Kussmaul type of breathing can develop when the condition leads to dehydration, hypernatraemia and hyperkalaemia, together

Table 3.6 Blood pH, TCO_2, PCO_2, $[HCO_3^-]$, respiratory rate and $[Cl^-]$ in a patient with hyperchloraemic acidosis resulting from uretero-colic anastomosis

	pH	TCO_2	PCO_2	$[HCO_3^-]$	Respiratory rate	$[Cl^-]$
a	7.21	9.6	23	8.9	20	122
b	7.23	10.8	25	10.0	21	118
c	7.25	10.6	23	9.9	20	120

TCO_2 = Plasma total CO_2 content (mmol/l).
PCO_2 = Plasma CO_2 tension (mmHg).
$[HCO_3^-]$ = Plasma bicarbonate ion concentration (mmol/l)
$\quad = (TCO_2 - 0.0301 \times PCO_2)$.
$[Cl^-]$ = Plasma chloride concentration in mmol/l (mEq/l).
Respiratory rate is in breaths/minute.

with a metabolic acidosis of great proportions. The patient is then liable to pass into coma and, because the blood urea is raised, the condition can sometimes be mistaken for uraemic coma or a terminal malignant state. Intravenous infusions of fluid and alkali rapidly reverse this process.

Hepatic coma
Hyperventilation almost invariably occurs in hepatic coma, but the biochemical analysis of the plasma reveals that both a respiratory and a metabolic alkalosis are present.

Clinically, the reverse is often suspected and has sometimes been treated with infusion of alkali without benefit to the patient. The associated sodium retention and low plasma potassium level are worsened by this therapy. Table 3.7 shows the acid–base findings in four patients with liver disease. The first three patients were not jaundiced and their comas were reversed by intravenous infusions of glucose and potassium chloride. Patient No. 1, however, was given a small quantity of sodium bicarbonate solution after the blood sample was taken as it was assumed that the hyperventilation was due to a metabolic acidosis. A true metabolic acidosis can occur in cases of liver necrosis

Table 3.7 Blood pH, TCO_2, PCO_2, [HCO_3^-] and respiratory rate in four patients with hepatic coma

	pH	TCO_2	PCO_2	[HCO_3^-]	Respiratory rate
1	7.52	29.7	36	28.6	35
2	7.55	30.1	34	29.1	36
3	7.56	28.8	32	27.8	37
4	7.24	12.6	28	11.8	36

TCO_2 = Plasma total CO_2 content (mmol/l).
PCO_2 = Plasma CO_2 tension (mmHg).
[HCO_3^-] = Plasma bicarbonate ion concentration (mmol/l)
    = (TCO_2 − 0.0301 × PCO_2).
Respiratory rate is in breaths/minute.

(patient No. 4); this 42-year-old man was deeply jaundiced, the liver was tense, hard and tender on palpation. At post-mortem thrombosis of the hepatic veins was found. Many different factors had summated to produce hyperventilation in these circumstances, because widespread liver damage had produced a greatly altered biochemical pattern.

Haemorrhage

Hyperventilation occurs spontaneously after loss of blood. The oxygen saturation of the arterial blood is not reduced unless ventilation is impaired (see p. 178). In the terminal stages, gross hyperventilation gives place to hypoventilation and then a bradycardia precedes cardiac arrest. When this occurs the plasma PCO_2 rises and the blood oxygen saturation falls. The pH of the blood can then be expected to be 6.9 or less. The presence of a metabolic acidosis after haemorrhagic shock has long been recognized.[32,33] In the fit, healthy patient the gross metabolic acidosis may be of little consequence, even though the acidosis, which is the result of an accumulation of lactic acid, can reach major proportions. The presence of any other pathological condition, however, may make its correction essential.

Acid-citrate dextrose (ACD) blood has a low concentration of base and a pH in the region of 6.4. The rapid infusion of ACD blood may precipitate cardiac arrest as the pH is suddenly lowered further, or there may be no improvement in blood pressure after the transfusion. In this situation the infusion of hypertonic sodium bicarbonate may have dramatically beneficial effects[27] and, when profound hypotension has been present for 5 minutes or more, may be indicated prior to blood transfusion. It has been suggested that because the hyperventilation that occurs during haemorrhagic shock is a result of the metabolic acidosis that is present, the infusion of alkali during shock will depress respiration. This, in fact, occurs neither in man nor in the experimental animal.[25–28] This aspect is dealt with fully in the chapter on shock (see p. 194). Although the maintenance of hyperosmolality of the ECF may be a predominant factor in preventing tissue damage (see p. 195), both this and the metabolic acidosis can be corrected simultaneously by the use of hypertonic solutions containing sodium bicarbonate.

Diabetic coma

The type of respiration which Kussmaul described as 'air hunger'[82] and which occurs in this condition is distinctive and characteristic, so that it is easily recognized. It is simulated in disturbances of the central nervous system, the pre-terminal stages of haemorrhagic shock and in the comatose form of hyperchloraemic acidosis. In all these conditions numerous common factors summate to produce it.

In diabetic coma there is, in addition to the profound metabolic acidosis sometimes producing plasma bicarbonate levels as low as 6 mmol/l (mEq/l), dehydration; a raised plasma osmolality and ketone bodies are also present. There is often a low arterial blood pressure.

Resuscitative measures of hydration and insulin will reduce the respiratory rate without any marked alteration of pH.

Case history. A woman of 37 years presented in hospital as an undiagnosed case of diabetes mellitus. Her respiratory rate was 38/min, her blood sugar was 710 mg% (39.4 mmol/l). She was not hypotensive but there were the signs of dehydration. She was suffering from polyuria and on examination her urine was found to contain much sugar and ketone bodies. An arterial blood sample taken at time of admission demonstrated that she had a marked metabolic acidosis and respiratory alkalosis (Table 3.8, a and b). She was given insulin (100 units) and infused with 3 litres of fluid, 2 litres of glucose 5% and 1 litre of normal saline. An arterial blood sample taken 4 hours later showed little change in the metabolic component of acid–base equilibrium, but the PCO_2 had risen (Table 3.8b). The ventilation rate had fallen to 23/min; 24 hours later (Table 3.8c) a moderate metabolic alkalosis was present.

This case clearly demonstrates that the presence of a metabolic acidosis is not necessarily an essential part of the air-hunger type of ventilation seen in diabetic coma.

Hydration alone can greatly reduce the degree of hyperventilation without any marked change in

Table 3.8 Blood pH, PCO_2, 'standard bicarbonate', plasma [Na$^+$] and [K$^+$], blood sugar and respiratory rate in a patient with diabetic coma

	pH	St. bic	PCO_2	PCV (%)	[Na$^+$]	[K$^+$]	Blood sugar	Respiratory rate
a 11 a.m.	7.15	9.3	13	48	116	3.1	710 (39.4)	38
b 3 p.m.	7.26	13.4	29	42	128	2.4	209 (11.6)	24
c 11 a.m.	7.49	28.2	37	41	138	3.7	87 (4.8)	21

pH = Arterial blood pH at 38°C.
PCO_2 = Blood CO_2 tension (mmHg).
St. bic. = Standard bicarbonate (mmol/l).
PCV = Packed cell volume.
[Na$^+$] = Plasma sodium concentration in mmol/l (mEq/l).
[K$^+$] = Plasma potassium concentration in mmol/l (mEq/l).
Blood sugar is in mg% (figures in brackets = mmol/l).
Respiratory rate is in breaths/minute.

the acid–base state. It must be remembered, however, that when patients have developed a severe metabolic acidosis the intravenous infusion of sodium bicarbonate solution may produce a dramatic improvement in blood pressure and may be an essential part of treatment.[46]

Hypoventilation

Respiratory acidosis
This implies that the alveolar and therefore the arterial partial pressure of carbon dioxide (PCO_2) is raised above the normal (sea-level) value of 40 mmHg. The rate of diffusion of carbon dioxide across the alveolar membrane is some 20 times that of oxygen. Accumulation of CO_2 can therefore only occur in the presence of a low blood oxygen tension producing cyanosis, unless hypoventilation is present in an oxygen-enriched mixture, such as an oxygen tent, or the rebreathing of carbon dioxide from the oxygen-rich mixture of an anaesthetic circuit. Under these conditions a raised PCO_2 can be demonstrated in the presence of a normal or raised PO_2. Although it is well recognized that a moderate increase in the alveolar CO_2 tension produces an increase in respiratory rate, it was demonstrated by Scurr[107] that abnormally high levels can produce respiratory depression.

Retention of carbon dioxide can also occur when respiration is depressed as the result of an acute metabolic acidosis (see p. 134).

Unlike the mathematically predictable situation, hypoventilation can be seen quite commonly in clinical practice in the presence of both a respiratory and metabolic acidosis, and complete apnoea can be produced by both.

The two types of acute respiratory acidosis listed below have been termed primary (a) and secondary (b) acute CO_2 retention:[27]

(a) respiratory acidosis due to rebreathing CO_2,
(b) retention of CO_2 caused by impaired spontaneous ventilation resulting from a metabolic acidosis or other biochemical abnormality.

Several acute clinical conditions give rise to severe hypoventilation. It is seen when a patient with uncompensated respiratory acidosis is exposed to high tensions of oxygen (see p. 127) in postoperative failure to breathe, when there appears to be a syndrome of central nervous system depression (see p. 134), and after massive blood transfusion. It also occurs after cardiac arrest, haemorrhage of acute onset and prolonged haemorrhagic shock. The following account illustrates one of the circumstances in which 'secondary respiratory failure' and CO_2 retention can occur.

Case history. A 46-year-old woman underwent heart surgery for mitral value replacement. The pump-oxygenator was primed with 5% dextrose in water. Frequent blood-gas analyses were performed and, at the appropriate stages during the heart–lung bypass operation, 8.4% $NaHCO_3$ was added to the oxygenator to correct the metabolic acidosis which developed.

At the end of the operation, the patient was removed from the pump-oxygenator without difficulty, and she demonstrated no irregularities of rhythm once sinus rhythm had been restored. The blood pressure, which was monitored by intra-arterial catheter and electrical transducer, was visualized with the electrocardiogram on a cathode-ray oscilloscope. The blood pressure was 120/70 mmHg when the patient was placed in the intensive care ward.

The endotracheal tube was kept *in situ* and artificial ventilation of the lungs was maintained by means of a patient-triggered pressure-cycled ventilator using an oxygen/air mixture.

Very little bleeding occurred from the chest drainage tubes; blood which was lost was more than adequately replaced by transfusion. The central venous pressure (CVP) was 9 cmH$_2$O measured at the mid-axillary line with the patient laying flat (see p. 179). The urine output was also normal and of considerable volume, partly because of the priming of the pump-oxygenator and partly because of an associated infusion of saline containing KCl which provided K$^+$ 20 mmol/hour.

Soon after arriving in the intensive care ward, the patient was awake and well orientated and, approximately 45 minutes later, she was disconnected from the ventilator. The patient at that time had a tidal volume of 550 ml, as measured by a Wright Respirometer, when she was breathing spontaneously with the endotracheal tube *in situ*. This was 50 ml greater than the average tidal volume measured while the patient was on the ventilator. Humidified oxygen was given by means of a catheter and a chimney.

Approximately 1 hour later, an arterial blood sample was taken via the catheter and, after the catheter had been flushed with heparinized saline and reconnected to the transducer, the patient's blood pressure was observed to have fallen to 75/50 mmHg. There was also a reduction in pulse pressure. The patient was peripherally cyanosed and ventilation appeared to be laboured. The CVP was measured and found to be 17 cmH$_2$O.

The arterial blood sample obtained at that moment demonstrated a metabolic acidosis, a slight rise in PCO_2, no lack of oxygenation of the arterial blood and a normal plasma [Na$^+$] and [K$^+$] as shown in Table 3.9. Before these results were known, a self-inflating Ambu bag was attached to the endotracheal tube and 100% humidified O$_2$ was delivered to the bag.

As soon as ventilation was begun, the blood pressure fell precipitously so that it was close to 40 mmHg systolic. An infusion of metaraminol (Aramine), which was begun by means of a Y-connector attached to the intravenous infusion catheter, had no effect on the blood pressure, nor did an injection of 10 ml of 10% CaCl$_2$ i.v. An infusion of NaHCO$_3$ was begun by adding 150 ml of 4.2% NaHCO$_3$ to the Soluset chamber of a new giving-set; 50 ml were given to the patient over a period of a few minutes and the infusion was continued at a rapid rate. A rapid increase in blood pressure occurred; the blood pressure continued to increase until approximately 10 minutes later it was 105/70 mmHg. No vasopressor had been given because the bicarbonate infusion had replaced that which contained the metaraminol (Aramine). Injection of a further 10 ml of CaCl$_2$ through the saline infusion caused the blood pressure to rise to 115/80 mmHg, and the heart rate to increase to 110 beats/min for a brief period.

The tidal volume, which had fallen to 115 ml during the hypotensive period, was now 650 ml, and the patient was breathing oxygen-enriched air spontaneously, after 100 ml of 4.2% NaHCO$_3$ solution (50 mmol NaHCO$_3$) had been given. The blood gases reverted to normal; pH 7.38, [HCO$_3^-$] 18.4 mmol/l and PCO2 36 mmHg.

The patient, who had become semicomatose while the blood pressure was low, was once again alert and orientated, and a slow infusion of 4.2% NaHCO$_3$ was maintained over the next 6 hours so that a further 100 mmol were given. The CVP, which had been raised when the hypotensive episode occurred, fell to 8 cmH$_2$O. The patient's temperature was 37°C.

No further hypotensive event occurred and no further ventilation was required, although the endotracheal tube was not removed until

Table 3.9 Blood pH, 'standard bicarbonate', PCO_2, PO_2, plasma [K$^+$] and tidal volume in a 46-year-old woman following mitral valve replacement

	pH	St. bic.	PCO$_2^*$	PO$_2$	[K$^+$]	Tidal volume
Post operation, before disconnection from ventilator	7.39	23.4	39	380	4.2	500
Just before fall in blood pressure	7.21	17.4	42	96	4.6	115
During infusion of 4.2% NaHCO$_3$	7.58	29.8	33	180		650
After infusion of 4.2% NaHCO$_3$	7.42	28.2	40	120		450

pH = Blood pH at 37°C.
St. bic. = Standard bicarbonate in mmol/l (mEq/l).
PCO_2 = CO$_2$ tension in mmHg.
PO_2 = O$_2$ tension in mmHg.
[K$^+$] = Potassium concentration in mmol/l (mEq/l).
Tidal volume = Volume of air (gas) in ml measured by a Wright respirometer.
*Early intervention and ventilation of the lungs with an Ambu bag prevented the PCO_2 from rising to a high value.

the following morning. Urine output, which had decreased just prior to the hypotensive episode, returned to the expected excretion pattern.

Treatment of acid–base changes

Metabolic alkalosis

It is rarely necessary to use ammonium chloride to correct a metabolic alkalosis. In some cases of high gut obstruction with infection, or dilation of the stomach, the loss of chloride in the large volume of fluid, lost either by vomit or aspiration, may be so much greater than the sodium loss, that ammonium chloride infusions may be required.

However, we have seen how metabolic alkalosis does occur in the presence of abnormal liver function In these circumstances hepatic coma may be precipitated by the infusion of the ammonium salt and care must be taken to avoid this hazard. KCl, 20 mmol/hour (mEq/hour) should be infused in 0.9% NaCl.

Arginine HCl infusions may be used, but they may give rise to hyperkalaemia (see p. 38). Infusion of HCl can also be given in a 0.15 normal solution at 125 ml/hour.[2,16,61,127] Theoretically, hyperkalaemia could occur with infusions of HCl if renal function is impaired. Rowlands *et al.* have used dilute HCl with intravenous cimetidine to suppress gastric HCl secretion.[104]

When the associated potassium deficiency has been corrected together with adequate hydration and sodium chloride administration, it is possible to tide over most cases until a situation close to normality is reached and the patient is fit for surgery.

Metabolic acidosis

The best and most natural solution to use is sodium bicarbonate and the strength of solution will depend upon the condition being treated. In the grossly dehydrated diabetic coma it is usually advisable to use the isotonic solution. The safest and most universally applicable solution in medicine and surgical practice is that which has twice the osmolality of plasma, a 2.74% solution. Gross excess of both fluid and bicarbonate can then be avoided and, as a metabolic acidosis is so often associated with dehydration and sodium depletion, the latter can be repaired without greatly increasing the former.

In extracorporeal circulations the more hypertonic solutions of 4.2% and 8.4% have been used successfully. The 8.4% solution contains $NaHCO_3$ 1 mmol/ml (mEq/ml).

Sodium lactate does not alter the pH of blood when it is infused for some hours, because a considerable time is required before it is converted to bicarbonate and is able to raise the concentration of this anion in the plasma.

Estimation of $NaHCO_3$ requirements

We have seen that when a metabolic acidosis is present the base deficit found in the plasma reflects that which has appeared throughout the whole body. Because of this a total correction of a base deficit has to be based on total body water, i.e. the number of millimoles (milliequivalents) required = 0.6 × body weight (in kg) × base deficit (in mmol/l). For example, a 50-kg patient was found to have a total CO_2 content of 16 mmol/l (mEq/l), a blood pH of 7.08 at 38°C and a PCO_2 of 50 mmHg. The $[HCO_3^-]$ (PCO_2 × 0.0301, subtracted from the total CO_2) was 14.5 mmol/l (mEq/l).

The number of millimoles (milliequivalents) required by the patient

$$= (0.6 \times 50) \times (25 - 14.5) = 30 \times 10.5 = 315 \text{ mmol (mEq)}$$

A 2.74% solution of $NaHCO_3$ contains 166 mmol/500 ml (33 mmol/100 ml). It was necessary, therefore, to infuse 1 litre of this solution over a period of 3 hours. In conditions such as cardiac arrest, a much faster rate is necessary.

It is wrong to believe that the accurate titration of a metabolic acidosis in an individual patient is always possible, or indeed necessary. Much depends upon whether the abnormal process which is producing the metabolic acidosis is continuing, improving or becoming worse. It must be remembered that a measurement depicts only the conditions prevailing at that time and, therefore, the very nature of the disease process will also determine the rate at which infusions of sodium bicarbonate are made. Because the equilibration of the HCO_3^- between the extracellular fluid space and the cells is slow, sodium bicarbonate is initially confined to the ECF and because of this, high concentrations of sodium bicarbonate will be found after a relatively small infusion. As a result of these raised plasma HCO_3^- levels, myocardial and respiratory function may improve enormously, so that the oxygenation of the blood and perfusion of tissues are increased and the conditions which were producing the metabolic acidosis are reversed. In this way, spontaneous correction of the metabolic acidosis occurs. A marked improvement in the acid–base state may, therefore, often be observed after a relatively small infusion of alkali, but in very severe disease processes or where abnormal physiological conditions have prevailed for a considerable period, a very large infusion may be needed before any improvement is obtained. For these reasons it is probable that formulae which are based on correction of the metabolic acidosis with smaller volumes of sodium bicarbonate, such as that which would correct the deficit of base within the extracellular fluid space alone, are frequently effective, because of high $[HCO_3^-]$ produced in blood which follows the initial infusion. Mellemgård and Astrup[91] established that for man the number of milliequivalents required = $(0.3 \times body\ weight) \times (the\ base\ deficit)$. Without doubt, this quantity is essentially correct for a rapid infusion, but clinicians must be prepared to give greater amounts of alkali as time progresses and these amounts approach a figure based upon 60–70% or more of body weight.

It can be readily appreciated that in the case of phenformin lactacidosis (see p. 87) estimations based on the extracellular fluid volume would be quite inadequate for treatment. This is also true for some cases of diabetic ketosis. Ideally, correction of abnormalities of the acid–base state can only be made in the light of repeated measurements of pH, $[HCO_3^-]$ and PCO_2. The most common fault is to give insufficient treatment, especially in the adult; these measurements become more necessary when a patient is being artifically ventilated. In the absence of artificial ventilation, when a solution which has twice the osmolality of plasma is used (2.74% $NaHCO_3$), excessive quantities are rarely given.

Respiratory alkalosis

The treatment of a spontaneous respiratory alkalosis rests in treating the underlying cause, but prolonged spontaneous hyperventilation is in general a bad prognostic sign.

A gross respiratory alkalosis produced by unusually great hyperventilation during anaesthesia may produce arrhythmias and a fall in blood pressure.

Gross hyperventilation during anaesthesia may produce a metabolic acidosis and the origin of this is almost certainly an impaired cardiac output as a result of either obstructed venous return or the impairment of myocardial contraction.

Contrary to general acceptance, the loss of large quantities of bicarbonate in the urine is not a constant feature of respiratory alkalosis.

Respiratory acidosis

Because respiratory depression is caused by a high alveolar CO_2 tension (PCO_2) and can occur in the absence of anoxia by rebreathing carbon dioxide contained within an anaesthetic circuit, high flows of gas (e.g. in excess of 11 litre/min)[89] and hyperventilation are necessary to remove the accumulated CO_2.

When it is consequent upon a metabolic acidosis, the underlying base deficit must be treated with sodium bicarbonate and the period during which artificial ventilation has to be performed may be shortened. When CO_2 is retained because of lung pathology and insufficient time has passed for naturally occurring compensation to be developed by the retention of HCO_3^- by the renal tubules, infusions of $NaHCO_3$ may be necessary (see p. 130). In this way 'artificial compensation' is performed.

THAM (Tris hydroxymethyl amino-methane)

The buffer THAM (Nahas, 1959, 1962)[96,97] has been used with success in the presence of a respiratory and metabolic acidosis, but care has to be taken to maintain ventilation.

Although THAM is a substitute for sodium bicarbonate, it has different characteristics:

Methane   THAM

It can pass into the cells and become an intracellular buffer. In some circumstances this may be beneficial, but in others it can disturb enzyme action. Although it has been used successfully in clinial medicine in many different types of cases, its superiority to the readily available natural substance $NaHCO_3$ has not yet been confirmed.

Hyperventilation as a cause of lactate production

Voluntary hyperventilation in man can give rise to increased lactate production.[20,51] It can also be produced by passive hyperventilation in anaesthetized dogs[7,18,30,31,50,116,117,131] and in man.[34,99] Lactate production associated with a rise in blood lactate concentration occurs when hyperventilation is used, especially in the hypothermic patient or animal. It has been demonstrated that patients can be anaesthetized by hyperventilation alone following induction with anaesthetic in the normal way.

The mechanism by which lactate production occurs is interesting and can be due to more than one factor: (a) positive pressure ventilation alone can cause a fall in cardiac output and thus induce poor tissue perfusion, (b) the fall in PCO_2 associated with hyperventilation can produce impaired myocardial function so that there is a fall in cardiac output and thus a fall in blood pressure (see p. 97), and this is more likely to occur following and during hypothermia when endogenous CO_2 production is reduced. Hypotension can, however, occur at normal body temperature.

Certainly, it has been demonstrated that breathing 5% CO_2 during hyperventilation prevents the development of the lactacidaemia.[50,71] If CO_2 is added to the inspired gases, the lactacidaemia is reversed [131] and the author has demonstrated this in both animals and man following hypotension that has developed postoperatively in the hypothermic dog and patients.

Case history. A 12-year-old boy was operated upon for a ventricular septal defect (VSD) and the operation went well until the time came for the patient to be disconnected from the heart–lung bypass. Attempts to continue the operation on 'partial bypass' resulted in a fall in blood pressure so that the occlusive tapes around the canuli in the superior and inferior venae cavae had to be placed once again under tension. A blood sample taken at that time demonstrated a normal bicarbonate ion concentration (23.8 mmol/l) a high pH 7.56 and a low PCO_2. The rectal temperature of the patient, although reduced to approximately 32°C during the bypass, had now returned to 37.5°C. The PCO_2 was only 24 mmHg.

The patient was once again separated from the heart–lung bypass and carbon dioxide was added to the anaesthetic gases. This resulted in an almost immediate rise in blood pressure and the patient was disconnected from the heart–lung bypass without difficulty. Lactate concentration at that time was found to be 10.5 mmol/l. When measured 30 minutes after separation from the heart–lung apparatus, the level had fallen to 5.8 mmol/l.

From these figures it appears that the cause of the low cardiac output and impaired myocardial function was hypocapnoea and that this alone appeared to be the cause of the hypotension.

It should be noted that the lactacidaemia and metabolic acidosis produced by hyperventilation can give rise to the syndrome described on p. 134 so that hypoventilation and hypotension occur simultaneously.

The case described above demonstrates the importance of maintaining a normal acid–base state and that hyperventilation alone cannot compensate for a metabolic acidosis. It is only one of many cases that have been observed by the author, and only careful measurement and clinical observation prevent physiological changes occurring due to abnormalities, in this complex field of medical practice.

Acid–base balance is of immense clinical importance in medicine. It has its own characteristic physical signs, but they have no firm correlation with mathematical reasoning. When the acid–base state of the body is carefully measured and correction carefully applied, it results in a reduced morbidity and often the difference between life and death.

References

1. Aberman, A. and Fulop, M. (1972). The metabolic and respiratory acidosis of acute pulmonary oedema. *Ann. Int. Med.*, **76**, 173.
2. Abouna, G. M., Veatey, P. R. and Terry, D. B. (1974). Intravenous infusion of hydrochloric acid for treatment of severe metabolic alkalosis. *Surgery*, **75**, 194.
3. Agostini, A. (1967). Acid–base disturbances in pulmonary oedema. *Arch. Int. Med.*, **120**, 307.
4. Alberti, K. G. M. M., Corbett, J., Hockaday, T. D. R. and Williamson, D. H. (1971). Lactic acidosis. *Brit. med. J.*, **1**, 47.
5. Andersen, O. S. and Engel, K. (1960). A new acid–base nomogram. An improved method for the calculation of the relevant blood acid–base data. *Scand. J. clin. Lab. Invest.*, **12**, 177.
6. Anderson, J. and Mazza, R. (1963). Pyruvate and lactate excretion in patients with diabetes mellitus and benign glycosuria. *Lancet*, **ii**, 270.
7. Anrep, G. V. and Cannan, R. K. (1923). The concentration of lactic acid in the blood in experimental alkalaemia and acidaemia. *J. Physiol.*, **58**, 244.
8. Arieff, A. I. and Carroll, H. J. (1972). Non-ketotic hyperosomolar coma with hyperglycaemia; clinical features, pathophysiology, renal function acid–base balance, plasma-cerebrospinal fluid equilibria and the effects of therapy in 37 cases. *Medicine*, **51**, 73.
9. Assan, R., Heuclin, C., Girard, J. R. and Attali, J. R. (1977). Metformin-induced lactic acidosis in the presence of acute renal failure. *Diabetologia*, **13**, 211.
10. Assan, R., Heuclin, C., Girard, J. R., LeMaire, F. and Attali, J. R. (1975). Phenformin-induced lactic

acidosis in diabetic patients. *Diabetes*, **24**, 791.

11. Astrup, P. (1954). Om erkendelsen af forstyrrelser i organismens syre-base-stofskifte. *Ugeskr. f. Laeger*, **116**, 758.

12. Astrup, P. (1956). A simple electrometric technique for the determination of carbon dioxide tension in blood and plasma, total content of carbon dioxide in plasma, and bicarbonate content in 'separated' plasma at a fixed carbon dioxide tension (40 mmHg). *Scand. J. clin. Lab. Invest.*, **8**, 33.

13. Astrup, P., Jørgensen, K., Andersen, O. S. and Engel, K. (1960). The acid–base metabolism: a new approach. *Lancet*, **i**, 1035.

14. Avery, W. G., Samet, P. and Sackner, M. A. (1970). The acidosis of pulmonary oedema. *Amer. J. Med.*, **48**, 320.

15. Barnardo, D. E., Cohen, R. D. and Iles, R. A. (1970). 'Idiopathic' lactic and beta-hydroxybutyric acidosis. *Brit. med. J.*, **4**, 348.

16. Beach, F. X. M. and Jones, E. S. (1971). Metabolic alkalosis treated with intravenous hydrochloric acid. *Postgrad. med. J.*, **47**, 516.

17. Beatty, C. H. (1945). The effect of hemorrhage on the lactate/pyruvate ratio and arterio-venous differences in glucose and lactate. *Amer. J. Physiol.*, **143**, 579.

18. Berry, H. N. and Scheuer, J. (1967). Splanchnic lactic acid metabolism in hyperventilation, metabolic alkalosis and shock. *Metabolism*, **16**, 537.

19. Blume, R. S., MacLowry, J. D. and Wolff, S. M. (1968). Limitations of chloride determination in the diagnosis of bromism. *N. Engl. J. of med.*, **279**, 593.

20. Bock, A. V., Dill, D. B. and Edwards, H. T. (1932). Lactic acid in the blood of resting man. *J. clin. Invest.*, **11**, 775.

21. Boyd, J. D. (1931). Chronic acidosis secondary to ureteral transplantation. *Amer. J. Dis. Child.*, **42**, 366.

22. Brewin, E. G., Gould, R. P., Nashat, F. S. and Neil, E. (1955). An investigation of problems of acid–base equilibrium in hypothermia. *Guy's Hosp. Rep.*, **104**, 177.

23. Broder, G. and Weil, M. H. (1964). Excess lactate: An index of reversibility of shock in human patients. *Science*, **143**, 1457.

24. Brönsted, J. N. (1923). Einige Bemerkungen über den Begriff der Säuren und Basen. *Rec. Trav. chim. Pays-Bas*, **42**, 718.

25. Brooks, D. K. (1964). Osmolar, electrolyte and respiratory changes in hemorrhagic shock. *Amer. Heart J.*, **68**, 574.

26. Brooks, D. K. (1965). Physiological responses produced by changes in acid–base equilibrium following profound hypothermia. *Anaesthesia*, **20**, 173.

27. Brooks, D. K. and Feldman, S. A. (1962). Metabolic acidosis: a new approach to 'neostigmine resistant curarisation'. *Anaesthesia*, **17**, 161.

28. Brooks, D. K., Williams, W. G., Manley, R. W. and Whiteman, P. (1963). Respiratory changes in haemorrhagic shock. *Anaesthesia*, **18**, 363.

29. Brooks, D. K. and Wynn, V. (1959). Use of venous blood for pH and carbon dioxide studies especially in respiratory failure and during anaesthesia. *Lancet*, **i**, 227.

30. Cain, S. M. (1965). Appearance of excess lactate in anaesthetized dogs during anaemic and hypoxic hypoxia. *Amer. J. Physiol.*, **209**, 604.

31. Cain, S. M. (1968). Effect of PCO_2 on the relation of lactate and excess lactate to O_2 deficit. *Amer. J. Physiol.*, **214**, 1322.

32. Cannon, W. B. (1918). Acidosis in cases of shock, hemorrhage and gas infection. *J. Amer. med. Ass.*, **70**, 531.

33. Cannon, W. W. B. and Bayliss, W. M. (1919). Note on muscle injury in relation to shock. In Reports of the Special Investigation Committee on Surgical Shock and Allied Conditions. *Spec. Rep. Ser. med. Res. Coun. (Lond.)*, **26**, 19.

34. Chamberlain, J. H. and Lis, M. T. (1968). Observations of blood lactate and pyruvate levels and excess lactate production during and after anaesthesia with and without hyperventilation. *Brit. J. Anaesth.*, **40**, 315.

35. Clarke, L. C. Jr. (1956). Monitor and control of blood and tissue oxygen tensions. *Trans. Am. Soc. Artif. Int. Organs*, **2**, 41.

36. Clausen, S. W. (1925). Anhydremic acidosis due to lactic acid. *Amer. J. Dis. Child.*, **29**, 761.

37. Clowes, G. H. A., Alichniewicz, A., Del Guercio, L. R. M. and Gillespie, D. (1960). The relationship of postoperative acidosis to pulmonary and cardiovascular function. *J. thorac. cardiovasc. Surg.*, **39**, 1.

38. Cohen, R. D. and Simpson, R. (1975). Lactate metabolism. *Anesthesiology*, **43**, 661.

39. Cohen, R. D. and Woods, H. F. (1976). *Clinical and Biochemical Aspects of Lactic Acidosis*. Oxford: Blackwell.

40. Conley, L. A. and Loewenstein, J. E. (1976). Phenformin and lactic acidosis. *J. Amer. med. Assoc.*, **235**, 1575.

41. Cook, L. C. and Hurst, R. H. (1933). Blood lactic acid in man during rest. *J. Physiol.*, **79**, 443.

42. Cournand, A., Riley, R. L., Bradley, S. E., Breed, E. S., Bobel, R. O., Lauson, H. D., Gregersen, M. I. and Richards, D. W. (1943). Studies of circulation in clinical shock. *Surgery*, **13**, 964.

43. Cowan, R. A., Hartnell, G. G., Lowdell, C. P., McLean Baird, I. and Leak, A. M. (1984). Metabolic acidosis induced by carbonic anhydrase inhibitors and salicylates in patients with normal renal function. *Brit. med. J.*, **289**, 347.

44. Cruz, W. O., Baumgarten, A. and Oliveira, A. C. (1954). Objective evaluation of intensity of shock induced by antiplatelet serum in dog. *Amer. J. Physiol.*, **177**, 515.

45. Cubberley, P. T., Polster, S. A. and Schulman, C. L. (1965). Lactic acidosis and death after the treatment of obesity by fasting. *N. Engl. J. of Med.*, **272**, 628.

46. Cunningham, J. S. and Hilton, P. J. (1964). Bicarbonate therapy in diabetic acidosis. *Lancet*, **ii**, 758.

47. Daughaday, W. H., Lipicky, R. J. and Rasinski, D. C. (1962). Lactic acidosis as a cause of non-ketotic acidosis in diabetic patients. *N. Engl. J. of Med.*, **267**, 1010.

48. Davidson, M. B., Bozarth, W. R., Challoner, D. R., Goodner, C. J. (1966). Phenformin, hypoglycemia, and lactic acidosis. *N. Engl. J. of Med.*, **275**, 886.

49. Eggletone, M. G. and Evans, C. L. (1930). Lactic acid formation and removal with change of blood reaction. *J. Physiol.*, **70**, 261.

50. Eichenholz, A., Mulhausen, R. O., Anderson, W. E. and MacDonald, F. M. (1962). Primary hypocapnia; a cause of metabolic acidosis. *J. appl. Physiol.*, **17**, 283.

51. Eldridge, F. and Salzer, F. (1966). Effect of respiratory alkalosis on blood lactate and pyruvate in humans. *J. appl. Physiol.*, **22**, 461.

52. Emmett, M. and Narins, R. G. (1976). Hypermagnesaemia and hypotension. *Ann. Int. Med.*, **84**, 340. (Letter.)

53. Emmett, M. and Narins, R. G. (1977). Clinical use of the anion gap. *Medicine*, **56**, 38.

54. Ferris, D. O. and Odel, H. M. (1950). Electrolyte pattern of the blood after bilateral uretero-sigmoid-ostomy. *J. Amer. med. Ass.*, **142**, 634.

55. Friedemann, T. E., Haugen, C. E. and Kmieciak, T. C. (1945). Pyruvic Acid III. The level of pyruvic and lactic acids, and the lactic–pyruvic ratio, in the blood of human subjects. The effect of food, light muscular activity, and anoxia at high altitude. *J. Biol. Chem.*, **157**, 673.

56. Fulop, M., Harowitz, M., Aberman, A. and Jaffe, E. R. (1973). Lactic acidosis in pulmonary oedema due to left ventricular failure. *Ann. Int. Med.*, **79**, 180.

57. Fulop, M. and Hoberman, H. D. (1976). Phenformin-associated metabolic acidosis. *Diabetes*, **25**, 292.

58. Gevers, W. and Dowdle, E. (1963). The effect of pH on glycolysis *in vitro*. *Clin. Sci.*, **25**, 343.

59. Griffith, K. K., McKenzie, M. B., Peterson, W. E. and Keyes, J. K. (1983). Mixed venous blood gas composition in experimentally induced acid–base disturbances. *Heart and Lung*, **12**, 581.

60. Haldi, J. (1933). Lactic acid in blood and tissues following intravenous injection of sodium bicarbonate. *Amer. J. Physiol.*, **106**, 134.

61. Harken, A. H., Gabel, R. A., Fencl, V. and Moore, F. D. (1975). Hydrochloric acid in the correction of metabolic alkalosis. *Arch. Surg.*, **110**, 819.

62. Hartman, A. F. (1935). Treatment of severe diabetic acidosis. *Arch. Int. Med.*, **56**, 413.

63. Hasselbalch, K. A. (1916). Die Berechnung der Wasserstoffzahl des Blutes aus der freien und gebundenen Kohlensäure desselben, und die Sauerstoffbindung des Blutes als Funktion der Wasserstoffzahl. *Biochem. Z.*, **78**, 112.

64. Hasselbalch, K. A. (1916). Die 'reduzierte' und die 'regulierte' Wasserstoffzahl des Blutes. *Biochem. Z.*, **74**, 56.

65. Hasselbalch, K. A. (1917). Die Berechnung der Wasserstoffzahl des Blutes aus der freien und gebundenen Kohlensäure desselben, und die Sauerstoffbindung des Blutes als Funktion der Wasserstoffzahl. *Biochem. Z.*, **78**, 112.

66. Henderson, L. J. (1908). Concerning the relationship between the strength of acids and their capacity to preserve neutrality. *Amer. J. Physiol.*, **21**, 173.

67. Henderson, L. J. (1908). The theory of neutrality regulation in the animal organism. *Amer. J. Physiol.*, **21**, 427.

68. Henderson, L. J. and Haggard, H. W. (1918). Respiratory regulation of the CO_2 capacity of the blood. 111. The effects of excessive pulmonary ventilation. *J. Biol. Chem.*, **33**, 355.

69. Hockaday, T. D. R. and Alberti, K. G. M. M. (1972). Diabetic coma. *Clinics in Endocrinology and Metabolism*, **1:3**, 751.

70. Hopkins, R. W., Satga, G., Penn, I. and Simeone, F. A. (1965). Hemodynamic aspects of hemorrhagic and septic shock. *J. Amer. med. Assoc.*, **191**, 731.

71. Huckabee, W. E. (1958). Relationship of pyruvate and lactate during anaerobic metabolism. Effects of infusion of pyruvate or glucose and hyperventilation. *J. clin. Invest.*, **37**, 244.

72. Huckabee, W. E. (1961). Abnormal resting blood lactate. 2. Lactic acidosis. *Amer. J. Med.*, **30**, 840.

73. Huckabee, W. E. (1965). Metabolic consequences of chronic hypoxia. *Ann. N.Y. Acad. Sci.*, **121**, 723.

74. Irvine, W. T., Yule, D. H., Arnott, D. G. and Peruma, C. (1961). Reduction in colonic mucosal absorption with reference to the chemical imbalance of uretero-colostomy. *Brit. J. Urol.*, **33**, 1.

75. Jervell, O. (1928). Investigation of the concentration of lactic acid in blood and urine under physiologic and pathologic conditions. *Acta. med. Scand.*, **24** (Suppl.), 1.

76. Jewett, H. J. (1940). Uretero-intestinal implantation: preliminary report. *J. Urol. (Baltimore)*, **44**, 223.

77. Jewett, H. J. (1944). Uretero-intestinal anastomosis in two stages for cancer of the bladder: modification of original technique and report of 33 cases. *J. Urol. (Baltimore)*, **52**, 536.

78. Johnson, H. K. and Waterhouse, C. (1968). Lactic acidosis and phenformin. *Arch. Int. Med.*, **122**, 367.

79. Jørgensen, K. and Astrup, P. (1957). Standard bicarbonate, its clinical significance, and a new method for its determination. *Scan. J. clin. Lab. Invest.*, **9**, 122.

80. Kenyon, J. R., Ludbrook, J., Downs, A. R., Tait, I. B., Brooks, D. K. and Pryczkowski, J. (1959). Experimental deep hypothermia. *Lancet*, **ii**, 41.

81. Kreisberg, R. A., Crawford Owen, W. and Siegal, A. M. (1971). Ethanol-induced hyperlacticacidemia: Inhibition of lactate utilization. *J. of clin. Invest.*, **50**, 166.

82. Kussmaul, A. (1874). Zur Lehre vom Diabetes mellitus. *Dtsch. Arch. Klin. Med.*, **14**, 1.

83. Litwin, M. S., Panico, F. G., Rubini, C., Harken, D. E. and Moore, F. D. (1959). Acidosis and lactic-acidaemia in extracorporeal circulation. The significance of perfusion flow rates and the relation to preperfusion respiratory alkalosis. *Ann. Surg.*, **149**, 188.

84. Loubatieres, A., Ribes, G., Blayac, J. P. and Valette, G. (1973). Effects of exogenous and endogenous insulin on phenformin-induced experimental hyperlactacidaemia in the dog. *J. Annu. Diabetol. Hotel Dieu*, **3**, 225.

85. Lowry, T. M. (1923). The uniqueness of hydrogen. *Chem. Ind.*, **1**, 43.

86. MacLean, L. D., Mulligan, W. G., McLean, A. P. H. and Duff, J. H. (1967). Patterns of septic shock in man—A detailed study of 56 patients. *Ann. Surg.*, **166**, 543.

87. Macleod, J. J. R. and Hoover, D. H. (1917). Studies in experimental glycosuria XII. Lactic acid production in the blood following the injection of alkaline solutions of dextrose or of alkaline solutions alone. *Amer. J. Physiol.*, **42**, 460.

88. Majoor, C. L. H. (1978). Alcoholism as a cause of beri-beri heart disease. *J. R. Coll. Phys.*, **12**, 143.

89. Mapleson, W. W. (1954). The elimination of rebreathing in various semi-closed anaesthetic systems. *Brit. J. Anaesth.*, **26**, 323.

90. Marliss, E. B., Ohman, J. L., Aoki, T. T. and Kozak, G. P. (1970). Altered redox state obscuring ketoacidosis in diabetic patients with lactic acidosis. *N. Engl. J. of Med.*, **283**, 978.

91. Mellemgärd, K. and Astrup, P. (1960). The quantitative determination of surplus amounts of acid or base in the human body. *Scand. J. clin. Lab. Invest.*, **12**, 187.

92. Mikulski, S. M. (1976). Anion gap and myeloma (letter). *N. Engl. J. of Med.* **294**, 111.

93. Mithoefer, J. C., Runser, R. H. and Karetzki, M. S. (1965). The use of sodium bicarbonate in the treatment of acute bronchial asthma. *N. Engl. J. of Med.*, **272**, 1200.

94. Moorhouse, J. A. (1964). Pyruvate-tolerance tests in healthy and diabetic subjects. *Lancet*, **i**, 689.

95. Murray, T., Long, W. and Narins, R. G. (1975). Multiple myeloma and the anion gap. *N. Engl. J. of Med.*, **292**, 574.

96. Nahas, G. G. (1959). Use of an organic carbon dioxide buffer *in vivo*. *Science*, **129**, 782.

97. Nahas, G. G. (1962). The pharmacology of tris (hydroxymethyl) aminomethane (THAM). *Pharmacol. Rev.*, **14**, 447.

98. Oliva, P. B. (1970). Lactic acidosis. *Amer. J. Med.*, **48**, 209.

99. Papadopoulos, C. N. and Keats, A. S. (1959). The metabolic acidosis of hyperventilation produced by controlled respiration. *Anesthesiology*, **20**, 156.

100. Peretz, D. I., McGregor, M. and Dossetor, J. E. (1964). Lactic acidosis: a clinically significant aspect of shock. *Canad. med. Assoc. J.*, **90**, 673.

101. Peretz, D. I., Scott, H. M., Duff, J., Dossetor, J. E., MacLean, L. D. and McGregor, M. (1965). The significance of lactacidaemia in the shock syndrome. *Ann. N.Y. Acad. Sci.*, **119**, 1133.

102. Peters, J. P. and Van Slyke, D. D. (1932). *Quantitative clinical chemistry II.* Baltimore: Williams & Wilkins.

103. Phillipson, E. A. and Sproule, B. J. (1965). The clinical significance of elevated blood lactate. *Canad. med. Assoc. J.*, **92**, 1334.

104. Rowlands, B. J., Tindael, S. F. and Elliot, D. J. (1978). The use of dilute hydrochloric acid and cimetidine to reverse severe metabolic alkalosis. *Postgrad. med. J.*, **54**, 118.

105. Ruggles, T. N., Lavietes, M. H., Miller, M., Woodward, H. and Treister, M. (1968). Effect of phenformin on the elevated blood lactic acid produced by hypoxia in normal and diabetic rats. *Ann. N. Y. Acad. Sci.*, **148**, 662.

106. Schnur, M. J., Appel, G. B., Karp, G. and Osserman, E. P. (1977). The anion gap in asymptomatic plasma cell dyscrasias. *Ann. Int. Med.*, **86**, 304.

107. Scurr, C. F. (1956). Pulmonary ventilation and carbon dioxide levels during anaesthesia. *Brit. J. Anaesth.*, **28**, 422.

108. Searle, G. L. and Siperstein, M. D. (1975). Lactic acidosis associated with phenformin therapy. *Diabetes*, **24**, 741.

109. Seligman, A. M., Frank, H. A., Alexander, B. and Fine, J. (1947). Traumatic shock. XV. Carbohydrate metabolism in hemorrhagic shock in the dog. *J. clin. Invest.*, **26**, 536.

110. Siggaard-Andersen, O. (1974). *The Acid–Base Status of the Blood*, 4th edn. Copenhagen: Munksgaard.

111. Singer, R. B. and Hastings, A. B. (1948). An improved clinical method for the estimation of disturbances of the acid–base balance of human blood. *Medicine (Baltimore)*, **27**, 223.

112. Sørensen, S. P. L. (1912). Über die Messung und Bedeutung der Wasserstoffionen-konzentration bei biologischen Prozessen. *Ergebn. Physiol.*, **12**, 393.

113. Strauss, F. G. and Sullivan, M. A. (1971). Phenformin intoxication resulting in lactic acidosis. *Johns Hopkins med J.*, **128**, 278.

114. Strauss, J., Fine, R. M., Medina, D. A. and Donnell, J. M. (1966). The use of THAM in the treatment of status asthmaticus. *Paediatrics.*, **28**, 655.

115. Sussman, K. E., Alfrey, A., Kirsch, W. M., Zweig, P., Felig, P. and Messner, F. (1970). Chronic lactic acidosis in an adult. A new syndrome associated with an altered redox state of certain NAD/NADH coupled reactions. *Amer. J. Med.*, **48**, 104.

116. Takano, N. (1966). Blood lactate accumulation and its causative factors during passive hyperventilation in dogs. *Jap. J. Physiol.*, **16**, 481.

117. Takano, N. (1968). Role of hypocapnia in the blood lactate accumulation during acute hypoxia. *Resp.*

Physiol., **4**, 32.

118. Tobin, R. B. (1964). *In vivo* influences of hydrogen ions on lactate and pyruvate of blood. *Amer. J. Physiol.*, **207**, 601.

119. Tranquada, R. E., Grant, W. J. and Peterson, C. R. (1966). Lactic acidosis. *Arch. Int. Med.*, **117**, 192.

120. Van Slyke, D. D. and Cullen, G. E. (1917). Studies of acidosis. 1. The bicarbonate concentration of the blood plasma: its significance and its determination as a measure of acidosis. *J. Biol. Chem.*, **30**, 289.

121. Van Slyke, D. D., Hastings, A. B., Heidelberger, M. and Neill, J. M. (1922). Studies of gas and electrolyte equilibria in the blood. *J. Biol. Chem.*, **54**, 481.

122. Van Slyke, D. D. and Neill, J. M. (1924). The determination of gases in blood and other solutions by vacuum extraction and manometric measurement. *J. Biol. Chem.*, **61**, 523.

123. Varma, S. K., Heaney, S. J., Whyte, W. G. and Walker, R. S. (1972). Hyperlactataemia in phenformin-treated diabetes. *Brit. med. J.*, **1**, 205.

124. Waters, W. C., Hall, J. D. and Schwartz, W. R. (1963). Spontaneous lactic acidosis. The nature of the acid–base disturbance and considerations on diagnosis and management. *Amer. J. Med.*, **35**, 781.

125. Watkins, P. J., Smith, J. S., Fitzgerald, M. G. and Malins, J. M. (1969). Lactic acidosis in diabetes. *Brit. med. J.*, **1**, 744.

126. Whitehead, T. P. (1965). Acid–base status, pH and PCO_2. *Lancet*, **ii**, 1015.

127. Williams, D. B. and Lyons, J. H. (1980). Treatment of severe metabolic alkalosis with intravenous infusion of hydrochloric acid. *Surg. Gynecol. & Obstet.*, **150**, 315.

128. Williamson, D. H., Lund, P. and Krebs, H. A. (1967). The redox state of free nicotinamide–adenine dinucleotide in the cytoplasm and mitochondria of rat liver. *Biochem. J.*, **103**, 514.

129. Wise, P. H., Chapman, M., Thomas, D. W., Clarkson, A. R., Harding, P. E. and Edwards, J. B. (1976). Phenformin and lactic acidosis. *Brit. med. J.*, **1**, 70.

130. Wrong, O. M. and Feest, T. G. (1981). Renal tubular acidosis. *N. Engl. J. of Med.*, **304**, 1548.

131. Zborowska-Sluis, D. T. and Dossetor, J. B. (1967). Hyperlactataemia of hyperventilation. *J. appl. Physiol.*, **22**, 746.

132. Zimmet, P. Z., Taft, P., Ennis, G. C. and Sheath, J. (1970). Acid production in diabetic acidosis: a more rational approach to alkali replacement. *Brit. med. J.*, **3**, 610.

Chapter 4
Acute Renal Failure

Oliguria and its Causes

This condition may follow any operative procedure or the processes of resuscitation of any origin. Each patient behaves differently, requires individual treatment and represents a new challenge. In most cases recovery can only be assured by the application of modern techniques, careful clinical and biochemical assessment and accuracy in all measurements. Acute renal failure rarely leads to complete anuria. Total absence of urine only occurs when there is mechanical obstruction. It is therefore essential that this condition should be defined in a recognizable form, as failure to appreciate the consequences of the altered body function may lead to early death or, at the very best, hamper treatment in the later stages. In health the normal output of urine varies between 1 and 2 litres per day; on a mixed diet it is obligatory to pass a minimum of approximately 500 ml in 24 hours. This entails perfect renal function and implies the ability to concentrate urine fully to a maximum specific gravity in the region of 1.030 (1155–1300 mosmol/l).

Oliguria has been defined as an output of urine of less than 700 ml in 24 hours. Where good renal function is present, the urine passed will be concentrated sufficiently to produce a specific gravity of 1.018 (595 mosmol/l) or more. When renal damage is present so that there is tubular malfunction, urine of low specific gravity will be passed; the specific gravity of such urine will be 1.008–1.014 (265–460 mosmol/l).

Severe oliguria may be defined as a urine output of 500 ml or less in 24 hours and, when the specific gravity of this urine is low, this will lead to a marked rise in the blood urea concentration. When there is a urine output of 300 ml or less, the kidneys will be unable to keep pace with the production of metabolites, and biochemical abnormalities will rapidly become manifest. Sometimes this condition is referred to as 'anuria by definition', but it is probably preferable to retain the term 'severe oliguria' and to quote the volume of urine voided so that assessment of the degree of severity can be made. The object of all treatment in oliguria and anuria is to tide the patient over until the kidneys have had time to recover their function. At this time, it is largely true to say that the suppression of urine output resulting from malignant hypertension, chronic nephritis and polycystic kidneys, which develops into oliguria and the comparatively rare condition of bilateral cortical necrosis is, in the main, not reversible. The treatment of this condition now rests solely on the developments in the field of renal transplant.

The reversible causes of acute suppression of urine are listed below.

1. Mechanical: obstruction of the ureters by operative procedures, bilateral renal calculi, carcinoma of the prostate or cervix and procedentia.
2. Dehydration and electrolyte depletion (e.g. the low salt syndrome (see p. 24), pre-renal azotaemia).
3. Tubular necrosis (lower nephron nephrosis) such as that which follows gross dehydration, prolonged hypotension, abortion, separation of the placenta (toxic and non-toxic accidental haemorrhage), haemorrhagic shock, crush syndrome, mismatched blood transfusions, and nephrotoxins (e.g. mercuric chloride, bismuth and sulphonamides).
4. Acute nephritis.
5. Low cardiac output and hypovolaemia (Table 4.1).

Differentiation Between Pre-Renal Azotaemia and Acute Renal Failure

The clinician is frequently faced with the problem of differentiating between oliguria, which is easily

Table 4.1 Conditions giving rise to acute renal failure

Hypovolaemic shock	Haemorrhage Burns Pancreatitis Dehydration Acute obstruction of the gut Peritonitis
Normovolaemic shock	Cardiogenic Neurogenic Toxic
Cardiovascular	Myocardial infarction Pulmonary embolism Aortic aneurysm Aortic dissection Hypertension[57] Surgery[16,26,46,48,56,61,77] Low flow perfusion with acidosis[2,59]
Septicaemia	Perforation of the gut Instrumentation of the bladder Septic abortion Drainage of intra-abdominal abscesses Ventilation of the lungs during acute respiratory infections
Haemolysis	Incompatible blood transfusion Damaged prosthetic aortic valve Hypophosphataemia Glucose 6-phosphate dehydrogenase deficiency Falciparum malaria
Nephrotoxic agents	Antibiotics Cytotoxic agents Paraquat Ethylene glycol Phenindione ϵ-amino-caproic acid Metal salts Urografin solution (angiography)[18] Mushroom poisoning CO poisoning[49] TAB and cholera vaccination[25] Fish gall bladder
Obstetric conditions	Septic abortion Eclampsia Uncontrolled post-partum haemorrhage
Intrinsic renal disease	Acute glomerulonephritis Acute interstitial nephritis Collagen diseases Polyarteritis nodosa Systemic lupus erythematosus Renal transplant Cortical necrosis
Blockage of the tubular part of the nephron	Crystalluria Dysproteinaemia Acute hyperuricaemia (e.g. in the treatment of leukaemia)
Blockage of the urinary tract	Calculi (Ca^{++} salts, urates, cysteine) Fibrosis Stricture Tumours, benign and malignant Congenital malformations plus the above Procidenture
Drugs	Ritodrine[23] Ibuprofen[7] Barbiturates[21,66]

reversible and not associated with a significant degree of renal damage, and acute renal failure. It was found in a prospective study[58] that potentially reversible pre-renal azotaemia was present when the osmolality of the urine was greater than 500 mosmol/l, the urine sodium concentration was less than 20 mmol/l (mEq/l), the urine : plasma urea nitrogen ratio was greater than 8, and the urine : plasma creatinine ratio was greater than 40. When acute renal failure was present, the urine osmolality was less than 350 mosmol/l, the urine [Na$^+$] was more than 40 mmol/l (mEq/l), the urine : plasma urea nitrogen ratio was less than 3, and the urine : plasma creatinine ratio was more than 20. On many occasions, however, it is difficult to make a firm diagnosis at the time of onset of oliguria (as stated in Table 4.2), so that careful monitoring is necessary and early precautionary measures should be taken.

When a case of acute renal failure is treated successfully, the history of this condition falls into four phases.

(*a*) The precipitating condition or cause.
(*b*) The anuric phase.
(*c*) The diuretic or pre-recovery phase.
(*d*) The recovery phase.

The diuretic phase, as a recognizable entity in the sequence of recovery following anuria, is much less commonly seen today. This is because of the improved control of fluid balance and early dialysis.

Let us look at these four phases in turn.

The precipitating condition or cause

A careful history and a careful clinical assessment to elucidate the cause of the anuria or oliguria are important because of the need to remedy quickly and fully any condition that is immediately treatable. The early treatment of dehydration, electrolyte imbalance and low blood pressure is almost always possible. There is some evidence that acute renal failure may be avoided during blood loss and trauma if hypertonic solutions are infused quickly. Anuria resulting from sulphonamides usually responds to the infusion of alkalis and an increased fluid intake. The onset of renal failure, which may follow poisoning with bismuth, mercuric chloride, lead, zinc and other salts, may be avoided by the early use of British Anti-Lewisite (BAL) (dimercaprol) or calcium disodium EDTA. Both these substances may, however, be toxic once anuria has been established. British Anti-Lewisite, for example, may give rise to tremors, coma, convulsions, marked vasoconstriction and capillary damage. It may contribute to the production of a metabolic acidosis and may also cause sweating, fever, vomiting and abdominal pain. The substances are available in the following forms.

British Anti-Lewisite (BAL) (dimercaprol) is available in solutions containing dimercaprol 100 mg/ml in peanut oil and benzyl benzoate. It is administered intramuscularly by deep injection.

Calcium disodium edetate (CaNa$_2$ ethylene-diamine-tetra-acetic acid) is a chelating agent which

Table 4.2 The characteristics of urine when oliguria is the result of physiological changes and acute renal failure

	Physiological oliguria	Acute renal failure
Urine volume	< 500 ml/24 hours	< 500 ml/24 hours
Sodium content	< 20 mmol/l (mEq/l)	> 60 mmol/l (mEq/l)
Urea content	> 250 mmol/l (1.5 g%)	< 160 mmol/l (1 g%)
Specific gravity	1.018 or greater	1.010–1.012
Urine osmolality	> 500 mosmol/l	< 480 mosmol/l
U/P osmolar ratio	> 1.3	> 1.1
Response to loop diuretics and mannitol	Almost always	Sometimes

(a) As described in the text, a clear picture does not emerge immediately on all occasions and constant monitoring is necessary.

(b) When oliguria is caused by hypovolaemia (shock), an inability to concentrate the urine may also be present and this will result in urine of low specific gravity and osmolality.

(c) When 'high output' acute renal failure is present, the characteristics of the urine are similar to the above (i.e. the urine has a low specific gravity, in the region of 1.010, but the volume is high).

(d) Loop diuretics or mannitol almost *always* produce a diuresis during physiological oliguria. An exception may be severe hypovolaemia for example, as a result of pancreatitis, haemorrhage or gut obstruction. When acute renal failure is present, loop diuretics *may* produce a diuresis when given in large doses (e.g. frusemide 400 mg i.v.).

may be given as a 0.5–1% solution in physiological saline or glucose in doses of 1–2 g spread over 24 hours.

Lead-induced kidney damage was reported in 1909 by Turner[74] when he recognized that albuminuria developed following an outbreak of lead poisoning in children in Brisbane. Yver *et al.*[79] described acute renal failure in a man who was exposed to lead during an industrial accident, and who developed the condition during calcium disodium edetate (EDTA) treatment. As calcium disodium edetate and D-penicillamine are both nephrotoxic, the patient was rechallenged with EDTA following recovery. Because there was no impairment of renal function on this occasion, Yver and his co-workers concluded that the lead, rather than the drug, was responsible for the development of acute renal failure. Acute tubular necrosis developed in two patients suffering from severe lead poisoning following self-injection of contaminated opium—a lead/opium suspension.

Penicillamine (β,β-*dimethylcysteine, Distamine, Cuprimine*) is an effective chelating agent for copper, zinc, mercury and lead and it increases the excretion of these metals in the urine. It is relatively non-toxic but pyrexia and skin reactions have been observed. Its long-term use has been associated with a lupus erythematosus-like reaction, and prolonged treatment has been associated with renal damage.

Raw fish gall bladder. It is the practice in the Far East and some parts of Europe to eat raw fish, and this may give rise to poisoning. Three cases of acute renal failure associated with hepatotoxicity have been reported from Hong Kong (Chan *et al.*, 1985).[19] The gall bladder was from the fresh water grass carp, and it represents one of the many toxins that may give rise to acute renal failure. Many of these toxins have not been identified (Yip, 1981).[1,78]

The pathogenesis of acute renal failure

The pathogenic processes that cause tubular cell damage and therefore acute renal failure are not fully understood.[8,41,45] In 1917, Borst postulated that the changes were caused by ischaemia,[6] but other workers, such as Bywaters and Dible,[15] who observed acute renal failure following crush injuries during the bombing of London in 1942, considered that other mechanisms were responsible. It was found that stimulation of the splanchnic nerve and infusion of adrenaline into the renal artery produced cortical ischaemia,[73] and that the renal blood flow in acute renal failure is reduced by approximately 40%[12] while the glomerular filtration rate

(GFR) is almost zero. Xenon wash-out studies have confirmed that cortical blood flow is markedly reduced in the presence of acute renal failure.[33,34,73] It has also been postulated that, because the renal renin levels are raised in acute renal failure, locally produced angiotensin II in the renal cortex is the cause of afferent arteriolar vasoconstriction.[11] Another interesting suggestion is that prostaglandins produced in the renal medulla and transported by the tubular urine in the loop of Henlé to the macula densa, inhibit afferent arteriolar vasoconstriction. When the tubular urine ceases in acute renal failure, prostaglandins are no longer able to affect the macula densa, so that afferent vasoconstriction occurs free from inhibiting forces.[62]

It is well known, however, that the gradients of osmolality that occur in the kidney, for which a flow of tubular urine in the loop of Henlé is essential if the counter-current multiplier system is to function, disappear rapidly in shock. It has been suggested that, because tissue damage can be prevented elsewhere in the body by maintaining a high osmolality of the tissue fluids by means of the infusion of hypertonic solutions, the prevention of acute renal failure can be successful in some cases. There is some supporting evidence for this. Acute renal failure rarely occurs, even in the presence of prolonged hypotension during diabetic ketosis, when there is a raised osmotic pressure of the blood and extracellular fluid (ECF). The incidence of acute renal failure since the introduction of the routine administration of sodium bicarbonate solutions in hypertonic form appears to be low following cardiac arrest; further investigation into the use of hypertonic solutions in preventing acute renal failure is, however, required.

Since 1963 it has been demonstrated that massive infusions of sodium bicarbonate solution do not impair renal function or cardiac output or blood pressure (Kanter, 1963).[37]

Acute interstitial nephritis

This form of reversible acute renal failure is frequently seen in association with antibiotic therapy. It can occur when a cephalosporin, for example cephaloridine,[28] or methicillin[29] is administered. In these circumstances acute renal failure would appear to be an 'allergic' or sensitivity reaction similar to that which follows the administration of non-steroidal anti-inflammatory agents, for example ibuprofen, analgesics and diuretics. The sensitivity reaction induces skin rashes, in addition to the acute renal failure; eosinophilia and raised serum IgE levels are present. Eosinophils are found in the urinary sediment.[29] Acute renal failure can also be precipitated by phenylbutazone[32] and cimetidine.[42,55,64]

Interstitial nephritis can be differentiated by the uptake of gallium citrate by the kidneys; in lower nephron nephrosis, the gallium is not absorbed by the kidneys and the scan is negative.[47] The diagnosis is important because treatment with steroids rapidly improves renal function when interstitial nephritis is a result of drug and antibiotic treatment.[29]

Prevention of acute renal failure

Intravenous mannitol has frequently been used to protect the kidney during open-heart surgery, trauma and other acute conditions. There are over 600 publications on the subject, but the results are conflicting. There are indications, however, that mannitol withdraws fluid from the tubular cells during hypotension,[27] and thus prevents cellular damage. Other investigators[22] have suggested that ischaemic acute renal failure may be prevented by mannitol because of the high intratubular pressure and flow rates that prevent intratubular obstruction.

Experiments have indicated that long-term saline loading in rats effectively prevents acute renal failure induced by glycerol[20,54] and mercuric chloride ($HgCl_2$).[24,44] However, ischaemic renal failure as a result of renal artery clamping was not prevented by this means.[51] Nevertheless, the protective effect of NaCl in some circumstances may be similar to the prevention of tissue damage that results from the infusion of hypertonic salt solutions during haemorrhage.[10]

Frusemide (Lasix) has been indicated to prevent acute renal failure in both experimental animals and man, and there seems to be a close correlation between the diuretic response and the increase in cortical blood flow, in acute renal failure induced by haemorrhagic shock in dogs.[50] However, no protection appears to result from frusemide following clamping of the renal artery,[52] or renal failure induced by gentamicin in rats.[71]

Infusions of prostaglandin (e.g. prostaglandin E1) have given varying results in the experimental animal.[53,60,75] However, there are indications that some substances, such as propranolol, clonidine and guanethidine, may be beneficial.[67,68] The vasopressor dopamine, which is being used increasingly, may also have protective effects.[35,36] Dopamine may be more effective in this respect when given in combination with frusemide.[69]

Hepatorenal syndrome

This term is used to identify the onset of oliguria associated with liver disease. However, many gastroenterologists specializing in liver disease confine the term to the unexplained renal failure that is associated with hepatic cirrhosis. Some clinicians therefore use the term 'pseudohepatorenal syndrome' to include almost any condition in which both hepatic and renal functions are simultaneously impaired. These include, in addition to acute liver failure and obstructive jaundice, conditions such as leptospirosis, eclampsia, hypernephroma with metastatic and cholestatic disease, and heart failure.

The onset of hepatorenal syndrome is usually abrupt and is characterized by a urine output of less than 500 ml in 24 hours,[76] acidaemia and metabolic acidosis develops (in place of alkalaemia), increasing azotaemia and rapidly changing blood biochemistry as described above. Although initially the urine osmolality may be high (600–900 mosmol/l) and the urine may contain less than 10 mmol/l (mEq/l) of Na^+, as the condition persists, the urine osmolality falls to approximately 300 mosmol/l and the urine [Na^+] increases to 40 or 50 mmol/l (mEq/l), indicating the development of acute tubular necrosis.

At post-mortem examination, however, the kidneys demonstrate no histological evidence of acute renal failure and, if the kidneys are transplanted into a patient suffering from chronic renal failure, they usually function normally.

While fluid is being administered and abnormal electrolyte concentrations are being corrected by infusions, it must be remembered that renal damage may have already occurred. Care must therefore be taken to ensure that treatment during a prolonged anuric phase is not made more difficult.

The anuric phase

The following factors emerge as consequences of the complete suppression of urine.

1. Retention of water.
2. Accumulation of the products of metabolism such as urea, uric acid, creatinine, phosphate, sulphate, etc.
3. Changes in total body metabolism arising from (1) and (2), which are still not well understood, but involve shifts of electrolytes from the cells to the extracellular fluid compartments and in the reverse direction.

When an unrestricted fluid intake is allowed (or, far worse, when fluids are forced in the misguided attempt to invoke a diuresis) the consequences of fluid retention rapidly become apparent. Cardiac failure, oedema, pulmonary congestion, hypertension, cerebral oedema, convulsions and other symptoms of water intoxication will result. It has been stressed that the most common cause of death within 14 days of the onset of oliguria due to renal disease is overhydration. Even when fluid intake is strictly controlled and overhydration is not a factor, the retained products of metabolism produce the gradual onset of lethargy, coma, vomiting, pericarditis and a lowered resistance to infection. The inability to excrete K^+ is reflected in the rising plasma K^+ levels, and this is associated with cardiac failure and muscle weakness.

Some return of renal function may be seen within 4 or 5 days, but adequate renal function may not return for as long as 6–8 weeks, and this may progress until there is no detectable abnormality. When the kidney begins to recover, it secretes a dilute urine of low concentration which does not begin to reduce the blood urea until the volume reaches 1 litre or more. At this stage the kidney still has an impaired tubular function and is unable to differentiate between electrolytes or to concentrate most substances that are filtered. The passing of a profuse, dilute urine may soon lead to dehydration, electrolyte imbalance and electrolyte depletion. Therapy, therefore, must be aimed at regulating essential factors until adequate kidney function returns.

The regulation of water
Because the temperature of the environment is so important in determining the amount of fluid lost insensibly through the skin and lungs, formulae for calculating this volume cannot be applied with confidence to every patient. The measured insensible loss of the average adult in a temperate climate such as Britain is now accepted to be less than 1 litre in 24 hours, but generally falls as time elapses from the onset of anuria, probably because of the endogenous production of water from fat metabolism. Unless the weather is particularly warm, the insensible loss of an oliguric patient is usually taken as being 400–500 ml in 24 hours. When the fluid requirements are being calculated this volume is added to the volume of urine lost in the previous 24 hours.

When it is borne in mind that some degree of overhydration may have occurred before the oliguric state was recognized and that the endogenous production of water has also to be taken into account, as little as 400 ml of fluid in 24 hours can be recommended as the treatment of choice in the very early stages.

The simplest and most accurate method is to record the daily change in weight, the weighing being performed at the same time each day with the bladder empty and on the same scales. Ideally, this is done on a bed weighing machine, but mobilization of the patient for weighing, when this is clinically possible, is by no means contraindicated.

An accurate record of all additions to the patient in the form of fluids, such as medicines, ion exchange resin etc., and all losses in the form of vomit, urine and faeces must be kept, in order that this assessment can be made.

The accurate measurement of urine output is of paramount importance, not only for the assessment of fluid replacement, but also for the determination of the progress of the patient, and the amount of urea and electrolytes excreted.

Although many people object to retaining a catheter within the bladder, the author has found that it is of immense benefit in maintaining an accurate balance in difficult patients, especially those who are incontinent, and he has not seen any difficulties arise from the pure retention of the catheter. Infection appears to be more likely when the catheter is repeatedly inserted. If it is essential to retain a catheter in the bladder so that urine output can be measured accurately, and if an infection is suspected, a measured volume of fluid containing an antibiotic may be reinserted into the bladder through the catheter after emptying; 30 ml of fluid containing 100 mg of chloramphenicol have been used successfully. This volume must be deducted from the volume of urine obtained when the catheter is released again.

To avoid the oral complications associated with oliguria and its treatment (i.e. parotitis, thrush and ulceration), part of the fluid intake should be by mouth. This regimen should be reinforced by the sucking of pure glucose sweets followed by bland antiseptic mouth washes.

The suppression of harmful products of metabolism
The main metabolic consequences which the anuric patient has to face arise from the metabolism of protein which produces a rising blood non-protein nitrogen, cardiotoxic levels of plasma potassium and release of unexcretable fixed acid.

Treatment therefore entails a completely protein-free intake and the reduction of endogenous protein metabolism. Advantage is taken of the protein-sparing effect of glucose and, owing to the necessity of restricting fluid intake, this entails the use of hypertonic solutions.

Hypertonic glucose or fructose in a 20% solution can be given by mouth, but quite often this is not tolerated and leads to vomiting and profuse diarrhoea. It is possible, however, to give small volumes of hypertonic solution through a Ryles tube when these solutions are dripped in *slowly* over 24 hours. When profuse loss of fluid occurs as a result of diarrhoea, the volume lost must be calculated when assessing the daily fluid requirements. Diarrhoea appears to occur more frequently if fructose is given orally, and glucose may therefore be preferred in some cases.

Up to 50% glucose can be safely injected into a large vein such as the SVC by means of a polythene catheter.[13] Although the procedure of passing the catheter is simple, in the condition of anuria the catheter may have to stay *in situ* for 3 weeks, and therefore maximum precautions for sterility should be enforced and complete sterility maintained each time the bottle is changed.

To each 500 ml of glucose solution 1000 units of heparin are added, and 1 unit of insulin is added for every 3 g of glucose. The slow infusion of not less than 200 g of glucose should be the objective in the adult, and this can be achieved in only 400 ml of water over 24 hours.

Changes in blood chemistry

Lowered pH and plasma sodium, calcium, bicarbonate concentrations, and raised phosphate and sulphate concentrations are all found in the uraemic state.

The reduced serum sodium level may be the result of either sodium depletion or dilution. Usually it results from dilution following an excessive water load. This can only be treated by water restriction. The movement of sodium from the plasma into the cells because of the poisoned cell phenomenon is also a possible cause.

When it is thought that sodium depletion has occurred or correction of the plasma sodium is advisable, small volumes of sodium lactate, bicarbonate or chloride can be administered, preferably in a hypertonic solution. If sodium lactate or sodium bicarbonate is given, some correction of the metabolic acidosis arising from the retention of fixed acid will result. If clinical improvement follows the infusion of sodium salts, further quantities can be administered until the deficit as calculated from the plasma deficiency and the total body water is corrected. When the onset of acute renal failure has been clearly established, it may be advisable to treat the metabolic acidosis, which will inevitably result, prophylactically by infusing hypertonic sodium bicarbonate (100 ml of 4.2% solution) during the first 1 or 2 days.

No marked clinical improvement is to be expected, in the later stages, from the attempts to modify acidosis resulting from accumulation of fixed acids, phosphate, sulphate etc., by administration of alkali in the form of bicarbonate or lactate. Also tetany, resulting from a further lowering of the already decreased plasma $[Ca^{++}]$, may occur on the administration of alkali.

Treatment of hyperkalaemia

A complete potassium-free intake should be instituted and maintained throughout the period of anuria. Milk, fruit etc. are banned. Tea without milk may relieve the monotony of glucose drinks.

A raised plasma $[K^+]$ occurs mainly as a result of its release from protein catabolism and probably partly as an inherent metabolic consequence of anuria. When toxic levels are reached, muscular weakness, cardiac irregularities and absence of tendon reflexes can be demonstrated. When plasma levels of 7 or 8 mmol/l (mEq/l) are reached, the electrocardiogram shows high-peaked T waves, absent P waves and slurred widened QRS complexes. Cardiotoxic levels of potassium vary with each individual, age and duration of the disease. Rapid onset of K^+ intoxication is expected following major operative procedures and when gross tissue damage has occurred.[14] Treatment for the control of K^+ intoxication should be instituted early, before pathological levels appear. Intravenous glucose tends to alleviate the condition by the uptake of K^+ in its metabolism. Ion exchange resins which exchange Na^+ for K^+ may be used.

Resin, 15 g, given in 30 ml of 5 or 10% glucose in water is well tolerated orally when given early in the course of the disease and, if necessary, it can be given three times a day: 100 g of ion exchange resin can be given rectally in 200 ml of water or 1% methyl cellulose. Resonium A is a suitable resin. It may be necessary to administer a glycerine or magnesium sulphate enema in order to obtain return of the resin, as retained resin is of only limited value. The rectal route can be combined with oral administrations or used alone when the patient is vomiting or unable to swallow.

Attempts to make use of the low K^+ content of stored packed cells have proved disappointing, and it must be remembered that transfusions of blood or plasma are followed by an increase in protein metabolism. Unless the haematocrit falls to below 25%, correction of anaemia should be avoided for this reason. Infusion of calcium gluconate may assist neutralization of the harmful effects of hyperkalaemia, and the infusion of 100 ml of 10% solution every 24 hours has been advocated. The danger of calcium blood levels resulting in arrhythmias and the possibility that renal calcification may occur suggest that these large volumes should be used with caution. Hyperkalaemia is an indication for dialysis. The rapid infusion of hypertonic saline or of sodium bicarbonate will temporarily (for 1 or 2 hours) reverse the cardiotoxic effect of potassium and may be used, for example, prior to dialysis.

The extrarenal removal of metabolites
When conservative treatment, as described above, is inadequate to control or maintain the patient until the pre-recovery stage develops, the extrarenal removal of metabolites becomes essential.

This requires strict biochemical and physiological control and a well-trained team. The indications for this procedure, which should be regarded as part of therapy and not as a substitute for the regimen described above, may be summarized as follows.

(*a*) General clinical deterioration—'the uraemic state'. No hard and fast rules can be laid down because individual tolerance to raised plasma nonprotein nitrogen levels appears to vary so much. A careful clinical assessment of the rate of progress as manifested by drowsiness, pericarditis, vomiting, and muscular irritability may have to be made. Because of the 'disequilibrium syndrome', lassitude, headache, drowsiness and mental confusion, present-day practice is to tend to perform dialysis early, when the blood urea is above 33 mmol/l (200 mg%). This syndrome is associated with a raised osmolality of the cerebrospinal fluid (CSF) because urea is retained within this space; this may be avoided by increasing the concentration of glucose in the diasylate.[38,39,40,63]

(*b*) Hyperkalaemia. Cardiotoxic plasma potassium levels of 7 mmol/l (mEq/l) or more as shown by electrocardiogram recordings.

(*c*) Metabolic acidosis. A plasma [HCO_3^-] of less than 15 mmol/l (mEq/l). The only effective treatment for this condition is dialysis.

(*d*) Gross overhydration.

High output acute renal failure
It is now well recognized that acute renal insufficiency can occur without the period of persistent oliguria being observed. It is not dissimilar to the diuretic phase of acute renal failure in which urine of low osmolality (specific gravity) is excreted but the ability to concentrate or dilute the urine further is lost. Electrolyte and fluid imbalance develops and there is an associated rise in the nitrogen-containing products in the blood. The increasing azotaemia which characterizes the condition can be associated with a normal and even increased daily urine output.[65] It has been reported after burns,[31] head injury[70] and soft tissue trauma.[65] Baxter *et al.*[3] described nine patients suffering from high output acute renal failure, seven of these patients had received gunshot wounds and two had blunt abdominal trauma. Baxter and his co-workers noted that the greater the urine volume, the higher the rise in blood urea nitrogen. In other words, the increase in blood urea nitrogen was paralleled by increasing 24-hour urinary volume. When the serum potassium rose to 6 mmol/l (mEq/l), the patients were treated with a cation exchange resin. When a metabolic acidosis developed, this was corrected by infusions of isotonic lactate solutions; however this failed to improve the acid–base state in two patients, who subsequently died. Treatment, therefore, largely entails the maintenance of fluid and electrolyte balance and the control of abnormally high plasma [K^+] and low plasma [HCO_3^-], the latter preferably with $NaHCO_3$. Dialysis may be necessary in order to reduce the plasma [K^+] and to remove the fixed acids and therefore raise the plasma [HCO_3^-].

The therapeutic methods available for the treatment of acute renal failure are: the restriction of fluid and suppression of harmful metabolites with glucose infusions, peritoneal lavage and haemodialysis. Intestinal irrigation is no longer performed. High dosage of diuretics is often used at an early stage.

Restriction of fluid and hypertonic glucose infusions
This is now used initially and only when dialysis is delayed for any reason.

Intestinal irrigation
The perfusion of hypertonic fluids of varying composition through the gut at a constant rate is difficult to perform and may be associated with complications of intestinal haemorrhage, perforation, ileus and pulmonary oedema. It is never used today.

Diuretics
Large doses of the diuretic frusemide (Lasix) given intravenously have sometimes been demonstrated to induce a diuresis.[17] As much as 2 g have been given and, although ototoxicity has been largely related to ethacrynic acid, it can occur transitorily with this substance. Bumetanide (Burinex) may also prove to be of value.

Peritoneal lavage
The use of the large peritoneal surface as a dialysing membrane is physiologically sound and clinically

valuable, but it cannot be used after injury to the abdominal organs and it is not the method of choice following abdominal surgery. It is a method which is rapidly gaining popularity when these factors are absent. However, in reporting a review of 48 patients stabilized in this way, Thomson et al.[72] included a patient who had been operated upon 10 days previously for an abdominal aortic aneurysm. The increased popularity of this treatment is mainly because of the ease with which it can be performed, the small amount of apparatus that is necessary and a realization that it is effective. Continuous ambulatory peritoneal dialysis for the treatment of chronic renal failure is being used with increasing frequency.[30]

Ideally, slightly hypertonic sterile solutions, varied according to the biochemical and fluid needs of the patient, are infused into the abdominal cavity through a cannula placed below the umbilicus. If it is necessary to remove water from the body, solutions of greater osmotic force are required. Two solutions that have been used successfully are supplied in convenient plastic packs. One is more hypertonic than the other by virtue of a higher glucose concentration.

It is to be noted that neither solution contains potassium and it will therefore be necessary to add this cation if its removal from the body is contraindicated (e.g. when peritoneal dialysis is being used to remove excess water from the digitalized patient who is already suffering from hypokalaemia).

Solutions containing KCl and sodium bicarbonate instead of sodium lactate have been described elsewhere.[9]

Solutions prepared by pharmaceutical firms are readily available in disposable plastic containers. Those made by Boots, Nottingham, England, contain the following concentrations of solutions:

In each case the fluid must be hypertonic compared with the patient's plasma and it can be kept so by the addition of glucose.

The amount of fluid withdrawn from the abdominal cavity will be greater than that infused when hypertonic solutions are used. The greater the osmolality of the fluid, the greater the volume of fluid lost by the patient. While this is effective in reducing the concentration of harmful metabolites, it is essential that the patient does not become grossly dehydrated and, in fact, a correct water balance should be maintained throughout the whole procedure. To keep pace with the water loss, it will therefore be necessary to continue the infusion of normal saline and glucose solution throughout the procedure. Proportionately more water than Na^+ will be removed. Therefore, if the volume of fluid removed is replaced by the same volume of isotonic saline, hypernatraemia will result.

The sterile fluid is allowed to drip into or perfuse the abdominal cavity at 2 or 3 litres per hour. Faster rates can be obtained if desired for the treatment of conditions such as gross overhydration. A metal cannula is passed through the abdominal wall, under local anaesthetic. When a single cannula is used it is usually inserted mid-line below the umbilicus. A plastic cannula is passed through a metal cannula in the abdominal cavity and the metal cannula is then withdrawn and removed. When 2 litres of fluid have entered the abdominal cavity, they are allowed to remain there for 30 minutes. The bottles are then lowered to floor level so that the dialysing solution, which has undergone exchange with the body fluids through the peritoneum, syphons out.

When this fluid has been recovered completely together with that volume of fluid extracted from the patient, the process is repeated. This

Sodium lactate	0.5%	$[Na^+]$	141 mmol/l (mEq/l)
Sodium chloride	0.56%	$[Ca^{++}]$	1.8 mmol/l (3.6 mEq/l)
Calcium chloride	0.039%	$[Mg^{++}]$	0.75 mmol/l (1.5 mEq/l)
Magnesium chloride	0.015%	$[Cl^-]$	100.8 mmol/l (mEq/l)
Dextrose BP	1.36% = 367 mosmol/l	$[HCO_3^-]$	
or Dextrose BP	6.36% = 648 mosmol/l	as lactate	44.6 mmol/l (mEq/l)

A low Na^+-containing solution is also available which can be used in the dehydrated patient.

Sodium lactate	0.50%	$[Na^+]$	131 mmol/l (mEq/l)
Sodium chloride BP	0.50%	$[Ca^{++}]$	1.8 mmol/l (3.6 mEq/l)
Calcium chloride BP	0.26%	$[Mg^{++}]$	0.75 mmol/l (1.5 mEq/l)
Magnesium chloride	0.015%	$[Cl^-]$	91 mmol/l (mEq/l)
Sodium metabisulphite BP	0.005%	$[HCO_3^-]$	
Anhydrous dextrose BP	1.36%	as lactate	45 mmol/l (mEq/l)

procedure is allowed to continue until the blood levels of urea and potassium have been reduced adequately and the metabolic acidosis has been corrected. When performed as a resuscitative procedure it is best to have the patient on a weighing bed and sedation is necessary. Abdominal pain may occur and if it is prominent during the peritoneal dialysis then 2 or 3 ml of 2% procaine can be injected with the dialysing fluid. Meteorism, intestinal haemorrhage, perforation of bowel and peritonitis are some of the obvious but rare complications of this procedure and they can be avoided by careful technique.

It has been shown that major protein loss into the diasylate can occur and amounts range from 10 to 207 g per dialysis. If this occurs, replacement may be necessary with plasma or fractionated human albumin.[4,72]

Peritoneal dialysis has a much slower clearance rate for urea[5] than that of the artificial kidney, as described below.

The artificial kidney
The extrarenal removal of metabolites can be performed by the more effective and sometimes safer procedure of dialysis through an artificial kidney. Various models for dialysis are in existence but the principles involved are the same.[43] In the older forms of apparatus, many of which are still being used, blood is pumped from an artery or large vein through cellophane and back into the patient through another vein. The cellophane tubes or sheets are bathed in a circulating fluid of composition suitably similar to that used for peritoneal dialysis and adjusted to the needs of the patient.

When dialysis is performed as a resuscitative procedure, a well-trained team, able to detect changes in circulating blood volume, and facilities for quick electrolyte and blood urea determinations are essential for a successful outcome. Blood pressure, and when necessary the electrocardiogram, should be recorded at frequent intervals. The patient may be dialysed for 6–10 hours.

More sophisticated forms of apparatus are now available which are more compact (Fig 4.1) and the dialysis fluid is prepared on a continuous basis using deionized tap water and concentrated dialyate fluid. The two solutions are pumped continuously in the appropriate proportions so that the correct concentrations of electrolytes are present in the dialysing fluid. This fluid is pumped in the reverse direction to flow of blood.

The blood is pumped through very small diameter tubes (internal diameter 2 mm; length 16–20 cm), and these tubes are bathed in the dialysate fluid which flows past them at 500 ml/minute. The volume of blood in an artificial kidney unit is approximately 70–100 ml, although with the connecting tubing, the priming volume of blood is approximately 200 ml.

Membrane dialyzers consisting of flat plates but based on the same principle are also available. These are sometimes used in preference to the cellulose acetate tubes, especially when a more

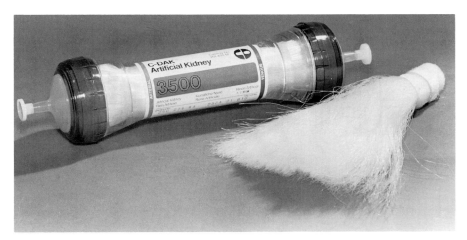

Fig. 4.1   One form of artificial kidney. It is composed of small diameter tubes (internal diameter 2 mm; length 16–20 cm) through which blood is pumped. The dialysate fluid is contained within the outer plastic cover and bathes the tubes at a flow rate of approximately 500 ml/minute.

rapid rate of ultrafiltration and removal of water is required.

When an arteriovenous connection between the radial artery and a large wrist vein is made, repeated dialysis may be performed with ease.

The diuretic or pre-recovery phase

When 1 litre of urine, or more, is produced, clinical improvement is expected and is reflected in falling plasma urea and non-protein nitrogen concentrations

A profuse dilute urine excretion soon leads to dehydration and electrolyte loss, so that daily weighing and plasma electrolyte recordings must be maintained. Infusions of appropriate solutions such as NaCl containing KCl, and perhaps $MgCl_2$, must be given

The recovery phase

As further recovery proceeds, intravenous therapy may be abandoned and dietary restrictions relaxed. Care must be taken, however, that each step towards a normal regimen, should be preceded by a careful biochemical assessment. When oral feeding begins a relatively low protein diet is to be recommended.

References

1. Anonymous. (1980). Fish poisoning. *Brit. med. J.*, **281**, 890.
2. Barker, E. S., Singer, R. B., Elkinton, J. R. and Clark, J. K. (1957). The renal response in man to acute experimental respiratory alkalosis and acidosis. *J. Clin. Invest.*, **36**, 515.
3. Baxter, C. R., Zedlitz, W. H. and Shires, G. T. (1964). The high output acute renal failure complicating traumatic injury. *J. of Trauma.*, **4**, 467.
4. Berlyne, G. M., Jones, J. H., Hewitt, V. and Nilwarangkur, S. (1964). Protein loss in peritoneal dialysis. *Lancet*, **i**, 738.
5. Boen, S. T. (1961). Kinetics of peritoneal dialysis: a comparison with the artificial kidney. *Medicine (Baltimore)*, **40**, 243.
6. Borst, M. (1917). Pathologisch—anatomische erfahrungen uber Kriegsverletzungen. *Sammlung Klinische Vortrage* (Volkmann), **735**, 297.
7. Brandstetter, R. D. and Mar, D. D. (1978). Reversible oliguric renal failure associated with ibuprofen treatment. *Brit. med. J.*, **2**, 1194.
8. British Medical Journal (1970). Leading article. Renin and renal failure. *Brit. med. J.*, **1**, 250.
9. Brooks, D. K. (1958). The modern treatment of anuria and oliguria. *Postgrad. med. J.*, **34**, 583.
10. Brooks, D. K., Williams, W. G., Manley, R. W. and Whiteman, P. (1963). Osmolar and electrolyte changes in haemorrhagic shock; hypertonic solutions in the prevention of tissue damage. *Lancet*, **i**, 521.
11. Brown, J. J., Gleadle, R. I., Lawson, D. H., Lever, A. F., Linton, A. L., Macadam, R. F., Prentice, E., Robertson, J. I. S. and Tree, M. (1970). Renin and acute renal failure: studies in man. *Brit. med. J.*, **1**, 253.
12. Brun, C., Crone, C., Davidson, H. G., Fabricius, J., Hansen, A. T., Lassen, N. A. and Munck, O. (1955). Renal blood flow in anuric human subject determined by use of radioactive Krypton 85 (21917). *Proc. Soc. Exp. Biol. & Med.*, **89**, 687.
13. Bull, G. M., Joekes, A. M., and Lowe, K. G. (1949). Conservative treatment of anuric uraemia. *Lancet*, **ii**, 229.
14. Bywaters, E. G. L. (1944). Ischemic muscle necrosis; crushing injury, traumatic edema, the crush syndrome, traumatic anuria, compression syndrome; a type of injury seen in air raid casualties following burial beneath debris. *J. Amer. med. Assoc.*, **124**, 1103.
15. Bywaters, E. G. L. and Dible, J. H. (1942). The renal lesion in traumatic anuria. *J. Path. & Bact.*, **54**, 111.
16. Calene, J. G., Weidman, W. H., Wakim, K. G., Rosevear, J. W., Kirklin, J. W. and Stickler, G. B. (1963). Renal function and hydrogen-ion excretion after open intracardiac surgery and whole body perfusion. *Ann. Surg.*, **157**, 336.
17. Cantarovitch, F., Galli, C., Benedetti, L., Chena, C., Castro, L., Correa, C., Perez Loredo, J., Fernandez, J. C., Locatelli, A. and Tizado, J. (1973). High dose frusemide in established acute renal failure. *Brit. med. J.*, **iv**, 449.
18. Catterall, J. R., Ferguson, R. J. and Miller, H. C. (1981). Intravascular haemolysis with acute renal failure after angiocardiography. *Brit. med. J.*, **282**, 779.
19. Chan, D. W. S., Yeung, C. K. and Chan, M. K. (1985). Acute renal failure after eating raw fish gall bladder. *Brit. med. J.*, **290**, 897.
20. Chedru, M. F., Baethke, R. and Oken, D. E. (1972). Renal cortical blood flow and glomerular filtration in myohemoglobinuric acute renal failure. *Kidney International*, **1**, 232.
21. Clark, J. G. and Summerling, M. D. (1966). Muscle necrosis and calcification in acute renal failure due to barbiturate intoxication. *Brit. med. J.*, **2**, 214.
22. Cronin, R. E., De Torrente, A., Miller, P. D., Bulger, R. E., Burke, T. J. and Schrier, R. (1978). Pathogenic

mechanisms in early norepinephrine-induced acute renal failure: Functional and histological correlates of protection. *Kidney International*, **14**, 115.

23. Desir, D., Van Coevorden, A., Kirkpatrick, C. and Caufreiz, A. (1978). Ritodrine-induced acidosis in pregnancy. *Brit. med. J.*, **2**, 1194.

24. Di Bona, G. F., McDonald, F. D., Flamenbaum, W., Dammin, G. J. and Oken, D. E. (1971). Maintenance of renal function in salt loaded rats despite severe tubular necrosis induced by HgCl₂. *Nephron*, **8**, 205.

25. Eisinger, A. J. and Smith, J. G. (1979). Acute renal failure after TAB and cholera vaccination. *Brit. med. J.*, **1**, 381.

26. Finsterbusch, W., Long, D. M., Sellers, R. D., Amplatz, K. and Lillehei, C. W. (1961). Renal arteriography during extracorporeal circulation in dogs, with a preliminary report upon the effects of low molecular weight dextran. *J. Thorac. & Cardiovasc. Surg.*, **41**, 252.

27. Flores, J., Di Bona, G. F., Beck, C. H. and Leaf, A. (1972). The role of cell swelling in ischemic renal damage and the protective effect of hypertonic solute. *J. Clin. Invest.*, **51**, 118.

28. Foord, R. D. (1975). Cephaloridine, cephalothin and the kidney. *J. Antimicrob. Chemother.*, **1** (Suppl.), 119.

29. Galpin, J. E., Shinaberger, J. H., Stanley, T. M., Blumenkrantz, M. J., Bayer, A. S., Friedman, G. S., Montgomerie, J. Z., Guze, L. B., Coburn, J. W. and Glassock, R. J. (1978). Acute interstitial nephritis due to methicillin. *Amer. J. Med.*, **65**, 756.

30. Gokal, R., McHugh,M., Fryer, R., Ward, M. K. and Kerr, D. N. S. (1980). Continuous ambulatory peritoneal dialysis: one year's experience in a UK dialysis unit. *Brit. Med. J.*, **281**, 474.

31. Graber, I. G. and Sevitt, S. (1959). Renal function in burned patients and its relationship to morphological changes. *J. Clin. Path.*, **12**, 25.

32. Greenstone, M., Hartley, B., Gabriel, R. and Bevan, G. (1981). Acute nephrotic syndrome with reversible renal failure after phenylbutazone. *Brit. med. J.*, **282**, 951.

33. Hollenberg, N. K., Adams, D. F., Oken, D. E. and Merrill, J. P. (1970). Acute renal failure due to nephrotoxins: renal chemodynamic and angiographic studies in man. *N Engl. J. of Med.*, **282**, 1329.

34. Hollenberg, N. K., Epstein, M., Rosen, S. M., Basch, R. I., Oken, D. E. and Merrill, J. P. (1968). Acute oliguric renal failure in man: evidence for preferential renal cortical ischemia. *Medicine (Baltimore)*, **47**, 455.

35. Iaina, A., Solomon, S. and Eliahou, H. E. (1975). Reduction of severity of acute renal failure in rats by beta-adrenergic blockade. *Lancet*, **ii**, 157.

36. Iaina, A., Solomon, S., Gavendo, S. and Eliahou, H. E. (1977). Reduction in severity of acute renal failure in rats by dopamine. *Biomedicine*, **27**, 137.

37. Kanter, G. S. (1963). Effect of massive sodium bicarbonate infusion on renal function. *Canadian J.*

Biochem. & Physiol., **41**, 1399.

38. Kennedy, A. C., Linton, A. L. and Eaton, J. C. (1962). Urea levels in cerebrospinal fluid after haemodialysis. *Lancet*, **i**, 410.

39. Kennedy, A. C., Linton, A. L., Luke, R. G. and Renfrew, S. (1963). Electroencephalographic changes during haemodialysis. *Lancet*, **i**, 408.

40. Kennedy, A. C., Linton, A. L., Luke, R. G., Renfrew, S. and Dinwoodie, A. (1964). The pathogenesis and prevention of cerebral dysfunction during dialysis. *Lancet*, **i**, 790.

41. Kerr, D. N. S. (1974). In *Acute Renal Failure*, p. 9. Edited by C. T. Flynn. London: Medical and Technical Publishing.

42. Kimberly, R. P., Weinberg, H. and Rudd, E. (1980). Great reduction in renal function associated with cimetidine. *Arthritis Rheum.*, **23**, 614.

43. Kolff, W. J. (1947). *New ways of treating uraemia: the artificial kidney, peritoneal lavage, intestinal lavage.* London: Churchill.

44. Lameire, N., Ringoir, S. and Leusen, I. (1976). Effect of variation in dietary, NaCl intake on total and fractional renal blood flow in the normal and mercury-intoxicated rat. *Circulation Research*, **39**, 506.

45. Lancet (1973). Leading article: Acute renal failure. *Lancet*, **ii**, 134.

46. Lefemine, A. A., Fosberg, A. M. and Harken, D. E. (1968). Prolonged partial extracorporeal perfusion. *Amer. Heart J.*, **75**, 531.

47. Linton, A. L. and Lindsay, R. M. (1979). Antibiotic nephrotoxicity. *Controversies in Nephrology*, **1**, 549.

48. Long, D. M., Folkman, M. J. and McClenathan, J. E. (1963). The use of low molecular weight dextran in extracorporeal circulation, hypothermia and hypercapnea. *J. Thorac. & Cardiovasc. Surg.*, **4**, 617.

49. Loughridge, L. W. Leader, L. P. and Bowen, D. A. L. (1958). Acute renal failure due to muscle necrosis in carbon monoxide poisoning. *Lancet*, **ii**, 349.

50. Manuel, C., Dubois, M., Beaufils, H., Guedon, J. and Chapman, A. (1973). Effet du furosémide à fortes doses sur le flux sanguin rénal au cours de l'insuffisance rénale aiguë expérimentale chez le chien. *J. d'urologie et de Néphrologie*, **79**, 948.

51. Mason, J. (1978). The effect of acute and chronic interruption of tubuloglomerular feedback upon the early course of experimental acute renal failure. In *Proceedings of the 7th International Congress of Nephrology* pD-44 Abstract.

52. Mason, J., Takabatake, T., Olbricht, C. and Thurau, K. (1978). The early phase of experimental acute renal failure III. Tubuloglomerular feedback. *Pflügers Archiv.*, **373**, 69.

53. Mauk, R. H., Patak, R. V., Fadem, S. Z., Lifschitz, M. D. and Stein, J. H. (1977). Effect of postaglandin E administration in a nephrotoxic and a vasoconstrictor model of acute renal failure. *Kidney International*, **12**, 122.

54. McDonald, F. D., Thiel, G., Wilson, D. R., Di Bona,

G. F. and Oken, D. E. (1969). The prevention of acute renal failure in the rat by long-term saline loading. A possible role of the renin angiotension axis. *Proc. Soc. Exp. Biol. & Med.*, **131**, 610.

55. McGowan, W. R. and Vermillion, S. E. (1980). Acute interstitial nephritis related to cimetidine therapy. *Gastroenterology*, **79**, 746.

56. McLeish, K. R., Luft, F. C. and Kleit, S. A. (1977). Factors affecting prognosis in acute renal failure following cardiac operations. *Surg. Gynecol. & Obstet.*, **145**, 28.

57. Meyrier, A., Laaban, J. P. and Kanfer, A. (1984). Protracted anuria due to active renal vasoconstriction in malignant hypertension. *Brit. med. J.*, **288**, 1045.

58. Miller, T. R., Anderson, R. J., Linas, S. L., Henrich, W. L., Berns, A. S., Gabow, P. A. and Schrier, R. W. (1978). Urinary diagnostic indices in acute renal failure: A prospective study. *Ann. Int. Med.*, **89**, 47.

59. Moore, D. and Bernhard, W. F. (1963). The prevention and treatment of acute metabolic complications associated with prolonged extracorporeal circulation. *J. Thorac. & Cardiovasc. Surg.*, **45**, 565.

60. Moskowitz, P. S., Korobkin, M. and Rambo, O. N. (1975). Diuresis and improved hemodynamics produced by prostaglandin E_1 in the dog with norepinephrine-induced acute renal failure. *Investigative Radiology*, **10**, 284.

61. Norman, J. C. (1968). Renal complications of cardio-pulmonary bypass. *Dis. Chest*, **54**, 50.

62. Oken, D. E. (1975). Role of prostaglandins in the pathogenesis of acute renal failure. *Lancet*, **i**, 1319.

63. Rosen, S. M., O'Connor, K. and Shaldon, S. (1964). Haemodialysis disequilibrium. *Brit. med. J.*, **2**, 672.

64. Rudnick, M. R., Bastl, C. P., Elfenbein, I. B., Sirota, R. A., Yudis, M. and Narins, R. G. (1982). Cimetidine-induced acute renal failure. *Ann. Int. Med.*, **96**, 180.

65. Sevitt, S. (1956). Distal tubular necrosis with little or no oliguria. *J. Clin. Path*, **9**, 12.

66. Sloan, M. F., Franks, A. J., Exley, K. A. and Davison, A. M. (1978). Acute renal failure due to polymyositis. *Brit. med. J.*, **1**, 1457.

67. Solez, K., d'Agostini, R. J., Stawowy, L., Freedman, M. T., Scott, W. W., Siegelman, S. S. and Heptinstall, R. H. (1977). Beneficial effect of propranolol in a histologically appropriate model of postischemic acute renal failure. *Amer. J. Pathol.*, **88**, 163.

68. Solez, K., Silva, C. B. and Heptinstall, R. H. (1978). Protective effect of clonidine or guanethidine in posti-schemic acute renal failure. *Kidney International*, **12**, 535a.

69. Talley, R. C., Forland, M. and Beller, R. (1970). Reversal of acute renal failure with a combination of IV dopamine and diuretics. *Clin. Res.*, **18**, 518(Abst).

70. Taylor, W. H. (1957). Management of acute renal failure following surgical operation and head injury. *Lancet*, **ii**, 703.

71. Thiel, G., De Rougemont, D., Konrad, L., Oeschger, A., Torhorst, J. and Brunner, F. (1978). Gentamicin induced acute renal failure in the rat. *Proceedings of the 7th International Congress of Nephrology*, pD-45 Abstract.

72. Thomson, W. B., Buchanan, A. A., Doak, P. B., and Peart, W. S. (1964). Peritoneal dialysis. *Brit. med. J.*, **1**, 932.

73. Trueta, J., Barclay, A. E., Daniel, P. M., Franklin, K. J. and Pritchard, M. M. L. (1947). *Studies of the Renal Circulation*. Oxford: Blackwell Scientific.

74. Turner, A. J. (1909). On lead poisoning in childhood. *Brit. med. J.*, **i**, 895.

75. Werb, R., Clark, W. F., Lindsay, R. M., Jones, E. O. P., Turnbull, D. I. and Linton, A. L. (1978). Protective effect of prostaglandin (PGE_2) in glycerol-induced acute renal failure in rats. *Clin. Sci. and Molecular Medicine*, **55**, 505.

76. Wilkinson, S. P., Blendis, L. M. and Williams, R. (1974). Frequency and type of renal and electrolyte disorders in fulminant hepatic failure. *Brit. med. J.*, **1**, 186.

77. Yeh, T. J., Brackney, E. L., Hall, D. P. and Ellison, R. G. (1964). Renal complications of open-heart surgery: predisposing factors, prevention, and management. *J. Thorac. & Cardiovasc. Surg.*, **47**, 79.

78. Yip, L. L. (1981). Toxic material from the gall bladder of the grass carp (Ctenopharyngodon idellus). *Toxicon*, **19**, 567.

79. Yver, L., Marechaud, R., Picaud, D., Touchard, G., Talin d'Eyzac, A., Matuchansky, C. and Patte, D. (1978). Insuffisance renale aiguë au cours d'un saturnisme professionnel. Responsabilité du traitement chélateur. *Nouveau Presse Méd.*, **7**, 1541.

Further Reading

Gabriel, R. (1981). *Renal Medicine*, 2nd edition. London: Baillière Tindall.

Myers, B. D. and Moran, S. M. (1986). Classic (oliguric) acute renal failure. *N. Engl. J. of Med.*, **314**, 97.

Chapter 5
Respiratory Failure

Pulmonary Circulation and Lung Function

In any process of resuscitation, and in the understanding of the pathophysiology of lung disease and respiratory failure, these two aspects of body function must be considered together. Changes in the pulmonary circulation produce changes in cardiac haemodynamics and lead to cardiac failure; conversely, both congenital and acquired myocardial and valvular disease cause pathological changes in the lung parenchyma. When treating patients with various drugs or when applying positive pressure ventilation, the interdependence of these two factors should never be forgotten and the clinician should not be satisfied until both aspects are responding correctly. This may be illustrated by a patient who is being artificially ventilated by means of a positive pressure ventilator with oxygen and who has an arterial oxygen saturation of 96%, a PO_2 of 250 mmHg but a systolic blood pressure of only 60 mmHg. An understanding of pulmonary haemodynamics may help to prevent this occurring.

The pulmonary circulation

The pulmonary vessels constitute a low-pressure distensible system. Anatomically the pulmonary circulation constitutes the blood that is in the pulmonary vessels, in the lungs and in the left atrium. Its exact volume is still unknown because it is so difficult to measure, but a variety of methods indicate that it lies between 10% and 20% of the total blood volume (i.e. between 500 and 1200 ml). The volume is greater in systole than in diastole. Blood enters the pulmonary artery during systole, but does not leave the left atrium until diastole. The homoeostatic mechanisms which control the pulmonary circulation are unknown as yet, but it has been pointed out that the stroke volume of the left ventricle, usually in the region of 70 ml, only needs to be in excess of the stroke volume of the right ventricle by 0.1 ml for the lungs to be emptied

within 2 hours. This may explain in part the hypotension and gradual deterioration of patients when they are placed on some forms of positive pressure respiration.

When the lungs are examined at *post mortem* it is found that, anatomically, approximately 510–580 ml of blood are probably contained within the lung parenchyma. In addition, the volume of blood within the oxygenating capillaries of the lung is approximately 80 ml. This very small volume of blood is spread over an oxygenating surface of 50–80 m², the area varies with expansion and therefore with exercise. The lung capillaries are so small that they can contain only one red cell placed across their lumen, thus diffusion of gases into and from the alveolar sac is facilitated by the individual exposure of the erythrocyte to the lining membrane. When the lungs expand, the cells comprising the capillary alveolar membrane are stretched, and elongation occurs so that they become thinner and the rate of diffusion of gases across the alveolar membrane increases. In the adult, when the cardiac output is 5 litres/minute, the rate at which the total capillary volume is exchanged is rapid; in fact an individual red cell traverses the lung parenchyma in just less than 1 second. The oxygenation of an individual red cell to 100% saturation can take place in less than 0.2 seconds and this allows much leeway in the ability of the pulmonary apparatus to produce full saturation of the blood when the cardiac output is increased in exercise to 30 litres/minute.

The volume of blood contained within the pulmonary circulation is altered by changes in the volume of blood in the systemic circulation. This in turn is controlled by mechanisms which determine the tone of the vessels. L-noradrenaline, for example, causes vasoconstriction, reduces the systemic blood volume and increases the pulmonary blood volume. Hexamethonium salts, on the other hand, produce vasodilatation, especially of the systemic arteriolar bed, and by this means reduce the quantity of blood in the pulmonary compartment and have therefore been used for the treatment of pulmonary oedema (see p. 365).

Similarly, the pulmonary circulation can be influenced by mechanical means. When venous tourniquets are applied to the limbs the pulmonary blood volume is reduced and, conversely, when special suits are worn to overcome the effects of gravity in high-speed vehicles by applying pressure externally, pulmonary blood volume is increased. Changes in posture from the upright to the horizontal position and changes in intrathoracic pressure produced by coughing or breath-holding etc., also influence this volume. The pulmonary blood volume is greatest when we are lying down and smallest when we are standing up. This change can have a therapeutic effect, as in acute left ventricular failure.

It can thus be seen that one of the ways in which control is maintained over a balanced pulmonary circulation is by alterations in the pulmonary blood volume and this can be achieved by various methods, such as sighing, breathing either more or less deeply, changing posture, as well as by varying the volume of blood ejected at each beat and, therefore, the volume retained within the ventricle before diastole. This last volume is also influenced by posture.

When man adopts the upright position, gravity exerts a force which, in many important organs such as the brain and the lungs and many of the abdominal viscera when the arterial supply is from below, is in the opposite direction to that imposed by the heart. Although it was postulated as long ago as 1887 by Johannes Orth[98] that a reduction of blood content in the apex of the lung when man was upright was the cause of tuberculosis being more prominent in those regions, it has been necessary to await more refined techniques in order to demonstrate that the distribution of blood in the normal lung is greater at the bases than in the apices. This has been done, using external counting techniques, by West.[140] It has therefore been clearly demonstrated that the distribution and regional flow of blood through the lungs are influenced by the negative pressure exerted by the weight of the column of blood in the pulmonary vessels, thus the ratio of blood flow to ventilation is unequal in different parts of the lung. The pulmonary circulation is of very low pressure so that gravitational forces have a much more important influence upon the circulation in the lungs than upon that in the rest of the body. The mean pulmonary artery pressure is 15 mmHg and the

systolic and diastolic pressures are approximately 25 mmHg and 5 mmHg respectively.

Alveolar ventilation

The most important function of the lungs is that of gas exchange. It is, therefore, always necessary to picture this function in precise terms of alveolar ventilation rather than in the more crude measurements of the volumes of gas that enter and leave. The degree of alveolar ventilation is determined by three factors: the frequency of respiration, tidal volume, and respiratory dead space.

A measurement of alveolar ventilation can be made using the numerical values of these three factors:

$$\text{Alveolar ventilation (ml/minute)} = \\ (\text{tidal volume} - \text{dead space}) \times \text{frequency}$$

If we take the respiratory dead space as being 150 ml, the tidal volume as being 500 ml, and the rate of breathing as 15/minute then:

$$\text{Alveolar ventilation} = \\ (500 - 150) \times 15 = 5250 \text{ ml/minute}$$

It can be seen that if air moves in and out of a tube with the same flat front that is presented when a piston moves backwards and forwards, then when the tidal volume is 150 ml, alveolar ventilation could be zero. In practice, however, gases do not move through a tube in this way; they have a pointed or conical front which, together with turbulence, ensures some alveolar ventilation even with very low tidal volumes. However, because of the inaccuracies that are present when the tidal volume is small, this method of calculation can only be used with tidal volumes greater than 300 ml and in the absence of lung pathology, when the anatomical and physiological dead spaces are very nearly equal. Another method of determination based on the ability of the lungs to remove CO_2 must be used when the tidal volume is less than 300 ml.

$$\text{Alveolar ventilation (ml/breath)} = \\ \frac{\text{volume of } CO_2 \text{ expired (ml)}}{\text{per cent } CO_2 \text{ in alveolar air}} \times 100$$

e.g.

$$\text{Alveolar ventilation} = \frac{18}{5.6} \times 100 = 321 \text{ ml/breath}$$

In the adult, if we add 150 ml to this figure, we have the tidal volume.

We have already mentioned that when the tidal volume is low, alveolar ventilation will decrease until it approaches very close to zero so that an increase in the rate of ventilation will have relatively little effect. Conversely, because the larger the tidal volume the greater the fraction of air available at each breath for alveolar ventilation, a small increase in the rate of respiration has a relatively large effect. Let us examine the degree of alveolar ventilation that is achieved under three different conditions of frequency of respiration and tidal volume when the volume of air breathed per minute ('minute volume') is the same.

Let us assume that the minute volume (MV) is 7 litres, but the tidal volume (TV) and respiratory rate (RR) vary. The respiratory dead space = 150 ml.

Case A

TV = 200 ml
RR = 35/minute MV = 200 × 35 = 7000 ml
Alveolar ventilation = (200 − 150) × 35
    = 1750 ml*

Case B

TV = 500 ml
RR = 14/minute MV = 500 × 14 = 7000 ml
Alveolar ventilation = (500 − 150) × 14
    = 4900 ml

Case C

TV = 700 ml
RR = 10/minute MV = 700 × 10 = 7000 ml
Alveolar ventilation = (700 − 150) × 10
    = 5500 ml

These figures readily demonstrate increasing alveolar ventilation in the presence of decreasing respiratory rate. It can be appreciated easily from these figures that a significant increase in alveolar ventilation can occur with consequent lowering of PCO_2 by an increase in respiratory rate and tidal volume that is virtually imperceptible by routine clinical observation.

Barbiturate intoxication

The converse is also true, and the following case illustrates the value of this simple calculation.

A 21-year-old man was admitted to the emergency room having taken a large dose of barbiturates. He responded poorly to stimuli and was cyanosed. His respirations were shallow and an endotracheal tube was passed without difficulty and without the use of relaxants or anaesthetic. The tidal and minute volumes were measured

using a Wright respirometer.

11.30 a.m.

TV = 215 ml
RR = 16/minute MV = 215 × 16 = 3440 ml
Alveolar ventilation = (215 − 150) × 16 = 1040 ml

This was associated with the following acid–base and blood gas data:

$$pH = 7.240, [HCO_3^-] = 21.8 \text{ mmol/l},$$
$$PCO_2 = 52 \text{ mmHg}, PO_2 = 73 \text{ mmHg}$$

The patient was artificially ventilated with a Bird pressure-cycled ventilator entraining air with a ventilation rate of 16 breaths/minute and a minute volume of 9.1 litres or tidal volume of 569 ml. Approximately 10 ml were added to the dead space by the endotracheal tube and its connections. If we calculate the alveolar ventilation from the simple formula, it was as follows:

11.55 a.m.

TV = 569 ml
RR = 16/minute MV = 16 × 569 = 9104 ml
Alveolar ventilation = (569 − 160) × 16 = 6544 ml

A marked improvement in the blood gas values was observed; there was a rise in blood pH, a fall in PCO_2 and a rise in PO_2.

$$pH = 7.52, [HCO_3^-] = 22.7 \text{ mmol/l},$$
$$PCO_2 = 28 \text{ mmHg}, PO_2 = 258 \text{ mmHg}$$

Ventilation: blood flow ratios

Now that we have examined how blood flows through the lung and the factors that govern alveolar ventilation in the absence of disease processes, we must now see how differences in the ratio of one to another will influence the oxygenation of blood and the removal of carbon dioxide.

The volume of air ventilating alveoli is denoted by V and the quantity of blood flowing through the capillaries by Q. In order to denote any measurement per unit time it is conventional to place a dot above the symbol so that the alveolar ventilation–blood flow ratio is commonly referred to as the $\dot{V}_A/\dot{Q}_C$ ratio where the suffix A refers to 'alveolar' and C to 'capillary'. It is extremely convenient for understanding ventilation–blood flow relationships that the ratio in health is very nearly unity:

$$\frac{\dot{V}_A}{\dot{Q}_C} = \frac{5000 \text{ ml/minute}}{5000 \text{ ml/minute}} = 1†$$

---

* Although this figure is inaccurate and should be a little higher, because the tidal volume is low, it serves to illustrate the point made.

† Many accounts give the average $\dot{V}_A/\dot{Q}_C$ ratio as being less than 1. Comroe *et al.*[35] give it as 0.8. While this may be more accurate, it is much easier in the first instance to look upon people with a $\dot{V}_A/\dot{Q}_C$ ratio of 1 as being in the majority.

That is to say, the cardiac output is approximately 5 l/minute and the alveolar ventilation is approximately 5 l/minute.

Blood enters the main pulmonary artery having an oxygen saturation of 70–75%. It enters the left atrium, through the pulmonary veins, with an oxygen saturation of 94–96%. If we imagine a virtually impossible situation in which the pulmonary artery to one lung was blocked while the main bronchus to that lung was fully open and all the blood pumped by the right ventricle flowed through the other lung, the bronchus of which was blocked, no gas exchange of the blood in the pulmonary circulation would take place and the

patient would rapidly die, even when the cardiac output and alveolar ventilation were normal (Fig. 5.1B and C). This situation can be related to the conditions that prevail in individual alveolar sacs during disease processes. It can, therefore, be seen that the degree of oxygenation of the desaturated mixed venous blood by the lungs will be determined by the ratio of alveolar ventilation to capillary blood flow as perfusion of the lungs takes place.

Respiratory dead space

The tension of oxygen in the atmosphere is approximately 150 mmHg and that of the alveoli

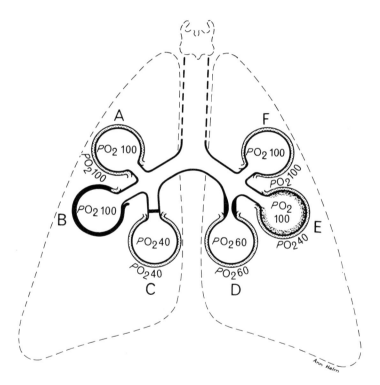

Fig. 5.1 Disturbances of alveolar ventilation and blood flow within the lungs.

A, normal; $\dfrac{\dot{V}_A}{\dot{Q}_C} = \dfrac{5}{5} = 1$.

B, ventilation normal; physiological dead space;

$$\dfrac{\dot{V}_A}{\dot{Q}_C} = \dfrac{5}{0} \text{ or } \infty.$$

C, no ventilation; normal blood flow; shunt;

$$\dfrac{\dot{V}_A}{\dot{Q}_C} = \dfrac{0}{5} = \text{blood } PCO_2 = \text{mixed venous } PCO_2.$$

D, ventilation reduced; blood flow normal; PO_2 rises after breathing O_2 for 10 min;

$$\dfrac{\dot{V}_A}{\dot{Q}_C} = \dfrac{2.5}{5} = 0.5; \text{ blood } PCO_2 \text{ high.}$$

E, alveolar capillary block = shunt; blood PCO_2 = mixed venous PCO_2.

F, increased ventilation; reduced blood flow;

$$\dfrac{\dot{V}_A}{\dot{Q}_C} = \dfrac{6}{2} = 3; \text{ blood } PCO_2 \text{ low.}$$

100 mmHg. This is because air has to flow along a series of channels and tubes before reaching the alveolar sacs. These comprise the anatomical dead space which is approximately 150 ml in the adult. The respiratory, or 'physiological', dead space is formed by the anatomical dead space together with: (1) the volume of gas that ventilates alveoli which have no capillary blood flow (Fig. 5. 1B), and (2) the volume of gas ventilating areas in excess of that required to produce maximum gas exchange (Fig. 5. 1F).[115]

It can thus be seen that when the flow of blood through a capillary is reduced or completely stopped, the alveolar, and therefore the respiratory, dead space is increased.

The pathological conditions that give rise to reduction or blockage of the flow of blood through the alveolar capillaries are fibrotic changes occurring in the pulmonary vessels, emboli arising from blood clots, air or fat following trauma, malignant tumours or parasites, degenerative and other disease processes such as endarteritis, collagen diseases and congenital abnormalities causing stenosis and atresia.

Causes of decreased PO_2 of the blood

Hydrothorax and pneumothorax are common causes of reduced capillary blood flow, but frequently the degree of alveolar ventilation is very nearly equally reduced so that there is little or no change in the $\dot{V}_A/\dot{Q}_C$ ratio.

When there is a decrease in the alveolar ventilation without any change in blood flow, the ratio becomes numerically smaller. This will also occur when there is a shunting of blood through an alveolus so that there is an increase in blood flow through the capillary in the absence of any increase in ventilation. Under these circumstances desaturation of the arterial blood will occur, although when the area of lung involved is small it may be detected only by the measurement of PO_2.

Conditions which cause a reduction in the $\dot{V}_A/\dot{Q}_C$ ratio are those which produce obstruction or increased resistance to the flow of air through the respiratory tract, such as pneumonia, asthma, emphysema, atelectasis and malignant growths. An acute change in the $\dot{V}_A/\dot{Q}_C$ ratio can occur with dramatic suddenness. This is being seen with increasing frequency following road traffic accidents during which the chest has hit the steering wheel. Usually, a small area of lung is affected when a subdivision of the main bronchus is occluded. The condition is similar to the case described below in which there was no apparent intrinsic damage to the lungs following abdominal surgery but a plug of viscid secretions caused almost complete occlusion of the left main bronchus and collapse of the lung.

Case history. A 54-year-old male underwent exploratory abdominal surgery. Immediately following the operation, automatic artificial ventilation of the lungs was maintained until spontaneous respiration returned soon after the cessation of the anaesthetic. One hour after the end of the operation the endotracheal tube was removed. Approximately 30 minutes later the patient was noticed to have marked respiratory distress with gasping, diaphoresis and cyanosis. Blood gas studies performed at that time showed severe hypoxia and, because of the tachypnoea, hypocarbia. Figure 5.2a reveals almost total collapse of the left lung with deviation of the mediastinum. Oxygen by mask was given at a high flow rate; there was no improvement of the cyanosis. While bronchoscopy was being arranged, endotracheal suction was performed using a small plastic catheter and the patient was encouraged to cough. One hour later the patient was able to clear the bronchial secretions and re-expand his lungs with marked improvement of his clinical condition (Fig. 5.2b). Bronchoscopy was therefore unnecessary and marked improvement in respiratory blood gas levels resulted.

This case is illustrated by Fig. 5.1C. Following occlusion of the bronchus, blood was suddenly shunted from the right to the left side of the heart without undergoing gas exchange. Almost 50% of the effective cardiac output with regard to oxygen transport was therefore lost, and it was thus not surprising that the condition of the patient changed dramatically from being a normal postoperative state one moment to being a state of severe respiratory distress a few seconds later. This circumstance is quite different from a pneumothorax in which, notwithstanding the severe changes in haemodynamics that occur, some blood is diverted from the collapsed lung so that there is increased perfusion of the non-collapsed lung and therefore increased effective gas exchange in the normally functioning lung. The right-to-left shunt of blood across the heart is then less severe.

Another condition in which an acute change in $V_A/\dot{Q}_C$ ratio can occur is the placement of an endotracheal tube so deeply that it extends past the bifurcation or carina. This gives rise to the same changes of ventilation and blood flow that are present in Fig. 5.1C. A radiograph of the lungs

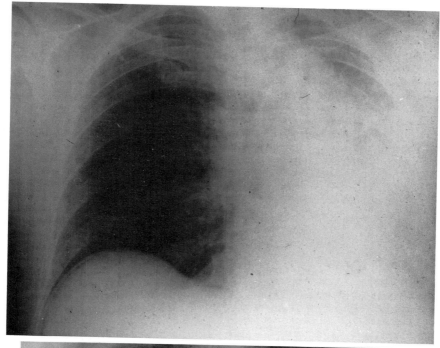

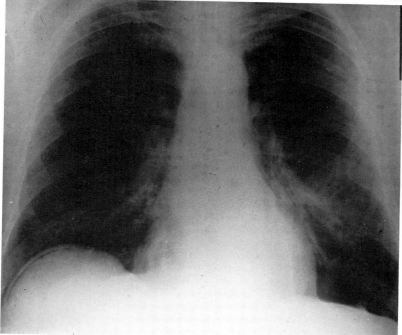

Fig. 5.2 (a) Radiograph of a 54-year-old patient who had undergone minor abdominal surgery (note air under diaphragm). Almost complete collapse of the left lung has occurred with consequent shunting of blood from the right to the left side of the heart. (b) Radiograph showing re-expansion of the lung in the same patient (note air under diaphragm) 1 hour later, after endotracheal suction. The patient coughed and removed a mucous plug.

Reproduced with permission from Brooks, D. K.: Organ Failure Following Surgery, in Hardy, J. D., *et al.* (eds): ADVANCES IN SURGERY, Volume 6. Copyright © 1972 by Year Book Medical Publishers, Inc., Chicago.

usually demonstrates the malpositioning of the endotracheal tube (Fig. 5.3). In this chest X-ray an 'air bronchogram' of the left main bronchus is visible but collapse of the left lung is progressing. There may be difficulty in detecting the condition by auscultation of the breath sounds. Ventilation of both lungs may occur intermittently, such as when the neck is extended, and breath sounds may then be heard from time to time in the non-ventilated lung in a misleading manner. Breath sounds may also be heard when the lungs are excessively inflated manually with a self-inflating (Ambu) resuscitator bag.

It will be readily appreciated that the changes occurring in large areas of lung can be present also in either very small groups of alveoli or single individual alveoli scattered throughout the lungs. Although the changes are a little more complicated, the principles involved are the same.

Another complication that can occur either spontaneously or postoperatively and can lead to most, if not all, of the abnormalities in alveolar ventilation–blood flow ratios is the inhalation of gastric contents. An inhalation pneumonitis can develop which has numerous immediate and long-term effects. All too frequently inhalation pneumonitis is caused by covering an endotracheal tube with an oxygen mask when the patient is unconscious. The mask channels vomit down the endotracheal tube. Anoxia can cause immediate cardiac arrest. However, in the very early stages, when the amount of vomit inhaled is small, acute anoxia is not marked and no ill-effects may be observed. During the following 24 hours, increasing respiratory dysfunction develops. This results in reduced oxygen and raised carbon dioxide levels in the blood. The capability of gas exchange in the lungs decreases as time progresses, until the hypoxia is so severe that it may be incompatible with life. It then becomes necessary to institute artificial ventilation of the lungs and sometimes to perform a tracheostomy.

In addition to normal supportive therapy, the regimen of treatment that is currently followed by most clinicians includes administration of antibiotics and large doses of corticosteroids.

Case history. A 56-year-old woman underwent a minor operation. While she was anaesthetized she suffered, undetected, a minor cerebrovascular accident. While recovering from the anaesthetic and breathing spontaneously, she inhaled some vomit. Although she was treated immediately following this episode by bronchoscopy and the removal of as much of the gastric contents as possible by suction, and although 6-methylprednisolone 21 sodium succinate (Solu-Medrone) was given intravenously in doses of 250 mg every 6 hours,

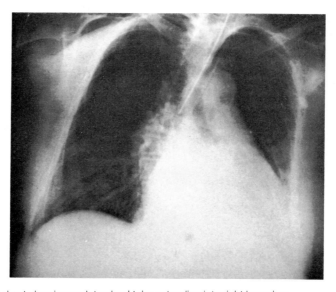

Fig. 5.3 Radiograph of chest showing endotracheal tube extending into right bronchus.

severe anoxia developed.

Three days later, severe dyspnoea suddenly appeared at a time when there was improvement in the blood gas values. A chest X-ray revealed a pneumothorax of the left lung cavity. An intrathoracic tube inserted for under-water drainage offered much relief. The following day the acute onset of dyspnoea occurred again. X-ray films of the chest demonstrated a pneumothorax on the right side. A tube was therefore inserted into the right side of chest, and this was once again followed by marked clinical improvement (Fig. 5.4a).

The patient's chest condition improved on the regimen of antibiotics and under reduced corticosteroid dosage so that the chest tubes could be withdrawn (Fig. 5.4b). Unfortunately, the patient died from a further cerebrovascular accident. However, her case serves to illustrate the possible dangers of inhalation pneumonitis as it is a known complication following surgery. Pneumothorax resulting from inhalation of gastric contents has also been observed in patients who have developed syncope following myocardial infarction.

The detection of a pneumothorax, in a patient who is being ventilated artificially, is sometimes very difficult by clinical examination. Pneumothorax should, however, be suspected when there are changes in the patient's haemodynamics and evidence of respiratory distress, for example suddenly 'fighting' the ventilator.

Ventilation may be generally reduced by diseases such as myasthenia gravis and the excessive administration of neostigmine in the treatment of this condition, the giving of muscle relaxants during anaesthesia, or the depression of the respiratory centre by the anaesthetic agents themselves (e.g. morphine and barbiturates). A metabolic acidosis, carbon dioxide retention, anoxia and damage to the brain and brainstem may also cause respiratory depression. In addition to the muscle relaxants used in anaesthesia, some antibiotics (see p. 137), botulinum and other toxins, nerve gases, nicotine poisoning, poliomyelitis, and damage to the thoracic cage may cause a reduction in overall ventilation of the lungs.

It can therefore be readily appreciated that when an alveolus is perfused with blood, but not ventilated, no change will occur in the gas content of the alveolus itself or the blood leaving it (see Fig. 5.1C). The blood has the same oxygen content as that of mixed venous blood in the right atrium, and desaturation of the arterial blood will result when this blood mixes with that which has passed through normally perfused and ventilated alveoli (see Fig. 5.1A). When the flow of air into and out of a single alveolus is impaired, but not completely blocked (see Fig. 5.1D), the degree of alveolar ventilation can be such that for the patient breathing air, the result in both cases is virtually identical. If, however, the patient is allowed to breathe oxygen of high concentration for 10–30 minutes, the mere process of diffusion will allow the nitrogen in the non-ventilated alveoli to be replaced with O_2. The arterial oxygen saturation then rises, very often to within normal values. This will only occur when blood flows from the right to the left side of the heart through alveoli that have a reduced ventilation and therefore a low $\dot{V}_A/\dot{Q}_C$ ratio. If a 'shunt' of this kind is caused by a congenital anomaly of the heart (e.g. tetralogy of Fallot), increasing the oxygen tension of the air breathed will not appreciably alter the PO_2 of the arterial blood, and anoxaemia will persist.

The two factors, alveolar hypoventilation and an abnormal (uneven) $\dot{V}_A/\dot{Q}_C$ ratio, may be present together. In certain conditions alveolar ventilation may be reduced to the same extent as capillary blood flow and a $\dot{V}_A/\dot{Q}_C$ ratio close to unity persists. The arterial blood is not desaturated, because of the reduced cardiac output that must be present, but the PO_2 of the mixed venous blood is reduced. When in disease processes, ventilation–blood flow ratios vary in different parts of the lung, then arterial anoxaemia must exist in a patient breathing air, and exacerbation of the anoxaemia will be readily apparent if a general reduction in ventilation is produced by the factors we have already noted, such as drugs, CO_2 retention and metabolic acidosis, or when the body's oxygen requirements are increased as during exercise and pyrexia.

A further cause of hypoxaemia is a reduced rate of diffusion of gases across the alveolar membrane, often referred to as alveolar capillary block. It can be caused by any material that lines the alveolar sac. It is present in diseases of the lung such as hyaline membrane disease of the newborn, asthma, bronchitis, bronchiolitis and broncho-pneumonia. Interstitial oedema and diffuse fibrosis, which causes pericapillary thickening as in pneumoconiosis and sarcoid, also give rise to alveolar-capillary block.

When a severe degree of alveolar capillary block is present, as in hyaline membrane disease, the arterial blood oxygen tension and saturation are low and the tension of CO_2 is high. The patient must breathe an oxygen-enriched gas mixture to maintain life. No difficulty is experienced in maintaining a high arterial blood oxygen tension if the

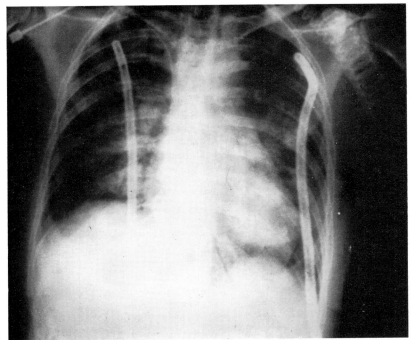

(a)

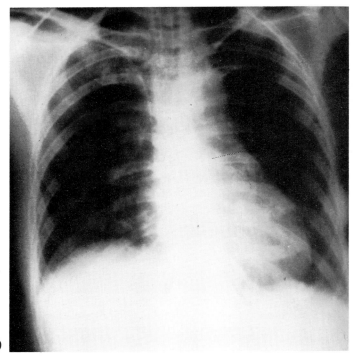

(b)

infants breathe an atmosphere containing 60% or more of oxygen. Carbon dioxide is not, however, eliminated, unless the lungs are artificially ventilated. In this condition all or nearly all the alveoli are affected.

In conditions other than hyaline membrane disease of the newborn the number of alveoli affected may be few, and desaturation of the arterial blood when the patient is at rest breathing air is not always present.

Some degree of alveolar-capillary block is always caused when a bronchogram is performed. A fall in the blood oxygen saturation is not an uncommon finding following this investigation. Normally, the degree of alveolar-capillary block is of little importance unless a bronchogram of both lungs is obtained at the same time or if the lung not under investigation has a grossly impaired function.

When alveolar–capillary block affects only a relatively small area of lung, hypoxaemia becomes apparent only in circumstances when the cardiac output has to increase during exercise or when the overall ventilation of the lungs is reduced.

When the rate of blood flow through the lungs increases, insufficient time is available for gas to diffuse through the exudate or thickened membrane, while any reduction in alveolar ventilation which causes a fall in the alveolar PO_2 reduces the gradient in oxygen tension between the alveolus and the blood and therefore the rate at which O_2 tends to diffuse.

The clinical picture of the patient suffering from impairment of diffusion across the alveolar membranes (alveolar-capillary block) is one in which there is dyspnoea either at rest or upon exercise; the depth and rate of ventilation increase and become more readily apparent with physical effort. The arterial blood oxygen saturation at rest may be normal or reduced and decreases with exercise. The reduced oxygen content of the blood can be more readily detected by the measurement of blood PO_2. Because of decreased cardiac output, the mixed venous oxygen saturation is frequently reduced at rest (e.g. in the region of 50%). A further fall is readily detected during exercise. Because CO_2 diffuses more rapidly than O_2, the PCO_2 of the arterial blood may be reduced. When the area of lung affected by alveolar capillary block is increased, a normal or raised PCO_2 is found.

Compensation for anoxia and hypercarbia

We can summarize the causes of hypoxaemia as being a result of hypoventilation, uneven ventilation–capillary blood flow ratios, the abnormal shunting of blood from the venous to the arterial circulation, and alveolar capillary block. All four conditions can exist in the same patient. We must now look at how a patient with chronic lung disease compensates for these changes.

In order to make the blood a more efficient oxygen-carrying system, the number of erythrocytes in chronic respiratory failure is increased. When the packed cell volume (PCV) is measured it is found to be raised from the normal 40–45%, to approximately 70%. This mechanism is very similar to that which occurs in the presence of cyanotic congenital heart disease and that which follows acclimatization to low oxygen tensions which are present at high altitudes. A relatively long period, extending over many days and even weeks, is required in order to achieve maximum increase in the red blood cell mass. An adequate supply of iron is also necessary. Because the process is so slow and because in the acute toxic state proliferation of erythrocytes is inhibited, it may sometimes be necessary to transfuse blood in the first instance. Because it is best to avoid expansion of the blood volume in the presence of cardiac failure, it is preferable to transfuse packed cells or blood which has been allowed to separate under gravity and has had the supernatant fluid and plasma removed or to combine the infusion with a rapidly acting diuretic such as ethacrynic acid or frusemide (see p. 365).

In all anoxic conditions the concentration of myohaemoglobin in the muscles is increased and this assists in the transfer of oxygen to the tissues when the tension in the blood is reduced.

When the lungs are unable to remove CO_2 so that the tension of this gas both in the blood and the alveoli is raised, then the pH of the arterial blood falls and there is a respiratory acidosis. Because of the characteristics and shape of the titration curve of H_2CO_3 with $NaHCO_3$ and the

Fig. 5.4 (a) Radiograph of a 56-year-old woman who postoperatively inhaled her vomit while unconscious as a result of a cerebrovascular accident. A pneumothorax developed while the lungs were being artificially ventilated, first on one side and then on the other. (b) Radiograph after removal of the intrathoracic drainage tubes following treatment with high doses of steroids and antibiotics.
Reproduced with permission from Brooks, D. K.: Organ Failure Following Surgery, in Hardy, J. D., et al. (eds): ADVANCES IN SURGERY, Volume 6. Copyright © 1972 by Year Book Medical Publishers, Inc., Chicago.

fact that within the body this buffer system is used within a range within which it is least effective (see p. 70), acute retention of CO_2 causes an abrupt fall in pH. The situation can therefore be referred to as an 'acute, uncompensated respiratory acidosis' (Table 5.1). As time passes, HCO_3^- is retained by the renal tubules, more Cl^- is excreted and the urine is also acidified. In this way the pH of the blood tends to return to more normal values. In practice, complete compensation to a normal pH is very rarely reached, although the $[HCO_3^-]$ may rise from its normal value of 24–25 mmol/l (mEq/l) to 38 mmol/l (mEq/l) or more. The process of retaining bicarbonate is characteristically relatively slow, requiring a minimum of 48 hours, and usually very much longer, before compensation in this respect has proceeded very far. Thus the acute onset of CO_2 retention, either in the uncompensated or partially compensated patient, may require treatment with infusions of $NaHCO_3$ so that the plasma $[HCO_3^-]$ is 'artificially' raised. During the time in which compensation is occurring spontaneously, the patient may be in great danger from central nervous system depression, and respiratory depression when allowed to breathe oxygen in high concentrations.

Functional changes in respiratory failure

The functional disturbances that develop in respiratory failure are determined very largely by the underlying lung pathology. Apart from the changes in biochemistry, red blood cells, the distribution of fluid and renal function, the two aspects that require most attention are those of the basic alterations that have occurred in respiratory function and the effects these changes have on the cardiovascular system.

The following changes are found: (a) impedance to the flow of air within the bronchial tree caused by constriction of the bronchioles or secretions; (b) impairment of gaseous diffusion across the alveolar capillary membrane; (c) changes in the ventilation–perfusion ratios because some blood flows through alveolar sacs which have a reduced or absent ventilation or through shunts across the bronchial artery pulmonary venous bed; and (d) reduction in overall ventilation because of movement of the thoracic cage and diaphragm.

Disease processes, present within the lung parenchyma, may increase the pulmonary vascular resistance so that to maintain the same output the right ventricle is forced to perform more work and, consequently to hypertrophy. The increased pulmonary vascular resistance may be caused by: (a) transitory constriction of the pulmonary arteriolar bed produced by the acute infective process; (b) reduction in the size of the pulmonary capillary bed in such conditions as emphysema and diffuse carcinomatous infiltration; and (c) direct obstruction of the pulmonary vascular bed by emboli, carcinoma, thrombosis, diffuse interstitial fibrosis, parasitic infiltration and rare conditions such as chorio-epithelioma.[11]

In the presence of chronic obstructive lung disease producing anoxaemia and therefore cyanosis, the respiratory centre becomes relatively insensitive to small changes in arterial PO_2. A new substance is now available, almitrine bimesylate (a triazine derivative), which stimulates the respiratory centre and improves blood flow and therefore the $\dot{V}_A/\dot{Q}_C$ ratio. There have been a number of

Table 5.1 Blood pH, 'standard bicarbonate' and oxygen saturation, plasma TCO_2, PCO_2, $[Cl^-]$ and PO_2 in five patients with respiratory disease

Sample	pH	St. bic. (mmol/l)	TCO_2 (mmol/l)	PCO_2 (mmHg)	$[Cl^-]$ (mmol/l)	O_2 sat. (%)	PO_2 (mmHg)
A	7.21	23.6		93	101	78	58
B	7.12		26.0	79	103	75	58
C*	7.03	15.6		105		90	100
D	7.27		34.8	74	100	77	61
E	7.39	30.0		71	96	81	79

*Samples A, B, D and E were obtained from arteries when the patients were not breathing oxygen-enriched mixtures; sample C was cord blood taken while the body was enclosed in an incubator and 80% O_2 was being inhaled.

A and B are examples of acute uncompensated respiratory acidosis in the adult.

C is taken from a case of hyaline membrane disease of the newborn. The patient in this case was born with an uncompensated respiratory acidosis.

D is an adult who has a partially compensated respiratory acidosis.

E is an adult who has, with the assistance of infusion of $NaHCO_3$, fully compensated respiratory acidosis.

pH = blood pH; St. bic. = standard bicarbonate; TCO_2 = plasma total CO_2 content; PCO_2 = partial pressure of CO_2; $[Cl^-]$ = plasma chloride concentration; O_2 sat. = oxygen saturation of whole blood; PO_2 = partial pressure of O_2 in arterial blood.

reports demonstrating an improvement in arterial PO_2 following its use.[94, 108, 127]

When respiratory failure is a result of severe bronchopneumonia superimposed upon chronic bronchitis and emphysema, the pathophysiology is one of obstruction to ventilation by constriction of the bronchioles, and profuse accumulations of secretions. There is impairment of diffusion across the alveoli and a general reduction in the ventilation–perfusion ratio.

When the prime pathology is that of pulmonary fibrosis, diffusion of gas across the alveolar membrane and obstruction to capillary blood flow are the most important disturbances of function. However, ventilation is also impaired when lung compliance is reduced. This is a progressive condition in which, in the early stages, normal saturation or desaturation of the arterial blood may be present with a reduced carbon dioxide tension. Later, desaturation of the arterial blood together with a raised PCO_2 are found.

Because of the resistance to blood flow caused by changes in the alveolar capillary bed, the right ventricle hypertrophies. We have seen how the normal pressure within the pulmonary artery is 25/5 mmHg with a mean pressure of 15 mmHg. It is usually accepted that a mean pressure greater than 25 mmHg is diagnostic of pulmonary artery hypertension. In any condition where the resistance to flow through the capillary bed is increased, the pulmonary artery mean pressure rises. In chronic lung disease, however, the pulmonary artery pressure when measured at rest may not be abnormally high, but rises to excessively high levels with exercise. In the normal healthy pulmonary circulation, no rise in the pulmonary artery pressure is associated with exercise. The degree of impairment of function and consequent rise in pulmonary artery pressure depends upon the length of time that the disease processes have been present and their severity. It will be apparent that it is these factors that determine the onset of right ventricular failure.

Shock caused by respiratory failure

It is not uncommon for patients who have developed respiratory failure and who have not had the benefits of medical and nursing care until the disease process is well advanced, to become severely dehydrated and malnourished. Also, in those patients who have been anoxic for a considerable period, the summation of different pathological processes produces cardiac failure and hypotension.

It is not uncommon for patients with severe bronchopneumonia to develop a bacteraemia following tracheal intubation and artificial ventilation of the lungs. The measures required for the treatment of toxic shock (see p. 210) then have to be instituted.

Shock can also be produced when the inflation pressure used to inflate the lungs is so great that blood flow through the lungs is impaired. Shock can also be induced by positive end-expiratory pressure (PEEP) (see p. 132).

It is often very difficult to diagnose a pneumothorax, during artificial ventilation of the lungs, by pure clinical observation. The clinician should therefore be on his guard and consider this complication when there is a fall in blood pressure. Frequent radiographs are sometimes necessary.

Two other complications are associated with respiratory failure. The first is hypotension caused by a severe metabolic acidosis (see p. 137). The second is stress ulceration in the stomach (see p. 199), sometimes associated with massive blood loss.

Carbon dioxide (CO_2) narcosis

There is one further pathophysiological response which is of prime importance in the treatment of patients with respiratory failure when anoxaemia is associated with hypercarbia. High tensions of carbon dioxide in the blood produce central nervous system depression. When they are extremely high the patients ventilate at a slow rate, are comatose or disorientated and have coarse twitching movements of the limb muscles. This is most commonly seen when the PCO_2 of the arterial blood is above 100 mmHg. The degree of severity depends, however, very largely upon the extent to which compensation, by means of a rise in plasma $[HCO_3^-]$, has occurred. When, for example, a patient, who is anoxic and has a PCO_2 in the region of 70 mmHg, is given high O_2 tensions to breathe, the anoxic stimulus to respiration is removed. As ventilation is depressed, so the PCO_2 rises to even greater values.

This situation is seen mainly in patients when in addition to very high CO_2 tensions in the arterial blood, there has not been sufficient time for the $[HCO_3^-]$ of the plasma to rise and compensate for the fall in blood pH. This is only seen when the onset of respiratory failure is acute or when there is an acute exacerbation of an existing disease process such as chronic obstructive lung disease (chronic bronchitis).

Summary of alterations in the arterial blood gas tensions

We have already mentioned how carbon dioxide diffuses at least 20 times more rapidly through tissues and solutions than oxygen. For this reason, reduced gas exchange will always be reflected in hypoxaemia long before it has any effect on the carbon dioxide tension of the blood. Normally speaking, therefore, mild degrees of reduced diffusing capacity produce hypoxaemia with hypocarbia (hypocapnia). However, in conditions where there is a massive accumulation of fluid or blood in the lungs, both hypoxaemia and hypercarbia will result.

Reduced alveolar ventilation

When a patient is breathing air, alveolar hypoventilation, which may be caused by drugs, insufficient ventilation during anaesthesia, damage to the thoracic cage, neuromuscular paralysis (e.g. poliomyelitis), pneumothorax, emphysema and idiopathic emphysema produce a condition of hypoxaemia associated with hypercarbia.

Reduction of the ventilation–perfusion ratio

The ventilation–perfusion ratio ($\dot{V}_A/\dot{Q}_C$) is reduced when (a) alveoli are underventilated, or (b) the capillary blood flow through alveoli is increased without any concomitant rise in ventilation. When blood passes through alveoli that are not ventilated at all, it retains the same characteristics as mixed venous blood that is contained within the right atrium; the $\dot{V}_A/\dot{Q}_C$ ratio is 0. The oxygen tension of this blood is low and the PCO_2 is high. When blood that has passed through normally ventilated alveoli mixes with the blood that has passed through non-ventilated alveoli, then the oxygen content of the blood flowing into the left atrium is reduced below normal values and its carbon dioxide tension (PCO_2) is raised above normal values.

When air is unable to enter some alveoli it may be diverted to other normal alveoli which are then overventilated. When blood that has passed through overventilated alveoli (where the $\dot{V}_A/\dot{Q}_C$ ratio is high) mixes with blood that has passed through underventilated alveoli (where the $V_A/\dot{Q}_C$ ratio is low), the reduced carbon dioxide tension of the blood from overventilated alveoli compensates for the raised carbon dioxide tension of blood from underventilated alveoli. The PCO_2 of the mixed blood may be normal or low depending upon the relative number of the two types of alveoli involved. The small increase of PO_2 in overventilated alveoli does not lead to any significant increase in oxygen content or saturation of the blood flowing through them because of the shape of the oxygen dissociation curve for whole blood. When, therefore, blood from underventilated alveoli mixes with blood from over-ventilated alveoli, there is no significant compensation for the reduced oxygen content of the blood that has passed through underventilated alveoli. When the mixed blood flows into the left atrium, hypoxaemia results.

It can be readily deduced that when there is uneven distribution of air within the lungs and uneven blood flow through the lungs, the tension of gas as measured in an arterial (mixed) blood sample will be different from the tension of gas in mixed alveolar air. These differences of gas tensions are referred to as alveolar–arterial tension gradients, or A–a differences. Because of the shape of the oxygen dissociation curve for blood, these gradients are more marked for oxygen than for carbon dioxide.

If a patient who has a large number of underventilated alveoli (see Fig. 5.1D), where the $\dot{V}_A/\dot{Q}_C$ ratio is low, is allowed to breathe high concentrations of oxygen for 10 minutes or longer, the oxygen tension within the underventilated alveoli will increase by diffusion alone. The oxygen tension and the oxygen saturation of the arterial blood will increase without any change in CO_2 tension. It must be assumed that respiratory depression is not provoked by breathing an oxygen-enriched mixture.

When the capillary blood flow through alveoli is increased without any concomitant rise in ventilation, the oxygenation of the blood when the patient is breathing air is incomplete and carbon dioxide is retained. The gas content is the same as that which is obtained if a portion of the blood is shunted across non-ventilated alveoli; anoxaemia and hypercarbia result. If the patient breathes an oxygen-enriched mixture, the anoxaemia decreases but the hypercarbia persists. In practice, most clinical conditions of this type consist of a mixture of the different types of altered ventilation–perfusion ratio.

Breathing low oxygen tensions

This normally occurs only in people at high altitudes and has been already described. It results in hypoxaemia and hypocarbia. It may also occur, however, accidentally during anaesthesia, especially during spontaneous ventilation. It also occurs in non-pressurized, high-flying aircraft, when supplementation with oxygen is necessary.

Management of respiratory failure caused by lung disease

Patients who fall into this category are most commonly those who have the pre-existing condition of chronic bronchitis. Usually, these patients have a variable degree of emphysema. They may be severely incapacitated by the primary lung condition and, in addition to a raised blood PCO_2 and low blood PO_2, there may be some measure of cardiac failure. An acute exacerbation of their bronchitis or the onset of bronchopneumonia produces a potentially lethal situation. The increased anoxia and increased work of breathing can cause the immediate onset of cardiac failure or increase its severity.

Not uncommonly, acute fulminating bronchopneumonia may appear acutely in patients of any age. A viral infection such as influenza often precedes the attack. In some respects these patients present an even greater immediate problem than those who have had chronic lung disease. This is because there has been no time for compensation for the abnormal gas tensions to develop. However, the management of both these groups is in principle very similar.

Treatment of respiratory failure

The prime causes of death in respiratory failure are anoxia and cardiac failure. Treatment is, therefore, directed as far as possible towards alleviating these conditions.

Sedation

This is often necessary in order to alleviate anxiety and discomfort. Care must be taken that respiration is not depressed and that allergic responses are not produced. The antihistamines, such as promethazine HCl (Phenergan) 25 mg/day, may be effective. The benzodiazepine group of drugs are also usually safe to give (e.g. diazepam, 5 mg).

Treatment of cardiac failure

In the severely anoxic patient, incipient cardiac failure is commonly present. During the period of severe respiratory failure no harm and much good may be achieved by digitalization. Quite often this is all that is required in order to maintain a correct water balance. Water retention is frequently associated with respiratory failure, even in the absence of obvious clinical signs of cardiac failure. Diuretic therapy is then necessary and the diuretics found to be most beneficial are of the thiazide group. In the presence of a high bicarbonate ion concentration, acetazolamide (Diamox) is often effective.

Removal of secretions

Active physiotherapy aimed at facilitating the removal of secretions contained within the bronchial tree is an essential part of treatment. This can be assisted by suction using a sterile catheter. Bronchoscopy and suction may be necessary. In the last resort a tracheotomy may have to be performed so that these secretions can be removed.

Oxygen therapy

It is essential that oxygen in adequate quantities is administered as early as possible. Most masks are inefficient and rarely allow an oxygen concentration of greater than 30%. Oxygen is often best administered through nasal catheters, at flow rates of 4 litre/minute. The oropharynx acts as a 'mask' and allows quite high concentrations of O_2 to be inhaled.

We have seen how, in these circumstances, a patient who has not compensated for the fall in blood pH resulting from the respiratory acidosis will ventilate at a slower rate and pass into coma because of the increase in CO_2 tension, when the arterial oxygen saturation rises. Much benefit can therefore be obtained by instituting 'artificial compensation' by infusing hypertonic (2.74%) $NaHCO_3$ solution. Care must be taken not to infuse the solution too rapidly because cardiac failure may be already present and in these circumstances it is essential to avoid expanding the vascular space too quickly. The importance of compensating for a fall of pH in respiratory failure is illustrated by the following case.

Case history A 57-year-old man had suffered from chronic bronchitis and emphysema for many years. He was admitted to hospital with acute bronchopneumonia. On examination he was cyanosed, extremely dyspnoeic and breathing at a rate of 38/minute. He had been given digitalis in adequate doses when he became breathless 3 days earlier. He was able to produce copious amounts of thick purulent sputum on coughing, but this required much effort and after a short while he became so exhausted that productive coughing occurred only at relatively infrequent intervals. Although his central venous pressure (CVP) was not raised, there was a slight degree of pitting oedema of the feet and ankles. When his arterial blood was analysed it was found to have an oxygen saturation, when he was breathing oxygen, of 75%. A markedly raised packed cell volume (PCV) was also present. The PCO_2 of

Table 5.2 Blood pH, 'standard bicarbonate', PCO_2, TCO_2, PCV, O_2 sat. and arterial PO_2 in a patient suffering from chronic obstructive lung disease with acute exacerbations

Sample	pH	St. bic. (mmol/l)	PCO_2 (mmHg)	TCO_2 (mmol/l)	PCV (%)	O_2 sat. (%)	PO_2 (mmHg)
1	7.24		85	38.6	71	75	46
2	7.18	27.5	115	—	55	72	45
3	7.42	40.2	91	—	62	84	87
4	7.35	31.2	78	—	63	89	96
5	7.38		55	33.5	62	88	92

pH = arterial blood pH at 38°C; St. bic. = standard bicarbonate; PCO_2 = partial pressure of CO_2; TCO_2 = plasma total CO_2 content; PCV = packed cell volume; O_2 sat. = oxygen saturation of whole blood; PO_2 = partial pressure of O_2.
Sample 1 was taken after bronchopneumonia, exactly 1 year before sample 2. Sample 2 shows that during the period of relatively good lung function, the bicarbonate content of the plasma and PCV had fallen so that decompensation was present when bronchopneumonia developed a second time. Sample 3 was taken 2 days after admission following an infusion of 800 ml of 2.74% $NaHCO_3$. Sample 4 was taken 9 days later, and sample 5 was taken 14 days later.

his arterial blood was 85 mmHg and a marked increase in plasma $[HCO_3^-]$ partially compensated the raised $[H^+]$ so that the pH of the blood was 7.24 (Table 5.2). Because of the increasing quantity of thick purulent fluid within the lungs which was causing a severe fall in oxygen saturation, it was decided that a tracheotomy should be performed so that better access was afforded to the bronchi and the purulent fluid could be removed by suction. This was carried out and a diuretic was given. The same day the oxygen saturation of the arterial blood had risen a little and the PCO_2 had fallen. Under continued digitalization and suction of the trachea and bronchi, a marked improvement occurred so that after 1 week, when the volume of fluid being sucked away was reduced, the tracheostomy was allowed to close. This patient left hospital approximately 3 weeks later and was maintained on tetracycline 1 g/day.

Just less than 1 year later, the patient stopped taking tetracycline because he was so greatly improved. Two weeks after stopping the antibiotic he once again developed bronchopneumonia. During the previous months his lung function had improved so markedly that a process of decompensation had taken place so that his PCV had fallen to 55% and his plasma $[HCO_3^-]$ had been reduced to just above normal values. When he was admitted to hospital with a PCO_2 of 115 mmHg he was, on inspection, comatose with weak twitching movements of the muscles. Ptosis was present and his respiratory rate was 41/minute. He was severely cyanosed. Although he had been given digitalis, since leaving hospital on the previous occasion, his CVP was raised. His arterial blood saturation was 72%. He was placed in an oxygen tent when he almost immediately became hypo-

tensive and even more comatose with shallow, slow respiration and increased twitching of the muscles. He was, therefore, infused with 800 ml of 2.74% $NaHCO_3$. The first 500 ml of this solution were given over a period of 4 hours, during which there was a marked increase in the patient's level of consciousness, a reduction in the severity of the muscular twitching, an improvement in the ventilatory activity and the degree of effort with which he could cough. He was, therefore, placed in the oxygen tent a second time with a decrease in the degree of cyanosis and improvement in cerebral activity. Two days later an arterial blood sample, taken while he was in the oxygen tent, showed an oxygen saturation of 84% and also that the rise in the $[HCO_3^-]$ of the plasma was so high that, in spite of a PCO_2 of 91 mmHg, the pH of the blood was within normal limits. Marked clinical improvement had occurred, the patient was eating well and maintaining a good urine volume and there was no rise in CVP. Improvement gradually continued so that 9 days later the oxygen saturation of the arterial blood while the patient was breathing oxygen was 89% and the large increase in $[HCO_3^-]$ had been in part reduced. This patient made further progress so that before leaving hospital the arterial PCO_2 was 55 mmHg.

Artificial ventilation

In the very severely afflicted patient with respiratory failure, conservative methods are not effective and artificial ventilation has to be performed. Although a plastic endotracheal tube may be kept *in situ* for many days, it is usually preferable to perform this method of treatment through a tracheostomy. The cuff of the tracheostomy tube should be deflated at regular intervals and the secretions should be removed by suction as far down the bronchial tree as possible, sometimes as frequently as every 15 minutes, but care must be taken not to collapse a segment of lung by suction which is too forceful (see p. 166). As recovery progresses, increasing lengths of time are allowed during which the patient is not ventilated but breathes humidified oxygen. Because of the combination of factors of respiratory and cardiac disease, the type of ventilator best suited for this purpose is the patient-triggered, pressure-cycled ventilator. Although aerosol humidification of the ventilating gases is usually achieved, further humidification can be obtained by placing 1–2 ml of isotonic (0.9%) saline, or preferably 0.45% saline, into the endotracheal or tracheostomy tube.

Artificial Ventilation of the Lungs: Changes of Pressure During Ventilation

Because flow, whether it is gas or blood, is dependent upon a pressure gradient, these aspects are of fundamental importance in understanding positive pressure ventilation of the lungs. In order to appreciate the changes caused by artificial inflation of the lungs, we have to be familiar with what happens during spontaneous ventilation, a condition that it is impossible to mimic artificially except with a Cuirass or other external negative pressure ventilator.

Pressure changes during spontaneous ventilation

Within the pleural cavity, throughout the whole of the respiratory cycle, there is a sustained negative pressure which varies between about $^-10$ cm H_2O at the peak of inspiration to about $^-2$ cm H_2O at the middle of expiration.

The intrapulmonary pressure during spontaneous ventilation results from the small resistance to flow produced by the bronchial tubes and amounts to a negative pressure of $^-2$ to $^-3$ cm H_2O during inspiration and a positive pressure of $^+2$ to $^+3$ cm H_2O during the peak of expiration.

The factors which tend to keep any blood vessel open are: (a) the pressure of blood within the vessel, and (b) the negative pressure outside the vessel. In most of the body vessels there is no negative pressure but a positive one, and the negative pressure which surrounds the capillaries of the lung is one of the factors that allows the blood in the pulmonary circulation to flow with such ease. The negative pressure environment of the pulmonary blood vessels is produced by the sum of the intrapleural pressure and the intrapulmonary pressure.

The factors which tend to close a vessel are: (a) the tone of the vessel itself, and (b) the positive pressure outside the vessel. Because the vessel tone of the alveolar capillaries is known to be so low that generally speaking it may be disregarded, it can be appreciated that during spontaneous ventilation there are no forces at any moment tending to close these vessels and that all pressures are tending to keep them open.

This state of affairs, therefore, can never be obtained by means of positive pressure ventilation. At some point in the cycle a force must be applied which is in excess of the 10–12 cmH$_2$O (7–9 mmHg), which is normally present within the alveolar capillaries. The flow of blood through the lungs and therefore the cardiac output must be reduced by the very nature of the forces imposed within the bronchial tree and thoracic cavity.

Pressures within the pulmonary circulation

If we follow the pressures through from the right atrium to the left atrium within the pulmonary circulation, we see that the pressure in the right atrium varies between 0 and 5 mmHg and that of the right ventricle between 25 and 0 mmHg. If there is no obstruction to the flow of blood through the pulmonary valve of the right ventricle, the systolic pressure in the pulmonary artery is very close to that of the right ventricle. The pressures within the pulmonary artery vary between 25 and 7 mmHg, so that the mean pressure, which determines the 'driving force' of blood through the lungs, is in the region of 13–15 mmHg. The exact pressure within the lung capillaries is not known, but if a small catheter is passed as far as it will go into the smallest pulmonary artery so that it is wedged in the lumen, it can be used to estimate the pulmonary venous pressure, assuming there is no obstruction to the flow of blood. This pressure, known as the 'wedge pressure', has a mean value in the region of 5 mmHg (6.8 cmH$_2$O). The left atrial pressure varies between 12 and 0 mmHg. When the mean pulmonary artery pressure is 15 mmHg and the mean left atrial pressure is 5 mmHg the 'driving pressure' of blood through the pulmonary circulation is 10 mmHg. In the presence of left ventricular failure and mitral incompetence, the pressure within the left atrium and, therefore, the pulmonary veins rises so that the mean pressure may be, for example, in the region of 20 mmHg. The force with which blood is propelled into the pulmonary artery then has to be increased so that the mean pressure within this vessel rises to the region of 30 mmHg. When the mean left atrial pressure rises above 30 mmHg, the hydrostatic pressure exceeds the osmotic pressure of the plasma proteins and pulmonary oedema is produced.

Intermittent positive pressure respiration (IPPR)

We have seen how the mean pressure within the pulmonary artery is in the region of 15 mmHg. It should be borne in mind that this is roughly equal to an inflation pressure of 20 cm H_2O (14.7 mmHg). When the lungs are inflated with this pressure, flow of blood through the lungs is temporarily blocked because the pressure within the capillaries is considerably lower. It must also be remembered that the heart may be beating at a rate of 70/minute or more while the lungs are being inflated at a rate which is usually in the region of 20/minute, so that the longer positive pressure is applied in excess of lung capillary pressure, the greater is the reduction in cardiac output. This subject has been well reviewed by Howells.[71] The application of a negative pressure during the expiratory phase of respiration so that the intrapulmonary pressure is rapidly lowered, should in theory assist the flow of blood through the pulmonary circulation and, therefore, increase the cardiac output. In clinical practice, the correct application of the positive pressure is the most important factor.

Artificial ventilation and cardiac output

Intermittent changes in the stroke volume and asynchronous ejection of blood from the ventricles are recognized as occurring during both spontaneous ventilation and intermittent positive pressure ventilation (IPPR) of the lungs,[68] but they are more marked during positive pressure ventilation.

The effect of IPPR in raising the intrathoracic pressure, reducing the ventricular stroke volume and the cardiac output has been demonstrated to be greater when the inspiratory phase is prolonged.[37,140] Experimentally, it has been demonstrated that the fall in cardiac output can be caused by increased pulmonary vascular resistance, reduced pulmonary blood volume and reduced venous return.[29] It can be predicted from the above that a reduction of blood volume would exacerbate the condition, and this can be observed clinically in man and has been clearly demonstrated experimentally in dogs.

PEEP

The use of positive end-expiratory pressure (PEEP) to increase the oxygenation of the blood in patients suffering from respiratory failure was introduced several years ago but has become more popular, and is used more frequently, following the report by Ashbaugh et al. (1967).[8] Although PEEP is of value in patients in whom the lung compliance has decreased markedly, there is, as might be predicted, a significant fall in cardiac output which becomes more marked as the intrapulmonary pressure increases.[130]

Sedation with morphine and other similar agents is often indicated during artificial ventilation of the lungs. Acutely ill patients who had no cardiovascular disease but who were being ventilated, were given morphine intravenously in doses of 0.15 mg/kg and 0.30 mg/kg (Rouby et al., 1979).[112] A very small and transitory decrease in systolic arterial blood pressure was observed with the smaller dose. However, an immediate and prolonged decrease in the cardiac index was observed together with decreases in heart rate, stroke volume index, arterial pressure and left ventricular stroke work index when the larger dose was given. Rouby and his co-workers concluded that in the adult the degree of haemodynamic impairment associated with an intravenous dose of 10 mg of morphine was negligible, but could be significant when 20 mg was administered intravenously.

Again, as might be predicted, the correction of any deficit in blood volume during PEEP, is associated with a rise in cardiac output.[109]

There are, however, factors other than the haemodynamic effects that the clinician has to bear in mind when the inspiratory phase is prolonged and PEEP is instituted. Even under experimental conditions with the chest open (and indeed with the chest wall removed), but the intrapulmonary pressure raised, PEEP decreases cardiac output. This cannot be explained by constriction of the pulmonary arteries.[85] Continued stretching of the alveoli can, however, modify prostaglandin metabolism,[15] and some prostaglandins (e.g. PGI_2) appear to have a negative inotropic effect. The possibility of the release of a humoral agent with negative inotropic properties could explain the fall in cardiac output during PEEP, even when the chest wall has been removed and the venous return is unimpeded but the stretch receptors are given an almost maximum stimulus.[85,91]

Although there may be factors, in addition to those of a purely mechanical and haemodynamic nature, which cause the fall in cardiac output and systemic blood pressure, and though PEEP may be of great value in conditions such as respiratory distress syndrome of the newborn, the reduction in cardiac output associated with PEEP may decrease any benefits to the patient as a whole, and a severe reduction in *total body* oxygenation may occur. The clinician should be aware that a fall in the central venous blood oxygen tension and saturation, a fall in urinary output and an increase in the degree of metabolic acidosis can result in the presence of cosmetically improved arterial blood oxygen tensions.

The use of PEEP must therefore be applied with great caution, and its continuance in the presence of a fall in blood pressure which is not responsive to volume replacement, an extremely high central venous pressure (CVP) and a deterioration in the biochemical parameters of the blood indicate that the degree of PEEP should be reduced, or that it should be discontinued altogether.

Some clinical improvement may, however, be obtained during PEEP by the infusion of the vasopressor dopamine.[67]

Artificial ventilators

As we have noted, it is impossible to mimic natural respiration accurately by artificial means, except perhaps when an external negative pressure ventilator, such as a Cuirass respirator, is used.

During natural, spontaneous, respiration, the intrathoracic pressure is negative for the whole of the respiratory cycle. During IPPR, the pressure within the thorax is positive for the whole of the cycle, even at its completion, unless a negative end-tidal pressure is specially applied. When positive end-expiratory pressure is used, even with all its benefits in suitable cases, the respiratory cycle is made more unnatural.

When possible, a system of ventilation which allows the patient some control over the respiratory rate, inflation pressure or tidal volume is preferable, and this may be achieved by means of a patient-triggered ventilator. When, because of the clinical circumstances, this is not possible and these parameters have to be controlled by the clinician, the nomogram relating body weight to tidal volume and frequency of ventilation produced by Radford *et al.* (1954)[110] can be used. This nomogram is designed to maintain a normal alveolar PCO_2 (Fig. 5.5).

It will be apparent that when IPPR has to be applied in clinical conditions in which there is some degree of cardiac failure and the pressure within the pulmonary artery is reduced by hypovolaemia and systemic hypotension, then the pressure used to inflate the lungs becomes of very great importance.

We can summarize the main cardiovascular consequences of artificial ventilation as follows: (*a*) a decrease in the venous return of blood to the right side of the heart, (*b*) a decrease in pulmonary circulation, (*c*) as a result of decreased cardiac output, a reduced systemic circulation, and (*d*) the direct effects of positive pressure upon the more rapidly beating myocardium and the possible direct effect of a large negative pressure on the relatively thin-walled right ventricle during systole.

There are three main types of ventilators which can serve as a basic classification.

1. *Time cycled.* The ventilator is set at a frequency of ventilation determined by the clinician, and further adjustments have to be made regarding the volume of gas delivered at each respiratory cycle. The inflation pressure will then be determined by the capacity of the lungs and the rate at which it is delivered. There are two methods by which the preset volume is forced from the ventilator into the lungs.

(*a*) A bellows is compressed by means of a powerful electric motor. In this way the set volume is compressed at a fixed rate no matter what obstruction is present in the tubing or to expansion in the lungs.

(*b*) Force is applied to the bellows by means of a falling weight which may or may not be varied. This is quite different from the previous method because if there is obstruction to the flow of gas in the lung, the rate of flow during inflation will be slower than when there is no resistance.

2. *Pressure cycled.* The inspiratory phase of the respiratory cycle is brought to a halt when a preset pressure is achieved and this is irrespective of the time taken or the volume of gas that has been delivered. In this way the pressure necessary to cycle the machine may be reached before an adequate volume of gas has inflated the lungs when there is resistance to flow in the airway. There is, therefore, no set tidal volume, and when the patient is being ventilated by means of a patient-triggered, pressure-cycled ventilator, the tidal volume required at each breath can be indirectly determined by the patient.

3. *Volume cycled.* In this type of machine a set volume is delivered at each respiratory cycle which is independent of the time required or the pressure achieved. The minute volume can therefore vary.

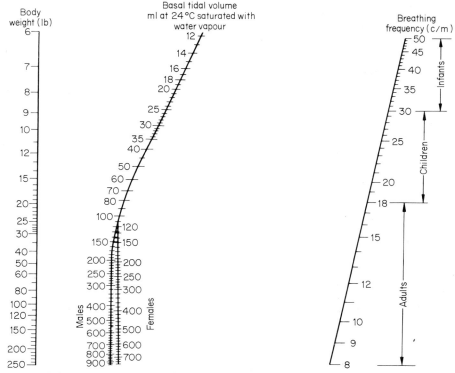

Fig. 5.5 Nomogram relating body weight, tidal volume and the frequency of respiration that will predictably produce a normal PCO_2 in the arterial blood (Radford, Ferris and Kriete, 1954).[110]

Patient-triggered respirators

When the patient makes an inspiratory effort, the negative pressure produced can be used to begin a respiratory cycle. Machines are available that are triggered by a negative pressure of 0.5 cmH₂O. Both pressure- and volume-cycled machines can be patient triggered. The most useful machines in resuscitation are those which are fitted with a device that allows artificial ventilation to be continued if the patient stops breathing spontaneously or if the patient's rate of breathing falls below a critical level (Fig. 5.6).

For a clear description of ventilators and artificial ventilation of the lungs, one should take advantage of the lucid specialized publications on this subject (Mushin *et al.*, 1980).[96]

Cyanosis

The colour of the skin in white races and the colour of the mucosa of the tongue and lips in all races are determined by the oxygen *saturation* of both the arterial and mixed venous bloods. In health, the oxygen saturation of the mixed venous blood is 70% or greater. It falls when the cardiac output falls and when the arterial oxygen saturation falls, as in anoxia and respiratory failure.

Although gross cyanosis is readily recognizable, in the early stages of an acute condition when recognition is most important this physical sign is almost as difficult to detect clinically (especially in artificial light) as depression of respiration in the patient who is covered with sheets and blankets. Even the experienced clinician sometimes has difficulty. The interpretation of cyanosis is also sometimes difficult when it has more than one cause. There are *three* main causes for cyanosis which are quite separate and distinct (see below); in appropriate clinical cases or during animal experiments they can be demonstrated separately. It is vitally important to establish the presence or absence of all three.

1. A low arterial oxygen *saturation* and therefore a low *arterial* blood PO_2.

2. A low cardiac output which causes a low *venous* blood O_2 *saturation*; this produces the appearance of cyanosis even when the arterial oxygen saturation (and PO_2) is normal and, in the

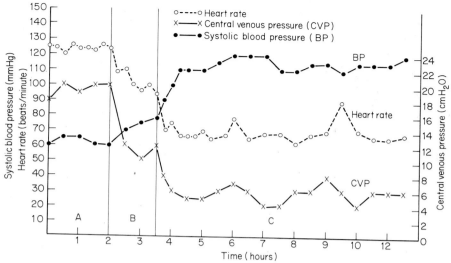

Fig. 5.6 The pulse rate, central venous pressure and blood pressure recorded in a patient who had undergone abdominal surgery which was followed by severe respiratory failure. The patient was ventilated initially using a volume-controlled, time-cycled ventilator (A) during which there was a very high pulse rate and central venous pressure (CVP) and a low blood pressure (BP). When the patient was allowed to initiate (trigger) each breath (B), the pulse rate fell and there was a significant fall in CVP and rise in BP. When the ventilator was changed to a Bird, patient triggered, pressure-cycled ventilator (C), so that the patient breathed at a spontaneous rate and the tidal volume was terminated by the pressure in the lungs, an even more significant rise in BP, fall in CVP and pulse rate occurred.

case of haemorrhagic shock, commonly raised above normal.

3. A low ambient temperature causing temporary peripheral cyanosis localized to the hands, feet, lips, etc., but both the cardiac output and the rectal temperature are normal. This condition is readily and spontaneously reversible. It can also be seen following major surgery, such as open-heart surgery following a return to normal body temperature and blood pressure, and occasionally after minor surgery or trauma and anxiety states.

As noted elsewhere, a fall in the arterial blood saturation occurs when blood is shunted from the right to the left side of the heart or when there is a failure to oxygenate the blood because of intrinsic lung disease.

A fall in cardiac output is produced either by failure of the heart to pump an adequate volume of blood or by a reduced blood volume. Both circumstances cause cyanosis.

A patient with a bleeding ectopic pregnancy, for example, is cyanosed, but the arterial blood oxygen saturation is 100% and the PO_2 is sometimes greater than 100 mmHg (e.g. 110 mmHg) because of hyperventilation when the patient is breathing air not enriched with O_2.

The patient suffering from myocardial infarction, however, is commonly cyanosed because of two factors. There is a reduction in ventricular stroke volume and cardiac output and this leads to desaturation of the venous blood. There is also commonly interstitial pulmonary oedema which reduces the O_2 tension and oxygen saturation of the arterial blood. The two factors together thus cause a significant degree of cyanosis.

'Central cyanosis'

This is a term that should never be used unless one uses it to mean desaturation of the arterial blood and a low arterial PO_2. Some people use the term to denote that the tongue is blue, but we know this occurs during haemorrhagic shock or when the cardiac output is low as a result of chronic valve disease (such as mitral stenosis with tricuspid incompetence) when, in both types of conditions, the arterial blood is fully oxygenated.

Postoperative Respiratory Failure

Postanaesthetic respiratory failure

Sometimes, after a short period of anaesthesia, patients fail to breathe. There may be a complete absence of respiration or respiration may be so inadequate that it is insufficient to maintain life.

These patients fall into six main classes.

1. Primary CO_2 retention produced either by lung pathology or by inadequate ventilation during anaesthesia.
2. A syndrome of central nervous system depression associated with hypoventilation and hypotension (secondary CO_2 retention).
3. Abnormal reaction to relaxants (latent myasthenia gravis, low pseudocholinesterase activity, overt myasthenia gravis).
4. Abnormalities of the thoracic cage and lung pathology causing impaired spontaneous ventilation (injuries to the chest).
5. Antibiotics.
6. Acute hyponatraemia.

Carbon dioxide retention (primary CO_2 retention)

It was first observed by Scurr in 1956[113] that retention of carbon dioxide during an anaesthetic could give rise to postoperative respiratory depression. When a patient is breathing oxygen-enriched mixtures, carbon dioxide can be retained without the advent of cyanosis or arterial oxygen blood desaturation. When the patient is breathing air, however, CO_2 retention can occur only in association with cyanosis. It can therefore be seen that if arterial blood desaturation occurs during the breathing of oxygen-enriched mixtures, marked hypoventilation must be present. Carbon dioxide retention can occur in three main ways.

1. Ventilation can be insufficient for the patient's needs (i.e. a minute volume that is too small may pass unnoticed because of the absence of cyanosis when the patient breathes oxygen-enriched mixtures). When an endotracheal tube is inserted too far so that is passes down one main bronchus and in this way only one lung is ventilated, severe hypoventilation may inadvertently occur.
2. Rebreathing can occur through a canister containing soda-lime which has been filled incorrectly. When a canister is filled incompletely in the vertical position and then placed on its side, which is the usual position for use, a gap appears between the upper surface of the soda-lime granules and the wall of the canister. Complete absorption of carbon dioxide does not occur because the gases pass to and fro through this channel of low resistance.
3. The use of an anaesthetic circuit which by its design permits rebreathing of carbon dioxide.

It has been stressed by Mapleson[92] that the commonly used anaesthetic circuits which are comprised of a rebreathing bag and a side arm delivering anaesthetic gases to the tubes leading to the patient frequently give rise to CO_2 retention unless a flow of fresh gas of 11 litre/minute or more is maintained throughout anaesthesia. If this large supply of fresh gas is not used, carbon dioxide accumulates within the rebreathing bag and the concentration of CO_2 rises with the length of time taken for the operation. This can produce very severe carbon dioxide retention.

It is convenient for descriptive as well as clinical purposes, because the treatment is different, to distinguish this form of carbon dioxide retention from that which is produced postoperatively from respiratory depression, caused by drugs, the presence of a gross metabolic acidosis, or abnormalities of the lungs and thoracic cavities.

When primary CO_2 retention causes respiratory depression and this in turn gives rise to a metabolic acidosis because of desaturation of the arterial blood, in the patient breathing air, a clinical picture not unlike that seen when respiratory depression is the result of a metabolic acidosis produced during the surgical procedure may then be observed. At a variable period of time after the end of an operation, the same acid–base state of the blood is found when analysis is made. It is necessary to separate primary and secondary CO_2 retention, because the initial management of the two conditions is different. Secondary CO_2 retention caused by the presence of a metabolic acidosis or other biochemical abnormality almost always follows a long period of anaesthesia involving major surgery. Primary CO_2 retention, however, can develop during a relatively short period of anaesthesia and is most likely to do so when it is least expected and when there are unsuspected abnormalities of the alveolar bed. Although in modern anaesthetic practice it is not commonly seen, and the work of Geddes and Gray[55] has demonstrated that hyperventilation during ordinary surgical procedures may be beneficial rather than harmful, the dangers of CO_2 retention occurring are such that its importance should not be ignored.

Detection of CO_2 retention

There are no reliable physical signs which can detect primary carbon dioxide retention. Peripheral vasodilatation occurs during anaesthesia without a raised PCO_2. The temperature of the soda-lime canister is also misleading because it is subject to so many variables. There are two reliable methods of detecting CO_2 retention. The first is blood gas analysis using the Severinghaus[114] PCO_2 electrode (see p. 76). This allows a rapid estimation to be made. Most machines now give all three components of acid–base balance. However, the Astrup[9] apparatus, in which the pH of two blood samples is plotted on a log PCO_2–pH graph having been equilibrated with O_2–CO_2 gas mixtures of known concentration, is still in use in many parts of the world. The second method requires a re-breathed sample of gas (using a small O_2 filled anaesthetic bag); this gas is analysed for CO_2 in an analyser such as that of Haldane or the more simple modified version of Campbell or the Dräger analyser.[27,33,107]

Although end-tidal gas sampling is reliable in those patients who have no lung pathology, this method gives misleadingly low results when the ventilation–perfusion ratios of parts of the lungs are abnormal. Accurate measurement of the end-tidal PCO_2 can, however, be made with a suitable continuously recording, electronic apparatus.

Treatment of primary CO_2 retention

At the end of the operation when respiratory depression is noted, CO_2 retention may be reversed by hyperventilating the patient actively through a CO_2 absorber. The cause of the hypoventilation is probably similar to that seen in cases of uncompensated respiratory acidosis resulting from chronic lung disease when the patient is given high oxygen tensions to breathe. Similarly, when the excess of CO_2 is removed by ventilation of the lungs, consciousness and respiratory effort return. If the condition has been allowed to develop so that hypoventilation has given rise to anoxia, then it may be necessary, in addition to hyperventilating the patient, to correct the metabolic acidosis. The infusion of sodium bicarbonate solution will help by compensating for the respiratory acidosis.

In the presence of lung pathology it may be difficult to hyperventilate to a degree that is necessary for CO_2 removal. It is then essential that 'artificial compensation' of the respiratory acidosis with sodium bicarbonate should be made in the same manner as that suggested for an acute infective process (see p. 129), because until this is done, it is unlikely that adequate spontaneous ventilation will return.

In the last resort, controlled artificial ventilation will be necessary.

A syndrome of central nervous system depression, hypotension and respiratory depression (secondary CO_2 retention)

At the end of an anaesthetic usually given for a major surgical procedure, some patients exhibit respiratory, circulatory and central nervous system depression. The patient remains unconscious or very confused at the end of the operation. Respiration may be absent or inadequate and is often gasping in character and is associated with tracheal or jaw tug. The abdominal and thoracic respiratory components are dissociated. Peripheral cyanosis is usually present and is most marked at the ear lobes and the nail beds, but commonly extends to the lips, hands and feet. The peripheral cyanosis is caused by a reduced cardiac output which produces a progressive hypotension, usually with a narrow pulse pressure. If the patient is allowed to breathe air spontaneously, desaturation of the arterial blood occurs. Cardiac arrhythmias are commonly present. The hypotension and peripheral cyanosis do not improve after blood transfusion and the central venous pressure (CVP) is raised. Little or no improvement is produced when vasopressor drugs are administered.

The overall picture of respiratory depression gives these patients the appearance of being partially paralysed, but no evidence of neuromuscular block is demonstrable when a motor nerve is stimulated. Death results from circulatory failure after adequate artificial ventilation, blood transfusion and the use of vasopressor drugs. The condition was first observed by the author in dogs (Kenyon et al., 1959)[80] (see p. 253) which had been rewarmed following profound hypothermia.

The clinical picture of an unconscious patient making inefficient respiratory effort who is cyanosed and hypotensive resembles the condition described as 'neostigmine resistant curarization'.[72] This condition in man was investigated by Brooks and Feldman (1962)[24] and it was found that patients who developed the complete syndrome revealed a common biochemical abnormality in that they all had a gross metabolic acidosis. The serum potassium concentrations in cases similar to those reported by Brooks and Feldman have since been investigated and found to have high, normal or low and to have no apparent correlation with the development of the syndrome or its severity.

When it had been established that the patients had no neuromuscular block when stimulated with a 'Medelec' stimulator along the ulnar nerve, that the syndrome was similar to that of neostigmine resistant curarization and that there was a measurable degree of metabolic acidosis, sodium bicarbonate solution was infused intravenously until the acidosis was corrected. The solution chosen was 2.74% $NaHCO_3$ which has 166 mmol/500 ml (mEq/500 ml) and approximately twice the osmolality of plasma. Initially, the solution was used only after conventional methods of treatment at the time had failed. These included the administration of carbon dioxide, nikethamide and vanilic acid diethylamide.

Vigorous spontaneous respiration was almost invariably re-established before the volume required to correct the acidosis had been infused, but quite frequently the improvement was not maintained unless the infusion was continued. A volume in excess of that which could be calculated from the base deficit on the basis of total body water had then been given. It has sometimes been necessary to give as much as 400 mmol (mEq) of $NaHCO_3$. This is probably because the base deficit, which results from prolonged tissue anoxia and depressed circulation, is only slowly reflected in the changes of $[HCO_3^-]$ in the plasma. The isotonic solution and more hypertonic solutions are also effective, although, because it is necessary to maintain the osmolality of body fluids while expanding the volume of the ECF, sodium bicarbonate has to be used most frequently in the 2.74% solution and has been preferred because it deals suitably with both these factors.

Since the publication of this paper,[24] many types of surgical patients have been found to develop secondary CO_2 retention. Most commonly it is seen in the severely ill and debilitated patient who has previously developed biochemical abnormalities as a result of disease processes. It may be seen, for example, after a relatively short period of anaesthesia (i.e. for the insertion of a tube into the oesophagus obstructed by carcinoma). The four main categories of patients who display this clinical syndrome need little revision.

1. *Prolonged gut obstruction:* e.g. strangulated hernia (abnormalities of hydration and biochemistry which are accentuated by anaesthesia and surgical intervention).

2. *Occlusion of large vessels:* e.g. obstruction resulting from emboli, aortic grafts, especially for leaking abdominal aneurysms. (A deficiency of base caused by reduction in blood flow through the tissues and the release of metabolic products from anoxic tissues following release of aortic clamps.) When there has been a gradual occlusion of the abdominal aorta so that anastomotic channels have developed (e.g. around the hip joint etc.), as in Leriche syndrome, the degree of 'washout acidosis' on release of the clamps is often small.

3. *Circulatory insufficiency:* e.g. low flow pump oxygenators, postoperative hypotension and haemorrhage. (Tissue hypoxia causing a metabolic acidosis.)

4. *Circulatory arrest:* e.g. following temporary cessation of an extracorporeal circulation for surgical procedures when some of the tissues are warm, cardiac arrest. (Metabolic acidosis resulting from total body anoxia.)

Table 5.3 gives the biochemical findings in five patients, four of whom presented with a clinical picture similar to that which has been described. All five patients died.

Now that we know that it is possible to obtain a quick response to the rapid infusion of alkali, the dangers associated with a postoperative metabolic acidosis are not as great. It is, however, necessary to point out that as hypotension increases when the metabolic acidosis is left uncorrected, the effects of artificial ventilation in the presence of myocardial inadequacy tend to impair tissue perfusion further. As the cardiac output is reduced, the pressure required to inflate the lungs has a more marked effect in impeding blood flow through the alveolar capillaries. This is because the perfusion pressure of the lungs is also decreased. A situation which is similar to that occurring in haemorrhagic shock with positive pressure ventilation then develops. An inflation pressure of $20 \, cmH_2O$ is equal to 14.7 mmHg. If this pressure is exerted directly on the capillary bed, marked impedance to flow results. When this happens the blood

Table 5.3 Arterial blood pH, PCO_2, plasma TCO_2 and $[HCO_3^-]$ in five patients demonstrating secondary CO_2 retention[24]

Patient	pH	TCO_2	PCO_2	$[HCO_3^-]$
1 Abdominal aortic graft	6.94	10.4	43.6	9.1
2 Small-bowel obstruction	7.12	11.3	29.6	10.4
3 Partial gastrectomy	7.15	12.4	30.5	11.5
4 Haemorrhage after partial gastrectomy	7.21	14.4	34.4	13.4
5 Repair of VSD pump oxygenator	7.08	11.4	37.0	10.3

pH = blood pH at 38°C; TCO_2 = plasma total CO_2 (mmol/l); PCO_2 = partial pressure of CO_2 (mmHg); $[HCO_3^-]$ = plasma bicarbonate (mmol/l): $(TCO_2 - 0.0301 \times PCO_2)$.

returning to the right side of the heart is almost completely desaturated and the opening of shunts across the lungs, which take no part in oxidative processes, contributes to the desaturation of blood entering the left atrium. It can be seen, therefore, that the syndrome represents a self-potentiating situation and arterial blood desaturation is found as a terminal event.

The value of treating this syndrome with infusions of sodium bicarbonate can be best illustrated by referring to cases which are typical of the categories that have been outlined.

A case of strangulated hernia

A 58-year-old man had suffered from an inguinal hernia for many years. Three days prior to admission he developed acute abdominal pain. He began to vomit and was unable to retain any form of solid or liquid food. On admission to hospital he was found to be moderately dehydrated and to have a strangulated hernia. At the end of the operation he remained unconscious and made little effort at spontaneous ventilation. He demonstrated both tracheal and jaw tug and his blood pressure remained at 90/75 mmHg. When his respiratory minute volume was measured with a Wright respirometer, it was found to be only 2.4 litres. Stimulation of his ulnar nerve with a Medelec stimulator revealed no neuromuscular block. His lips, toes and finger-nail beds were cyanosed. Examination of the acid–base status of his arterial blood revealed a metabolic acidosis (Table 5.4A). 200 ml of 2.74% sodium bicarbonate were infused over a period of 15 minutes and at the end of this period the patient began to cough and swallow on the endotracheal tube. The jaw and tracheal tug became less marked and the measurement of his respiratory minute volume showed that is had risen to 4.9 litres. A further 100 ml of solution were infused over a period of 10 minutes and at the end of this time his minute volume had risen to over 8 litres and consciousness was rapidly returning. Measurement of the acid-base status of his blood revealed an improvement in the metabolic component [HCO_3^-] (Table 5.4B). The infusion was continued and the tracheal tube was removed a few minutes later when the minute volume had increased to a value in excess of 9 litres. During this period the peripheral cyanosis disappeared and the blood pressure rose to 140/95 mmHg. Although the physical signs demonstrated a marked improvement and the blood acid–base status was returning to values approaching those of normality,

the infusion of sodium bicarbonate was maintained until 500 ml of a 2.74% solution had been given over a further period of 2 hours when the patient had been returned to bed to make an uneventful recovery.

Table 5.4 Acid–base data from a case of strangulated hernia exhibiting postoperative respiratory depression

	pH	St. bic. (mmol/l)	PCO_2 (mmHg)	Minute volume (l/min)
A	7.24	16.8	42	2.4
B	7.32	19.5	39	8.1

pH = arterial blood pH at 38°C; St. bic. = standard bicarbonate; PCO_2 = partial pressure of CO_2.
Sample B was taken when the patient had received 300 ml of 2.74% $NaHCO_3$ (100 mmol).

When patients undergo grafting of the abdominal aorta it is always advisable that hypertonic $NaHCO_3$ solution (2.74%) should be infused throughout the procedure. This is even more important when there is major blood loss. The infusion of 500 ml of the solution does no harm and is rapidly excreted following the operation if it is not required. The solution is, however, available should it be needed if clamping of the vessels, for the purposes of applying the graft, produces a marked fall in the loss of base when a normal circulation is re-established. When there has been some impairment of renal function prior to surgery in a leaking abdominal aneurysm and the operation is performed as an emergency procedure, then the practice of infusing a hypertonic solution of $NaHCO_3$ from the beginning of the anaesthetic may be an essential part of the procedure.[81]

The following case illustrates the effect of the occlusion of the lower part of the aorta so that the limbs have become ischaemic and the circulation impaired. During this operation there was no major blood loss; the patient received only 3 units (1.5 litres) of blood during the whole operation.

A case of aortic endarterectomy

A 75-year-old woman underwent the operation for abdominal aortic endarterectomy because of occlusion close to the bifurcation of the central aorta. She had discoloration of the left foot and lower half of the left leg and also of the right foot and ankle. The endarterectomy was performed with comparative ease and very little blood loss, but when the abdomen had been closed and attempts were made to allow the patient to breathe spontaneously, it was evident that she was suffering from severe respiratory depression. Although she was being ventilated with 100% O_2, she demonstrated the clinical signs of hypotension (blood pressure 80/60 mmHg), tracheal and jaw tug, peripheral cyanosis, especially marked at the fingers and the ear lobes and the toe-nail beds. Her venous pressure was raised. She was slow to respond to stimuli and shouted commands. After 1–2 minutes of attempted spontaneous ventilation she was unable to open her eyes, although initially she had been able to do so. Analysis of her arterial blood revealed a metabolic acidosis (Table 5.5A). Her clinical state appeared to be that of a case of neostigmine-resistant curarization, but no neuromuscular block could be demonstrated. 200 ml of 2.74% sodium bicarbonate were infused over a period of 10 minutes. Almost immediately she regained consciousness and the tracheal tug became less marked and the jaw tug disappeared completely. The blood pressure rose to 120/70 mmHg and the peripheral cyanosis disappeared. Because respiratory effort increased markedly, the endotracheal tube was removed and she was allowed to breathe spontaneously. At this point also the infusion of sodium bicarbonate solution was stopped. Ten minutes later the respiratory depression was seen to have returned, together with the tracheal and jaw tug, and there was a marked reduction in the level of consciousness. The infusion of alkali was, therefore, begun once more with the same effect as on the previous occasion. The plasma acid–base values measured in an arterial blood sample at this time are shown in Table 5.5B. It can be seen that there was no significant improvement of the [HCO_3^-] following the previous infusion. It must be assumed, therefore, that there was a gradual diffusion of acidotic products from the previously anoxic tissues into the general circulation and that neutralization of these products had been incomplete. The infusion was continued slowly throughout the night until altogether 550 ml of the 2.74% solution had been given.

Calcium chloride 10% had been given in an attempt to restore the blood pressure, with no effect, and neostigmine was given in therapeutic doses, but failed to correct what was thought to be a neuromuscular block produced by d-tubocurarine. Although blood loss had been minimal, approximately 250 ml of blood had been infused rapidly after the closing of the abdomen when the blood pressure was low,

but this had no effect and appeared to produce a further fall in arterial blood pressure and rise in central venous pressure.

Table 5.5 Acid–base data from a case of aortic endarterectomy exhibiting the syndrome of postoperative central nervous system depression with inadequate ventilation

	pH	St. bic. (mmol/l)	PCO_2 (mmHg)
A	7.25	18.6	45
B	7.28	19.5	44

pH = arterial blood pH at 38°C; St. bic. = standard bicarbonate; PCO_2 = partial pressure of CO_2.
Sample B was taken when the patient had received 200 ml of 2.74% $NaHCO_3$. It can be seen that the metabolic acidosis was not greatly improved.

Hypothermia induced by extracorporeal circulation
Although the following case does not illustrate the effects of low flow extracorporeal circulation because it was performed by the technique of Drew and his co-workers[42,43] whereby a virtually unlimited supply of fully oxygenated blood is available for perfusion because oxygenation takes place within the lungs, it does illustrate the effects of perfusion of the body with desaturated blood, especially in the early stages of the operation, and the effects of infusing ACD (acid-citrate-dextrose) blood in a patient who already has a marked metabolic acidosis. If great care is not taken, overtransfusion can be produced and respiratory impairment, which is already present, can be exacerbated.

Case history. A boy of 4 years suffering from tetralogy of Fallot had undergone profound hypothermia with circulatory arrest using autogenous lung perfusion for complete repair of his defect. He was an unusual case in that the left atrium was so small and inaccessible that in the early stages of cooling the cannula that was normally inserted into the left atrium was inserted into the right atrium, together with the cannula that was normally inserted in that chamber. It was not until the nasopharyngeal temperature had reached 28°C that it was considered safe to place the left atrial cannula in the relatively inaccessible, small left atrium. In the early stages of cooling, therefore, before reduction in the metabolism of many of the body tissues had reduced the uptake of O_2, relatively desaturated blood perfused the body via the femoral artery at a rate of 80 ml/kg of body weight. Heparinized blood was used to prime the apparatus, and intermittent positive pressure ventilation was maintained with nitrous oxide and oxygen during the procedure. The administration of nitrous oxide was stopped when the nasopharyngeal temperature reached 30°C and restarted during the rewarming period when the nasopharynx had returned to that temperature. At the end of the perfusion a metabolic acidosis was present and, because of hypotension, some difficulty was experienced in stopping the extracorporeal circulation, even after transfusion with blood in excess of blood loss. After further perfusion and therefore rewarming, a systolic blood pressure of 90–100 mmHg was finally obtained and the extracorporeal circulation terminated. One and a half hours after the end of the perfusion little change had occurred in the acid–base state.

The patient was returned to bed still maintaining the same pressure, but 2 hours later his blood pressure and pulse became unrecordable. During this time and during the period of hypotension, blood was tranfused rapidly until more than 200 ml of blood in excess of requirements had been given. The transfusion produced no improvement, but a marked rise in venous pressure was noted. Ventilation was poor and marked peripheral cyanosis was evident even though oxygen was being administered continuously by means of an anaesthetic mask. Consciousness was also depressed. 80 ml of a solution of isotonic sodium bicarbonate were then infused slowly over a period of 35 minutes and the pulse became palpable and the blood pressure could be recorded. When the systolic blood pressure had reached 60–70 mmHg blood was transfused again as the venous pressure had fallen a little and hypovolaemia was considered to be a contributory cause. The same level of the blood pressure was maintained for 45 minutes, the pulse rate during the blood transfusion increased a little, but when the rate of transfusion was increased the blood pressure became unrecordable for the second time. Sodium bicarbonate solution was again infused; this resulted in improvement in both the pulse pressure and the systolic pressure and a lowering of the venous pressure which had again become markedly raised during the previous transfusion. Thereafter a slow infusion of sodium bicarbonate was maintained which alternated with the transfusion of blood to keep pace with further drainage from the chest. Gradually, the blood pressure rose, the pulse rate fell and the pulse pressure increased.

It was evident that the infusion of alkali not only raised the blood pressure, but also increased both the rate and depth of ventilation. Quite typically, this patient did not respond to noise or painful stimuli until infusions of alkali had been given. In all, 250 ml of isotonic sodium bicarbonate solution were infused. This patient made a good recovery and the period of hypotension in no way affected the function of other organs. The sequence of events relating to blood transfusion, pulse rate, blood pressure and pulse pressure are depicted in Fig. 5.7.

It can be seen that this was a case in which overtransfusion could so easily have been produced if the rise in venous pressure had not been noted or had been ignored. It is this situation that frequently leads to extravasation of blood into the lungs, especially in those patients who are treated with a pump-oxygenator (sometimes called 'pump lung') or who receive a rapid transfusion following major haemorrhage. The effects of haemorrhage upon ventilation are dealt with fully in the chapter on shock (see Chapter 6), but it is well to note at this stage that after a prolonged period of hypotension resulting from haemorrhage, respiratory failure ensues giving rise to desaturation of the arterial blood. A sudden massive haemorrhage gives rise sometimes to complete apnoea so that, unless immediate steps are made for artificial ventilation, cardiac arrest occurs from this cause alone and predominates in importance over blood replacement. A case of respiratory failure following prolonged haemorrhagic hypotension has been described by Brooks and Feldman.[24] Almost any strength of sodium bicarbonate solution is effective, and it is sometimes beneficial to use the more concentrated form (8.4% or 1 mmol/ml) commonly used during the treatment of cardiac arrest.

Case history. A 42-year-old man underwent open-heart surgery for a mitral valve replacement. The pump-oxygenator was primed with 5% glucose in water. Because a metabolic acidosis developed during the procedure, 50 ml (50 mmol) of sodium bicarbonate was given in an 8.4% solution. At the end of the operation the blood pressure was 130/70 mmHg, the patient was in sinus rhythm and the heart rate was 72 beats/minute. The endotracheal tube was kept *in situ* and the patient was ventilated artificially with a pressure-cycled ventilator. Blood gas measurements at that time were normal (Table 5.6), considering that the patient was breathing an oxygen-enriched mixture. Approximately 90 minutes later the ventilator

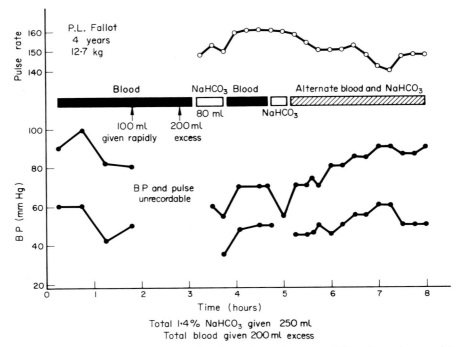

Fig. 5.7 The postoperative course of a patient with Fallot's tetralogy who successfully underwent a complete repair of the defect under profound hypothermia. Infusions of isotonic NaHCO$_3$ solution reversed the hypotension which excess blood transfusion failed to correct. A total volume of 250 ml of 1.4% NaHCO$_3$ was given.

was disconnected and the patient was allowed to breathe spontaneously because he was awake and alert. The patient's tidal volume was 530 ml and he was capable of taking a deep breath, when urged to do so, of more than 1 litre.

After approximately 40 minutes of spontaneous respiration, it was observed that the arterial pressure had fallen and the systolic value was in the region of 80 mmHg. The patient had become semicomatose and was barely responsive. The tidal volume had fallen to 210 ml. Blood gas analysis performed at that time indicated a slight rise in PCO_2 and a marked metabolic acidosis. Hypoxia was also present. The central venous pressure (CVP) had risen from 8.5 cmH$_2$O to 12 cmH$_2$O. No analgesia had been given.

The ventilator was reconnected to the endotracheal tube and the blood pressure fell

Table 5.6 Successive blood-gas determinations in a patient following open-heart surgery

Time reading taken	pH	[HCO$_3^-$] (mEq/l; mmol/l)	PCO_2 (mmHg)	PO_2 (mmHg)	Tidal volume (ml)
1 Immediately postoperatively	7.42	24.4	38	294	540
2 130 min postoperatively (ventilator disconnected 90 min postoperatively)	7.20	16.3	43	80	210
3 10 min after disconnection of ventilator for the second time and injection of 100 mmol/l (mEq/l) sodium bicarbonate	7.46	26.1	37	135*	600

pH measured at 37°C; [HCO$_3^-$], derived value for plasma bicarbonate concentration; PCO_2, partial pressure of CO$_2$ in blood; PO_2, partial pressure of O$_2$ in blood; Tidal volume measured using a Wright respirometer.
*PO_2 value obtained when inspired air was enriched with O$_2$ by means of a chimney attached to the endotracheal tube.

to a systolic value of 65 mmHg, probably because of the effect described below. Because this syndrome was recognized, 50 mmol of sodium bicarbonate in an 8.4% solution were given intravenously. The blood pressure rose immediately and an increased rate of ventilation was also observed. The patient once again became alert and responsive. The blood pressure at that time was 125/75 mmHg and the CVP was 7 cmH$_2$O. Calcium gluconate (0.5 g) was also given intravenously; this produced a dramatic rise in blood pressure to 145/90 mmHg, which fell rapidly to 130/75 mmHg. A second intravenous injection of 50 mmol of sodium bicarbonate was given.

Ten minutes following the second injection of NaHCO$_3$ another blood gas analysis was performed, as shown in Table 5.6. The patient was then conscious and alert, breathing spontaneously without the ventilator at a rate of 26 inspirations/minute at a tidal volume of 600 ml. He began to find the endotracheal tube irritating and it was removed. The patient continued to progress well with no further repetition of this incident.

Treatment of syndrome of postanaesthetic central nervous system depression

Whenever possible, it is advisable to begin the treatment of a patient exhibiting the syndrome of nervous system depression by infusing a volume of sodium bicarbonate solution that is calculated from the base deficit found in blood samples and the total body water content (see p. 96). However, as the infusion proceeds and an increase in cardiac output occurs, assisted by increased respiratory excursion or the abandonment of positive pressure ventilation, spontaneous correction of the base deficit becomes more rapid. A smaller volume than was indicated initially by blood analysis must be infused. Conversely, we have already seen that blood analysis may not indicate the true degree of total base deficit within the body, probably because of the slow diffusion of fixed acids into the extracellular fluid (ECF). A much greater volume of sodium bicarbonate solution than was initially indicated by blood analysis has to be infused in order to maintain functional improvement. In both these situations repeated blood analyses are therefore necessary but are not always available. For this reason the following regimen is recommended, it has proved to be safe and therapeutically reliable in a large number of cases.

The infusion of 200 ml of 2.74% NaHCO$_3$ solution (66 mmol) over a period of 15–20 minutes is quite safe in the average adult patient. This represents approximately 1 mmol/kg (mEq/kg) body weight in a 60-kg patient. Because the bicarbonate is initially restricted to the extracellular fluid (ECF) compartment, high values of plasma bicarbonate concentration may be obtained during the infusion. A further 100 ml (33 mmol) can be given safely over the next 30–60 minutes. This rate of infusion can be repeated until 500 ml of the solution have been given.

In some conditions it may be necessary to increase the rate of infusion and this has often been done with no ill-effects. More concentrated solutions have also been used, especially 4.2% NaHCO$_3$, which has approximately three times the osmolality of plasma and contains 0.5 mmol/ml (mEq/ml) of bicarbonate, and 8.4% of NaHCO$_3$ which has six times the osmolality of plasma and contains 1 mmol/ml (mEq/ml) of bicarbonate. Care must be exercised, however, to prevent gross overexpansion of the ECF, because the dangers that are present when sodium bicarbonate is infused are similar to those of any electrolyte-containing fluid. Most patients presenting for surgery are usually slightly underhydrated and, because of movements of fluid between the compartments, the dangers are minimized if there has been no large infusion of non-electrolyte-containing solutions such as 5% glucose. The most common circumstance is that of undertreatment, so that after initial improvement the patient lapses back into respiratory depression, which can too often pass unnoticed by the medical attendants.

Abnormal reaction to muscle relaxants

Some patients behave in such a way during anaesthesia that either they may be suspected of having a latent form of myasthenia gravis or they have an abnormal sensitivity to muscle relaxants. Agents used for muscle relaxation during anaesthesia can be divided into two groups: (a) those that are non-depolarizing, such as d-tubocurarine and gallamine, and (b) those that have a depolarizing effect at the muscle end-plate, such as decamethonium and suxamethonium. It is therefore sometimes possible, by a combination of agents, to produce a 'mixed' neuromuscular block.

When there is abnormal sensitivity to relaxing agents, apnoea may persist for many hours after the cessation of the operation, and artificial ventilation is necessary either by hand or with a non-patient-triggered artificial ventilator.

Sometimes prolonged apnoea is associated with a low pseudocholinesterase concentration in the blood. The normal level lies between 55 and 125 units/ml, with little variation occurring from day to day between the sexes or age-groups.[28] It has been shown that prolonged apnoea after suxamethonium is associated with a pseudocholinesterase level that is half the normal value.[18] A low pseudocholinesterase level may be found in the presence of parenchymatous liver disease, malnutrition often associated with anaemia, malignant growths and in some apparently normal people. The subject has been well reviewed by Lehmann and Liddell.[84]

Even with an improved understanding of the myasthenic state (see p. 154), the abnormal reaction to muscle relaxants is still complicated. For example, it was established a considerable time ago (Churchill-Davidson and Richardson, 1953)[31] that the muscles in myasthenia were not blocked by decamethonium given in doses that usually produced a 90% block, and that the more diseased the muscles, the more readily this effect was obtained. Even so, the block was readily reversible in most cases by the administration of edrophonium (see p. 156).

The metabolic state of the patient is also important, and a considerable amount of knowledge has been accumulated with regard to the influence played by the ionic composition (especially Mg^{++} and K^+) of the fluid bathing the neuromuscular junction. Calcium has been shown to decrease the degree of muscle depolarization produced by acetylcholine,[57] and to change the affinity of the receptor site for tubocurarine.[75] All these effects occur *post*-synaptically. *Pre*synaptically, the electrical nerve impulse releases a greater quantity of acetylcholine if the $[Ca^{++}]$ is increased.[79] The importance of Ca^{++} and K^+, their influence on blockade of the muscle receptor site, and the interaction of these two cations has been reviewed by Waud and Waud (1980).[138]

In some patients, prolonged apnoea may be found after small doses of relaxants, even when the pseudocholinesterase level is not found to be markedly abnormal. In these patients the question of the possibility of latent myasthenia gravis arises, but the exact aetiology and pathophysiology of this condition are not known.

An example of sensitivity to muscle relaxants in a patient who had no apparent metabolic disturbance other than a pseudocholinesterase activity that was just within the normal range, is illustrated by the following case.

Case history. A woman of 44 years was anaesthetized for the removal of a lump in her right breast. Anaesthesia was induced with thiopentone 315 mg and suxamethonium 50 mg. An endotracheal tube was inserted and she was maintained on gas and oxygen together with gallamine 80 mg. Postoperatively there was complete apnoea. Nalorphine (Lethidrone) 20 mg and edrophonium (Tensilon) 10 mg and hyperventilation with CO_2 were all tried, but without effect. The patient was placed on an artificial ventilator for 2 hours and at the end of that time was given a further dose of edrophonium (Tensilon) and then atropine with neostigmine. Spontaneous respiration returned, and the patient was taken back to the ward. She made an uneventful recovery, and it was suspected that a mixed block had been produced by administering the gallamine before the suxamethonium had ceased to act.

Almost 1 year later the patient was again anaesthetized for the removal of a lump from her left breast. On this occasion she was given thiopentone 225 mg and only 10 mg of suxamethonium. An endotracheal tube was inserted, and she was maintained on N_2O, O_2 and halothane. It was noticed that complete relaxation was obtained from this small dose of suxamethonium. At the end of the operation, respiratory depression was not present and a satisfactory recovery was made.

Six months later she was anaesthetized for the biopsy of a lump on her tongue. Anaesthesia was induced with thiopentone 450 mg and maintained with N_2O, O_2 and halothane. No relaxant was given and apnoea was not present at the end of the operation. Three years later she was again anaesthetized for the removal of another lump from her right breast. Induction was performed with 275 mg of thiopentone and 10 mg of suxamethonium. She was intubated and maintained on N_2O, O_2 and halothane. Complete relaxation for intubation was obtained on this occasion, complete apnoea lasting for just over 3 minutes.

The following month a total hysterectomy was performed. She was induced with thiopentone 375 mg and *d*-tubocurarine 30 mg. An endotracheal tube was passed and she was maintained on gas and oxygen, the ventilation being controlled. While the skin was being prepared for surgery, it was noted that there was a marked erythema and vasodilatation of the skin from the mandible to the knees and an allergic reaction to thiopentone or *d*-tubocurarine was questioned at that time. At the end of the operation there was still complete apnoea which did not reverse when neostigmine and atropine were given. Nikethamide was also given and she was hyperventilated with CO_2, but to no avail. One hour after the operation there was still no improvement in muscle tone and the 'Medelec' stimulator showed post-tetanic facilitation. Edrophonium (Tensilon) 10 mg was given with very little improvement and the patient was unable to maintain adequate oxygenation on air. Artificial ventilation was continued for a further 4 hours when a second dose of edrophonium (Tensilon) was given. A marked improvement in muscle tone and spontaneous ventilation followed. Atropine and neostigmine were then given once more and full respiratory function returned. Thus, more than 5 hours after the cessation of the operation, the endotracheal tube was removed and the patient was able to breathe without assistance. The patient was in good general health and had a haemoglobin of 80% and a pseudocholinesterase level of 56 units. No metabolic disturbance was detected and it is apparent that this patient was sensitive to relaxants of both the non-depolarizing and depolarizing type.

Injuries to the chest

Respiratory failure may develop after either surgery to the chest wall or trauma which has fractured the ribs or sternum.

The fracture of ribs causes pain so that the patient finds it difficult to maintain an adequate tidal volume. The rough sharp edges of the fractured ribs may pierce the lung giving rise to a pneumothorax or haemopneumothorax. Damage to the lung may produce blood and exudate which obstruct the bronchioles. When part of the lung is collapsed by either air or blood in the thoracic cavity or by compression of the chest wall, shunting of blood flowing through parts of the lung occurs and arterial oxygen desaturation develops. To this must be added the effects of overall hypoventilation. For these reasons, artificial ventilation of the lung may be necessary for many days, frequently with oxygen-enriched gas mixtures. Patients who belong to this category as a result of trauma require many of the aspects of the most modern forms of resuscitative treatment. These include treatment of shock, early surgical intervention, controlled ventilation, attention to fluid and electrolyte balance and frequent blood-gas analyses. When the lung has been punctured, surgical emphysema becomes widespread (Fig. 5.8a and b) as air tracks through the tissues. This is well illustrated by the following case.

Case history. A lorry crashed into the back of a stationary car which contained a 52-year-old man who was sitting in the front seat. He was admitted to hospital suffering from severe

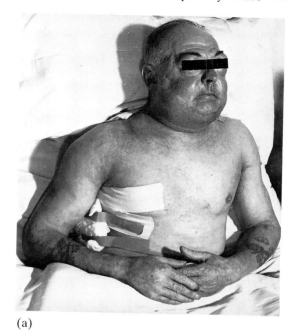

(a)

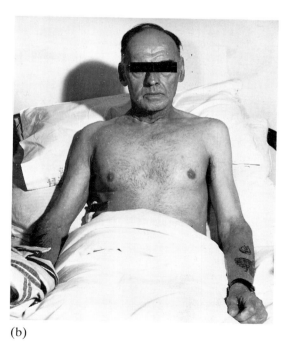

(b)

Fig. 5.8   (a) The appearance of a man with gross surgical emphysema 'Michelin man' following the leakage of air from the lung into the subcutaneous tissue. The appearance is similar to that of the patient who suffered trauma to both lungs from a car accident (see *Case history*). (b) The same patient when the air had been reabsorbed.

dyspnoea and subcutaneous emphysema. He suffered fractures to eight ribs in the right and four ribs in the left hemithorax just lateral to the vertebral bodies. A pneumothorax was produced in the right chest and a haemo-pneumothorax in the left chest (Fig. 5.9). When he was examined there was depressed respiration and he was cyanosed and hypoten-sive. Artificial ventilation, by means of a mask and rebreathing bag containing oxygen, was begun. The metabolic acidosis found on blood analysis was corrected with infusions of hyper-tonic sodium bicarbonate and the blood volume was restored by blood transfusion. A tension pneumothorax was treated by releasing the air in his right chest and both thoracic cavities were opened surgically so that damage to the lungs could be repaired. Under-water drainage of the thoracic cavities was then main-tained. A tracheotomy was performed and positive pressure ventilation continued. At the end of the anaesthetic, when spontaneous respiratory effort returned, intermittent posi-tive pressure respiration was continued by means of a patient-triggered, pressure-cycled ventilator. Sedation with morphine was necessary. The patient continued to drain blood for a further 24 hours and this was replaced. Air was aspirated from the thoracic cavities for a further week. The day following the accident, examination of the arterial blood revealed a slightly reduced oxygen saturation, a moderate metabolic acidosis and a respiratory acidosis. Consciousness had returned during the night, but mental disorientation persisted for 2–3 days. Because of surgical emphysema, his appearance was similar to that of the man in Fig. 5.8(a). Gradual weaning from the venti-lator was begun after 8 days and the patient slowly recovered; he left hospital 5 weeks later.

This type of case requires great care in all aspects of management, especially experienced nursing. In spite of a strict fluid regimen, the patient developed moderate hyponatraemia and a raised blood urea. This is a commonly observed bio-chemical response following major trauma (treatment given in Chapter 2).

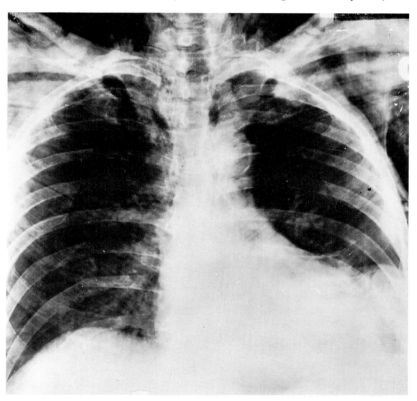

Fig. 5.9 Chest X-ray of the patient described above. The mottled appearance is because of widespread surgical emphysema, similar to that of the patient in Fig. 5.8.

Antibiotics as a cause of respiratory failure

The rapid absorption into the bloodstream of antibiotics from that group which includes streptomycin,[52] neomycin,[41,50,51,59,88,105,106] kanamycin, polymixin, lincomycin and clindamycin,[54,103,104] can give rise to respiratory depression, in some cases producing complete apnoea and therefore resulting in cardiac arrest.[111] These antibiotics produce a neuromuscular block of the non-depolarizing type that is identical to that produced by d-tubocurarine. This effect usually only occurs when the antibiotics are given intravenously or are inserted into the pleural or peritoneal cavity[105] where the large serous surface allows rapid diffusion of the substances into the bloodstream. While respiratory paralysis has been reported following a large dose of streptomycin, neomycin is the next most common antibiotic to cause this condition. Other aminoglycosides are now being used increasingly when organisms are isolated that are insensitive to the more commonly used antibiotics. Complete apnoea followed by cardiac arrest in a 16-year-old girl has been reported following the rapid intravenous infusion of kanamycin.[111] This patient had previously been treated with streptomycin and it was considered that this may have reinforced the neuromuscular-blocking action of the kanamycin.

It has been well established that the skeletal muscle paralysis that occurs both in man and in experimental animals and which has been investigated both *in vivo* and *in vitro*, is potentiated by muscle relaxants.[2,36] Studies have indicated that the predominant mechanism by which muscle paralysis is produced is that of a magnesium-like depression of the release of acetylcholine.[47,120,121,135,144] However, when Singh *et al.* (1979)[122] investigated the condition, they found that there appeared to be a difference of action between different antibiotics. Streptomycin, for example, resembled magnesium in its action on the end-plate potentials, while lincomycin, clindamycin and polymixin B resembled tubocurarine in abolishing miniature end-plate potentials. Their investigations tended to confirm that which had been observed clinically, that the neuromuscular block produced by some antibiotics (e.g. streptomycin), could be reversed by Ca^{++}, whereas that produced by other antibiotics has no known mechanism of reversal (when both Ca^{++} and neostigmine are ineffective) and the condition has to be treated with artificial ventilation until the effects of the antibiotic have been dissipated and an adequate tidal volume has been maintained spontaneously for a significant period.

Antibiotics are most commonly inserted into the thoracic and peritoneal cavities during surgery and, therefore, anaesthesia, and it has been considered that ether anaesthesia especially may be implicated in the production of a neuromuscular block.[106] These effects can, however, be produced when no anaesthetic is used (e.g. kanamycin given intravenously). It is therefore possible that the emphasis on an anaesthetic agent playing a part in the production of respiratory depression is a result of the mode of administration rather than a clearly definable pharmacological effect. The neuromuscular blocking action can be reversed by calcium gluconate. Ream[111] found that the effects produced by kanamycin could only be antagonized by neostigmine.

Treatment

Ventilation must be maintained from the moment respiratory insufficiency begins to appear and, because complete apnoea may be produced, a patient-triggered ventilator cannot be used with safety. Calcium gluconate should be given intravenously to the adult in doses of 10 ml of a 10% solution. Because the group of antibiotics in question has been known to produce systemic hypertension and a tachycardia and because calcium gluconate can, in its own right, produce these physiological changes, the intravenous injection of this substance must be given slowly and with caution. The hypertension and tachycardia observed may, however, be the result of anoxia alone. Because the curare-like action of this group of antibiotics can be reversed by neostigmine, this substance should also be given intravenously, at the earliest possible moment. Doses of 0.25 mg i.v. can be given in repeated doses until the desired effect is produced. If the dose of neostigmine is slowly increased, its muscarine-like action may be avoided without the administration of atropine. If larger doses of neostigmine have to be used, it is advisable to administer atropine in doses of 0.4 mg i.v. in order to avoid these effects.

Acute hyponatraemia

The accidental insertion of distilled water into the peritoneal cavity during diathermy of the bladder has given rise to acute, postoperative respiratoy depression. Treatment is the slow infusion of 6% NaCl i.v. (see p. 31).

Inhaled solvents

In the United Kingdom there are approximately 80 deaths each year from solvent abuse (Anderson *et al.*, 1985).[4] Most of these deaths occur when no medical attendant is present, and the cause of death, when sudden, may be cardiac arrhythmias or respiratory depression. A lucid account has been given of a patient who developed reversible respiratory arrest after glue sniffing. The adhesive contained toluene and the authors (Cronk *et al.*, 1985)[38] considered respiratory arrest to be an important, and perhaps major cause of death due to solvent abuse. A sinus tachycardia only was present on the electrocardiogram (ECG).

Postoperative respiratory infection and failure

The consequences of respiratory failure after surgery are frequently horrendous. Excellent surgery is very often vitiated because of inadequate preparation and poor standards of postoperative care. Minor respiratory disturbances are allowed to develop into serious respiratory failure, because of inadequate and inappropriate treatment, administered too late.

In spite of the best care, however, serious respiratory failure can develop, especially when the patient has smoked cigarettes on the day of the operation, up to the time of receiving the pre-medication therapy. Certainly, spirometry indicates impaired performance in smokers.[95]

At the very least, respiratory dysfunction prolongs recovery, sometimes for long periods of time (as described below, see p. 149) when serious infection develops and the medical and nursing effort must be increased, thus straining resources and leaving the patient mentally and physically scarred. This is made worse by the development of acute renal failure, stress ulceration and toxic shock.

Some indication of impending respiratory failure can be obtained by preoperative respiratory function tests.[6,40,65,125,126] However, severe respiratory failure develops in non-smokers with no history of respiratory disease, and some authors consider that clinical examination prior to surgery is still the most important factor, to which can be added simple spirometric tests.[26]

How, therefore, can postoperative respiratory failure be avoided or reduced in severity? In addition to the general measures, chronic lung disease can be treated pre-operatively with antibiotics such as tetracycline or erythromycin.

Damage to the lungs by microaggregates in the blood can be avoided by the use of the Swank blood transfusion filter (see p. 197), and the insertion of a similar filter into the extracorporeal circuit when open-heart surgery is performed.

When infection has developed early, treatment with antibiotics of wide spectrum is essential. Treatment with intravenous amino acids and other forms of parenteral hyperalimentation should be discontinued if they have been begun, as they reach high concentrations in the small volume of blood in the pulmonary circulation and nourish the organisms in the lungs rather than the patient during this catabolic phase.

Patients suffering from severe postoperative respiratory failure incubate numerous organisms in the stomach.[21,22] This is most marked when a paralytic ileus is present, or during artificial ventilation of the lungs. Bacteria can grow in the fluid within the stomach when the secretion of HCl ceases and the pH rises above 2. When the pH is 3.5 or higher, organisms can be found in the nasogastric drainage and identical organisms are found in the tracheal aspirate.[21,22,23,25]

Virus infections are sometimes the initiating cause and they can be the source of respiratory failure. It has been demonstrated that inhalation of the antiviral agent *ribavirin* following correct atomization is an effective form of treatment (Knight *et al.*, 1981).[82]

Great care must be taken that overhydration and excessive expansion of the vascular compartment are not allowed to occur. This can be avoided by carefully taking note of the CVP measurement and the wedge pressure measurement using a Swan-Ganz catheter. Excessive hydration is most likely to occur following tracheal intubation, when a bacteraemia commonly causes toxic shock, the blood pressure falls and this is mistaken for hypovolaemia. Care must then be taken with the correct measurement of CVP (see pp. 179–183) so that this mistake is avoided.

Adult respiratory distress syndrome (Adult hyaline membrane disease)

It is unfortunate that 'adult respiratory distress syndrome' is now being used as a generic term for all forms of respiratory failure. If there is to be any order in defining the many different pathological changes that occur in the lungs, the term should be reserved for hyaline membrane disease, whatever the aetiology.

In addition to respiratory distress syndrome in the newborn, hyaline membrane formation occurs as a result of influenza, radiation injury, exposure to volatile chemical substances, uraemia, high-altitude sickness in which the inspired and alveolar PO_2 is low, and is said to occur during oxygen therapy where the PO_2 is high.[7,10,70,124,137] The last-mentioned, however, has never been proved to occur, in isolation, in man. Hyaline membrane disease does not occur in all animals. Hyaline membrane was found in six patients at post-mortem,[123] all these patients had received 100% O_2 as a terminal event during IPPR which failed to increase the arterial PO_2. However, one patient had suffered toxic shock, another had convulsed because of eclampsia and had vomited during the convulsion, a third was admitted with fulminating pulmonary oedema, a fourth had experienced cardiac arrest twice during surgery for a recurrence of cervical carcinoma, and the fifth was decerebrate after a road traffic accident. The last-mentioned patient underwent a tracheostomy, and stress ulceration occurred after 5 days and recurred at 10 days. He was ventilated with 100% O_2 after 15 days of poor respiratory function following a sudden severe rise in CVP. The sixth case was an 8-year-old child with Fallot's tetralogy who, following surgery, had pulmonary oedema, a tracheostomy, intravascular clotting and acute renal failure. To those of us who have treated similar patients successfully with well-humidified 100% O_2 for long periods of time, including those that have suffered stress ulceration, the conclusion that the high tensions of inspired PO_2 alone caused the hyaline membrane disease is difficult to accept.

Only when hyaline membrane disease is observed in adult man following exposure to 100% O_2 and all other factors are absent, will it be possible to establish a causal relationship. Meanwhile, astronauts appear to have been exposed to 100% O_2 at approximately 1/3 atmospheres without experiencing lung damage. However, by entraining atmospheric air during artificial ventilation of the lungs, at least partial humidification of the inspired gases occurs. The O_2 content of the inspired gases should, therefore, be maintained at the lowest concentration conducive with the establishment of a satisfactory arterial PO_2, approximately 70 mmHg in the patient who has a normal haemoglobin concentration.

All gases delivered from cylinders contain no water vapour. If patients are ventilated with *air* from a cylinder, problems develop which are the same as those associated with the use of dry O_2.

Case history. The patient, a 61–year-old Caucasian woman, was admitted to the hospital via the accident and emergency department complaining of severe epigastric pain. She had, 3 days previously, undergone endoscopy which demonstrated the presence of a peptic ulcer. When examined, a diagnosis of acute perfora-

tion was made, and surgery revealed perforation of a duodenal ulcer, which was repaired. It was then June 26th. Three days after the operation, bowel sounds had returned and the nasogastric tube was removed. The patient vomited four or five times that evening and the nasogastric tube was replaced and intravenous infusions were re-commenced. Eight days after the operation the patient complained of pain in the chest which was worse on breathing deeply. Chest X-ray revealed shadowing on the left basal region and a pleural effusion on the right side of the chest. X-ray of the abdomen showed gross gaseous distension. The patient had a leucocytosis of 19 000/cm³. Haemoglobin was 13.6 g%, PCV was 42%.

Ampicillin and gentamicin, which had been given the previous day, following examination of the sputum, were continued. The arterial blood PO_2 was 57 mmHg and PCO_2 was 30 mmHg. O_2 was administered by mask. Because the patient's condition deteriorated the following day, she was artificially ventilated using a time-cycled, volume-controlled 'Radcliffe' ventilator following the insertion of a cuffed endotracheal tube. It was necessary to use humidified 100% O_2 (see Table 5.7).

The patient did not improve markedly with this type of ventilator. A serious tachycardia developed and it was suspected that she had suffered a myocardial infarction, which might have accounted for some of the pulmonary congestion and cyanosis. This was treated with diuretics and digitalization with 0.75 mg digoxin. Digoxin was then continued 0.125 mg/day. It should be noted that the patient was grossly cyanosed and grossly anoxic on this first day of artificial ventilation of the lungs.

Because of the tachycardia and low systemic blood pressure, the ventilator was changed to a patient-triggered, pressure-cycled, Bird ventilator. Although there was no improvement in oxygenation, the patient's haemodynamics improved markedly. The peripheral cyanosis was reduced and the venous distention decreased. When air was entrained via the Bird ventilator so that the O_2 content of the inhaled gases was 40%, the arterial PO_2 fell to 24 mmHg. There was an associated fall in blood pressure and an increase in heart rate. There was therefore no alternative but to continue with 100% O_2, although care was taken to ensure maximum humidification. The need to administer 100% O_2 could not have been due to O_2 toxicity or O_2 damage to the lungs because, prior to ventilation and endotracheal intubation, O_2 had been administered only by low-concentration mask. It was due largely to the

Table 5.7   The blood pH, PCO_2, PO_2, $[HCO_3^-]$, and base excess in a patient who developed respiratory failure following the repair of a perforated duodenal ulcer and was artificially ventilated for 47 days, sometimes with 100% O_2

Days ill		Days on ventilator	pH	Blood-gases		$[HCO_3^-]$	Base excess	Ventilation O_2 per cent	
				PCO_2	PO_2				
24		1	7.38	50	50	29	+3	100%	
25	2 a.m.	2	7.45	37	55	25	+2	100%	
	5 a.m.		7.30	63	26	30	+1	40%	
			7.35	42	75	23	−3	100%	
	6 a.m.		7.30	51	24	24	−3	40%	
	7 a.m.		7.47	31	69	22	0	100%	
26	1 p.m.	3	7.45	32	78	22	0	100%	
	8 p.m.		7.48	37	87	27	+4.5	100%	
	1.45 a.m.		7.41	37	40	23	−1	100%	
27		4	7.52	35	47	27	+6	100%	
28		5	7.56	28	169	24	+5	100%	
29		6	7.38	41	131	24	−1	100%	
30		7	7.45	37	55	25	+2	40%	
31		8	7.44	59	136	39	+11	40%	
32		9	7.50	65	52	50	+19	40%	
34		11	7.50	44	79	33	+10	40%	
35		12	7.44	48	23	32	+7	100%	Off ventilator
									Transfusion of 2 units of blood
42		19	7.50	61	58	48	+17	100%	On Radcliffe ventilator
44		21	7.43	58	67	37	+10	100%	On Bird patient triggered ventilator
45		22	7.30	76	150	36	+7	100%	
46		23						100%	
47		24	7.32	74	58	39	+5	40%	
48		25	7.34	73	164	38	+8	40%	
			7.29	79	150	37	+6	40%	
52		29	7.31	94	163	46	+8	40%	On Bird ventilator
			7.45	54	89	36	+10.5		On Radcliffe ventilator
53		30	7.47	42	125	31	+6		
54		31	7.25	65	67	28	−2		
63		40	7.62	60	220	60	+30	100%	
			7.48	70	150	55	+25	40%	
64		41	7.40	78	173	52	+18	100%	
65		42	7.37	66	173	37	+9	100%	
67		43	7.36	85	128	48	+16		Off ventilator 15 minutes every hour
70		47	7.49	56	106	41	+15	40%	

primary infection and possibly the added sequelae of pulmonary oedema and the pathological changes in the lungs that follow perforation of the gut. This form of ventilation was continued for 9 days.

The patient was given diazepam (Valium) 5 mg i.v. while being ventilated with the Bird ventilator. However, on the morning of the following day, the patient suddenly obstructed a bronchus, failed to trigger the ventilator, which was incorrectly set so that it failed to take over the ventilation of the lungs spontaneously. After endotracheal suction, the insertion of 2 ml of isotonic NaCl down the endotracheal tube every hour and careful humidification of the inspired oxygen, the PO_2 of the arterial blood rose to 87 mmHg by the evening of the same day.

During the following day, the same regimen was followed, the humidification of the inspired gases was continued and 0.9% NaCl solution was inserted into the endotracheal tube every half-hour. Endotracheal suction was continued half-hourly. It became evident during that day, in which low arterial PO_2 values were obtained, that in this patient's circumstances it was not possible to remove the secretions produced by the lungs in an adequate manner. The following day, therefore, a tracheotomy was performed (Day 28, Table 5.7), and careful suction of both bronchi could then be ensured. This resulted in a rise in the arterial PO_2 to 169 mmHg, using initially 100% O_2, and later adequate oxygenation was obtained with entrained air (40% O_2) but this was not sustained and a return to 100% O_2 was necessary.

By this time, colliforms and *Pseudomonas* organisms had been isolated from the tracheal aspirate, and these were sensitive to ampicillin and gentamicin so that treatment with these antibiotics was maintained. Improvement in the patients's condition continued, although when she was disconnected from the ventilator she became grossly cyanosed within 1 or 2 minutes so that the arterial blood PO_2 fell to 23 mmHg (Day 35, Table 5.7).

The improvement that was maintained on the ventilator was not without careful management of the fluid balance and electrolytes. Both hyponatraemia and hypokalaemia occurred, the plasma $[K^+]$ falling to 2.6 mmol/l (mEq/l), and this was associated with a rising metabolic alkalosis. Intravenous KCl, 120 mmol in 1 litre of saline, was given over periods of 8 hours. The blood urea concentration rose to 16.6 mmol/l (100 mg%), indicating that there was some degree of renal impairment, although the urine volume was maintained satisfactorily at over 1.5 l/24 hours. There was virtual identity of plasma (290 mosmol/l) and urine (350 mosmol/l) osmolality. This is referred to as high output acute renal failure (see p. 55). Hypophosphataemia 0.45 mmol/l (1.4 mg%) developed which possibly caused gradual haemolysis (see p. 55), resulting in a fall of Hb to 7.8 g%. No massive bleed had occurred, although red cells had been found in the gastric aspirate, which had a pH of 5.6. Two units of packed cells were therefore transfused over 6 hours.

By 5 August (Day 39) the patient could tolerate short periods breathing spontaneously and could swallow liquids orally. When not ventilated, her arterial PO_2 was 50 mmHg and PCO_2 56 mmHg.

However, following the transfusion of 2 units of whole blood 2 days later, on the 40th day of her illness, having been ventilated for 17 days, she passed into congestive cardiac failure and had to be placed on the time-cycled, volume-controlled Radcliffe ventilator using 100% O_2 for 5 days. She became unconscious, her blood pressure fell and an infusion of metaraminol (Aramine) had to be given to maintain the blood pressure. Recovery, however, gradually took place and by 13 August, 47 days after the onset of her perforation and 21 days of artificial ventilation, the patient tolerated short periods breathing air spontaneously off the ventilator and 40% O_2 when on the ventilator. Diuretics meanwhile had controlled the congestive cardiac failure (CCF) but no improvement occurred initially in lung function.

Following tracheostomy, the organisms within the trachea could be identified by inserting a sterile sputum trap between the suction catheter and the mechanical suction apparatus. At various times, colliforms, *Pseudomonas aeruginosa* and *Klebsiella* sp. were present in the sputum.

Pseudomonas aeruginosa persisted until the middle of September in spite of appropriate antibiotic therapy.

Measurements of the pH values of the gastric aspirate were obtained and, when the samples were taken before the administration of dilute HCl via the nasogastric tube, these were in the region of 6.5. The highest value measured was 8.5, but this sample was obtained 30 minutes after giving the liquid diet. Following insertion of the HCl through the nasogastric tube, the pH of the gastric contents fell to between 1.0 and 2.0. The specimens with the low pH proved to be sterile. However, when the pH was 6.5, an abundant growth of colliforms was found and when the pH was 8.5 an abundant growth of both colliforms and *P. aeruginosa* was demonstrated. These were similar findings to those obtained earlier from other patients.[21] Prior to insertion of HCl, the gastric aspirate contained a small number of red cells, but following its use none was seen.

The patient was only semiconscious for the greater part of this period. By 14 August, 1 month after the commencement of artificial ventilation of the lungs, bowel function had been normal for some days and the patient was taking sips of water. A nasogastric tube was again passed and a high-protein diet was administered in doses of 100 ml/hour. Methylprednisolone was also given intravenously, initially in a dose of 500 mg and then 6-hourly in doses of 40 mg.

Methylprednisolone was given because there had been no improvement in the patient's condition, and episodes of hypotension associated with bronchoconstriction had occurred, making ventilation of the lungs difficult. The bronchoconstriction responded only partially to aminophylline in doses of 500 mg i.v.; 100% O_2 had to be given during these episodes to maintain oxygenation. Some improvement occurred in nasogastric feeding with either a commercially available diet or meat and vegetables, blended to make them liquid.

Because the organisms which were found in the drainage from the stomach were identical to those present in the tracheal aspirate, dilute HCl was given via the nasogastric tube just prior to administering the diet.

The patient remained semiconscious (18 August, 29 days of ventilation) and a pleural rub was noted in the left chest. Three days later, however, the patient was not only conscious but in good spirits and tolerated a few minutes off the ventilator. The chest X-rays showed the right lung to be clearing, although there was still consolidation present of approximately two thirds of the left lung. The methylprednisolone (Solu-Medrone) was reduced to 20 mg/day.

A sudden attack of bronchoconstriction occurred 4 days later, 32 days after the beginning of ventilation, which was treated with aminophylline, with little effect, and intravenous frusemide. The patient was again ventilated with the Radcliffe ventilator using 100% O_2 and was given methylprednisolone 120 mg i.v. and an infusion of metaraminol (Aramine) when the blood pressure fell. By 29 August (40 days) the patient was again ventilated using the patient-triggered Bird ventilator, and even though 100% O_2 had been given during the previous 8 days for most of the time, spontaneous improvement continued and by 2 September (43 days) the chest X-rays showed a marked improvement and the patient was allowed to breath O_2 spontaneously through a humidifier for 15 minutes every hour. Three days later, 46 days after artificial ventilation began, the cuffed tracheostomy tube was replaced with a metal tube and this was removed after a further 2 days. The tracheostomy was covered and allowed to heal. The steroids were reduced gradually.

The patient had one further attack of CCF which was treated with frusemide; ampicillin, and flucloxacillin were given orally. She complained bitterly and increasingly of being unable to breathe and this was due to a fibrous stricture of the trachea which was removed surgically. Although this was a prolonged traumatic period, the patient became active very quickly and returned to a completely normal life.

Only the salient aspects have been recorded in the above account. The successful outcome for this patient was because of attention to detail by nursing staff, devoted physiotherapy and tracheal toilet, responding to changes in the patient's condition immediately. Even so, severe hypokalaemia developed and was corrected with KCl administered intravenously at a rate of 20 mmol (mEq)/hour. Hypophosphataemia was corrected by oral feeding. The fall in [PO_4] may have contributed to the congestive cardiac failure (see p. 55) and the fall in haemoglobin, although this was not recognized at the time. It may also have contributed to the respiratory failure. A fungal infection of the bladder developed and was treated with nystatin. This anti-fungal agent was used to irrigate the bladder and the catheter was clamped for 4 hours so that there was sufficient time for it to act. The problems in fluid balance were legion, and over such a long period of time mistakes were made. It was wrong to infuse two units of blood without giving a rapidly acting diuretic such as ethacrynic acid, 50 mg, which can be added to the blood. A patient attached to a ventilator for this length of time has to be fed, but it is the author's opinion, based on a large number of cases, that intravenous alimentation in the presence of parenchymatous lung infection should be avoided. Although steroids appear to reduce the period of paralytic ileus following surgery, they cannot always be used, but where possible oral alimentation should be started as soon as possible.

Although 100% O_2 was administered to this patient for considerable lengths of time humidification was maintained and it was without ill-effect. This was similar to the experience of McCaughey et al. (1973)[87] who ventilated a patient with 100% O_2 for 25 days following blast injury to the lungs and that of Hastleton et al. (1981)[64] and Hastleton and Penna (1981)[63] who also question the danger of oxygen toxicity, especially when the period of artificial ventilation of the lungs is restricted to a few days.

In what way was this patient different from others that have been reported?

1. The patient survived just over 7 weeks of continuous ventilation of the lungs for a severe infection and did not develop anuria or uncontrollable stress ulceration or irreversible toxic shock. If hyaline membrane disease developed, it was obviously reversible.

2. Oxygen 100% was given continuously for periods of 3–9 days and for shorter periods at other times. The need to administer 100% O_2 was precipitated initially by acute respiratory insufficiency and not by a gradual decline following the use of high O_2 tensions in the inspired gases. When 100% O_2 was administered at numerous times subsequently, it was not related to previously administered high O_2 tensions, and each time the patient improved spontaneously.

3. Corticosteroids were given 1 month after the beginning of IPPR, initially in very high doses which were later reduced and eventually discontinued.

4. The reservoir of organisms in the stomach that appear to be related to stress ulceration (see p. 199) and the continuance of the respiratory infection were treated with dilute HCl, B.P.

Bleeding at slow rate from the gastro-intestinal tract may have occurred on one occasion and was corrected by transfusion of packed cells. Following this, dilute HCl was administered hourly, through the nasogastric tube.

5. All feeding was performed by nasogastric tube and no intravenous alimentation was given, so that enhancement of the respiratory infection was avoided.

6. Constriction of the trachea developed very shortly after removal of the tracheostomy tube and required surgery for its relief.

Fat Embolism

A clinical condition that gives rise to severe and prolonged respiratory failure is the dissemination of fat globules following severe injury and fracture of bones. Although fracture of the long bones usually gives rise to the condition, it is recognized that it can follow fracture of the ribs and other conditions.

The earliest sign of fat embolization is a fall in arterial PO_2 with a low or normal PCO_2.

As fat blocks the lung capillaries, the compliance of the lungs decreases, spontaneous ventilation becomes increasingly difficult for the patient and artificial ventilation becomes necessary. This entails endotracheal intubation in the first instance and later a tracheostomy if necessary.

The very earliest physical sign, therefore, other than dyspnoea is cyanosis. This is commonly associated with restlessness of the patient who becomes abusive and frequently noisy, shouting vituperative insults at the attending staff. The body temperature rises and a tachycardia often develops. Petechial eruptions are sometimes observed and present on the anterior aspects of the neck, axillae and in less obvious places such as the buccal cavity and the conjunctival sacs (Fig. 5.10), when they can be seen by depressing the lower lid. The petechiae last 4–24 hours and appear in groups or crops.

Fat emboli can sometimes be observed in the retinal vessels. Convulsions can occur and these, as well as the restlessness and abusive behaviour, are almost certainly caused by emboli occurring within the brain. Cardiac arrhythmias sometimes occur including heart block. Cardiac failure can develop. In one of the author's patients, acute

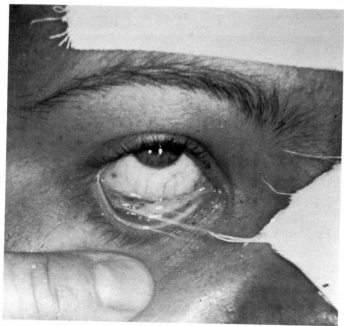

Fig. 5.10 Sublachrymal petechial haemorrhages that developed as a result of fat emboli. (Reproduced by kind permission of Dr John Kennedy).

right heart failure developed, although in other ways the patient was not severely affected. Fat globules had been identified in the urine and sputum following a road traffic accident in which the ribs were fractured on both sides of the thoracic cage. Digitalization produced a dramatic clinical improvement.

Investigations

Blood investigations frequently allow the earliest identification of fat emboli. In addition to the fall in arterial PO_2, there is a reduction in the platelet count associated with the fall in lung compliance. There is frequently an associated metabolic acidosis and, because of hyperventilation due to the anoxia, a fall in the PCO_2. The pH therefore may be normal or raised. At a later stage there is a reduction in the plasma [Ca^{++}] which is considered to be caused by the formation of calcium soaps. Fat globules may be found in the urine; these can be seen on microscopy and can be stained with Sudan III (red).

A chest X-ray should be taken early and this reveals a 'cotton-wool' or snow-storm appearance which is quite classic, but can be mistaken for pulmonary oedema. The development of pulmonary oedema can also occur, espcially if the myocardium is severely affected.

The following should be performed.

Arterial blood gases
Chest X-ray
Full blood count
Platelet count
Examination for fat in the urine
Electrocardiogram
Sputum for fat
Serum lipase estimation (may be raised)
Skin biopsy in which a fat globule can be identified by appropriate staining
Clotted venous blood which can be sectioned and stained for fat

In addition to the early changes in blood gases, an early fall in the platelet count and plasma [Ca^{++}] can be measured when there are no outward physical signs of fat emboli other than those of dyspnoea and respiratory failure. The identification of fat in the urine and the above tests are of some help in making the correct diagnosis and instituting the correct treatment.

Treatment

Early treatment with oxygen is most essential, together with correction of hypovolaemia and a base deficit. Artificial ventilation of the lungs, when it becomes necessary, should be instituted early, and delay until the patient is *in extremis* should be avoided. Steroids should be given in large doses intravenously in the early stages of the condition and continued until improvement in the lung condition and arterial blood oxygenation occurs.

Myasthenia Gravis

This is a condition in which there is gradually increasing fatigue of the muscles which is associated with an enlarged abnormal thymus or carcinoma, especially carcinoma of the bronchus.

When Dr Mary Walker treated a patient suffering from myasthenia gravis with an anticholinesterase when she was a house physician at St Alfege's Hospital in 1934, the beneficial effects were so impressive the results were considered 'to be miraculous'.[136]

For a long period it was considered that the abnormal transmission of the chemical stimulus from the motor nerve ending to the muscle fibre was due to competitive blocking or the release of abnormally low concentrations of acetylcholine.[46] Certainly, electrophysiological recordings of the motor end-plate potentials revealed that these were smaller than normal.[46] However, more recently it has been demonstrated that the responsiveness of the post-synaptic acetylcholine receptors is decreased and the quantity of acetylcholine released is probably normal.[61] The reduced responsiveness appears to be due to degenerative changes in the post-synaptic folds, loss of acetylcholine receptor sites, and widening of synaptic clefts.[48,49]

While these changes in the ultrastructure of the muscle end-plate have emerged, as in the contraction of the myocardium (see p. 300), help in understanding the pathophysiology of myasthenia gravis has been obtained by using extraneous agents. The venom from the snake *Bungarus multicinctus* (α bungarotoxin) binds specifically to the acetylcholine receptor sites. This has been used to isolate the receptor sites in the electric organ of the electric eel (*Torpedo californica*) as these organs are homologous to motor end-plates. Repeated immunization of rabbits with purified receptor site material has induced a myasthenia-like disease.[101]

An initial phase of macrophage invasion of the muscle end-plate is followed by degeneration of the post-synaptic cleft, without cellular invasion and the onset of chronic disease.*

The condition has also been produced by immunization of syngeneic muscle acetylcholine receptor protein in rats.[86] Physiologically and pathologically, the chronic condition in animals appears to be similar to the chronic condition in man,[117] and it can be transferred from one animal to another using appropriate antibodies.[86]

The autoimmune nature of myasthenia gravis had been postulated by Simpson in 1960,[119] and had been indicated by lymphocytic infiltration and antibodies identified by immunofluorescent techniques by Strauss et al.[129] in patients with thymic hyperplasia. It has now been demonstrated that 87% of patients with myasthenia gravis have antigens to acetylcholine receptor protein and these are absent in normal people or non-myasthenic patients.[3,13,86]

These facts have an important influence on treatment and management. Now it is known that myasthenia gravis results from an immune mechanism, early thymectomy is rapidly gaining acceptance and it is realized that the pharmacological treatment (described below) is largely palliative until this can be achieved.

This approach is not new. It has long been recognized that the earlier thymectomy was performed, the better the prognosis.[83,118] There was, however, a reluctance to subject patients to an operative procedure, associated with significant mortality, when control with anticholinesterases could, in most cases, be readily achieved, especially in the early stages of the disease.

Much progress has, however, been made in artificial ventilation of the lungs, biochemical control and maintenance of fluid balance so that the risks of thymectomy have been greatly reduced. Also, as time passes, the possibility of a remission following thymectomy increases. A combined study in Boston and New York reported that of 45 women suffering from myasthenia gravis, 84% had either complete remission or significant improvement following thymectomy, although they did not have a thymic tumour. Similar findings have been reported by other workers,[44] while Papatestas et al. (1971)[99] found improvement or remission in 90% of patients 5 years following thymectomy.

In Britain, Havard (1973)[66] advocated thymectomy for all patients except those in whom the

---

* A full review of myasthenia gravis is available from the Proceedings of the Symposium held at the New York Academy of Sciences in 1981.[60]

disease is confined to the ocular form. Similar findings and approach to early thymectomy have been reported elsewhere.[56] This approach may, however, be modified by the findings of Davis et al. (1979)[39] and Behan et al. (1979).[12] Behan et al.[12] found that, following a course of plasma exchange using a continuous-flow cell separator and immunosuppression with azathioprine (150 mg/day) and prednisolone (100 mg/day), a dramatic clinical improvement took place. Although 6 of their 21 patients had a recurrence of their symptoms 3–9 months later, 9 patients required no further anticholinesterase agents for as long as 19 months following the plasma exchange. The benefits of plasma exchange and immunosuppression for the short-term control of severe myasthenia gravis has therefore been demonstrated by Davis and his co-workers,[39] but because plasma exchange has no cumulative long-term benefit, early thymectomy followed by careful postoperative management are probably still indicated.

Classification

Myasthenia gravis can be classified according to the degree of muscle involvement and the period of time that has elapsed following its onset. The classification helps with management and treatment.

Type 1

The disease involves ocular movements alone. Usually, if the condition is confined entirely to the ocular muscles for 2 years after its onset, there is only a small probability of the disease progressing into the generalized form.

Type 2

This form of the disease is usually benign and, although there is a mild generalized myasthenia, the response to drug treatment is satisfactory.

Type 3

There is a moderately severe generalized myasthenia with the onset usually characterized by weakness of the ocular muscles, but gradual progression occurs to involvement of the bulbar area, therefore necessitating periodic artificial ventilation of the lungs.

Type 4

An acute fulminating form of myasthenia that develops with rapid progression to involvement of the bulbar area, associated with generalized muscle weakness and weakness of the respiratory muscles at an early stage. The response to drug treatment is poor and the mortality rate is high. These patients require immediate treatment in the emergency department and then transfer to a critical care unit.

Type 5
Severe life-threatening myasthenia which develops from the relatively minor forms seen in patients who could be classified as type 2 or type 3, but who rapidly develop ocular and bulbar manifestations, generalized muscle weakness and respiratory insufficiency.

Treatment
The therapeutic substances used most commonly in the treatment of this condition are neostigmine (Prostigmine), pyridostigmine (Mestinon) and edrophonium (Tensilon).

Neostigmine (Prostigmine)
This is usually given with atropine to suppress its action on other acetylcholine-motivated organs, such as the gut and the bladder. For routine treatment, therefore, neostigmine 1.5 mg is given subcutaneously together with atropine 0.6 mg. The preparation is also effective orally when 15 mg is given every 4 hours or when necessary. The two forms of treatment may have to be given in unison and an intramuscular or subcutaneous injection of neostigmine may be necessary before eating or muscular effort.

The condition may give rise to episodes in which there is severe weakness of all muscles. There is then a difficulty in swallowing so that saliva may be inhaled and paralysis of the respiratory muscles may give rise to cardiac arrest from anoxia. In these circumstances, neostigmine may be required in doses of 0.5–2 mg every 20–30 minutes, or it can be given by continuous intravenous infusion, 5 mg or 10 mg in 500 ml of 5% dextrose given over 8–24 hours. Preparations for artificial ventilation have to be made. The muscarine effects of neostigmine may be avoided by giving small doses of atropine at the same time. It must be borne in mind that if neostigmine is given in excess, it may produce respiratory and other paralysis by depolarization of the muscle end-plate brought about by the excessive accumulation of acetylcholine. Neostigmine administration should, therefore, be kept to the minimum that is required.

The administration of neostigmine by continuous subcutaneous infusion has been described by Bingle et al. (1979)[16] in a woman with severe myasthenia gravis following thymectomy and radiotherapy for carcinoma of the thymus. Initially, the electrically driven constant-infusion pump was used in hospital, but later the patient was allowed home with a battery-operated infusion pump (Syringe Driver Type MS—Pye Dynamics Ltd., UK). The patient described by Bingle et al.[16] required up to 50 mg/day, but this enabled her to drive a car, perform light housework and removed all difficulties of swallowing. The syringe contained 2.5 g of neostigmine/litre.

Pyridostigmine (Mestinon)
This preparation has a longer action than neostigmine and may be more suitable and effective in some cases. It is given orally in doses of 60 mg.

Edrophonium (Tensilon)
This preparation, like pyridostigmine, is an analogue of neostigmine, but its pharmacological action is shorter and much more rapid than either of the other two preparations. Its use is largely diagnostic. When myasthenia gravis is suspected, an injection of 10 mg is given and the effect of muscle activity is noted. An increase in muscle power and activity is indicative of myasthenia gravis. We have already noted that overdosage with neostigmine in the treated case of myasthenia gravis may itself produce a condition which is so similar to a myasthenic crisis that it may be difficult to distinguish the two conditions. Because the action of edrophonium lasts for such a short time (1 or 2 minutes), it may be given with relative safety. A third use is at the end of an anaesthetic when it is sometimes necessary to distinguish between the continued action of depolarizing agents producing a neuromuscular block and metabolic disturbances.

The action of all these substances with anticholinesterase activity may be enhanced by administering ephedrine 30–60 mg, either orally or intramuscularly, and KCl.

Ambenonium chloride (Mytelase)
This is prepared in a 10-mg tablet and is given in doses of 5–25 mg daily. It can be used in place of pyridostigmine.

ACTH and steroid therapy
In recent years steroid therapy has been found to be effective in severely ill patients suffering from a generalized myasthenia gravis.[116] Frequently, there is a transitory worsening of the myasthenia so that artificial ventilation of the lungs becomes necessary if it is not already being used. After the first few days of treatment, improvement occurs.

Treatment with ACTH appears to be effective in doses of 100 units/day for 10 days. When prednisolone is given, it is prescribed in doses of 100 mg/day, if necessary for several weeks.

The patient is best treated in hospital so that transient periods of muscle weakness can be noted and infection, if it develops, can be treated. The course of ACTH can be repeated at intervals and, when improvement with prednisolone has been obtained, a reduction in dosage and alternate-day treatment can be instituted.

Overdosage with anticholinesterase drugs

This condition is difficult to distinguish from a myasthenic crisis because the patient demonstrates the same clinical signs (i.e. respiratory depression, inability to swallow, raise the eyelids, or move the eyes and limbs effectively). The patient is in danger because obstruction to the airway can easily occur, and a further dose of neostigmine will produce complete apnoea and, subsequently, cardiac arrest.

When a patient presents possibly suffering from this condition, it is therefore essential that in the first instance ventilation of the lungs should be assisted by artificial means. The diagnosis may be made by giving a small dose of edrophonium (Tensilon) 5–10 mg i.v. If the condition is one of overdosage, no improvement in muscle tone occurs and the patient may be made temporarily worse, but the action of the drug is so short that the dangers associated with its use are slight. Artificial ventilation, if not already started, must be made available before edrophonium is given. The effects of overdosage may last longer than a week, and controlled ventilation with an artificial ventilator may be necessary during this time. If the condition coincides with a myasthenic crisis, then the patient will show temporary improvement following the administration of edrophonium, but this will not be sustained.

Peripheral Polyneuritis

Peripheral neuritis, such as postinfectious polyneuritis (Guillain–Barré–Stroll syndrome), gives rise to respiratory failure similar to that seen in myasthenia gravis and is probably the more commonly observed. This syndrome and chronic or relapsing polyneuritis may progress so rapidly to respiratory failure that the clinician may be taken unawares unless careful monitoring of the patient is maintained. In the case of relapsing polyneuritis, rapid onset of respiratory failure can occur when the disease has been chronic for some

time. Diphtheria, although rare in the UK, still occurs elsewhere and can also cause respiratory failure.

Other forms of peripheral neuropathy can be induced by diabetes, porphyria, uraemia, neoplasms and various toxins. All can give rise to respiratory failure.

Tracheal intubation, *under an anaesthetic,* has to be performed and the patient must be placed on an automatic ventilator. Once the tube has been inserted, discomfort is not as marked as might be expected, but the process of insertion in the conscious patient can be agonizingly painful if an anaesthetic is not given.

Asthma

It is quite apparent that deaths from asthma are not decreasing in the UK and may be increasing a little in other parts of the world. There has been a complete failure to make any significant reduction in mortality in Britain during the past 20 years (Johnson *et al.*, 1984; Jackson *et al.*, 1982; Wood and Baker, 1984).[74,76,143] When the British Thoracic Association studied deaths from asthma in 1982, they found that in 83 out of 90 patients who died *serial* peak flow measurements had not been made. Also Ormerod and Stableforth (1980)[97] and Wilson *et al.* (1981)[142] demonstrated that the majority of patients who died from asthma had not received corticosteroids during their final attack.

It is apparent that many patients die without the benefit of other forms of treatment, such as simple rehydration, correction of the metabolic acidosis with $NaHCO_3$ infusions, intravenous salbutamol or isoprenaline and artificial ventilation of the lungs.

Pathological changes

At autopsy following death from asthma, the lungs appear to be over distended and fail to deflate when the chest is opened. Grey mucous plugs which are infiltrated with eosinophils and often bacteria are found to have sealed many of the bronchi producing a complete obstruction to airflow as in Fig. 5.1 C. Partial obstruction of the airway Fig. 5.1 D is also present due to marked bronchial muscle hypertrophy and hyperplasia, thickening of the epithelium and mucous exudate in addition to bronchoconstriction. Spontaneous removal of the mucous plugs is not only difficult because of bronchial constriction and the tenacity of the material, but also because of the shedding of the bronchial epithelium causing damage to the lining of the bronchi. This latter effect may of course be reduced by steroid therapy.

Although it is probably an oversimplification, two types of asthma are generally recognized which allow a broad assessment with regard to treatment in the short term and prognosis in the long term.

These are: (a) the allergic form in which exogenous influences cause and affect the condition, which tends to occur early in life; and (b) the non-allergic form which is usually of late onset and is affected by endogenous influences.

The allergic (exogenous or extrinsic) form has the following characteristics.

1. It appears in childhood.
2. Attacks are caused by an external agent frequently referred to as a 'trigger' agent.
3. It has atopic features, such as hay fever, eczema and other skin manifestations.
4. It is frequently precipitated by infections.
5. It is episodic in character.
6. Commonly a family history of asthma is evident.
7. It may improve or disappear with age.
8. Steroids are required less frequently for treatment.

The prognosis of childhood asthma was reviewed in 1977.[17] The observations of Blair[17] were noted which indicated that only approximately 50% of children suffering from childhood asthma were found to be symptom free in adult life. Three of the group died and 21% suffered from chronic asthma. The prognosis appeared to be unaltered by the positivity of the skin tests performed when first seen.

The non-allergic (endogenous or intrinsic) form can be said to be quite different and has characteristics which can differentiate it from the extrinsic form, although, of course, intermediate forms exist.

1. Onset occurs in adult life.
2. No 'trigger' mechanism is required to cause an attack.
3. There are commonly no atopic features or skin manifestations.
4. It is frequently caused or exacerbated by infections.
5. Although sometimes episodic in character, it generally becomes chronic and the prognosis tends to be poor.
6. It most frequently requires treatment with steroids.
7. There is often no family history.

'Trigger' mechanisms

'Trigger' mechanisms can be considered to be due to allergic factors which vary between pollen and the house mite (*Dermatophagoides pteronyssinus*). Following exposure to the antigen, which in most circumstances is impossible to avoid, the patient becomes sensitized. The reaction to preformed circulating antibodies causing bronchoconstriction is now considered to be produced by *mediators* contained within the mast cells which are situated in the walls of the bronchial mucosa. These mediators include histamine and other substances. Inhibition of these mediators is considered to occur when the therapeutic agent disodium cromoglycate (Intal) is used.

Infections of all types appear to act as important 'trigger' mechanism, especially in intrinsic asthma. The early use of broad-spectrum antibiotics, such as the tetracyclines, and semisynthetic penicillins, such as ampicillin, talampicillin and amoxicillin, given early in the attack are therefore commonly beneficial. Sensitization may occur as an industrial hazard such as exposure to epoxy resins used in making plastics and adhesives, a perfect example of sensitization of a patient who would otherwise be free from disease.[19] This aspect has been well reviewed.

There are also non-specific 'trigger' mechanisms, such as exercise, deep breathing, passing from a cold to a warm atmosphere, and the inhalation of irritants such as tobacco smoke.

Bronchodilators

Recent work has shed some light on the method by which some of the bronchodilators in use function. Two cyclic nucleotides play a part in this mechanism. Cyclic AMP (cyclic 3' 5'-adenosine monophosphate) and cyclic GMP (cyclic 3' 5'-guanosine monophosphate) are the nucleotides which play an important part.

Cyclic AMP is produced by the conversion of adenosine triphosphate (ATP) by the enzyme adenylcyclase. Increased concentration of cyclic AMP in the mast cells of the bronchi inhibits the release of chemical mediators. The increased concentration of cyclic AMP in the smooth muscle of the bronchi produces relaxation.

Cyclic GMP is produced by the action of guanylcyclase on ATP and produces the converse effects of cyclic AMP bronchoconstriction.

Beta-adrenergic agonists

The beta-2-adrenoreceptors are situated in the bronchial smooth muscle and in mast cells. Beta-receptor agonists have been developed which have a selective action at these receptor sites, for example terbutaline (Bricanyl) and salbutamol (Ventolin). These substances are less likely to produce changes either in heart rate or rhythm, although other undesirable effects have been noted. Amongst the side-effects that have been observed are hyperglycaemia and muscle tremor.

Stimulation of the beta-receptors initiates an increase in concentration of intracellular ATP, and the activation of adenylcyclase leading to an increase in cyclic AMP and therefore broncho-dilatation. It should be noted that the nonspecific beta agonist isoprenaline is still the most potent and most rapidly acting bronchodilator available, although because of its nonspecificity it causes an increase in heart rate. In serious cases it is best to give isoprenaline by infusion, 5 mg of isoprenaline sulphate (Isuprel) in 1 litre of 5% dextrose, infused at 5–10 drops/minute. Subcutaneous adrenaline 1 ml of 1/1000 solution can be given at a rate of 0.1 ml/min. Orciprenaline may also be of value in mild cases. The concurrent administration of ipratropium bromide and fenoterol produces greater broncho-dilation than either agent used alone.

Methylxanthines

The breakdown of cyclic AMP (which is active) to 5'-AMP, (which is inactive) is achieved by the enzyme phosphodiesterase. The methylxanthines, such as aminophylline and its derivatives, inhibit the action of phosphodiesterase and therefore reduce the rate of degradation of cyclic AMP.

Parasympathetic antagonists

The activity of guanylcyclase is enhanced by cholinergic preparations and thus leads to an in-crease in the concentration of cyclic GMP, which (as described above) has a competitive and antag-onistic effect on cyclic AMP.

Anticholinergic substances are therefore of value in the maintenance of a patent bronchial tree. The substance most studied—atropine—is the most important but, because of its action on other organs, its use is limited. The isopropyl-substituted deriva-tive of atropine, ipratropium bromide (Atrovent), is now being investigated for intravenous use, with advantageous results. It has been used to date only as an inhalant.

Degrees of incapacity

The degree of severity of the asthma attack can be assessed in the following ways, although one may merge into another.

Mild	The patient is able to speak whole sentences, and is not cyanosed when breathing air.
Moderate	The patient speaks haltingly in incomplete sentences. He does not like to move very much as exercise causes breathlessness. He is not cyanosed when breathing O_2.
Severe	The patient is unable to talk. He may be semiconscious or unconscious. He is cyanosed even when breathing O_2, and is obviously dyspnoeic. Adult peak flow is 120 or less than 20% of predicted value, or unobtainable. Pulsus paradoxus may be present.

Management of life-threatening asthma

Oxygen

It is essential, whenever possible, that a blood gas estimation should be made. As the patient is suf-fering from severe O_2 lack, a high tension of O_2 in the inspired gases is essential. However, if the PCO_2 is high, it is possible for further respiratory depression to occur (see p. 127). In a large number of cases, because CO_2 diffuses twenty times faster than O_2, the PCO_2 is either reduced or normal. Even when the PCO_2 is raised, it is not increased to a significant degree. Under these circumstances it is quite safe to give high tensions of O_2, taking into account that it must be adequately humidified.

When oxygenation by mask or through nasal catheters is inadequate, the patient must be venti-lated artificially.

Hydration and acid-base balance

Many patients rapidly become dehydrated, especially following a prolonged period of severe asthma. Adequate hydration with 5% glucose or glucose/saline solutions given intravenously is often necessary. This is because these patients find it difficult to swallow and are unable to take an adequate volume of fluid orally. The degree of dehydration is frequently indicated by the increase in PCV and the plasma [Na^+].

In the very severe asthmatic, it is essential to estimate the blood gas levels for a further reason. In several cases there is a rise in the serum lactate which results in a marked degree of metabolic acidosis. It is well recognized that in these patients bronchodilator agents are frequently ineffective, and the rapid i.v. injection of aminophylline may give rise to serious cardiac arrhythmias.

If an i.v. infusion is given, correction of the acid–base balance with sodium bicarbonate (e.g. 100 mmol i.v.) sometimes produces marked relief.

Aminophylline

In the severe asthmatic attack this should be given intravenously as a bolus of 500 mg over a period of 5–6 minutes. This may produce a tachycardia and a feeling of light headedness. The rate of intravenous administration should be reduced in cases of severe anoxia and in patients who have liver disease. It can also be given as an intravenous infusion at approximately 1 mg/minute.

The rate of metabolism of theophylline varies greatly from one patient to another. Also the effective blood concentration of theophylline required to produce a therapeutic effect, is a variable entity. There are, therefore, numerous recommendations made by various authors in order to avoid the adverse reactions produced by overdosage. In the presence of a metabolic acidosis, slower rates of intravenous injection are advisable if cardiac arrhythmias are to be avoided.

The measurement of blood theophylline levels is of little value, the result being obtained long after the event. Jusko *et al.*,[78] having studied 72 patients, therefore produced a nomogram based on body weight. The nomogram indicated the quantity of aminophylline required both for immediate treatment (or 'loading dose') and for maintenance therapy. They also subdivided the nomogram so that it would be applicable to the young, vigorous patient who metabolizes theophylline rapidly, the older patient who would metabolize it more slowly, and those with liver disease in whom the rate of metabolism is very slow.

Salbutamol

This preparation is available in tablet form and as a syrup for children, and also for injections. In status asthmaticus it may be given as an intravenous dose of 0.5 mg over a period of 5–10 minutes and as a continuous infusion of 10 μg/minute.[77,133]

Many clinicians would agree with Collins *et al.*[34] that corticosteroid treatment in asthma sometimes requires several hours before an effective change in airway resistance is produced. Nevertheless, sensitivity to salbutamol can be restored by means of intravenous hydrocortisone.[69]

Williams *et al.*[141] examined 20 patients in hospital with severe asthma who had a pulse rate greater than 120/minute and a peak flow rate (PFR) of less than 25% of that which should have been predicted for their body size and weight. Their arterial O_2 tension (PaO_2) was less than 69.8 mmHg. While all the patients were given hydrocortisone intravenously and O_2 by a 28% O_2 Ventimask, either aminophylline 0.5 g or salbutamol 500 μg was given intravenously. Both medications were administered over 1 hour by means of a constant-rate infusion pump. Response to treatment was assessed by changes in performance using a Wright peak flowmeter. They found that salbutamol was at least as effective as aminophylline in the doses used and by this method but had fewer side-effects.

There are different views with regard to the mode of treatment with salbutamol. May *et al.*[93] concluded that salbutamol infused at 4 μg/minute provided adequate bronchodilatation with no cardiovascular effects. Fitchett *et al.*[53] gave a bolus injection over a period of 1 minute. Salbutamol provides an important mode of treatment in those patients who are severely ill with asthma and it appears to be especially effective in patients in whom aminophylline fails to act when injected intravenously. Early treatment at home with salbutamol by means of nebulization may help to reduce mortality (Wood and Baker, 1984),[143] and can be given prior to, and while the patient is being transferred to hospital.

Corticosteroids

Very large doses of corticosteroids are given to patients suffering from other severe conditions, for example toxic and cardiogenic shock. Severe asthma can be of the same order of danger as these conditions; death occurs from the gross anoxia that develops. Cardiac arrhythmias are also more common because of the metabolic changes produced by anoxia and, of course, due to the anoxia itself.

Experience with organ transplants has demonstrated that very large doses of steroids can be given without any great danger if the period of administration is limited to 3–4 days. Beyond this, the dangers from infection increase greatly.

An intravenous loading dose of 1 g of hydrocortisone diluted in saline or glucose saline to avoid damaging the vein is effective. Further doses of methylprednisolone, 250 mg i.v. 6-hourly, appear to be highly effective. This dose can be rapidly reduced and treatment with corticosteroids stopped, if necessary completely, after a period of 5 days without problems because of withdrawal. It is common, however, following an attack of status asthmaticus, to maintain the patient on low doses of corticosteroids following a severe attack. The dose chosen is the lowest that is compatible with keeping the patient free from an attack. Alternate-day therapy is one of the methods by which the problem associated with steroid treatment can be reduced or avoided.

Calcium antagonists
Calcium antagonists may be of value in exercise-induced asthma.[100] Patel used verapamil and nifedipine, substances which retard or block the entry of Ca^{++} into the cell. The possible value of calcium blocking agents in asthma has been clearly reviewed (McFadden, 1981).[89]

Legionnaire's Disease

Another form of fatal respiratory failure caused by bacterial infection is that which has now become known as Legionnaire's disease. It derives its name from the fact that an epidemic of acute fatal respiratory failure developed when, in the late summer of 1976, a meeting of the American Legion consisting of some 4500 people gathered in a hotel in Philadelphia.

It was first considered to be a new disease entity which affected 182 members of the Pennsylvania American Legion, although retrospective investigations into antibodies have revealed that epidemics have occurred before the Philadelphia outbreak. Since the identification of the organism, numerous centres have reported sudden outbreaks of the disease, including the author's hospital. One patient was aged 22 years and died. Of the 123 patients admitted to hospital, 26 died and 111 had radiographically proven pneumonia. It was found that the severity of the condition could vary between a generalized fulminant disease affecting many different organs and a mild influenza type of infection. When severe, there was extensive pneumonia, diarrhoea, hepatic dysfunction, shock and renal failure.[132]

There are a number of characteristics of the disease.

Respiratory failure
The patients commonly presented with pain in the chest and dyspnoea. Examination of the blood gases revealed hypoxia of the arterial blood, the PO_2 sometimes being less than 50 mmHg, even when O_2 was being supplied by mask or nasal catheters. Compensatory hyperventilation causing a fall in the PCO_2 was found so that values of 29 mmHg with an alkalaemia giving a pH of 7.50 was also found. This was in the early stages, but progression into more severe respiratory failure and death occurred in a number of people.

X-ray changes initially demonstrated infiltration of the lungs, either unilaterally or bilaterally. An air bronchogram was sometimes present and the changes progressed to consolidation of both lungs. Nineteen patients required artificial ventilation of the lungs.

Renal failure
Some degree of renal failure and insufficiency appears to have occurred in 18 of the 123 patients admitted to hospital. Although toxic shock occurred, as is commonly recognized following respiratory failure, renal failure was evident before this developed in some patients. The majority of patients who died suffered from renal failure, and urinalysis demonstrated casts, both granular and erythrocyte, even when renal function was not impaired. Leucocytes were also found in significant numbers.

Serum sodium
The serum sodium concentration of 130 mmol/l (mEq/l) or less was found in 38 patients: 19 of these had no evidence of renal insufficiency and in all patients hyponatraemia was observed within 6 days of admission to hospital. Even in the absence of overt renal failure, hyponatraemia would appear to be due to retention of H_2O.

Central nervous system
Severe headache and serious mental disturbances, including confusion and dilirium with periods of unconsciousness, have been observed in Legionnaire's disease. No serious changes in the cerebrospinal fluid have been identified. No consistent diagnostic changes are therefore available.

Presenting symptoms and signs
The illness frequently begins as if it were an attack of influenza with the onset of malaise, pyrexia, rigors and muscle pain. The early changes of respiratory tract involvement were similar to those seen in a simple coryza. Pleuritic chest pain occurred in only 11 of the patients in the Philadelphia epidemic. The changes in the cerebrum were seen sometimes at a relatively early stage, with slurring of speech, mental confusion and ataxia. Abdominal pain was present in some, but neither diarrhoea nor vomiting was conspicuously present. Respiratory distress was indicated by a tachypnoea and an increased temperature and pulse rate. The temperature, however, rarely rose above 40.0°C (104°F). The pulse rate rose most markedly in those with the more serious degree of illness, and was highest in those who died.

Epidemiology
In 1979, Eickhoff[45] identified at least 10 epidemics

of Legionnaire's disease, some associated with no mortality whatsoever and running a benign course. The identity of the disease has been well established from serum stored for more than a decade at the Center for Disease Control in the USA. It is noticeable that, as in the case of the first recorded epidemic, investigated at St Elizabeth's Hospital in Washington DC, USA in 1965, extensive soil excavations had taken place in the area. This would appear to be a frequent finding in many of the epidemics, although the cause is not known. In addition to the epidemics, a number of sporadic cases have been identified. These have run a varying course of mortality and morbidity. Air-conditioning cooling systems have been identified as a source.

Causative organism

The Legionnaire's disease bacterium has now been isolated with certainty, and serological tests for its identification are now well established.[73] It appears to be a short pleomorphic rod and is now called *Legionella pneumophila*, which, *in vivo*, is best treated with either erythromycin (Erycen, Erythrocin, Pediamycin) or antibiotics of the tetracycline group, for example oxytetracycline (Terramycin, Berkmycen, Clinimycin). Since the isolation of *Legionella pneumophila*, a number of additional species that are phenotypically similar have been isolated, for example *Legionella pittsburgensis* and, more recently, *Legionella longbeachae*.[90]

Treatment

The general treatment for severe respiratory failure accompanied by hypotension, fluid and water balance changes, hyponatraemia and the possibility of acute renal failure is well described elsewhere (Chapter 2). Hypotension due to endotoxic shock and impairment of cardiac output due to positive pressure ventilation has to be carefully monitored, as it is well recognized as a complication of positive pressure ventilation following intubation of the trachea. Antibiotic therapy would appear from the published reports to be best conducted by intravenous medication as described above. The treatment of choice appears to be erythromycin.

RESPIRATORY DISTRESS SYNDROME IN THE NEWBORN

Impairment of gas exchange in lungs of the newborn can be caused by hyaline membrane disease,

atelectasis, infection, intrapulmonary haemorrhage and occasionally by the aspiration of a large volume of amniotic fluid. The affected infant may breathe normally at first and show the signs of respiratory distress 2 or more hours after birth.

The incidence of respiratory distress syndrome has fallen with the introduction of medication of the mother with steroids 1 or 2 days before the birth of the infant, when prematurity is suspected. The probability of the condition may be indicated by the amniotic lecithin/sphingomyelin ratio.[62]

Hyaline membrane disease

The respiratory rate is rapid. At each inspiration there is retraction of the sternum and rib cage. The degree of retraction reflects the severity of the disease and the intrapleural pressure. There may be tracheal tug and a grunting type of respiration. Periods of apnoea may occur which can be terminated by physical stimulation, such as bending the lower limbs so that the knees move towards the chest. Noise may also be effective in stimulating respiration. While periods of apnoea are usually a bad prognostic sign, they are not necessarily indicative of a fatal outcome. The condition is often associated with persistant hypothermia. X-ray of chest shows a reticulogranular infiltration of the lung fields which may be associated with cardiomegaly.

The mortality from fully developed hyaline membrane disease is very high, probably in excess of 50%. The membrane has been shown to contain fibrin,[58] and this, together with possible changes in the alveolar membrane, produces the condition of alveolar capillary block. Adequate arterial oxygen saturation can only be maintained by placing the infant in a greatly oxygen-enriched atmosphere. There is, however, so gross an impairment of gas diffusion that carbon dioxide is retained. Usher (1960)[134] demonstrated that there is a continuously progressing increase in the metabolic acidosis from the time of birth, and this is confirmed by the author's own observations. It is apparent, therefore, that the infant is born not only with an uncompensated respiratory acidosis, but also with an impaired ability to compensate by producing and retaining bicarbonate. Table 5.8 shows the results from two samples of blood taken, 24 hours apart, from the umbilical cord of a 5 lb 1 oz baby.

In the intervening period between samples A and B, 35 ml of 2.74% sodium bicarbonate solution had been infused through a catheter, that had been passed via the cord vein, and this had been followed with a slow drip of 10% glucose solution

Table 5.8 Blood pH, 'standard bicarbonate' and PCO_2 of blood taken from the umbilical cord of a baby suffering from respiratory distress syndrome

	pH	St. bic. (mmol/l)	PCO_2 (mmHg)
A	7.10	19.0	135
B	7.24	25.6	86

pH = blood pH; St. bic. = standard bicarbonate; PCO_2 = partial pressure of CO_2.
Sample B was taken 24 hours after sample A.

in the volumes recommended by Usher (65 ml/kg). Gradual improvement continued so that a complete recovery was made.

Some cases are less fortunate in that a pneumothorax may develop, there may be shunting of blood through the lungs so that cyanosis still persists in spite of an atmosphere of 100% oxygen. The condition may be associated with congenital cardiac abnormalities which add to the problem of management, and digitalization may be necessary because of cardiac failure. A raised plasma [K$^+$] is not an uncommon finding. A raised plasma [Na$^+$], together with a low blood glucose level, is found in association with pathological changes of the central nervous system.

The regimen recommended by Usher,[134] of infusing sodium bicarbonate glucose solutions at the rate of 65 ml/kg, would appear to lower the mortality in this condition. It is possible, however, that some benefit may be gained by raising the osmolality of the solutions.

The following case illustrates the effectiveness of treatment in this condition and, because of excessive hydration at birth, the danger of producing oedema thus making fluid restriction necessary. The volume of urine passed by a premature infant is in the region of 30 ml in 24 hours. This urine may contain 1–2 mmol (mEq) of potassium, and replacement of this cation may become necessary; it should be given orally as KCl. If an alkalosis is to be avoided, the chloride ion is most essential when sodium bicarbonate is infused. It must be remembered that 3 mmol (mEq) of KCl will raise the plasma [K$^+$] by approximately 1.5 mmol/l (mEq/l) in these very small infants. Caution must therefore be exercised in the administration of this cation.

Case history. A premature infant weighing 5 lb 1 oz developed the signs of hyaline membrane disease very soon after birth. Cord blood obtained 4 hours after birth had a pH of 7.19

(Table 5.9A). The infant was placed in an incubator with an atmosphere of 85% O_2. 20 ml of $NaHCO_3$ (2.74%) were infused through the cord over a period of 3–4 hours with improvement of respiration. The pH and standard bicarbonate of the blood, taken 8 hours after birth, had improved and the PCO_2, although still raised, was not dangerously high for this condition (Table 5.9B). 100 ml of glucose 5% were infused during the night.

The following morning, 24 hours after birth, the blood pH and standard bicarbonate had again fallen and oedema of the limbs was apparent. The plasma sodium concentration was 138 mmol/l (mEq/l), and the plasma potassium concentration was 8.3 mmol/l (mEq/l) (Table 5.9C).

Table 5.9 The blood pH, 'standard bicarbonate' and PCO_2 of umbilical cord blood taken over a period of 48 hours from a premature baby with respiratory distress syndrome

	pH	St. bic. (mmol/l)	PCO_2 (mmHg)
A	7.19		
B	7.39	18.8	62
C	7.10	15.1	66
D	7.37	18.5	28

pH = blood pH; St. bic. = standard bicarbonate; PCO_2 = partial pressure of CO_2.

During the next 24 hours, 36 ml of fluid were infused containing 20 ml of 2.74% $NaHCO_3$ and 16 ml of laevulose (fructose) 15%. By the afternoon of the same day, respiration had improved greatly and cyanosis was not present when concentrations of O_2 in the incubator were lowered. The following day the infant had much improved, a good urine output had been maintained and the oedema had regressed. The cord blood revealed a moderate metabolic acidosis and a respiratory alkalosis. It was apparent that the infant had to hyperventilate to maintain adequate oxygenation (Table 5.9D). A few millilitres of glucose water were given orally during that evening, and the following day normal oral feeding was begun.

Not all cases respond as well as the one described above, and an increasingly high PCO_2 may develop even with adequate treatment. A metabolic acidosis that persists after attempted correction with sodium bicarbonate is a bad prognostic sign.

The introduction of artificial ventilation of the lungs using PEEP (see p. 132) has made the management of the respiratory factor in respiratory distress syndrome very much easier.

It has been noted that a marked right-to-left shunt in idiopathic respiratory distress syndrome is an important factor in the severe hypoxia and the metabolic acidosis.[128] There is, therefore, a reduced pulmonary perfusion and a high pulmonary vascular resistance.[30] In view of this, Abbot et al.[1] infused sodium nitroprusside, which resulted in an improved and sustained increase in the arterial oxygen tension and a rise in pH as the PCO_2 fell. It should be noted that sodium bicarbonate was also given. Positive airway pressure was instituted initially, followed by intermittent positive pressure respiration (IPPR) using 100% O_2 via an endotracheal tube with a PEEP of 6 cmH$_2$O. When the acidosis did not respond to alkali and the arterial PO_2 remained low, sodium nitroprusside was infused via the umbilical artery at 2 mg/kg per minute, as previously described by Bennett and Abbott (1977).[14] This may represent an advance in treatment.

TRACHEOTOMY

Positioning the patient

This is important if the operation is to be performed with ease. The patient should lie in the supine position with the head extended. This is achieved by placing a sandbag or other pad under the shoulders and lowest part of the neck, and care should be taken that the head does not deviate from the midline and that the neck is not hyperextended.

The skin incision

A transverse (collar) incision 5 cm in length is made midway between the cricoid cartilage, palpable just above the first ring of the trachea, and the suprasternal notch. The incision is continued down through subcutaneous tissue until the investing layer of the deep cervical fascia is reached. A self-retaining retractor is then inserted into the wound so that a diamond-shaped opening in the skin and superficial fascia is obtained.

The investing layer of deep cervical fascia is then incised vertically between the two sternothyroid muscles, which are in turn separated and held apart laterally. Care must be taken not to damage the internal jugular veins which are in close proximity.

The exact position of the trachea can now be defined by palpating with the index finger through the pretracheal fascia above the isthmus of the thyroid gland. Normally, the trachea lies along the midline, but may be deviated by mediastinal shift or diseased gland masses. If there is any difficulty in locating the exact position of the trachea relative to the midline, then the pretracheal fascia should be opened and dissected upwards until the cricoid cartilage is revealed. The anatomy of the area will then become clear. The pretracheal fascia is always opened because when this is done the thyroid isthmus can be lifted away from the trachea by blunt dissection and it may then be divided between clamps which are inserted from above.

A window in the trachea is then made. The first ring of the trachea must be left undamaged if perichondritis of the cricoid cartilage is to be avoided. If the trachea is opened below the fourth ring, difficulty may be encountered because at this point the trachea lies deeply and is in close proximity to the great vessels. In addition, mediastinal emphysema is more likely to occur and displacement of the tracheostomy tube is more common.

We are therefore, left with rings 2, 3 and 4 as the most satisfactory area in which to make the window. In practice, it is only necessary to resect parts of one or two of these rings. The window should be round and is made with a number 15 Bard Parker blade. Before the incision is completed, the fragment of anterior tracheal wall to be removed should be grasped with forceps to avoid it being lost into the trachea and sucked down the bronchial tree. Care must be taken to avoid making the window too small, and the size of the tube to be inserted must be kept in mind. There is an ever-present danger that, in the process of making the window, the posterior wall of the trachea can be damaged, and this is more likely in the non-anaesthetized, restless patient. Such damage may lead to a tracheo-oesophageal fistula.

An alternative method of opening the anterior wall of the trachea is to make a cruciate incision without removing any tissue. The tracheostomy tube is forced through the opening. A vertical incision is made in the midline, approximately 1 cm in length, and a transverse incision, again approximately 1 cm long, is made between the two tracheal rings that bisect the vertical incision. Inserting the cuffed tracheostomy tube is slightly more difficult and requires a little more force, but this incision is said to be less frequently associated with constriction of the trachea after the tracheostomy tube has been removed and healing has taken place.

As soon as the window has been made, the lumen of the trachea is thoroughly aspirated and, if an endotracheal tube has already been inserted for the purposes of anaesthesia or ventilation, a suction catheter should be passed through it and suction maintained as it is withdrawn in order to allow entry of the tracheostomy tube. If the purpose of the tracheotomy is for aspiration alone, a silver metal tube is inserted, but when it is made for the purposes of positive pressure ventilation, or for the protection of the lungs from the pharyngeal secretions, then a cuffed rubber tube must be inserted. Although the rubber tubes may cause severe reactions to occur to the mucosal lining of the trachea and may become coated with crusts and inspissated secretions, they can in practice be retained for many months when they are looked after carefully.

When the bleeding points have been ligated, the wound is closed loosely. Usually, it is sufficient to place one stitch at either end of the incision and to place a piece of gauze, which has a slit in it, around the tracheostomy tube. This loose and simple closure avoids the production of surgical emphysema and facilitates the rapid withdrawal, changing and re-insertion of the tube if it becomes necessary. Most metal and some rubber tracheostomy tubes have flanges to which tapes can be tied and then joined round the neck. When these are applied, the tapes should be tied with a fair degree of tightness. Loosely tied tapes, apart from being of no value, are dangerous because they allow displacement of the tube so that obstruction can occur, but leave insufficient room for the patient to remove the tube entirely.

When a tracheostomy has been performed it is apparent that the normal humidification of the inspired air or gases which occurs through the nasal and oral tracts is absent. If unattended, this will lead to crusting and erosion of the tracheal mucosa. It is an important part of tracheal toilet that the mucous membranes should be kept moist with isotonic $NaHCO_3$ or isotonic $NaCl$; 1 ml may be inserted into the tracheal opening every half-hour, except in conditions such as pulmonary oedema when excessive volumes of wet secretion are being applied to the endotracheal lining. Humidification of the inspired air must be arranged. It is to be noted that when the inhaled gases are contained in cylinders they are completely dry and do not contain even the quantity of water which is present in the atmospheric air.

When the tracheostomy tube is finally removed the wound is covered with sterile gauze and then with waterproof sticking plaster so that the patient may talk without difficulty and the area is allowed to granulate and close spontaneously.

Dangers and disadvantages associated with tracheostomy

Bleeding
Loss of blood can occur as a result of the initial surgery so that blood loss, if unchecked, can be severe. It care is not taken, some blood may be lost into the bronchi and this is inhaled giving rise to alveolar–capillary block and sometimes to consolidation of the lung. Trauma of the lining of the trachea may be caused by the insertion of the endotracheal tube, especially when the tube is made of metal. When a cuffed rubber tube is kept *in situ* for a long period of time with the cuff inflated, ulceration of the mucosa commonly takes place. This frequently gives rise to haemorrhage and is most commonly seen in patients who have an increased bronchial circulation, such as those suffering from tetralogy of Fallot. Ulceration of the trachea can develop so that it extends through the whole wall, and even into the innominate artery causing a fatal haemorrhage. Bleeding may also be produced from trauma that is caused by catheters that are used for sucking away endobronchial secretions.

Obstruction of the airway
The endotracheal and endobronchial secretions are dried and give rise to crusting when the air breathed is of low humidity. Slowly, occlusion of the airway takes place and complete obstruction can occur within a few hours, especially in children. Then only expert bronchoscopy will give relief. If the gases entering the trachea are both warmed and humidified, this danger is completely avoided. Crusting of secretions may occur within the lumen of the tracheostomy tube, but this is easily remedied when the tracheostomy tube is large by changing the tube.

A not uncommon form of obstruction is caused by overinflation of the cuff around the tracheostomy tube. The cuff herniates over the end of the tube obstructing its lumen.

Infection
Although relatively rare, infection may occur at the tracheostomy site. A relatively more important danger is caused by the conditions that prevail when a tracheostomy replaces a normal airway. Filtering of the inspired air so that dust particles and bacteria are removed is no longer possible so that the lungs are left vulnerable to pathogenic

organisms. Because glottic control is lost, the effectiveness of coughing is reduced. In addition, the cilia function less well when they are cold, dry or overwhelmed with local infective processes resulting from organisms which may be airborne or introduced on a suction catheter. Active physiotherapy with assisted coughing helped by intermittent positive pressure inflation, or the temporary application of a Cuirass respirator so that the volume of air entering the lungs is increased prior to the cough, assists in reducing the incidence of local or generalized lung disease.

Misplaced tracheostomy tube

A rubber tracheostomy tube that is too long may cause complications in two ways. In the first place, it may curl so that it rubs the trachea posteriorly at the point of greatest convexity. Also at its lower end, which may be sharp, it may rub against the anterior wall of the trachea. A tracheostomy tube of excessive length passed through a tracheostomy made too low in the trachea can enter one of the main bronchi, usually the right. In this way one lung only is ventilated. Displacement of the tracheostomy tube in this way is most likely to occur when the neck is hyperextended during surgery.

Dilatation of the trachea

If a cuff is excessively inflated and does not herniate over the end of the tracheostomy tube, it causes pressure to be exerted so that the trachea dilates. This is most likely to happen when there is a 'kink' or obstruction in the side tube leading to the inflatable cuff. A ball valve system is then produced so that air will pass into the cuff under pressure from a syringe, but does not leak away when the clip or spiggot is removed. In this way deflation of the cuff does not occur and this may well pass unnoticed by the nursing staff and medical attendants. When the time comes to reinflate the cuff, more air is pushed into the already overfilled space and, if this is done repeatedly, the trachea may be so stretched that eventually a tight fit with existing tubes is difficult to obtain. It is important, therefore, that all attendants are informed of this danger and care should be taken to make sure that the cuff deflates whenever the clips are removed from the side tube. When the cuff is deflated the tracheostomy tube lies more loosely within the lumen of the trachea.

Atelectasis

The inadequate removal of pus and secretions will in itself lead to the blocking of a bronchiole and,

therefore, atelectasis of part of the lung. It can, however, be induced when a suction catheter is inserted so far that it occludes the bronchiole. In this way the whole of the suction force is transmitted along the tube, collapsing that segment of lung. Although it is essential in some cases to pass the catheter as far as possible, this danger must be borne in mind. The danger is reduced by using catheters which have small side holes at their tips. Atelectasis may also be produced in the non-inflated lung when the tracheostomy tube is misplaced down one main bronchus.

Inadequate physiotherapy and nursing

A freshly made tracheostomy requires constant attention, especially in patients who have had this particular operation so that fluid, pus and secretions can be removed. It may be necessary to insert a suction catheter every 10–15 minutes during the initial period. Therefore, in addition to constant humidification or adjustments that have to be made to a ventilator, the full benefit of a tracheostomy will only be achieved if there is constant physiotherapy and nursing care. It is not uncommon for this to be performed in an excellent manner during the day, but to become almost nonexistent during the night; in no circumstances should this be allowed. Ideally, this sort of patient should be looked after in a special unit.

Loss of glottic control

In addition to the fact that loss of glottic control makes coughing less effective unless associated with suction and active physiotherapy, gas exchange in the lungs may be decreased. This is most likely to occur in the emphysematous patient who has a very large respiratory dead space. We have seen in the chapter dealing with gas exchange in the lungs that in normal man diffusion across the alveoli increases with exercise, and this is considered to be partly because when the lungs are fully expanded, the walls of the alveolar capillaries are thinned, thus creating a smaller barrier to gas diffusion. Some patients with respiratory disease use their glottis to produce a state of affairs similar to that used by patients suffering from residual poliomyelitis when they perform 'frog breathing'. By temporarily restricting deflation of the lungs and by increasing the intrathoracic pressure by raising the diaphragm, these patients are able to compress emphysematous bullae while at the same time expanding some alveoli still further. In this way they are able to increase the diffusion of gas. When glottic control is lost this is no longer possible and a fall in the oxygen saturation of the blood follows.

Care of patient following tracheostomy

Humidification
The oldest and simplest method of humidifying the atmosphere is by means of a steam kettle, but more elegant methods are now available. Air or oxygen can be bubbled through water kept at 45°–50°C. Machines which blow air over water that is warmed by means of a small immersion heater are also avaiable. Porous wicks increase the surface area of water exposed so that maximum humidification is achieved. In a patient who is not being ventilated artificially, the simplest method of humidification is to place a piece of wet gauze over the mouth of the tube. However, the gauze dries very rapidly and requires continuous attention if constant humidification of the inspired air is to be achieved. It is on this principle that the 'Swedish nose', consisting of layers of stainless steel wire, has been developed. A very slow drip of isotonic saline or isotonic sodium bicarbonate, 2–4 drops/minute, is an effective way of keeping the trachea moist. It also tends to make the patient cough and, in some circumstances, this may be beneficial.

Liquefaction and removal of secretions
Detergent preparations, such as Alivaire which decreases the surface tension of mucus and other secretions, can be injected into the trachea at intervals of an hour. A few drops are inserted each time and then removed by suction a short time later. A mixture of isoprenaline and chymotrypsin (Lomudase) is now available and dispensed in the form of a nebulizer so that a fine powder may be blown through the tracheostomy opening. This assists in the dilatation of the bronchioles and in the liquefaction of secretions. A suction catheter must be pased 6–7 inches (2.4–2.8 cm) before adequate clearance of the air passages is effected, and it is necessary to train nursing staff in this respect.

Patients who have tracheostomies must have antibiotics, especially in the early stages, even when infection is not already present.

Feeding
A patient with a tracheostomy tube in place has some difficulty in swallowing. If positive pressure ventilation is being applied through a tracheostomy tube the cuff of which is inflated, it is sometimes very difficult for patients to swallow even finely chopped solid food. In these circumstances it is necessary to feed them with pulverized food.

Body water and electrolytes
Respiratory disease accompanied by anoxia frequently causes a severe upset in water balance and body biochemistry. Careful note should, therefore, be made of this aspect of management, especially when oral replacement and normal feeding cannot be maintained.

References

1. Abbott, T. R., Rees, G. J., Dickinson, D., Reynolds, G. and Lord, D. (1978). Sodium nitroprusside in idiopathic respiratory distress syndrome. *Brit. med. J.*, **1**, 1113.

2. Adams, H. R., Mathew, B. P., Teske, R. H. and Mercer, H. D. (1976). Neuromuscular blocking effects of aminoglycoside antibiotics on fast- and slow-contracting muscles of the cat. *Anesth. Analg. (Cleve.)*, **55**, 500.

3. Aharanov, A., Abramsky, O., Tarrab-Hazdai, R. and Fuchs, S. (1975). Humoral antibodies to acetylcholine receptor in patients with myasthenia gravis. *Lancet*, **ii**, 340.

4. Anderson, H. R., Macnair, R. S. and Ramsey, J. D. (1985). Epidemiology: Deaths from abuse of volatile substances: a national epidemiological study. *Brit. med. J.*, **290**, 304.

5. Anonymous (1985). Almitrine in chronic airflow obstruction. *Lancet*, **i**, 796.

6. Appleberg, M., Gordon, L. and Fatti, L. P. (1974). Preoperative pulmonary evaluation of surgical patients using the vitalograph. *Brit. J. Surg.*, **61**, 57.

7. Arias-Stella, J. and Kruger, H. (1963). Pathology of high altitude pulmonary edema. *Arch. Path.*, **76**, 147.

8. Ashbaugh, D. G., Bigelow, D. B., Petty, T. L. and Levine, B. E. (1967). Acute respiratory distress in adults. *Lancet*, **ii**, 319.

9. Astrup, P., Jørgensen, K., Andersen, O. S. and Engel, K. (1960). The acid-base metabolism: a new approach. *Lancet*, **i**, 1035.

10. Avery, M. E. and Mead, J. (1959). Surface properties in relation to atelectasis and hyaline membrane disease. *Amer. J. Dis., Child.*, **97**, 517.

11. Bagshawe, K. D. and Brooks, W. L. W. (1959).

Subacute pulmonary hypertension due to chorion-epithelioma. *Lancet*, **i**, 653.

12. Behan, P. O., Shakir, R. A., Simpson, J. A., Burnett, A. K., Allan, T. L. and Haase, G. (1979). Plasma-exchange combined with immunosuppressive therapy in myasthenia gravis. *Lancet*, **ii**, 438.

13. Bender, A. N., Ringel, S. P., Engel, W. K., Daniels, M. P. and Vogel, Z. (1975). Myasthenia gravis: a serum factor blocking acetylcholine receptors of the human neuromuscular junction. *Lancet*, **i**, 607.

14. Bennett, N. J. and Abbott, T. R. (1977). The use of sodium nitroprusside in children. *Anaesthesia*, **32**, 456.

15. Berry, E. M., Edmonds, J. F. and Wyllie, J. H. (1971). Release of prostaglandin E_2 and unidentified factors from ventilated lungs. *Brit. J. Surg.*, **58**, 189.

16. Bingle, J. P., Rutherford, J. D. and Woodrow, P. (1979). Continuous subcutaneous neostigmine in the management of severe myasthenia gravis. *Brit. Med. J.*, **1**, 1050.

17. Blair, H. (1977). Natural history of childhood asthma. *Arch. Diseases in childhood.*, **52**, 613

18. Bourne, J. G., Collier, H. O. J. and Somers, G. F. (1952). Succinylcholine (succinoylcholine); muscle-relaxant of short action. *Lancet*, **i**, 1225.

19. British Medical Journal (1977). Leading article: Asthma induced by epoxy resin systems. *Brit. Med. J.*, **II**, 655.

20. British Thoracic Association. (1982). Death from asthma in the regions of England. *Brit. med. J.*, **285**, 1251.

21. Brooks, D. K. (1972). Organ failure following surgery. *Advances in Surgery*, **6**, 289.

22. Brooks, D. K. (1978). Stomach as a reservoir for respiratory pathogens. *Lancet*, **ii**, 1147.

23. Brooks, D. K. (1978). Gastrointestinal bleeding in acute respiratory failure. *Brit. med. J.*, **1**, 922.

24. Brooks, D. K. and Feldman, S. A. (1962). Metabolic acidosis; a new approach to 'neostigmine resistant curarisation'. *Anaesthesia*, **17**, 161.

25. Brooks, D. K. and Ghilchik, M. (1974). Unpublished observations.

26. Cain, H. D., Stevens, P. M. and Adaniya, R. (1979). Preoperative pulmonary function and complications after cardiovascular surgery. *Chest*, **76**, 2.

27. Callaway, S., Davies, D. R. and Rutland, J. P. (1951). Blood cholinesterase levels and range of personal variation in a healthy adult population. *Brit. med. J.*, **2**, 812.

28. Campbell, E. J. M. and Howell, J. B. L. (1959). The determination of mixed venous and arterial CO_2 tension by rebreathing techniques. In *A symposium on pH and blood gas measurement: methods and interpretation*, p. 101 Edited by R. F. Woolmer and J. Parkinson. London: Churchill.

29. Charlier, A. A. (1968). Beat to beat haemodynamic effects of lung inflation and normal respiration in anaesthetised and conscious dogs. *Presses Academiques Europeennes, Brussels.*

30. Chu, J., Clements, J. A., Cotton, E. K., Klaus, M. H., Sweet, A. Y., Tooley, W. H., with the assistance of Bradley, B. L. and Brandorff, L. C. (1967). Neonatal pulmonary ischaemia Part 1: clinical and physiological studies. *Pediatrics*, **40**, 709.

31. Churchill-Davidson, H. C. and Richardson, A. T. (1953). Neuromuscular transmission in myasthenia gravis. *J. Physiol, Lond.*, **122**, 252.

32. Cohen, I. M., Warren, S. E. and Skowsky, W. R. (1984). Occult pulmonary malignancy in syndrome of inappropriate ADH secretion with normal ADH levels. *Chest*, **86**, 929.

33. Collier, C. R. (1956). Determination of mixed venous CO_2 tensions by rebreathing. *J. appl. Physiol.*, **9**, 25.

34. Collins, J. V., Clarke, T. H. H., Brown, D. and Townsend, J. (1975). The use of corticosteroids in the treatment of acute asthma. *Quart. J. Med.*, **44**, 259.

35. Comroe, J. H., Forster, R. E., Dubois, A. B., Briscoe, W. A. and Carlsen, E. (1962). *The Lung*, 2nd ed. Chicago: Yearbook Medical Publishers.

36. Corrado, A. P., Ramos, A. O. and De Escobar, C. T. (1959). Neuromuscular blockade by neomycin, potentiation by ether anesthesia and tubocurarine and antagonism by calcium and prostigmine. *Arch. Int. Pharmacodyn. Ther.*, **121**, 380.

37. Cournand, A., Motley, H. L., Werko, L. and Richards, D. W. (1948). Physiological studies of the effects of intermittent positive pressure breathing on cardiac output in man. *Amer. J. Physiol.*, **152**, 162.

38. Cronk, S. L., Barkley, D. E. H. and Farrell, M. F. (1985). Respiratory arrest after solvent abuse. *Brit. Med. J.*, **290**, 897.

39. Davis, J. N., Wilson, S. G., Vincent, A. and Ward, C. D. (1979). Long-term effects of repeated plasma exchange in myasthenia gravis. *Lancet*, **i**, 464.

40. Diament, M. L. and Palmer, K. N. V. (1967). Spirometry for preoperative assessment of airways resistance. *Lancet*, **i**, 1251.

41. Doremus, W. P. (1959). Respiratory arrest following intraperitoneal use of neomycin. *Ann. Surg.*, **149**, 546.

42. Drew, C. E. and Anderson, I. M. (1959). Profound hypothermia in cardiac surgery: report of three cases. *Lancet*, **i**, 748.

43. Drew, C. E., Keen, G. and Benazon, D. B. (1959). Profound hypothermia. *Lancet*, **i**, 745.

44. Edwards, F. R. and Wilson, A. (1972). Thymectomy for myasthenia gravis. *Thorax*, **27**, 513.

45. Eickhoff, T. C. (1979). Epidemiology of Legionnaires' Disease. *Ann. Int. Med.*, **90**, 499.

46. Elmqvist, D., Hofmann, W. W., Kugelberg, J. and Quastel, D. M. J. (1964). An electrophysiological investigation of neuromuscular transmission in myasthenia gravis. *J. Physiol.*, **174**, 417.

47. Elmqvist, D. and Josefsson, J. O. (1962). The nature of the neuromuscular block produced by neomycin.

Acta. Physiol. Scand., **54**, 105.

48. Engel, A. G., Lindstrom, J. M., Lambert, E. H. and Lennon, V. A. (1977). Ultrastructural localisation of the acetylcholine receptor in myasthenia gravis and in its experimental autoimmune model. *Neurology*, **27**, 307.

49. Engel, A. G., Tsujihata, M., Lindstrom, J. M. and Lennon, V. A. (1976). The motor end plate in myasthenia gravis and in experimental autoimmune myasthenia gravis. A quantitative ultrastructural study. *Ann. N. Y. Acad. Sci.*, **274**, 60.

50. Engel, H. L. and Denson, J. S. (1957). Respiratory depression due to neomycin. *Surgery*, **42**, 862.

51. Ferrara, B. E. and Phillips, R. D. (1957). Respiratory arrest following administration of intraperitoneal neomycin. *Amer. Surg.*, **23**, 710.

52. Fisk, G. C. (1961). Respiratory paralysis after a large dose of streptomycin: report of a case. *Brit. med. J.*, **1**, 556.

53. Fitchett, D. H., McNicol, M. W. and Riordan, J. F. (1975). Intravenous salbutamol in management of status asthmaticus. *Br. med. J.*, **1**, 53.

54. Fogdall, R. P. and Miller, R. D. (1974). Prolongation of a pancuronium-induced neuromuscular block by clyndamycin. *Anesthesiology*, **41**, 407.

55. Geddes, I. C. and Gray, T. C. (1959). Hyperventilation for the maintenance of anaesthesia. *Lancet*, **ii**, 4.

56. Genkins, G., Papatestas, A. E., Horowitz, S. H. and Kornfeld, P. (1975). Studies in myasthenia gravis: early thymectomy: electrophysiologic and pathologic correlations. *Amer. J. Med.*, **58**, 517.

57. Ginsborg, B. L. and Jenkinson, D. H. (1976). Transmission of impulses from nerve to muscle. In *Hefter's Handbuch der experimentellen Pharmakologie, New Series*, Vol. 42, p. 229. Edited by E. Zaimis. London: Springer.

58. Gitlin, D. and Craig, J. M. (1956). The nature of the hyaline membrane in asphyxia of the newborn. *Pediatrics*, **17**, 64.

59. Gliedman, M. L., Sellers, R. D., Spier, N., Grant, R. N., Vestal, B. L. and Karlson, K. E. (1959). Respiratory arrest following intraperitoneal administration of neomycin, an experimental study. *Surg. Forum.*, **9**, 404.

60. Grob, D. (1981) (Editor). Myasthenia gravis: pathophysiology and management. *Ann. N.Y. Acad. Sciences*, **337**.

61. Grob, D. and Namba, T. (1976). Characteristics and mechanism of neuromuscular block in myasthenia gravis. *Ann. N. Y. Acad. Sci.*, **274**, 143.

62. Harvey, D. R., Parkinson, C. E., Campbell, S. (1975). Risk of respiratory distress syndrome, *Lancet*, **i**, 42.

63. Hastleton, P. S. and Penna, P. E. (1981). Oxygen toxicity. *Lancet*, **i**, 1159.

64. Hastleton, P. S., Penna, P. and Torry, J. (1981). The effect of oxygen on the lungs after blast injury and burns. *J. Clin. Pathol.*, **34**, 1147.

65. Hatch, H. B., Bradford, J. K. and Ochsner, A. (1957). The value of routine pulmonary function studies in thoracic surgical cases. *J. Thorac. Surg.*, **34**, 351.

66. Havard, C. W. H. (1973). Progress in myasthenia gravis. *Brit. med. J.*, **3**, 437.

67. Hemmer, M. and Suter, P. M. (1979). Treatment of cardiac and renal effects of PEEP with dopamine in patients with acute respiratory failure. *Anesthesiology*, **50**, 399.

68. Hoffman, J. I. E., Guz, A., Charlier, A. A. and Wilcken, D. E. L. (1965). Stroke volume in conscious dogs: effect of respiration, posture and vascular occlusion. *J. appl. Physiol.*, **20**, 865.

69. Holgate, S. T., Baldwin, C. J. and Tattersfield, A. E. (1977). Adrenergic agonist resistance in normal human airways. *Lancet*, **ii**, 375.

70. Hopps, H. C. and Wissler, R. W. (1955). Uremic pneumonitis. *Amer. J. Path.*, **31**, 261

71. Howells, T. H. (1963). Automatic pulmonary ventilators. *Wld. med. Electron. Instrumentation*, **1**, 106.

72. Hunter, A. R. (1956). Neostigmine-resistant curarization. *Brit. med. J.*, **2**, 919.

73. Isenberg, H. D. (1979). Microbiology of Legionnaires' Disease bacterium. *Ann. Int. Med.*, **90**, 502.

74. Jackson, R. T., Beaglehole, R., Rea, H. H. and Sutherland, D. C. (1982). Asthma mortality: a new epidemic in New Zealand. *Brit. med. J.*, **285**, 771.

75. Jenkinson, D. H. (1960). The antagonism between tubocurarine and substances which depolarize the motor-end plate. *J. Physiol. (Lond.)*, **152**, 309.

76. Johnson, A. J., Nunn, A. J., Somner, A. R., Stableforth, D. E. and Steward, C. J. (1984). Circumstances of death from asthma. *Brit. med. J.*, **288**, 1870.

77. Johnson, A. J., Spiro, S. G., Pidgeon, J., Bateman, S. and Clarke, S. W. (1978). Intravenous infusion of salbutamol in severe acute asthma. *Brit. med. J.*, **1**, 1013.

78. Jusko, W. H., Koup, J. R., Vance, J. W., Schentag, J. J. and Kuritzky, P. (1977). Intravenous theophylline therapy: nomogram guidelines. *Ann. Int. Med.*, **86**, 400.

79. Katz, B. and Miledi, R. (1965). The effect of calcium on acetylcholine release from motor nerve terminals. *Proc. R. Soc. B.*, **161**, 496.

80. Kenyon, J. R., Ludbrook, J., Downs, A. R., Tait, I. B., Brooks, D. K and Pryczkowki, J. (1959). Experimental deep hypothermia. *Lancet*, **i**, 41.

81. Knight, P. F. (1963). Anaesthesia for the leaking abdominal aortic aneurysm. *Anaesthesia*, **18**, 151.

82. Knight, V., Wilson, S. Z., Quarles, J. M., Greggs, S. E., McClung, H. W., Waters, B. K., Cameron, R. W., Zerwas, J. M. and Couch, R. B. (1981). Ribavirin small-particle aerosol treatment of influenza. *Lancet*, **ii**, 945.

83. Lange, M. J. (1960). The preparation for and the results of surgery in myasthenia gravis. *Brit. J. Surg.*, **48**, 285.

84. Lehmann, H. and Liddell, J. (1962). The cholinesterases. In *Modern trends in anaesthesia*, **2**. p. 164. Edited by F. T. Evans and T. C. Gray. London: Butterworth.

85. Liebman, P. R., Patten, M. T., Manny, J., Shepro, D. and Hechtman, H. B. (1978). The mechanism of depressed cardiac output on positive end-expiratory pressure (PEEP). *Surgery*, **83**, 594.

86. Lindstrom, J. M., Engel, A. G., Seybold, M. E., Lennon, V. A. and Lambert, E. H. (1976). Passive transfer of experimental autoimmune myasthenia gravis in rats with anti-acetylcholine receptor antibodies. *J. Exp. Med.*, **144**, 739.

87. McCaughey, W., Coppell, D. L. and Dundee, J. W. (1973). Blast injuries to the lung: a report of two cases. *Anaesthesia*, **28**, 2.

88. McCorkle, R. G. (1958). Neomycin toxicity: a case report. *Arch. Pediat.*, **75**, 439.

89. McFadden, E. R. (1981). Calcium-channel blocking agents and asthma. *Ann. Int. Med.*, **95**, 232.

90. McKinney, R. M., Porschen, R. K., Edelstein, P. H., Bissett, M. L., Harris, P. P., Bondell, S. P., Steigerwalt, A. G., Weaver, R. E., Ein, M. E., Lindquist, D. S., Kops, R. S. and Brenner, D. J. (1981). Legionella Longbeachae species nova, another etiologic agent of human pneumonia. *Ann. Int. Med.*, **94**, 739.

91. Manny, J., Patten, M. T., Liebman, P. R. and Hechtman, H. B. (1978). The association of lung distention, PEEP and biventricular failure. *Ann. Surg.*, **187**, 151.

92. Mapleson, W. W. (1954). The elimination of rebreathing in various semi-closed anaesthetic systems. *Brit. J. anaesth.*, **26**, 323.

93. May, C. S., Spiro, S. G., Johnson, A. J. and Paterson, J. W. (1975). Intravenous infusion of salbutamol in the management of asthma. *Thorax*, **30**, 236.

94. Melot, C., Naeije, R., Rothschild, T., Mestens, P., Mols, P. and Hallemans, R. (1983). Improvement in ventilation-perfusion matching by almitrine in COPD. *Chest*, **3**, 528.

95. Morris, J. F., Koski, A. and Johnson, L. C. (1971). Spirometric standards for healthy non-smoking adults. *Am. Rev. Respir. Dis.*, **103**, 56.

96. Mushin, W. M., Rendell-Baker, L., Thompson, P. W. and Mapleson, W. W. (1980). *Automatic Ventilation of the Lungs*. p. 381. Oxford: Blackwell Scientific Publications.

97. Ormerod, L. P. and Stableforth, D. E. (1980). Asthma mortality in Birmingham 1975–7: 53 deaths. *Brit. med. J.*, **281**, 687.

98. Orth, J. (1887) *Aetiologisches und Anatomisches über Lungenschwindsucht*. p. 20. Berlin: Hirschwald.

99. Papatestas, A. E., Alpert, L. I., Osserman, K. E., Osserman, R. S. and Kark, A. E. (1971). Studies in myasthenia gravis: effects of thymectomy: results on 185 patients with nonthymomatous and thymomatous myasthenia gravis, 1941–1969. *Amer. J. Med.*, **50**, 465.

100. Patel, K. R. (1981). Calcium antagonists in exercise-induced asthma. *Brit. med. J.*, **282**, 932.

101. Patrick, J. and Lindstrom, J. (1973). Autoimmune response to acetylcholine receptor. *Science*, **180**, 871.

102. Pearce, J. L. and Wesley, H. M. M. (1985). Children with asthma: will nebulised salbutamol reduce hospital admissions. *Brit. med. J.*, **290**, 595.

103. Pittinger, C. B. and Adamson, R. (1972). Antibiotic blockade of neuromuscular function. *Ann. Rev. Pharmacol.*, **12**, 169.

104. Pittinger, C. B., Eryasa, Y. and Adamson, R. (1970). Antibiotic-induced paralysis. *Anesth. Analg. (Cleve.)*, **49**, 487.

105. Pittinger, C. B. and Long, J. P. (1958). Danger of intraperitoneal neomycin during ether anesthesia. *Surgery*, **43**, 445.

106. Pittinger, C. B., Long, J. P. and Miller, J. R. (1958). The neuromuscular blocking action of neomycin; a concern of the anesthesiologist. *Anesth. Analg. Curr. Res.*, **37**, 276.

107. Plesch, J. (1909). Hämodynamische Studien. *Z. exp. Path. Ther.*, **6**, 380.

108. Powles, A. C. P., Tuxen, D. V., Mahood, C. B., Pugsley, S. O. and Campbell, E. J. M. (1983). The effect of intravenously administered almitrine, a peripheral chemoreceptor agonist, on patients with chronic airflow obstruction. *Ann. Rev. Resp. Des.*, **127**, 284.

109. Qvist, J., Pontoppidan, H., Wilson, R. S., Lowenstein, E. and Laver, M. B. (1975). Hemodynamic responses to mechanical ventilation with PEEP: the effect of hypervolemia. *Anesthesiology*, **42**, 45.

110. Radford, E. P., Ferris, B. G. and Kriete, B. C. (1954). Clinical use of a nomogram to estimate proper ventilation during artificial respiration. *New Engl. J. Med.*, **25**, 877.

111. Ream, C. R. (1963). Respiratory and cardiac arrest after intravenous administration of kanamycin with reversal of toxic effects by neostigmine. *Ann. Int. Med.*, **59**, 384.

112. Rouby, J. J., Glaser, P., Simmoneau, G., Gory, G., Guesde, R. and Viars, P. (1979). Cardiovascular response to the I.V. administration of morphine in critically ill patients undergoing IPPV. *Br. J. Anaesth*, **51**, 1071.

113. Scurr, C. F. (1956). Pulmonary ventilation and carbon dioxide levels during anaesthesia. *Brit. J. Anaesth.*, **28**, 422.

114. Severinghaus, J. W. and Bradley, A. F. (1958). Electrodes for blood pO_2 and pCO_2 determination. *J. appl. Physiol.*, **13**, 515.

115. Severinghaus, J. W. and Stupfel, M. (1957). Alveolar dead space as an index of distribution of blood flow in pulmonary capillaries. *J. appl. Physiol.*, **10**, 335.

116. Seybold, M. E. and Drachman, D. (1974). Gradually increasing doses of prednisone in myasthenia gravis. *N. Engl. J. of Med.*, **290**, 81.

117. Seybold, M. E., Lambert, E. H., Lennon, V. A. and

Lindstrom, J. M. (1976). Experimental auto-immune myasthenia: clinical neurophysiological and pharmacologic aspects. *Ann. NY. Acad. Sci.*, **274**, 275.

118. Simpson, J. A. (1958). An evaluation of thymectomy in myasthenia gravis. *Brain*, **81**, 112.

119. Simpson, J. A. (1960). Myasthenia gravis: a new hypothesis. *Scott. Med. J.*, **51**, 419.

120. Singh, Y. N., Harvey, A. L. and Marshall, I. G. (1978). Antibiotic-induced paralysis of the mouse phrenic nerve-hemidiaphragm preparation, and reversibility by calcium and neostigmine. *Anesthesiology*, **48**, 418.

121. Singh, Y. N., Marshall, I. G. and Harvey, A. L. (1978). Some effects of the aminoglycoside antibiotic amikacin on neuromuscular and autonomic transmission. *Br. J. Anaesth.*, **50**, 109.

122. Singh, Y. N., Marshall, I. G. and Harvey, A. L. (1979). Depression of transmitter release and postjunctional sensitivity during neuromuscular block produced by antibiotics. *Brit. J. Anaesth.*, **51**, 1027.

123. Soloway, H. B., Castillo, Y. and Martin, A. M. (1968). Adult hyaline membrane disease: relationship to oxygen therapy. *Ann. Surg.*, **168**, 937.

124. Soto, P. J., Brown, G. O. and Wyatt, J. P. (1959). Asian influenza pneumonitis. *Amer. J. Med.*, **27**, 18.

125. Stein, M. and Cassara, E. L. (1970). Preoperative pulmonary evaluation and therapy for surgery patients. *J. Amer. med. Assoc.*, **211**, 787.

126. Stein, M., Kouta, G. M., Simon, M. and Frank, H. A. (1962). Pulmonary evaluation of surgical patients. *J. Amer. med. Assoc.*, **181**, 765.

127. Stradling, J. R., Nicholl, C. G., Cover, D., Davies, E. E., Hughes, J. M. B. and Pride, N. B. (1984). The effects of oral almitrine on pattern of breathing and gas exchange in patients with chronic obstructive pulmonary disease. *Clin. Sci.*, **66**, 435.

128. Strang, L. B. (1966). The pulmonary circulation in the respiratory distress syndrome. *Ped. Clin. N. America*, **13**, 693.

129. Strauss, A. J. L., Seegal, B. C., Hsu, K. C., Burkholder, P. M., Nastuk, W. L. and Osserman, K. E. (1960). Immunofluorescence demonstration of a muscle binding complement-fixing serum globulin fraction in myasthenia gravis. *Proc. Soc. Exp. Biol. Med.*, **105**, 184.

130. Suter, P. M., Fairley, H. B. and Isenberg, M. D. (1975). Optimum end-expiratory airway pressure in patients with acute pulmonary failure. *N. Engl. J. of Med.*, **292**, 284.

131. Tal, A., Pasterkamp, H. and Leahy, F. (1984). Arterial oxygen desaturation following salbutamol inhalation in acute asthma. *Chest*, **86**, 868.

132. Tsai, T. F., Finn, D. R., Plikaytis, B. D., McCauley, W., Martin, S. M. and Fraser, D. W. (1979). Legionnaires' Disease: clinical features of the epidemic in Philadelphia. *Ann. Int. Med.*, **90**, 509.

133. Turner-Warwick, M. (1977). On observing patterns of air flow obstruction in chronic asthma. *Brit. J. Dis. Chest*, **71**, 73.

134. Usher, R. H. (1960). Management of metabolic changes in the respiratory distress syndrome of prematurity. *Amer. J. Dis. Child.*, **100**, 485.

135. Vital Brazil, O. and Prado-Franceschi, J. (1969). The nature of neuromuscular block produced by neomycin and gentamicin. *Arch. Int. Pharmacodyn. Ther.*, **179**, 78.

136. Walker, M. B. (1934). Treatment of myasthenia gravis with physostigmine. *Lancet*, **i**, 1200.

137. Warren, S. and Spencer, J. (1940). Radiation reaction in the lung. *Amer. J. Roentgenol.*, **43**, 682.

138. Waud, B. E. and Waud, D. R. (1980). Interaction of calcium and potassium with neuromuscular blocking agents. *Brit. J. Anaesth.*, **52**, 863.

139. Wërko, L. (1947). The influence of positive pressure breathing on the circulation of man. *Acta. Med. Scand.*, **193**, (Suppl) 1.

140. West, J. B. (1963). Distribution of gas and blood in the normal lungs. *Brit. med. Bull.*, **19**, 53.

141. Williams, S. J., Parrish, R. S. and Seaton, A. (1975). Comparison of intravenous aminophylline and salbutamol in severe asthma. *Brit. med. J.*, **4**, 685.

142. Wilson, J. D., Sutherland, D. C. and Thomas, A. C. (1981). Has the change to beta-agonists combined with oral theophylline increased cases of fatal asthma? *Lancet*, **i**, 1235.

143. Wood, N. and Baker, R. H. (1984). Deaths from asthma. *Brit. med. J.*, **289**, 186.

144. Wright, J. M. and Collier, B. (1976). Characterisation of the neuromuscular block produced by clindamycin and lincomycin. *Canad. J. Physiol. Pharmacol.*, **54**, 937.

Further Reading

Anonymous. (1986). Acute asthma. *Lancet*, **i**, 131.

Lancet (1985). Surfactant therapy in the newborn. *Lancet*, **ii**, 867.

Mehtar, S., Drabu, Y. J., Vijeratnam, S. and Mayet, F. (1986). Cross infection with *Streptococcus pneumoniae* through a resuscitaire. *Brit. med. J.*, **292**, 25.

Mossman, S., Vincent, A. and Newsom-Davis, J. (1986). Myasthenia gravis without acetylcholine-receptor antibody: a distinct disease entity. *Lancet*, **i**, 116.

Chapter 6
Shock

Definition and the Distribution of Blood Volume

Shock is a generic term covering a multitude of different conditions and is subject to many different interpretations. When we speak of shock in clinical practice we reserve the term to mean a fall in systemic blood pressure and this is usually associated with the general physical collapse of the patient. In the majority of cases it is a potentially lethal state requiring immediate treatment. In everyday language, however, shock is often used to describe a person's reaction to an unpleasant situation, for example, when he hears bad news, or is frightened by either being involved in or witnessing an accident. The term is also used for the sensation and results of a current of electricity passing through the body. The use of this term in these circumstances is not without foundation; we know that a fall of blood pressure and syncope can result from all the causes mentioned above. Death itself can be caused by electric currents of relatively low voltage and amperage; and it is known that a young girl, who was walking along the road at night, died suddenly when a quite innocent man, who had lost his way, blundered through the bushes onto her path. There is also the classical story of the unpopular college janitor who was blindfolded, made to climb some steps and place his head on a 'block', and who died immediately after being hit on the back of the neck with a wet towel. In both cases it must be presumed that ventricular fibrillation resulted from hyperactivity of the endocrine and autonomic nervous systems. It is essential, therefore, that fear developing into terror should never be accepted as being of no consequence. Alleviation of pain and anxiety is of the greatest importance in preventing the tragic consequences of severe trauma.

When we describe shock, therefore, it is necessary to qualify the term in such a way that it is made more precise. In some descriptions it is not easily understandable whether hypotension has been produced by a psychological upset or pain or whether the term 'shock' is merely describing the emotional aspects of the situation. When hypotension resulting from an emotional disturbance is profound, syncope results, but after major surgery a fall in blood pressure which does not respond to conventional treatment is sometimes observed to improve following sedation with morphine. We therefore have to speak of emotional or psychogenic shock with hypotension or without hypotension.

If in clinical practice we place non-hypotensive psychogenic shock in a completely separate category, we can confine the term shock to conditions which are associated with a reduced systemic arterial blood pressure. It is necessary to subdivide hypotension into two categories. The first is hypotension associated with a normal or near-normal blood volume. This occurs in cardiac failure, neurogenic disorders, bacteraemia (especially that due to *Eschericia coli* or staphylococci), impaired function of the suprarenal gland and positive pressure ventilation wrongly applied with a mechanical ventilator. The second is hypotension associated with a low blood volume, and this implies either gross dehydration or loss of blood from the body or into closed cavities, such as damaged muscle mass, the thorax, the abdominal cavity or fracture sites, or the loss of plasma and fluid into the lumen of the gut or from the skin following burns.

The reactions of the body to all these forms of shock have much in common. This may be seen in the cardiovascular aspects, the changes in respiration, the alterations in the body's biochemistry and the differences in function of some organs, such as the spleen, liver and kidney. In order to understand the importance of changes in blood volume we must see how it is distributed within the body.

The total blood volume is calculated to be between 70 and 100 ml/kg body weight. It varies with age, the amount of subcutaneous fat, the state of nutrition and normal physiological variations. The average 70-kg man has approximately 6 litres of blood in the circulation, of which only

1 litre is contained within the arteries. A further 300 ml of blood is contained within the capillaries of the body excluding those of the lungs. The veins and venules contain very nearly 70% of the blood volume, that is to say approximately 4 litres. Because the venules and small veins have the ability to contract and reduce their lumen, the redistribution of blood within the body by this means is of great importance because such a large volume is contained within this part of the vascular system. Venous constriction, although not as powerful as that which occurs within the arterial tree, is an important physiological mechanism.

The remainder of the blood lies within the pulmonary circulation; the volume changes with posture, respiration, contractility of the systemic vessels, exercise and many other variables. The volume of blood within the pulmonary circulation therefore varies between 500 and 1200 ml, altering in balance with the volume of blood in the systemic circulation; on average it probably lies in the region of 800 ml. The distribution of blood to organs other than the lung is also subject to much variation. In the resting state, especially after eating, a large part of the blood flow is distributed to the gut, liver and kidneys. During exercise, however, the blood flow to the muscles, which in the resting state, receive only one-fifth of the total blood flow, is increased ten times or more and comprises a much larger proportion of the total cardiac output. The repartitioning of cardiac output and blood volume during shock is subject to numerous factors depending upon whether the type of shock is normovolaemic or hypovolaemic, the maintenance of a normally beating myocardium, the redistribution of fluid within the body fluid compartments, as well as the severity of the shock state itself. Because redistribution of blood can be produced only by vasoconstriction, it is essential that the contractility of the vessels is not impaired by toxins or anaphylactoid reactions. Even after much investigation, many of the processes involved and even the basic physiology of the various types of shock still require elucidation.

Maintenance of Arterial Blood Pressure

It is readily apparent that a large number of different factors influence and maintain a normal arterial blood pressure. These include a normal endocrine function and water balance, autonomic nerve function and maintenance of cardiac output. As is well recognized, haemodynamic control is complicated and involved, and widely differing entities influence cardiac output.

Fundamentally, however, the blood pressure is maintained by a relatively fixed volume of blood being pumped through a resistant vascular bed, the resistance of which is controlled.

The arterial compartment is closed at its proximal end by the aortic valve and the distal end by the arterioles. In the absence of other haemodynamic changes, the competence of the aortic valve determines the diastolic pressure; the degree of impedence of the arterioles determines the systolic pressure.

In spite of this simple concept, the management of shock is difficult and is associated with a high mortality and morbidity. The reasons for this are that all three principles—the pump, blood volume and peripheral resistance—may be abnormal, to a *differing* degree, at *varying* time intervals, and from *more than one* cause, so that a great number of different factors have to be corrected before a rise in blood pressure and normal tissue perfusion can be obtained.

Much progress has been made in the understanding of the pathophysiology and metabolic abnormalities of these conditions. Two main groups of conditions cause hypotension (Brooks, 1967)[20] (Fig. 6.1).

1. Those associated with a reduced blood volume (hypovolaemic shock).
2. Those associated with a normal blood volume (normovolaemic shock).

The first may be superimposed upon the second and, until hypovolaemia has been corrected, the contribution made by other factors cannot be assessed. Unfortunately, the simple correction of a reduced blood volume sometimes induces alterations in the body biochemistry that have their own hypotensive effect.

Haemorrhage may be readily apparent or concealed within fracture sites and body cavities, but every time we see a patient with a low blood pressure we need to know whether it is because of a low blood volume or something else.

Plasma is lost into the gut during gut obstruction and paralytic ileus and following the development of peritonitis or pancreatitis, both into the gut and the peritoneal cavity. Ischaemic or bruised muscle tissue is also a site of marked plasma loss and occurs as a result of trauma, aneurisectomy and endarterectomy. Embolic occlusion of a major blood vessel, for example the profunda femoris,

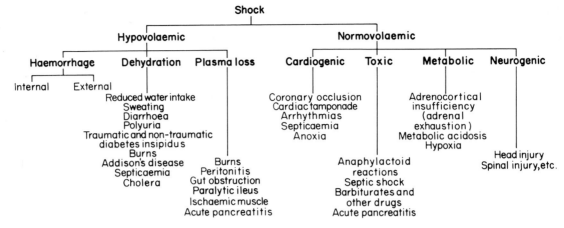

Fig. 6.1   Causes of shock. After Brooks (1967). *British Journal of Surgery.*[20]

which supplies the thigh muscles, can induce a massive and rapid sequestration of plasma, a fall in arterial blood pressure and a rise in packed cell volume (PCV). Both plasma and water loss occurs, from the body surface, after burns.

A number of different conditions give rise to water loss (Fig. 6.1). Severe diarrhoea, from infection, oral hyperalimentation, oral antibiotic therapy (especially the non-absorbable group of antibiotics); or in babies and young children, other non-related diseases, such as otitis media, can rapidly give rise to dehydration. Renal loss of water occurs during diabetic ketosis, hyperosmolar non-ketotic diabetic coma, and following cranial or traumatic diabetes insipidus which comes on at variable intervals following head injury in all ages.

The volume of fluid that must be replaced is commonly underestimated in patients suffering from peritonitis, paralytic ileus and pancreatitis.

The three forms of fluid loss (Table 6.1) produce characteristic changes in PCV, plasma [Na$^+$] and protein concentration, indicating the fluid to be infused (Table 6.1).

Fluid replacement is sometimes performed to excess, especially in the treatment of burns and when renal insufficiency is present. This can give rise to pulmonary oedema.

Table 6.1   Changes occurring in the plasma [Na$^+$], packed cell volume and protein concentrations during hypovolaemic shock

Cause of hypotension	Plasma [Na$^+$]	Packed cell volume (PCV)	Plasma protein concentration
Blood loss	Reduced	Reduced or unchanged	Reduced or unchanged
Dehydration	Increased*	Increased	Increased
Plasma loss	Reduced or unchanged	Increased	Unchanged

*This only applies when there is a pure water loss. The PCV may be increased and [Na$^+$] decreased in early diabetic coma and established Addison's disease. The [Na$^+$] may fall also in patients with gut obstruction, peritonitis and paralytic ileus, so that the [Na$^+$] and protein concentration are decreased.

IRREVERSIBLE SHOCK

The term 'irreversible shock' is used to describe a condition of hypotension which does not respond to the normal methods of treatment such as blood transfusion and vasopressors. There are many causes of irreversible shock.

In man, simple blood loss alone rarely gives rise to irreversible shock. Fluid and blood replacement usually causes a return of blood pressure to normal values when an adequate volume is transfused. There are, however, exceptions to this general rule.

Cardiac failure

When the heart pump fails to function adequately, the arterial blood pressure falls. Acute coronary occlusion can lead to irreversible shock at any time and can appear during any illness or surgical procedure. Acute anoxia, a gross metabolic acidosis, or citrate intoxication, can also lead to myocardial failure. Hypothermia and the sudden overfilling of the vascular compartment with fluid or blood can exacerbate the impairment of function of an already failing heart, thus overt cardiac failure is precipitated.

Septic shock

An acute infection, usually associated with a bacteraemia, may give rise to irreversible shock. Its various aspects are described in different parts of this chapter.

Haemorrhage

If an animal is subjected to a prolonged period of haemorrhagic shock so that the blood pressure is in the region of 60 mmHg or less in the central aorta, after some hours the replacement of all the blood lost will not cause a rise in blood pressure. Numerous factors contribute to this condition. The dog, in common with many other animals, but unlike man, undergoes haemorrhagic necrosis of the bowel after a relatively short period of hypotension as a result of blood loss. This is considered by some to be the main cause of irreversible shock. The author, like other investigators, has found that large areas of haemorrhagic necrosis of the bowel can be present and the animal can still maintain a normal blood pressure when the blood that has been lost is returned after a period of 1 hour or more.

The gut is unique as far as body organs are concerned because it has a constant bacterial content. In health, the relationship of bacterial flora in the gut to the body as a whole is one of symbiosis. If the organisms leave the gut and enter the bloodstream, the exotoxins of clostridia and staphylococci and the endotoxins of *Eschericia coli* have a profound effect upon the cardiovascular system. Hypotension is caused by the relaxation of tone of the arterioles in 'warm septic shock', and by inadequate myocardial function and movements of body fluids in 'cold septic shock'. When haemorrhagic necrosis of the bowel is produced by

haemorrhagic shock in the animal, bacteria can gain access to the vascular system. Some workers believe that irreversible shock in these conditions is primarily a result of endotoxins.[61] Although in man the bowel does not appear to react in the same way to haemorrhagic shock, a bacteraemia can be observed after abdominal surgery, after occlusion of the superior mesenteric artery and after other forms of intestinal ischaemia. Toxins causing hypotension which are derived from bacterial infection are dealt with later in this chapter.

Metabolic acidosis

A gross metabolic acidosis sometimes occurs in man during haemorrhagic shock, without any evidence of irreversible shock developing. When blood is returned, the blood pressure rises. It has been shown that an animal may live for some weeks following an experiment in which the blood pressure has been maintained at 40 mmHg for 90 minutes and the bicarbonate ion concentration of the plasma has fallen to low levels, for example, a total $CO_2(TCO_2)$ of 3.2 mmol/l (mEq/l). In clinical practice, however, it has been frequently observed that a moderate base deficit in some patients, amounting sometimes to a decrease of only 4 or 5 mmol/l (mEq/l) of bicarbonate in the plasma, may have a pronounced effect upon the blood pressure. It must be assumed, therefore, that some other factors, in addition to the metabolic acidosis, must be acting, but when the metabolic acidosis is corrected the other factors become of little significance. The main action of a metabolic acidosis on the cardiovascular system appears to be upon the myocardium. This action may vary from causing a moderate rise in the central venous pressure to producing such marked hypotension that the blood pressure cannot be recorded on a sphygmomanometer. In these circumstances it is usually associated with some degree of respiratory failure. When attempts are made to ventilate a patient in this condition, the pressure in the pulmonary arteries and in the lung capillaries may be so low that the inflation pressure exceeds that which is perfusing the lungs. The cardiac output in these circumstances is reduced even further and the very action of positive pressure ventilation may precipitate peripheral circulatory collapse.

If the venous pressure is not measured or observed to be raised by other means, there is a real danger that blood is transfused in excess of requirements because of the persisting low systemic arterial blood pressure. When this is done a fatal outcome commonly results from pulmonary oedema and extravasation of blood in the lungs so that at *post mortem* they may have a consolidated haemorrhagic appearance like that of liver. This appearance is sometimes referred to as 'pump lung' because it is sometimes seen after heart–lung bypass using a pump oxygenator, but it can also be seen after massive rapid blood transfusion has been necessary (e.g. during difficult, major vessel surgery).

The cause of the metabolic acidosis may be ischaemia from the clamping of the vessels, haemorrhagic shock causing reduced tissue perfusion and therefore tissue anoxia, inadequate ventilation, inadequate cardiac output, and the massive transfusion of old stored blood containing much acid and little bicarbonate. This danger may be avoided by correcting the metabolic acidosis by infusions of sodium bicarbonate solution, either before or during major blood transfusion. The importance of correcting the metabolic acidosis was recognized long ago by Cannon (1918 and 1923).[32–34]

Citrate intoxication

The rapid infusion of acid citrate dextrose (ACD) blood, by lowering the Ca^{++} fraction of plasma, may produce hypotension which does not respond to further blood transfusion. This may be avoided by giving calcium salts intravenously (i.e. calcium gluconate or calcium chloride 5 ml) after every unit of rapidly transfused blood.[108]

Anoxia

We have seen how the heart must have an adequate supply of oxygen in order to function normally and, if anoxia is superimposed upon other conditions, it can become one of the major factors in irreversible shock. Inadequate ventilation is a common association of traumatic conditions and great care has to be taken to see that this aspect is not forgotten. In some cases, however, water may be absorbed into the lung parenchyma, and this may be exacerbated by the infusion of electrolyte-containing fluid.[64–68]

Endocrine causes

It is well recognized in surgical practice, that patients who have been receiving adrenocortical hormones for any length of time, and therefore have suprarenal glands with a depressed function, are liable to undergo severe hypotension if supplements of corticoids are not given. Similarly, the natural function of the suprarenal glands may be impaired by toxins, infection and numerous other factors, so that during major trauma or surgery a similar form of treatment is necessary if irreversible shock is to be avoided.

It can be seen that some causes of 'irreversible' shock are in fact preventable and, if recognized sufficiently early, can be treated.

Physiology of Haemorrhagic Shock

As blood is lost from the vascular space, the reduction in volume within the arterial tree is partially compensated by constriction of vessels in other parts of the body, especially within the splanchnic area and the skin. To make the most use of the blood available for tissue oxygen transport, the heart rate increases. The patient is forced to adopt the horizontal position so that gravity no longer impedes the return of blood to the heart. The return of blood is further enhanced by increasing respiration so that the negative pressure within the thorax acting upon the thin-walled veins is transmitted along the venous system and the 'thoracic pump' becomes more effective.

Urine flow either ceases or becomes markedly reduced, partly as a result of a reduced glomerular filtration rate (GFR) and partly because of a secretion of antidiuretic hormone (ADH) in response to a reduced blood volume.

The volume of blood within the pulmonary circulation depends upon the volume of blood in the systemic circulation, and the pulmonary artery pressure falls when the systemic arterial blood pressure falls. The distribution of blood within the lungs is also altered so that ventilation–perfusion ratios are disorganized. Blood tends to leave the uppermost parts of the lungs and to accumulate in the lower regions so that increasing numbers of alveoli receive no capillary blood flow. Increase in ventilation, therefore, is stimulated in three ways:

1. as a result of the necessity for an increased use of the thoracic pump assisting the return of blood to the right side of the heart,

2. as a result of the tissue anoxia that is produced because of an inadequate volume of blood available for tissue oxidation,

3. because of an increase in the physiological (respiratory) dead space.

The physiological respiratory dead space consists

of the anatomical dead space (i.e. that part of the pulmonary tree in which no gas exchange occurs, such as the trachea, the main bronchi and bronchioles) together with: (1) the volume of gas that ventilates alveoli which have no capillary blood flow, and (2) the volume of gas ventilating areas in excess of that required to produce maximum gas exchange. In the normal person, the anatomical and physiological dead spaces are very nearly identical, but this is not so during haemorrhagic shock. On theoretical grounds alone, an increase in the physiological dead space should occur and experiments on animals have shown this to be so.[63,69]. It can therefore be seen that any failure in ventilation associated with haemorrhage is a potentially lethal combination of circumstances. It is also apparent that acid–base changes appear to play no part in producing hyperventilation, and in fact it has been demonstrated that it is independent of alterations in the acid–base state.[28] In the very late stages of haemorrhagic shock, correction of the metabolic acidosis prevents respiratory failure.

Another important factor in resuscitation is that as acidosis increases, and the pH of the circulating blood falls, the pulmonary vascular resistance increases[96] so that the output of the heart is further impaired.

Cardiac output

Although the heart rate increases, the cardiac output falls because the stroke volume is reduced by the very fact that the volume of blood returning to the heart is less than that which is present during normovolaemia. This is because the venous pressure is low and the veins collapse. Raising the foot of the bed facilitates the venous return by gravity flow and thus raises the systemic blood pressure. Because limitations upon cardiac output are set by the venous return, any interference with the thoracic pump mechanism of metabolic, anaesthetic, or neurogenic origin causing hypoventilation, will reduce the effective beating of the heart to a serious degree. It can also be seen that if positive pressure ventilation is applied incorrectly to a patient with haemorrhagic shock, the presence of increased concentrations of oxygen in the ventilating gases will afford little or no benefit. Certainly the presence of oxygen in the gases will not compensate for even a minor degree of reduction in the cardiac output. Because of the physiological mechanisms that help to increase the venous return to the heart, the cardiac output does not fall when the blood volume is first diminished. A critical pressure approximately 90–70 mmHg must be

reached before there is a significant reduction in the cardiac output. Different conditions are present in hypotension resulting from circulating toxins.

As the cardiac output falls and the volume of blood within the pulmonary circulation decreases, the pulmonary artery and lung capillary pressures are reduced. In this way occlusion of the pulmonary capillary bed during intermittent positive pressure ventilation occurs more easily and for a longer period even when the pressures used to inflate the lungs are low.

Oxygen saturation and PO_2 of arterial and venous blood

We have seen how the ventilation rate increases spontaneously after the onset of haemorrhagic shock so that the minute volume is very nearly doubled. In this way, the arterial oxygen saturation is maintained at normal values when the patient is breathing air. Because the cardiac output is reduced and the volume of blood perfusing individual tissues is markedly decreased, the amount of oxygen extracted is greater. As haemorrhage progresses, the oxygen content of the venous blood decreases so that when a comparison is made between blood in the right atrium and that in the left atrium, the difference in oxygen saturation gradually increases (Table 6.2). The venous blood oxygen saturation may fall to below 20% in the presence of an arterial oxygen saturation of 98% so that almost complete extraction of oxygen has occurred.

When the patient or experimental animal is breathing air during spontaneous respiration, the arterial PO_2 may rise to as high as 110 mmHg. This is the result of the increased alveolar ventilation achieved by both an increase in respiratory rate and the increase in tidal volume. When factors that can depress respiration (e.g. drugs, anaesthetics, head injury, damage to the thoracic cage etc.) are absent, this rise in the arterial PO_2 during haemorrhagic shock occurs, even though there is an increase in the physiological dead space caused by blood accumulating in the dependent parts of the lungs.

Full or increased oxygenation of blood therefore can be achieved only when cardiac output is not impaired by extraneous factors and the maximum degree of hyperventilation is present. It can be seen that any fall in the arterial PO_2 and oxygen saturation under these circumstances will give rise to severe tissue anoxia in essential organs. When alveolar ventilation is maximal, the blood leaving

Table 6.2   Blood pH, standard bicarbonate (St. bic.), PCO_2, oxygen saturation (O_2 sat.) and blood pressure in arterial (A) and central venous (V) blood samples in a dog with progressing haemorrhagic shock

Time (minutes)	pH		St. bic. mmol/l		PCO_2 mmHg		O_2 sat. %		BP mmHg
	A	V	A	V	A	V	A	V	
0	7.380	7.340	22.5	22.4	39	45.5	96	67	175
15	7.420	7.320	20.3	19.7	29	39	98	39	125
47	7.469	7.240	20.0	16.9	21.3	40	97	34	55
85	7.439	7.078	15.3	14.4	15.5	67	98	27	40

pH = blood pH at 38°C; PCO_2 = plasma carbon dioxide tension; Time = time in minutes from the beginning of bleeding; BP = mean blood pressure.

Note the increasing arteriovenous difference of pH, PCO_2 and oxygen saturation with increasing hypotension and time. Similar values and even greater arteriovenous differences have been observed in isolated blood samples in man. Remember (see p. 134), it is the fall in oxygen saturation of the venous blood that determines the degree of cyanosis in man, even in the presence of 100% saturation (100 mmHg PO_2 or more) of the arterial blood.

the lungs is almost completely saturated and the addition of oxygen to the air breathed has relatively little value. When there is inadequate ventilation because of lung pathology, high oxygen tensions in the inspired air will have a beneficial effect. For these reasons, therefore, while stress must be placed on the maintenance of an adequate cardiac output and respiratory minute volume, oxygen should not be withheld in doubtful cases.

Systemic arterial blood pressure

We have now examined how changes in ventilation, cardiac output and posture may affect blood pressure. If positive pressure ventilation is applied incorrectly, hypotension may occur, even in the absence of blood loss. It will therefore be realized that in the presence of trauma involving the heart and lungs, a moderate degree of blood loss (i.e. less than 10% of the total blood volume) may produce a precipitate fall in blood pressure. When more than 20% of the blood volume has been lost a marked decline in blood pressure follows. When the loss is in excess of 40%, it is usually impossible to measure blood pressure by means of a sphygmomanometer or oscillometer. If a conscious patient is lying down, 40% of the total blood volume can be removed before syncope occurs.[80] The two organs which receive most blood during haemorrhagic shock are the heart and the brain, together with the spinal cord. The blood flow to other organs such as the kidneys, gut, skin and most of the muscles is reduced. The intercostal muscles and diaphragm are relatively well supplied with circulating blood.

In a normal person with a normal blood volume, the arterial blood pressure is maintained by the systolic pressure exerted by the left ventricle and the resistance to flow exercised by the arterioles, the calibre of which can be altered. This is similar to placing a piece of rubber tubing on the end of a water tap. No pressure is exerted within the rubber tube until the end of it is partially occluded by pinching when a fine projectile jet is obtained. There is a differential change in calibre of vessels in various parts of the body. For example, those in the skin and splanchnic areas are made to contract while those in certain muscles and the brain are made to dilate. It is this ability to differentiate flow that permits the continuous partitioning of blood flow so that those organs that are essential for the immediate maintenance of life obtain the maximum amount of blood that is available. Because of their characteristics, which are different from most other body tissues and which give them a specialized function, the kidneys do not escape damage unless special steps are taken (see p. 188). The liver also may undergo tissue change when hypotension resulting from hypovolaemia is prolonged during surgery. This is reflected in abnormal liver function tests and sometimes postoperative jaundice.

In many animal experiments it has been possible to demonstrate that in the early stages of haemorrhagic shock the peak systolic pressure is maintained at a high level (e.g. 100 mmHg) when the mean aortic blood pressure is less than 50 mmHg. This only occurs in the healthy heart when the force of contraction during systole is increased. By maintaining this large pressure gradient, some capillaries will open when their critical closing pressure is exceeded. While this is a further method of maintaining blood flow, the systolic blood pressure may be a misleading measurement when assessing the degree of blood loss.

In summary, therefore, we can see that when the blood pressure is reduced by a reduction in the volume of circulating blood it is important that no action should be taken that will in any way impair the cardiac output or the flow of blood through the lungs or, on theoretical grounds, alter the differential flow of available blood within the body. It has been suggested that α-receptor-blocking agents, for example phenoxybenzamine (Dibenyline, Dibenzyline) which cause generalized vasodilatation, may be of value in haemorrhagic shock. In practice this aspect of treatment has not gained wide acceptance.

Central Venous Pressure

As the blood reservoirs become depleted, the central venous pressure (CVP) falls. The main reservoirs of blood consist of the splanchnic area, the venous plexuses in the skin, the large veins, the spleen (relatively unimportant in man), the pulmonary vessels and to a small extent the heart. By calling on these blood reservoirs, a reduction in blood volume of as much as 10% can occur without the appearance of circulatory changes. When this amount is exceeded, a systemic arterial blood pressure can only be maintained by means of increased function of the sympathetic system. Before the loss of 10% of the blood volume, the cardiac output, systemic arterial blood pressure and central venous pressure (CVP) remain the same. When blood loss is in excess of 10%, but reflex sympathetic activity mediated through baroreceptors maintains a normal systemic arterial blood pressure, the venous pressure is found to be reduced. As further haemorrhage reduces the volume of blood available to the arterial vascular tree and there is a further decline in cardiac output, the systemic blood pressure falls. Because the venous reservoir of blood is so large, in that it accommodates 60–70% of the blood volume, a moderate degree of constriction of the veins and venules results in a large volume of blood being made available for oxygenation within the pulmonary system and circulation through the body. Another factor that is important in the assessment of the degree of blood loss is the fact that initially no change in venous pressure may occur and further loss of blood is followed by a catastrophic fall in both arterial blood pressure and CVP.

Normal central venous pressure (CVP)
An isolated measurement of CVP is always of limited value and, if a clear interpretation of results

is to be obtained, frequent measurements repeated at short intervals should be made. In general it can be stated that when the pressure falls below 4 cmH$_2$O,* a reduced blood volume is probably present and some guide as to the degree of blood volume deficiency may be obtained by observing the response to transfusion. When the transfusion of a small volume of blood is followed by a marked rise in CVP it is indicative of obstruction to the venous outflow in addition to hypovolaemia. A slow rise in CVP following transfusion is indicative of either marked hypovolaemia or continued blood loss. A fall in CVP is usually observed long before a fall in the arterial pressure.

When the CVP rises above 15–17 cmH$_2$O,* the onset of cardiac failure or overtransfusion is indicated. It may also indicate obstruction of flow from the right side of the heart. This may be caused by positive pressure ventilation, especially when the inflation pressure is too high, when blood or fluid is enclosed within the pericardium, a tension pneumothorax and when shifting of the mediastinum occurs following injury to the lungs or chest wall.

In some circumstances a raised venous pressure is desirable, for example, in the postoperative state which is present after a complete repair of a patient suffering from tetralogy of Fallot. To maintain an adequate arterial blood pressure, under these circumstances, blood transfusion may be necessary to such a degree that the CVP in the region of 15–17 cmH$_2$O,* is maintained in the early postoperative period.

Measurement of central venous pressure
Indirect measurements of CVP can be made by observing the level of maximal distension of the external jugular veins. During cardiac failure the patient is placed in a position so that the thorax and abdomen are at an angle of 45° to the horizontal. A measurement is then taken from the manubrio-sternal angle. Instruments to make this measurement easier and more accurate have been devised. In almost all cases this method is of no practical value following trauma, surgery and toxic shock.

The CVP is measured by inserting a cannula into the superior vena cava (SVC). It can also be measured when the tip of the cannula is located in the subclavian vein, the brachiocephalic (innominate) vein and sometimes even the lower end of the internal jugular vein, but the measure-

---

* Measured from the mid-axillary line.

ment at these sites is commonly damped and inaccurate. The inferior vena cava (IVC) should never be used (see p. 181), although a cannula can be passed in an emergency, for example following extensive burns to the upper part of the body. A long cannula is passed via the femoral vein, through the IVC and right atrium, into the SVC. In ordinary circumstances, this is a hazard that is unacceptable for routine use, although it can be readily performed using a portable image intensifier.

Patency of the cannula is maintained by means of an intravenous infusion. The nature of the infusion fluid is unimportant, and many types of fluid, including hypertonic solutions, can be used. Blood, however, should never be used because it is too viscous, and it obscures the manometer making measurement of the CVP difficult.

Cannulation of the SVC can be achieved by passing the cannula through an antecubital vein in the forearm, the external jugular vein in the neck, the internal jugular vein from above the head of the clavicle between the two heads of sternomastoid,

and the subclavian vein from below the clavicle just lateral to its inner one-third. The last method, through the subclavian vein, is the one most commonly used.

Although CVP can be measured by means of an electrical transducer, the apparatus most commonly used consists of an intravenous infusion set connected to a three-way tap, which is in turn connected to the cannula that has been inserted into the SVC (Fig. 6.2). An upright tube or manometer is connected to the remaining arm of the three-way tap. Before CVP is measured, the tap is turned so that the infusion fluid is able to drip slowly through the venous cannula into the vein. When a measurement of CVP is required, the tap is again turned in such a way that the infusion fluid is allowed to flow into the manometer until the meniscus is close to the top of the tube and the manometer is almost full. The three-way tap is then turned once more so that the manometer and the intravenous cannula are in continuity, and the level of fluid in the manometer gradually falls until a measurement of CVP can be made.

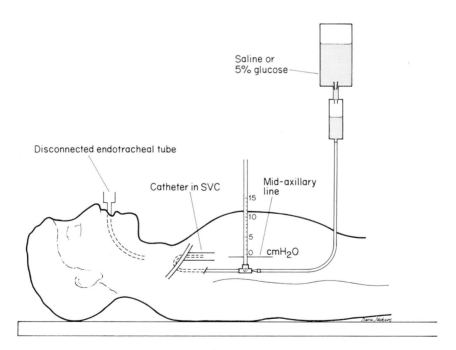

Fig. 6.2   Measurement of central venous pressure (CVP). This measurement is made with the patient lying flat with no pillow. The zero point of the manometer is placed at the midaxillary line. A mark can be drawn with a felt tipped pen. Fluid is allowed to run into the manometer via the three-way tap. The tap is then turned so that the fluid in the manometer runs into the SVC. A 'respiratory swing' should be observed. If the patient is receiving intermittent positive pressure respiration (IPPR), the fluid level in the manometer is allowed to fall. The patient is then momentarily disconnected from the ventilator and the final reading taken. Only the SVC is used.

(This figure has been drawn from an illustration by Diana Jackson.)

The manometer is usually calibrated in centimetres. The figure 0 does not appear at the bottom of the column, but a little way along its length. Below the figure 0 the numbers run in a reverse direction, usually 0 to minus 12, so that a negative pressure can be measured. Zero pressure is obtained by raising and lowering the column until the figure 0 is at the level of the mid-axillary line. This is denoted by a line drawn with a felt-tipped pen horizontally along the chest. A long rule fitted with a spirit level is usually used for this purpose.

Normal values

The normal value will depend upon the site from which the pressure is measured and the position of the zero point.[99]

As demonstrated by Rushmer,[135] posture and the position of the body will also affect the CVP measurement. Measurements should be made using a wide-bore catheter inserted into the superior vena cava. The patient should be lying flat without a pillow. If artificial ventilation of the lungs (IPPR) is being maintained, the ventilator should be disconnected from the patient for the very brief period that is required for the measurement to be made. When ventilation cannot be stopped except for a very brief period, the column of fluid is allowed to fall until the meniscus has reached its lower level before disconnecting the ventilator. The final lower reading is then obtained as quickly as possible and the ventilator is then reconnected.

During both spontaneous and assisted ventilation of the lungs, a change in the position of the meniscus occurs with inspiration and expiration when the cannula is patent and correctly located. This is sometimes referred to as the 'respiratory swing'. It is not uncommon for positive pressure ventilation to increase the CVP by as much as 10 cmH_2O.

Repeated measurements can be made at very short intervals by turning the three-way tap so that there is continuity between the fluid in the venous catheter and that in the column which measures the pressure. More than one measurement should be made. The apparatus can be kept sterile in a plastic container until required (see Fig. 6.2). Plastic, disposable, intravenous drip sets with venous pressure recording columns are now available.

The pressure measurement is made from a zero point which is taken at the mid-axillary line (Fig. 6.2) or 5 cm posterior to (below) the sternum. The normal CVP, measured from the mid-axillary line, is usually approximately 5–8 cmH_2O.

A number of factors can, however, modify a normal CVP. These include inaccurate positioning of the patient, positive pressure ventilation of the lungs, and a raised intra-abdominal pressure, especially when measurements are taken from the IVC.

During clinical practice it has become apparent that the measurement of CVP can sometimes be grossly misleading. One patient who had undergone abdominal surgery was found to have a systolic blood pressure of 60 mmHg in the presence of a CVP measurement of 17 mmHg. The catheter had been inserted via the femoral vein into the IVC. A Dacron prosthesis had been placed in the abdominal aorta and dilatation of the bowel had developed in the early postoperative period. When seen, the abdomen was greatly distended and a second catheter was inserted via the subclavian vein into the SVC. When the measurement was repeated, it was found that the CVP was only 2 cmH_2O. Saline and blood were infused rapidly and this caused an immediate increase in blood pressure, and a rise in the CVP to normal values. The CVP measured in the IVC rose at times to 35 mmHg, but fluctuated in a grossly misleading manner. A comparison of CVP in 12 patients showed marked discrepancies between the values obtained using catheters located at the two different sites; the results are shown in Table 6.3.

Table 6.3 Postoperative central venous pressure (CVP) as measured simultaneously in subclavian and femoral veins of 12 patients

Operation	CVP (cmH_2O)	
	Subclavian vein	Femoral vein
Partial gastrectomy	8	21
Aortofemoral bypass	7	14
Aortofemoral bypass	5	15
Aortofemoral bypass	7	11
Aortic valve prosthesis	8	15
Mitral valve prosthesis	12	17
Aortic abdominal aneurysm	8	19
Aortocoronary bypass	7	11
Aortocoronary bypass	15	23
Aortocoronary bypass	11	14
Aortocoronary bypass	9	11
Resection of small bowel	6	17

Interpretation of central venous pressure (CVP)

Because measurement of CVP can be performed easily, it is frequently carried out postoperatively, especially following surgery to the heart and great vessels. It is, however, a measurement that is a product of many factors, and a change in venous pressure has to be subjected to interpretation.

We have seen how the arterial tree contains only approximately 15% of the total blood volume and that the major part is contained within the venous system. It is also necessary to recall that an increase of 10–15% of the volume of blood contained within the venous system may be achieved without an increase in CVP. For this reason CVP does not respond to changes in blood volume in a linear manner. A further factor is the alterations in venous tone that occur as a result of changes in blood volume, cardiac output and the secretion of adrenaline and noradrenaline.

Fundamentally, the venous pressure is dependent upon the balance between the amount of blood flowing into the venous system and the volume removed by the heart in a given period of time. The inflow of blood, both in volume and in rate, is a function of the gradient of pressure that exists when blood leaves the capillaries to enter the venous system and of the cross-sectional diameter of the arterioles. As the lumen of the smaller vessels of the arterial tree diminishes, so the pressure drop across them is increased.[135]

The outflow of blood from the venous system varies with the cardiac output and this is very closely related to venous pressure. In this way a reduction in CVP produces a lowering of cardiac output unless, as in congestive cardiac failure, an overwhelming volume of blood is contained within the venous system, when a reduction in venous pressure results in an increase in cardiac output.[136]

The factors affecting venous pressure were reviewed by Landis and Hortenstine (1950),[99] and the use of venous pressure in a number of different clinical conditions has been discussed by Wilson *et al.* (1962).[161] Among the factors affecting pressure within the central venous system are the contractility of the veins, the pressure caused by skeletal muscle movement, the pressure of tissues surrounding the veins, the intrathoracic and intra-abdominal pressures (which vary with respiration), blood volume and capillary pressure. In clinical practice, therefore, measurements of CVP must be interpreted with these factors, which cause variation in its value, clearly in mind.

When cardiac failure and blood loss occur together, for example following trauma or open-heart surgery, measurement of CVP is of great value. As the blood volume is corrected the venous pressure rises, but the arterial pressure may not increase to a satisfactory level. If the arterial pressure alone is measured, there is a great danger that the volume of blood or fluid given will be too large and pulmonary oedema will be induced; cardiac failure does not need to be present for this to occur. The same situation can be observed following trauma when, in addition to blood loss into fracture sites or abdominal and thoracic cavities, the skull is fractured resulting in neurogenic (normovolaemic) shock. If CVP is not measured, excessive transfusion and lung damage can occur.

After trauma to the chest wall or following open-heart surgery, blood or fluid may collect within the pericardium and produce cardiac tamponade. This will normally cause a raised venous pressure. When cardiac tamponade is associated with a large volume of blood loss, a raised venous pressure is not found. Blood replacement is then accompanied by a dramatic rise in CVP without any rise in arterial pressure. A raised CVP also occurs together with hypotension in some cases of postoperative metabolic acidosis; the hypotension does not respond to blood transfusion. There is then the danger of over-transfusion which causes pulmonary oedema and extravasation of blood into the lungs. It is also important to note that when cardiac tamponade is present in combination with hypovolaemia so that the venous pressure is reduced, an increase in heart rate may be absent.

Complications of central venous pressure catheters

There are a number of complications associated with central venous pressure (CVP) measurement that, with care, can be avoided. The catheter can fracture and, if the distal portion comes to rest in the right atrium or ventricle, open-heart surgery becomes essential. If the CVP catheter becomes disconnected from the infusing fluid, massive air embolism can develop because of the negative intrathoracic pressure in the spontaneously breathing patient. A further complication is that of cardiac tamponade. The tip of an intravenous catheter can perforate the vein wall or right atrium. If the catheter is placed in a vein outside the pericardium, this may lead to a hydromediastinum or a hydrothorax. When the catheter is placed within the pericardial sac, cardiac tamponade can occur either within minutes following its insertion or many days later. The reports on 16 patients were reviewed by Greenall *et al.* (1975);[81] they found that 14 of these patients had died. The case history they reported was that of a 35-year-old man who developed cardiac tamponade 18 days after surgery and 8 days after the insertion of a second central venous catheter. At necropsy, the pericardium was distended with 400 ml of opaque yellow fluid, the composition of which was consistent with the parenteral diet that he was receiving.

Cardiac tamponade can largely be avoided by using a soft catheter and placing the tip of the catheter in the SVC proximal to the reflection of the pericardium. If the blood pressure falls and the venous pressure rises, infusion via the cannula should be stopped. The cannula should then be aspirated with a syringe, and failure to obtain a return of blood along the catheter is an absolute indication that the infusion should cease. If the catheter appears to be blocked, 2 ml of heparinized saline (2 drops of 5000 unit heparin in 10 ml of isotonic solution) should be used to free the end, and the aspiration should be repeated. If the free flow of blood backwards along the catheter is still not possible, the catheter should be withdrawn a short distance because it is possible that the tip is lodged against the internal surface of the vein. It is important that only a moderate degree of pressure is used during aspiration so that the intima is not damaged.

A CVP line can be inserted accidentally into the internal jugular vein. If the metal needle used for insertion has a bevel, then this should be turned medially after the subclavian vein has been punctured, and this helps to guide the plastic catheter away from the internal jugular vein. The placement of the CVP line in the internal jugular vein can be detected by placing a finger over the vein low down in the neck and applying pressure so that the vein is occluded. Following this manoeuvre a rise in CVP of 8 cmH$_2$O or more indicates the malpositioning of the catheter.

There is, however, in all these complications, no substitute for an immediate X-ray of the chest, and this should be mandatory when problems with the CVP line are suspected, and even when an X-ray has been taken only a few minutes earlier.

Changes in respiration

As haemorrhage progresses, the volume of blood within the pulmonary circulation falls as the total blood volume is reduced. The normal gravitational forces become of greater importance because blood is able to collect in the more dependent parts of the lungs as the pulmonary artery pressure diminishes. Some parts of the lungs are supplied with very little blood and in this way the respiratory physiological dead space is increased.

Hyperventilation is caused by the increase in the respiratory dead space, the reduction of pulmonary blood flow and the need to maintain the thoracic pump which, by its negative pressure, increases the venous return to the right side of the heart. The minute volume increases gradually as haemorrhage progresses until it is more than double the resting value. This degree of increase in ventilation leads to a marked rise in the ventilation–perfusion ($\dot{V}_A/\dot{Q}_C$) ratio described on page 139, because as the capillary blood flow per unit time ($\dot{Q}_C$) diminishes, the ratio becomes numerically greater, even in the absence of an increased volume of air per unit time ventilating the alveoli ($\dot{V}_A$).

When hyperventilation occurs as a result of blood loss, it is independent of acid–base changes in man. In a series of experiments it was also demonstrated that by infusing hypertonic solutions of saline or sodium bicarbonate when the pH of the circulating blood and ECF was either markedly alkaline, with a high pH and high bicarbonate concentration, or markedly acidotic, with a low pH and low bicarbonate concentration, an increase in ventilation occurred to the same degree. It was found that at the end of 90 minutes hypotension in dogs, an increase in the minute volume of 85% occurred when the dogs were acidotic and an increase of 90% occurred in the minute volume when the animals were made to have a high blood pH by the infusion of sodium bicarbonate. It was, therefore, demonstrated that forces other than acid–base balance determined the rate and degree of ventilation during and following haemorrhagic shock.[28,87,107] An inability to maintain adequate alveolar ventilation may occur in the following ways. If a metabolic acidosis arising from causes other than haemorrhagic shock is superimposed upon the condition, a state of central nervous system depression, similar to that described on page 137, may ensue. In these circumstances it may be necessary to infuse sodium bicarbonate to maintain ventilation. A case where this occurred in a patient with cirrhosis of the liver and oesophageal varices has been described by Brooks and Feldman (1962).[26]

A rapid transfusion of a large volume of acid-citrate-dextrose (ACD) blood may, in the severely acidotic patient, precipitate sudden respiratory failure and increase the hypotension. Large volumes of electrolyte-containing fluid, given at a rapid rate, may have a similar effect.[93]

Biochemical Changes in Haemorrhagic Shock

Many of the fundamental biochemical changes that occur during haemorrhagic shock have been known for some time. Their interpretation, however, has been the cause of much discussion and controversy. Some substances that have been incriminated in the cause of shock or irreversible shock have now been largely abandoned, but controversy still reigns over subjects such as acid–base balance, the repartitioning of the fluid within the tissue spaces, and the importance of the osmolality of tissue fluids. The pattern of biochemical change is in practice a very complex one and, because it is superimposed upon changes occurring within the neurological, cardiovascular, endocrine and respiratory systems, the significance of major changes tends to be obscured. If the circumstances are further complicated by the presence of circulating toxins, disease processes, anaesthesia, and positive pressure ventilation, then interpretation of events is made even more difficult. We shall, therefore, look at a number of biochemical changes in turn.

Acid–base changes

The presence of major alterations in the acid–base state following haemorrhage and shock has been recognized for a long time. In 1918, one year after Van Slyke produced his concept of CO_2 combining power or 'alkali reserve', Cannon et al.[34] demonstrated that soldiers wounded in the trenches developed a metabolic acidosis. They considered that treatment with sodium bicarbonate was beneficial and enthusiastically advocated that it should be given in all cases of shock, even when it could only be given orally.[33,34] Although this view had some impact at that time, it was soon forgotten when blood transfusion became more readily available. Experimental work at that time also was inconclusive as to the benefits of administering sodium bicarbonate. It is only recently that the findings in experimental animals are being compared with those obtained from shocked patients in whom other abnormal factors are superimposed upon blood loss. As haemorrhage progresses the bicarbonate ion concentration of the extracellular fluid (ECF) falls so that there is a decrease in the blood pH. Hyperventilation lowers the PCO_2 which in part compensates for this fall in pH. In this way the extremely low values of blood pH obtained when hyperventilation is prevented from occurring are not reached.

It is not possible to make serial estimations in man suffering from haemorrhagic shock because treatment is instituted as soon as it is recognized. It is possible, however, to reproduce these conditions experimentally. Figure 6.3 illustrates the findings in a dog which was kept hypotensive by

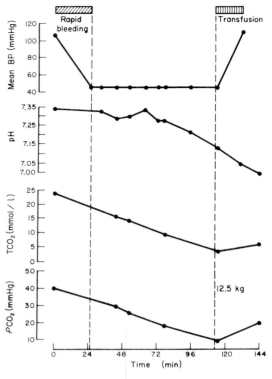

Fig. 6.3 The mean blood pressure, blood pH, total CO_2 (TCO_2) and partial pressure of CO_2 (PCO_2) in a dog subjected to haemorrhagic shock at a blood pressure of 40 mmHg. Note continued fall of pH as acid–citrate–dextrose (ACD) blood is returned to the animal. (Reproduced by permission of the *Lancet*.)[27]

bleeding into a reservoir for 90 minutes. The central arterial pressure was maintained at 40 mmHg. It can be seen that the pH, total CO_2 and PCO_2 fell throughout the whole of the 90-minute period. In the early stages of the hypotension the pH remained at relatively high levels because of respiratory compensation. Later, however, although there was an even greater increase in ventilation, the decrease in the metabolic component of acid–base balance (HCO_3^-) was so large that this was insufficient to maintain the pH at its previous values. A further point to note is that when the blood, which had been prevented from clotting by adding the same amount of acid-citrate-dextrose (ACD) solution that is used in clinical practice, was returned to the animal, little change in the metabolic component of acid–base balance was observed once the blood pressure had returned to normal values. Because the pH of the ACD blood was so low (in the region of 6.8), the pH of the blood within the animal fell even further. This is of immense importance when we consider the effects of transfusion with stored 'bank' blood in order to restore the blood pressure. It is one of the causes of irreversible shock and over-transfusion.

So far we have only considered the acid–base changes occurring in a person breathing spontaneously who is able to increase the respiratory rate and minute volume as haemorrhage progresses. In surgical practice, however, massive blood loss is encountered when a patient is being artificially ventilated, often at a constant rate by means of a mechanical ventilator. Under these circumstances a fall in PCO_2 does not occur as it is a function of ventilation. In practice it is found to remain constant when the ventilation is constant and may rise a little if there is a marked change in the respiratory physiological dead space. In these circumstances the pH of the blood falls to much lower levels, for example 6.5, and the oxygen saturation of both the arterial and venous blood is reduced unless very high concentrations of oxygen are supplied to the ventilating gases when the arterial oxygen saturation may increase, with little change in the venous oxygen saturation. Just as the arteriovenous difference in oxygen saturation increases with haemorrhage, so does the arteriovenous difference of pH and PCO_2. This is because of the reduced cardiac output and the decreased supply of circulating blood to the tissues (see Table 6.3). The very large arteriovenous difference of pH is greater during positive pressure ventilation than during spontaneous ventilation. In both man and animals, inadequate ventilation during haemorrhagic shock is lethal. When the arterial blood pressure is measured correctly and accurately, for example with a saline manometer, animals will not, as a rule, survive for 90 minutes when their blood pressure is kept at 40 mmHg and positive pressure ventilation is maintained. In addition to a reduction in the arterial oxygen saturation and pH values of the blood, the body temperature when measured in the rectum or oesophagus falls rapidly and death soon ensues. The same occurs in man. It is to be noted that the rate of onset of a metabolic acidosis and the degree to which it is produced for any given amount of blood loss is much greater when a constant rate of ventilation by means of a mechanical ventilator is performed at what are considered normal values for that size of patient. These values may be obtained, for example, from the nomogram devised by Radford (see p. 134), to maintain the PCO_2 of the normal patient at 40 mmHg. We have seen that this is an unnatural state of affairs during haemorrhagic shock, and to

this must be added impairment of cardiac output that must be produced by positive pressure ventilation under circumstances when the volume of blood in the pulmonary system and the pressure in the pulmonary artery are reduced.

Plasma sodium concentration

In all severe and prolonged haemorrhagic shock, the plasma sodium level falls. The degree of fall is largely dependent upon the volume of blood lost, the blood pressure and the duration of the hypotension. If the degree of blood loss is great so that a pressure of approximately 40–50 mmHg can be recorded in the central aorta, the onset of the fall of plasma sodium is early. If the blood loss is of such a degree that pressure in the central aorta is at 60 mmHg or above, a change in the plasma sodium may not be detected for some time and only becomes apparent when some degree of tissue damage has occurred as a result of hypotension or prolonged tissue anoxia. The more marked the tissue anoxia, the more marked the fall in serum sodium. It must be borne in mind that when we measure changes in the plasma this reflects changes that are occurring in the whole of the ECF. If we look at Figs. 6.4 and 6.5 we see the biochemical results from a dog who was kept at a central aortic blood pressure of 60 mmHg for many hours. Blood was drained from the left femoral artery into a reservoir so that it could be returned to the animal if the blood pressure fell below 60 mmHg and removed if it rose above this value. It is well known that after a period of time a condition known as irreversible shock develops so that all the blood lost by the animal can be returned without causing any rise in blood pressure. The transfusion of fresh blood obtained from a donor animal also has little effect in this respect. The phenomenon of experimental irreversible shock is discussed on page 159. It will be seen that in the initial stages of hypotension there was little change in the plasma [Na$^+$], until after approximately 150 minutes of haemorrhagic shock (175 minutes from the beginning of the experiment) had been experienced. There was then a marked fall in the plasma [Na$^+$] and this continued even when some of the blood that had been lost was returned to the animal. This blood contained NaCl, 167 mmol/l (mEq/l). The fall in plasma [Na$^+$] was temporarily checked when a large volume of the blood which had been lost was returned, but the downward trend of the [Na$^+$] continued and no rise was observed when almost all the blood had been replaced together with the ACD solution. The fall

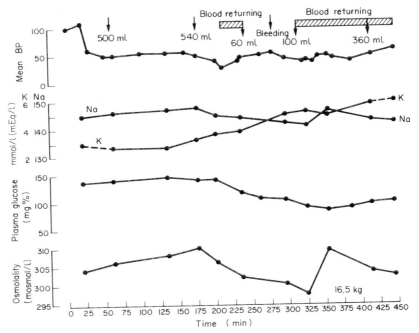

Fig. 6.4 Graph showing the mean blood pressure, plasma [Na⁺], [K⁺], glucose and osmolarity in a dog during prolonged hypotension. Blood was free to return to the animal when the blood pressure fell to low levels. Note the fall of plasma osmolarity after 175 minutes. BP = mean blood pressure measured using a catheter placed in the aorta with reference to the sternal angle. A pressure of 50 mmHg in this animal corresponded to a pressure in the central aorta of 62 mmHg. (Reproduced from *Anaesthesia*.)[28]

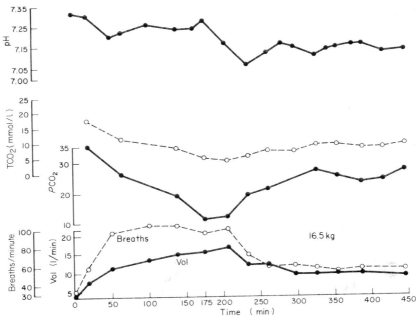

Fig. 6.5 Graph showing pH, TCO_2 and PCO_2, minute volume and respiratory rate in the same animal as in Fig. 6.4. Note the fall of osmolarity, pH, TCO_2 and PCO_2 precedes respiratory failure. (Reproduced from *Anaesthesia*.)[28]

in the plasma [Na$^+$] under these circumstances is, as we shall see later, associated with other biochemical changes, the onset of macroscopic tissue damage and the beginning of those conditions that go together to form the state of irreversible haemorrhagic shock. The decrease in the [Na$^+$] of the ECF may be as much as 10 mmol/l (mEq/l). This fall causes a decrease in the effective osmolality of the plasma and the interstitial fluid. Experimental and clinical evidence is accumulating that this is of importance in the prevention of tissue damage in the experimental animal and the protection of the kidney from acute tubular necrosis in man.

Plasma potassium concentration

In acute haemorrhagic shock of marked proportions the plasma [K$^+$] fluctuates in an unpredictable manner except when haemorrhage is accompanied by other disease processes and by anoxia. The general tendency, however, is for the plasma [K$^+$] to rise even in the absence of anoxia. When positive pressure ventilation at a constant rate is maintained the plasma [K$^+$] begins to rise after a relatively short period of haemorrhagic shock, even when oxygen is added to the inspired gases and only moderate desaturation of the arterial blood is present. It may, therefore, be related to the venous oxygen saturation, for when this is markedly reduced, in the region of 20% (PCO_2 40 mmHg), a marked rise in the plasma [K$^+$] rapidly follows. It can be inferred therefore that it is related directly to tissue anoxia and the exact exchange of K$^+$ for Na$^+$ is a subsidiary process. In Fig. 6.4 the gradual rise in the plasma [K$^+$] can be seen and this rise begins before the marked decrease in the plasma [Na$^+$]. Values for plasma [K$^+$] as high as 11 mmol/l (mEq/l) have been found in man after a period of haemorrhagic shock associated with respiratory inadequacy leading to anoxia. These levels are similar to those found following cardiac arrest. On the other hand, low plasma [K$^+$] are found in man after prolonged hypovolaemia, when the blood pressure is maintained at normal levels with large volumes of ACD blood, but, because of fibrinolysins, the patient continues to bleed. After 28 units (12.7 litres) of stored ACD blood one patient had a plasma [K$^+$] of 3.1 mmol/l (mEq/l). It would appear, therefore, that some K$^+$ enters the intracellular compartment.

Plasma glucose concentration

Glycosuria was observed by Goolden[78] in 1854, and the rise in plasma glucose concentration that followed haemorrhagic shock and other conditions was observed by Claude Bernard[14] in 1877. Hyperglycaemia was observed by Cannon in 1918, by Aub and Wu in 1920 and by Thomsen in 1938.[6,34,154] Thomsen found this to be more common below 30 years of age. During the Korean war, Howard[89] found that wounded soldiers had a diabetic response to glucose and that the decreased response to insulin roughly correlated with the extent of the injury.

In man the blood glucose concentration rises steeply as haemorrhage progresses, reaching values of 25 mmol/l (450 mg%) or more. The exact cause of this marked rise in plasma glucose is still obscure, but it is probably a response to adrenaline secretion causing glycolysis. It tends to compensate for the fall in plasma osmolality produced by the decrease in the plasma sodium concentration. 22 mmol/l (396 mg%) of glucose is osmotically equivalent to 11 mmol/l (mEq/l) of cation such as Na$^+$. Initially, the rise in blood glucose contributes to the low plasma [Na$^+$], as in diabetes. After a period of time the production of glucose becomes impaired and it is no longer possible to maintain raised levels in the ECF, and the plasma glucose concentration falls. This may be observed in the dog in Figure 6.4 where, in response to prolonged haemorrhage, the plasma glucose is maintained at a high level until the onset of the phase of irreversible shock. It then begins to fall steeply and does not rise very much even when glucose is infused in the form of ACD blood. An inability to raise the plasma glucose concentration by very much is seen in some elderly patients and sometimes in the newborn.

Hyperglycaemia has been reported in numerous other conditions, for example in burn shock. Evans and Butterfield[59] have described a condition of pseudodiabetes in which glycosuria and hyperglycaemia were present without ketonuria. Hyperglycaemia and glycosuria occur with acute anoxia. Loss of fluid from the ECF into the cells causes haemoconcentration so that initially the plasma osmolality is raised. The packed cell volume (PCV), plasma protein, plasma [K$^+$], and glucose concentration rise. The increase in blood glucose level is therefore exaggerated during this phase.

Plasma lactate concentration

In the absence of a large blood transfusion, when unmetabolized citrate may be present, the main cause of the decrease in plasma bicarbonate ion concentration is the accumulation of lactic acid. Repeated experiments in animals have demonstrated that when there is a fall in the [HCO$_3^-$]

there is an equivalent rise in lactic acid concentration (Table 6.4).

Table 6.4 The blood pH, TCO_2, PCO_2 and blood lactate concentration in a dog subjected to haemorrhagic shock taken at approximately 20-minute intervals

	pH	TCO_2 (mmol/l)	PCO_2 (mmHg)	Lactate (mmol/l)
I	7.36	22.5	41	3.2
II	7.31	18.8	36	5.9
III	7.32	15.6	30	10.4
IV	7.29	7.7	16	16.6
V	7.02	7.0	27	19.8
VI	7.16	6.9	18	19.2

Note how the rise in blood lactate concentration is quantitatively very similar to the fall in bicarbonate concentration.
pH = blood pH; TCO_2 = plasma total CO_2;
PCO_2 = plasma carbon dioxide tension.

Very high concentrations of lactate are found in the blood following a prolonged period of haemorrhage in man. These may not disperse completely for 24–48 hours. The lactacidosis, which persists long after the haemorrhage has been corrected, is of interest because its significance is still obscure. Lactacidosis, a plasma lactate level of 5–7 mmol/l (mEq/l), may also persist for some days after major surgery, especially open-heart surgery and hypothermia.

Plasma osmolality

We have seen how, in certain parts of the body, some cells have a raised osmotic pressure relative to the surrounding fluid. At the present time the main organs in which this is considered to occur are the tubules and surrounding tissues of the kidney. However, similar conditions may prevail in some of the specialized cells of the liver and perhaps the secreting layers of the gut. The main constituents which maintain the osmolality of the ECF are the sodium ions and the glucose content, which is not readily diffusible into the cells in the non-phosphorulated form. The plasma proteins contribute to the effective osmolality of the fluid within the vascular space, but when compared with the osmotic force exerted by glucose and electrolytes their influence is small. Nevertheless, even when the force they exert is of a minor degree, they control the movement of fluid between the vascular space and the interstitial fluid space. When we look at Fig. 6.4 we see that it is the very factors that contribute to raising the osmolality of the ECF that begin to fall after shock has continued for a period of time. This results in a

reduction in effective osmolality which precedes the onset of irreversible haemorrhagic shock. The association between the onset of tissue damage and the fall in the osmolality of the body fluids is of some significance. In 1963 it was also demonstrated that treatment with solutions which had twice the osmolality of plasma prevented tissue damage in dogs subjected to haemorrhagic shock, so that the blood pressure was maintained at 40 mmHg in the central aorta for 90 minutes. All the untreated animals developed haemorrhagic necrosis of the bowel and areas of degeneration in the liver and kidney and some subendocardial haemorrhages in the ventricles. All these were prevented when either 1.8% NaCl or 2.74% $NaHCO_3$ was infused throughout the experimental period; 10% glucose was less effective and isotonic solutions were of no value even when infused in excessive quantities. It became clear, therefore, that in the spontaneously breathing, shocked animal the osmolality of the tissues, rather than the acid–base state, was of prime importance in protecting vital organs from the tissue changes that accompanied profound haemorrhagic shock. This observation, of course, applied only to the fit healthy animal in which no extraneous disease processes were present. Since that time, much clinical evidence has been accumulated of the effectiveness of maintaining a raised osmotic pressure in the circulating plasma and ECF, in addition to the case quoted in the addendum to that report.[27] Patients undergoing emergency surgery for a leaking abdominal aneurysm have been treated with hypertonic saline, hypertonic sodium bicarbonate or the solution devised to correct the metabolic changes in shock with good results.

When these experiments were performed there was little evidence, except that indicated by Shires *et al.* (1960), that haemorrhagic shock was accompanied by contraction of the extracellular fluid space and that this contraction occurred when there was only a moderate degree of blood loss and hypotension was not a marked feature.[44,121,141,142] This work has led to the use of Ringer-lactate for the treatment of haemorrhagic shock by those working in Dallas, Texas. In the recommendations given in their paper, Brooks *et al.*,[27,28] recommended that, in addition to raising the osmolality of the ECF and correcting the acid–base deficit, it was probably necessary to provide fluid for expanding the volume of the extracellular fluid space so that fluids having twice the osmolality of plasma were recommended rather than solutions of greater tonicity. In addition, because it seemed that the blood sugar was always raised, the addition of this substance to the circulating blood might afford some benefit.

As a result of these biochemical findings, a solution was prepared[27] which was designed to maintain the osmolality of the extracellular fluids, correct the acidosis without producing a gross alkalosis, and supply sufficient water to meet the fluid requirements of the body, including that for expansion of the ECF. The solution contains:

$NaHCO_3$	166 mmol/l (mEq/l)	1.40 g%
NaCl	75 mmol/l (mEq/l)	0.44 g%
Glucose	21.2 g/l	2.12 g%
Osmolality	600 mosmol/l	

Some Aspects of Experimental Haemorrhagic Shock

The reports concerning the effects of haemorrhagic shock in man are by no means numerous. There are notable exceptions such as those of Beecher and his colleagues.[10] Most of the information that is published is derived from experiments on dogs and other animals. We have already examined the physiological changes that occur during the process of shock. It is, therefore, important to make clear from the very beginning that any experimental preparation is dependent upon a number of factors. For example, in some animal preparations the animals are anaesthetized and ventilated by means of a mechanical positive pressure ventilator. We have seen how this factor alone will modify the results of experiments by the influence of the inflation pressure upon venous return and lung capillary blood flow and, therefore, upon cardiac output. It is well recognized by people experienced in the field of experimentation that many of the anaesthetic agents used for animal work lower the blood pressure when used in therapeutic doses. It is therefore not uncommon for reports to be obtained from animals that have some degree of normovolaemic shock induced before haemorrhage. When an animal is anaesthetized in this way a smaller volume of blood loss is required in order to reduce the blood pressure to a given level than is required when an anaesthetic which does not induce hypotension is used.

Other factors which can make the interpretation of reports very difficult are blood pressure measurements which are inaccurate or which are made by manometric means, using a reference point that is either open to variation or is not readily definable. For example, if the blood pressure is measured from the sternal angle in a dog that has a large thorax, a much lower pressure will be recorded than if it is measured with reference to the central aorta. This latter site is less open to variation through a wide range of body weights. In their paper on experimental haemorrhagic shock, Brooks et al.[27] measured the central aortic blood pressure in three ways and obtained three different readings. The most accurate method at low pressures was a saline manometer where half an inch (1.27 cm) of saline is roughly equivalent to 1 mmHg pressure, but by accurate measurement and the use of conversion tables a precise measurement may be made at all times. An electrical transducer which was calibrated against a mercury manometer usually agreed with this reading to within 3 or 4 mmHg. It was also possible to measure the height of the column of blood in the cannula placed in the femoral artery and the animal could be bled to a preset pressure. It is this pressure which is reported in numerous publications, usually with reference to the sternal angle. Brooks et al. (1963)[27] found that this pressure could be 10 mmHg below that measured by the transducer or saline manometer. This demonstrated the fallacy of attempting to measure these very low levels of blood pressure through a cannula placed in a peripheral vessel. There are, however, many reports based on this form of measurement. It is of interest to note that when the blood pressure was measured accurately in the central aorta and the animals were subjected to a blood pressure of 30 mmHg they all died within very few minutes whether they breathed spontaneously or were artificially ventilated. Furthermore, when the blood pressure was raised to 40 mmHg many of the animals were able to survive for the period of hypotension even though irreversible tissue damage appeared sometimes before 30 minutes, but when these animals were ventilated artifically with a mechanical ventilator, once again all the animals died. These experiments illustrate the importance of accurately defining and measuring blood pressure and of reporting the method and type of ventilation used if comparable results are to be obtained by people working in different centres.

The experimental animal behaves very differently from man. Involvement of the bowel and liver is a characteristic tissue change in many of the animals used for investigations. The bowel does not appear to be affected in the same way in man in uncomplicated cases of haemorrhagic shock. However, in cases of haemorrhage and toxicity such as may be produced during surgical relief of bowel obstruction, the part played by the gut may be of extreme importance.[113]

Changes in cellular ultrastructure

Investigations have demonstrated that when tissue cells become anoxic, because of the impaired circulation, there is disruption of some subcellular particles. For example, the lysosomal membrane loses its continuity and hydrolytic enzymes including proteases, esterases and phosphatases are released. When these powerful agents are released intracellularly, they destroy the fine complex structure of the cell contents.[53]

The intracellular enzymes have been detected in the circulating blood after trauma and shock and may play a part in the problems of blood coagulation and tissue damage. Janoff et al.[92] found that animals made tolerant to shock, by graded exposure, had more stable lysosomes. This is of great therapeutic interest because Weissmann and Thomas (1962)[159] demonstrated that treatment with corticosteroids stabilized the lysosome membrane and prevented the release of the lysosomal enzymes.

Some Aspects of Haemorrhagic Shock in Man

If we bear in mind the great importance that the physiological and biochemical changes may have in the successful resuscitation of a patient, both in diagnosis and in treatment, the understanding of the sequence of events in widely different conditions is made very much easier. In subsequent pages we will examine haemorrhage of slow onset and gradually increasing severity, haemorrhagic shock which develops rapidly, septic shock caused by infections and shock caused by the release of fluid from a hydatid cyst. This last condition is similar to an anaphylactoid reaction. We must remember that factors such as simple dehydration, endocrine disturbances and cardiac failure, analgesic drugs and d-tubocurarine in large doses may cause hypotension by themselves and may be superimposed upon any other conditions we have to treat.

Slowly progressing haemorrhage in man

This form of haemorrhage is almost invariably 'internal'. It can arise from damage to a viscus such as the spleen, kidney, liver or gut. Superficial bruising may even be absent, for example after a car accident. Haemorrhagic shock of slow onset

also occurs from a bleeding peptic ulcer, when a malaena is often the first overt sign. A continuously bleeding tooth socket following an extraction may cause haemorrhagic shock of slow onset, and the patient may arrive in the emergency department of a hospital having bled continuously for many hours so that admission and blood transfusion are necessary. The author has treated one patient, a window cleaner, who fell 30 ft (9 m) to the ground after fainting. He had bled for 6 hours from a single tooth socket and the syncopal attack occurred before he had time to fasten his safety belt.

Signs and symptoms

When there is a slow continuous leak from a vessel so that blood is lost faster than it can be replaced, there is increasing pallor of the skin and of the lips. Both may appear grey as peripheral vasoconstriction develops. The finger tips and ear lobes become cyanosed. A tachycardia develops and the radial pulse is of poor volume and is usually described as being weak and thready. The blood pressure is usually either normal or only slightly reduced until the sudden onset of profound hypotension, which may be precipitated by a change of posture, a sudden increase in the rate of breathing, an increase in physical effort in order to gain assistance, or the sudden conscious awareness of being seriously ill. A high-pitched systolic murmur may be heard on listening to the heart. The rate of respiration slowly rises, but may be so gradual that it passes unnoticed until just before a syncopal attack occurs. There is a gradual onset of tiredness and lethargy followed by the development of undisguised weakness. It is at this stage that the patient may seek medical attention. It is not uncommon for a malaena to be passed or a haematemesis to occur just when the feeling of weakness becomes unbearable.

Case history. A lorry driver, 40 years of age, who took pride in keeping physically fit, had just completed loading his lorry 160 miles from London when a large bale of wool fell from the top. It hit him in the chest and abdomen so that he was knocked over onto the ground and stunned for a few seconds. He got up, drank a cup of tea and, accompanied by his co-driver, started on his journey towards London. He was in the habit of taking part of his physical exercise by swinging himself into the driving cabin from an overhead bar placed above the door instead of using the step provided. In order to demonstrate that all was well he did this before moving off. When he had travelled 60 miles he had a feeling of discomfort in his lower abdomen and a desire to micturate. He therefore stopped and was able to pass urine in the normal manner and of normal colour, but he was unable to defaecate. The small amount of physical exercise and movement appeared to alleviate the discomfort and made him feel much better and he ate a sandwich, but on getting back into the driving cabin did not feel strong enough this time to swing from the bar and climbed up in the normal manner. He drove on another 50 miles by which time he was feeling much weaker and more unwell, although the abdominal discomfort was no worse. He stopped the lorry again in order to drink some beer, but although his co-driver ordered a pint and drank it, he himself was unable to drink half that quantity. When they returned to the lorry his co-driver had this time to help him to climb into the driving cabin and from then on drive the lorry to London. When they arrived at their destination it was quite apparent to the co-driver that his friend was ill, and therefore without stopping to unload he drove towards the hospital. Before they arrived, however, the patient had a sudden desire to defaecate and on doing so passed frank blood.

On examination in hospital he was observed to be moderately dyspnoeic with extreme pallor, peripheral cyanosis and a blood pressure of 90/60 mmHg. He had moderate tenderness in the lower abdomen and relatively no guarding. At laparotomy it was found that his gut was ruptured at the rectosigmoid junction and that blood and gas had tracked retroperitoneally. He made an uneventful recovery following a temporary colostomy.

This typifies the gradual onset of haemorrhagic shock produced by the slow but continuous leakage of blood. The picture is, therefore, quite different from that found when a large volume of blood is lost rapidly.

Rapidly progressing haemorrhage in man

The physical signs depend upon the volume of blood that is lost over a given period. If a massive haemorrhage occurs within a few seconds, such as that which may follow the loss of a ligature over a pulmonary vessel or from a leaking abdominal aneurysm, then cardiac arrest may occur. It is not uncommon for a sudden massive haemorrhage to be followed by a complete cessation of respiration. The mechanism of this is not clear, but cardiac arrest or ventricular fibrillation must, under these circumstances, always follow unless assistance is at hand to apply artificial ventilation. This situation may arise, for example, following rupture of an abdominal aortic aneurism, although early surgery applied to small aneurisms can prevent this situation (Ruckley, 1985).[133] Under these circumstances it is necessary to institute the procedure for cardiac arrest (see Chapter 11) as well as to take steps to stop the flow of blood.[26]

If a large volume of blood is lost over a slightly longer period, then the physical signs are clearly discernible. There is pallor of the skin and tongue, the extremities are cold, there is peripheral cyanosis and the tongue is cyanosed; profuse sweating is present all over, as the sympathetic system is stimulated to maintain the circulation, and there is marked dyspnoea. Hyperventilation is the general accompaniment to massive blood loss. The blood and pulse pressures are reduced. The pulses at the wrist may be impalpable or difficult to feel, even at the brachium. The pulses over the femoral and carotid arteries are usually palpable but are of reduced volume. When a large volume of blood has been lost it may be impossible to measure the blood pressure by means of a sphygmomanometer. The intrinsic biochemical changes that are associated with haemorrhagic shock described by serial observations in the dog have also been found in isolated blood samples obtained from patients. These have an important influence upon the function of organs and the maintenance of the cellular integrity of tissues. In some cases these changes in biochemistry may be made worse by the transfusion of ACD or CPD blood when restoration of blood volume has been delayed for some time.

Care of a Patient with Haemorrhagic Shock

In clinical practice, patients who require treatment for acute haemorrhage fall into two main groups. The first group includes those patients who have experienced trauma, usually of an accidental nature, and have suffered blood loss while breathing spontaneously. The second group comprises those who have experienced unavoidable blood loss during a surgical procedure and are therefore almost always being artificially ventilated. We shall deal with the two groups in turn.

Haemorrhage during spontaneous ventilation

Trauma is one of the major causes of death, being exceeded only by cancer and diseases of the cardiovascular system. Deaths from road accidents increase yearly, and as buildings grow in number and in height, so there are more fatal falls amongst the people building them. Sometimes there are no superficial signs following a road accident when there is severe damage to a viscus. This can include a ruptured spleen, a lacerated kidney, liver or even pancreas, rupture of the small bowel, colon or stomach, with or without tearing of the mesentery. Sometimes there is rupture of the bladder. Occasionally, severe contusion of the bladder may give rise to haematuria even when true rupture is not present. Haemorrhage into the stomach may also occur from contusion and be associated with acute dilatation so that a large volume of blood of 4 or 5 litres may be contained within it. In this way the volume of blood that it is necessary to transfuse may be severely underestimated. The author has seen one patient in whom the diagnosis of intragastric bleeding was not made until it was too late. It is, therefore, always wise to pass a stomach tube following suspected trauma to the abdomen, especially in cases of unexplained hypotension associated with tachycardia, cyanosis, tachypnoea and sweating.

Any fracture site involving any bone may contain as much as 1 litre of blood. Multiple fractures almost always lead to hypovolaemia, the degree depends upon the severity of the fracture, the amount of movement that has been permissible following the accident, and the length of time since the fracture occurred. Damage to the skeletal system has its most profound effect in producing hypotension in those groups of people who are least well able to compensate for a change in blood volume. These include the elderly, people with concomitant disease processes, especially of the cardiovascular system and respiratory system, and people who are anaemic.

We have seen how spontaneous ventilation plays a large part in compensating for the effects of a reduction in blood volume. Damage to the thoracic cage may itself limit ventilation to such an extent that gas exchange is impaired and the thoracic pump producing its negative pressure is unable to function adequately. Injury to the lung may produce a pneumothorax, sometimes with extravasation of blood into the thoracic cavity (a haemopneumothorax). When this occurs, compensatory changes of respiration are impaired and the degree of shock is more profound.

Immediate requirements
When the severely injured person is first seen, the skin will be pale and, when there is major blood loss, the lips, finger tips, ear lobes, tongue and nose will be cyanosed. At this stage it is difficult to know whether this cyanosis is entirely due to inadequate tissue perfusion alone or whether inadequate ventilation is also a cause. In some cases blood from an arterial puncture revealing either full oxygenation or desaturation of the arterial blood is required to allow a true diagnosis to be made. It is therefore important to examine the respiratory excursion. In some cases violent agonal movements will result from anoxia, and this may be diagnosed by attendants as restlessness resulting from pain, anxiety and terror or a result of brain damage. When these movements are because of anoxia they disappear once inadequate ventilation is treated. It is important to make sure of the correct diagnosis because if at this stage morphine is given in large doses, the hypotension may be exacerbated and the respiration further depressed.

Expired air resuscitation (mouth-to-mouth ventilation, see p. 392) should not be confined to cases of cardiac arrest. It is a valuable means by which cardiac arrest may be prevented.

It is, however, important to relieve pain. If a patient has to be moved in order to obtain medical care, broken limbs should be immobilized as much as possible. This is of greater importance than giving analgesic drugs which may take some time to act, and in any case they should be administered to the shocked patient in relatively small quantities until expert medical care is at hand. Following the use of analgesic drugs, even greater care and attention must be given to the maintenance of adequate ventilation. The transfer of the patient from the site of injury to hospital must be performed in such a way that there is the minimum of pressure to sites of injury and the minimum movement of broken limbs. Once in hospital, and the techniques of intravenous infusion and artificial ventilation are available, analgesic drugs can be given in greater quantities and, once the processes for the relief of hypovolaemia and the effects of blood loss are in motion, the opening of wounded areas and the setting of limbs in plaster, even of a temporary nature, become of primary importance. This is so that the patient can be turned and moved for nursing procedures without increasing the degree of pain. Anyone who has experienced a broken limb will well appreciate the relief that is obtained once it has been immobilized or placed in a well-padded plaster.

Treatment of blood loss
The same basic biochemical changes are found whether the blood is lost from a superficial wound

and frank bleeding can be observed, or when blood is lost internally into fracture sites, the peritoneal or thoracic cavities, into the lumen of the gut or into the areas of severely bruised muscle tissue that may be present. When the blood is examined it will be found that the [Na$^+$] has fallen, the [K$^+$] probably risen a little, the [HCO$_3^-$] undergone a marked fall and that there has been a rise in blood sugar. Lactic acid concentrations will have risen to an amount equal to the fall in the bicarbonate ion concentration. If the thorax has not been damaged and ventilation not impaired, increase in respiratory rate will have reduced the PCO_2. This last factor will modify the degree of reduction in pH which accompanies the induced metabolic acidosis. The packed cell volume (PCV) will be either unchanged or reduced a little. Even in the absence of damage to the renal apparatus, urine flow will have ceased.

It is now the duty of the clinician to do two things: (a) to correct the biochemical changes that are associated with hypovolaemic shock, and (b) to repair the hypovolaemia as rapidly as possible.

In all cases of haemorrhagic shock there is never any excuse for not setting up an intravenous drip with whatever fluid there is available, but preferably using electrolyte solutions of increased tonicity. All patients who have a low blood pressure following trauma will require transfusion, and while blood is being taken for cross-matching and grouping it is possible to set up an infusion intravenously. Ideally, a solution such as that described on page 189 should be given, but this requires careful preparation and may not always be available. As a second choice, sodium bicarbonate, having twice the osmolality of plasma, 2.74%, should be given in volumes of 1 unit (540 ml) to a shocked patient in the first instance. When there is a marked fall in blood pressure this solution may be run in rapidly. If further bleeding is not occurring, then this solution alone, by its expansion of the ECF, will tend to raise the blood pressure. If bleeding persists and hypotension continues, a further unit of the hypertonic solution (540 ml) may be given with good effect. This should be followed by transfusion of blood wherever possible, but if this is delayed, a plasma expander such as Hemaccel in 0.9% saline or dextran 6% in 0.9% saline can be given. These solutions are highly effective in restoring blood volume.

Blood transfusion

In the fit healthy patient with unimpaired ventilation, the transfusion of an adequate volume of blood will very quickly restore the arterial blood pressure to its normal value. If, therefore, only a short time has elapsed between the onset of haemorrhage and its treatment, blood transfusion alone will suffice to return the arterial blood pressure and the body biochemistry to normal values. It must be remembered that in this sort of circumstance a relatively small volume of transfused blood will produce a marked rise in blood pressure long before the blood volume has been restored. The central venous pressure (CVP) if measured at this time will still be low, even though a prehaemorrhage value for arterial pressure is repeatedly obtained. This is because the compensating systems of vasoconstriction are still present. Any further haemorrhage, however, is followed by a profound fall in arterial blood pressure. During this period of partial blood volume replacement, the arteriovenous differences in oxygen saturation do not return to their prehaemorrhage values, although some rise in venous oxygen saturation is observed. Also the rate at which other biochemical changes are improved is slowed. If further haemorrhage is superimposed upon these long-standing biochemical changes without the protective influences of a corrected acid–base state and hyperosmolality of the ECF, tissue damage in the form of tubular necrosis and the production of fibrinolysins is more likely to occur.

Let us turn now to the aspects of stored bank ACD and CPD blood. Two forms of stored bank blood are available: that in which the anticoagulant is acid-citrate-dextrose (ACD) and the other in which the anticoagulant is citrate-phosphate-dextrose (CPD). The most commonly used bank blood is prevented from coagulating by means of 120 ml of acid-citrate-dextrose (ACD) solution. Although this volume of liquid assists in the expansion of the ECF, only a small fraction of it is available for expansion of the intravascular space. It is therefore essential that in any assessment of blood loss this volume should be subtracted from the volume of bank blood transfused. To determine the volume of whole anticoagulated blood which will effectively expand the vascular compartment, 1 unit (500 ml) of blood has to be estimated as being 380 ml when ACD blood is transfused, and 400 ml when CPD blood is transfused. This is of major importance when the blood loss, as measured from a chest drain into an underwater seal bottle, or similar device, has to be replaced. The rate at which the anticoagulation fluid equilibrates with the rest of the ECF after entry into the vascular space is extremely rapid, and equilibration with the rest of the body water contained within the cellular compartment also occurs at a fast rate.

Even when prolonged major blood loss is followed by rapid transfusion, it must be assumed that blood alone is lost from the body and the water containing electrolytes is retained. The transfusion of 8 units of blood involves the addition to the body of approximately 1 litre of isotonic saline administered as anticoagulant fluid. More correctly the anticoagulant fluid should in the long term be considered to be isotonic $NaHCO_3$ because the citrate is converted into HCO_3^-. Approximately 24 hours after a massive transfusion, the plasma $[HCO_3^-]$ is raised.

The pH of stored bank blood is approximately 6.8, and after prolonged storage it is in the region of 6.5. The bicarbonate ion concentration varies between 15 mmol/l (mEq/l) when it is fresh and 5 mmol/l (mEq/l) or less when it has been stored for 2 or 3 weeks. It can thus be seen that even when it is freshly taken, a large transfusion of ACD blood will contribute to the metabolic acidosis. It is also apparent that a very large transfusion will dilute the existing bicarbonate content of the ECF so that further transfusion makes the situation worse rather than better. It has been shown that a metabolic acidosis in itself will produce hypotension because of a fall in cardiac output. When this occurs the transfusion of further quantities of blood produces a lowering of blood pressure instead of a rise. If the clinician is unaware of this, he will interpret the situation as being a result of hypovolaemia, and gross overtransfusion can occur. In this situation the venous pressure may be raised, but in the severely injured patient might well pass unnoticed unless special care is taken. Because there is an inadequate cardiac output, the peripheral cyanosis is maintained and a syndrome similar to that described following anaesthesia (see p. 137) develops. When a patient has been overtransfused, haemorrhagic pulmonary oedema develops. A frothy bloodstained sputum is found in the bronchial tree. The cyanosis found peripherally increases in intensity. This is because the oxygen saturation of the arterial blood falls markedly even when ventilation of the lungs is maintained with pure oxygen. Patients rarely recover when there is marked parenchymatous lung damage resulting from overtransfusion. For this reason the greatest care should be taken to avoid this situation developing. The importance of infusing hypertonic sodium bicarbonate solution in the early stages of haemorrhagic shock cannot, therefore, be stressed excessively.

The action of citrate in the ACD solution is to neutralize the effect of ionized calcium so that the processes of coagulation cannot proceed. There is approximately twice the volume of solution present within the container that is required for anticoagulation because this facilitates the taking of blood from donors while avoiding the production of clots. In every container, therefore, there is an excess of free citrate. In this way the ionized Ca^{++} of the circulating blood may be reduced if blood transfusion is rapid. The contractility of the myocardium is influenced by the ratio of the concentrations of Ca^{++} and K^+. If the calcium ion concentration of the circulation is reduced, then myocardial function is impaired. If, therefore, it is necessary to infuse a unit of blood in less than 5 minutes, it is essential that each unit should be accompanied by the intravenous injection of either 5 ml of 10% calcium gluconate or 5 ml of 10% calcium chloride. Probably, only 7 ml of 10% $CaCl_2$ is required, but in clinical practice a slight excess of calcium ions appears to be beneficial. The latter preparation provides a higher concentration of Ca^{++}. When large transfusions are given and there is some impairment of hepatic function, it is sometimes necessary to administer calcium salts when large volumes of blood are given at a much slower rate. Both calcium gluconate and calcium chloride are highly effective in improving cardiac output and raising the blood pressure when body temperature is reduced. They may, however, be ineffective in the presence of a gross metabolic acidosis when they may produce no effect at all or may raise the blood pressure for only a few seconds. An abrupt rise of blood pressure is followed immediately by an abrupt fall.

The potassium concentration of the plasma fraction of stored blood rises very soon after storage and increases further as time passes.[138] Even after 48 hours, the plasma $[K^+]$ may be 11 mmol/l. When this is transfused into a patient, the plasma $[K^+]$ does not rise to a degree that would be expected from this level of cation found in stored blood. This may be because the K^+ returns to the red cell on rewarming, but most probably because it is taken up by certain organs within the body. Although a raised $[K^+]$ has often been incriminated as a cause of cardiac arrest during massive transfusion, a much more common cause is a gross metabolic acidosis and citrate intoxication. In any case, both these factors contribute to and exacerbate any degree of K^+ intoxication. The greater the degree of either respiratory or metabolic acidosis, the higher the plasma K^+ concentration following transfusion. It is also raised by injury to tissues.

In addition to the free citric acid that is present in stored ACD blood, there is a high concentration of lactic acid. This in part depends upon the content and degree of oxygenation of blood when it is first taken and also upon the length of time it has been stored. In the condition of haemorrhagic shock when the lactic acid level of the circulating blood is already raised, this free acid contributes to the degree of metabolic acidosis. Similar changes occur with CPD (citrate-phosphate-dextrose) blood. The plasma [K$^+$] of CPD blood rises with storage, and samples of CPD blood examined at 21 days gave values of 9–17 mmol/l (mEq/l).[118]

To summarize, therefore, the metabolic effects of blood transfusion are as follows:

1. the addition of 120 ml of water which must be added to the fluid balance chart (100 ml in the case of CPD blood);
2. the addition of varying quantities of K$^+$;
3. the infusion of lactate (as well as citrate) which produces an initial fall in the plasma [HCO$_3^-$] followed by a rise in plasma [HCO$_3^-$] when these acids are metabolized;
4. a decrease in the ionized plasma [Ca^{++}].

The care of the patient who has undergone trauma and a fall in circulating blood volume should be based on the physiological principles we have examined. The following case illustrates the steps that can be taken following severe trauma.

Case history. A woman of 75 years was hit by a car. In addition to superficial bruising of the abdomen and elsewhere, she also suffered a Colles' fracture of one wrist, a fracture of the shaft of the radius in the opposite arm and fractures of the tibia and fibula of one leg. On admission to hospital she was hyperventilating and her systolic blood pressure was 75 mmHg. While blood was being taken for grouping and cross-matching her blood pressure fell to 60 mmHg and an intravenous drip was set up through the same needle so that twice normal sodium chloride could be infused. Her condition was so poor that she was considered unfit for anaesthesia so that when 500 ml of 1.8% saline had been infused over a period of 20 minutes and her blood pressure had risen to 75 mmHg she was given 50 mg of pethidine (Demerol) i.v. The 1.8% NaCl was replaced with Dextraven 6% in 0.9% saline and the blood pressure rose to 80 mmHg when 200 ml of this solution had been infused. A further 50 mg of pethidine (Demerol) was given i.m. Under the analgesic action of pethidine, the lower limb fracture was reduced and set in plaster. The fractured radius was similarly treated with a subjective improvement in the degree of pain experienced. The blood pressure, however, had once again fallen to below 70 mmHg systolic and a second

bottle of 6% Dextraven 0.9% saline was begun. The blood pressure then rose above 80 mmHg. The wrist which had suffered the Colles' fracture was then cleansed with alcohol and the haematoma injected with 2% procaine (HCl). After a few minutes, when it had been ascertained that no pain followed pressure over the fracture site, the Colles' fracture was reduced and the wrist supported by means of a padded plaster slab. The blood pressure had not risen above 85 mmHg and she was, therefore, transfused quickly with 2 units of ACD blood. The blood pressure rose to 110 mmHg following this transfusion and a further 2 units were infused over the next 2 hours, when the blood pressure rose to 140/90 mmHg. The following morning only a small volume of urine was passed (200 ml), but the specific gravity of this urine was 1.026. This demonstrated that, in spite of a prolonged period of hypotension, renal function was not impaired. She made a relatively rapid recovery without complications.

This case is of interest because the prolonged period of hypotension which responded to intravenous fluid is the sort of circumstance in which acute tubular necrosis is to be expected. It is to be noted, however, that pain might also have contributed to the degree of hypotension and that, therefore, an element of normovolaemic shock may also have been present. Intravenous pethidine (Demerol) especially will also produce a lowering of blood pressure and this is another form of hypotension which may be induced in a patient with a normal blood volume. However, experience has shown that the combination of hypotensive agents and hypovolaemia can cause a severe acute renal failure. The infusion of hypertonic solutions followed by a plasma expander containing an adequate concentration of electrolyte, followed by blood transfusion was sufficient to protect the kidneys from the effects of hypotension.

Haemorrhagic shock during controlled ventilation

We have seen how it is impossible to mimic exactly spontaneous ventilation when intermittent positive pressure ventilation is used (see p. 177). This method of inflating the lungs tends to impair the venous return and reduce cardiac output, although in part this may be overcome by means of a negative pressure phase on the ventilator. Even when the blood volume is normal, there is a limit to the assistance a negative pressure phase can give, and when the pulmonary artery pressure is low the effect of the inflation pressure is increased both in degree and in the length of time occlusion of the capillaries occurs. We have also seen how positive pressure ventilation during haemorrhagic shock causes anoxia so that the arterial oxygen saturation falls even when breathing oxygen, and the already increased arteriovenous difference is further widened. If a constant ventilation is maintained in dogs who have been bled in such a way that an accurately measured central aortic pressure of 40 mmHg is obtained, the majority of dogs will die within a 90-minute period. This tendency to die within this relatively short period can be prevented by raising the blood pressure to 60 mmHg. At this new and raised pressure the oxygen tension and saturation of the arterial blood is, however, increased only by a little, even when breathing oxygen.

We have also seen how haemorrhagic shock occurring in the spontaneously breathing subject causes hyperventilation with a resultant lowering of the PCO_2. If, before producing haemorrhage, an animal is ventilated in such a way that the PCO_2 is maintained at 40 mmHg and this constant artificial ventilation is maintained, when hypotension is induced by means of haemorrhage, the PCO_2 remains relatively constant throughout the period of hypotension. It may rise a little initially, for example from 40 mmHg to 45 or 50 mmHg, but no tendency to fall can be found. The arteriovenous difference of PCO_2 and PO_2 is much greater during ventilation with a mechanical ventilator than during spontaneous ventilation and this can be interpreted as being caused by an impaired cardiac output and, therefore, further impairment of tissue perfusion.

The packed cell volume (PCV) of the circulating blood has less tendency to fall, and in some cases terminally to rise, following haemorrhage. The greater the degree of tissue anoxia, the higher the PCV. This indicates a shift of fluid from the extracellular to the intracellular space. The fall of plasma [Na^+] which was detected in the spontaneously breathing animal occurs much more rapidly in the animal that is being artificially ventilated, but later, when there is a rise in PCV, the plasma [Na^+] together with the plasma [K^+] and protein concentration rise. Conversely, the rise in blood sugar is less marked, except for the initial period when it may rise to levels which are higher than would be expected in the animal undergoing haemorrhagic shock during spontaneous ventilation. This might indicate that the reserve of glycogen in the body are more rapidly depleted than during spontaneous ventilation. A marked fall in body temperature also occurs.

Particulate matter in stored blood

In 1961, during studies to measure blood viscosity, Swank discovered that a very high pressure was needed to force stored blood through a 20-μm metal mesh screen. The normal constituents of blood are usually no greater than 15 μm. He therefore concluded that the raised pressure was due to microaggregates in the blood that had accumulated during storage. He perfected a method based on this observation for measuring the quantity of microaggregates present.[149,152] Since then, improved electronic methods have been developed.[164]

It was demonstrated that microaggregates were lower in the venous line of a pump oxygenator during perfusion than in the arterial line, and it was concluded that this was due to filtration by the patient's tissues. Numerous studies have demonstated the cerebral and sometimes lethal effects of microaggregates during extracorporeal circulation. The benefits of the Swank disposable filter (Fig. 6.6) have also been clearly demonstrated.[1,4,8,16,54–56,83–85,125,129,145,146]

It is however, during the rapid blood replacement for conditions other than extracorporeal circulation that the correct filtration of stored blood becomes of the greatest importance, especially when the volume of blood transfused, due to trauma or surgery, is large. In 1966, Blaisdell et al.[15] reported that pulmonary microembolism was a major cause of lung pathology and death in patients who had vascular surgery. It was also found that soldiers from the Vietnam War, who received excellent surgery, died later from pulmonary insufficiency following massive blood transfusions.[109,111,112,114] It was also demonstrated that there was a correlation between the quantity of microaggregates and the oxygen tension of the arterial blood.[112,119] The smaller the total volume of blood transfused, the less the degree of pulmonary damage.[30] The rate of resolution of pulmonary damage was also more rapid. It is not surprising, therefore, that the use of micropore filters in trauma units has resulted in a reduction of pulmonary complications.[132]

The use of micropore filters for blood transfusion

In stored blood the accumulation of particulate matter consisting of platelets, white cells and fibrin deposits (microaggregates) was reported in 1940, and the effect upon the encephalogram was reported in 1948. The lack of evidence with regard to the quantity present or to the harmful effects, and the many patients receiving large volumes of blood with no apparent ill effects, led to the view that

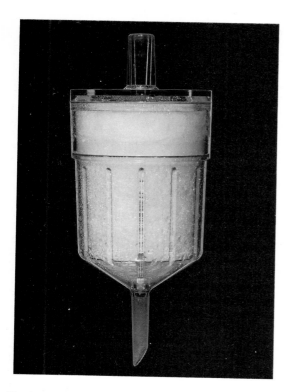

Fig. 6.6 A model of a Swank micropore filter which is used to remove the micro-aggregates in stored blood when it is necessary to transfuse a large volume of blood.

a filter with a pore size of 125–250 μm was satisfactory.

It is now well established that both ACD and CPD blood, stored at 4°C, accumulate microaggregates[2,3,70,71,103,109,111,112] that vary in size between 15 and approximately 200 μm. The longer the period of storage, the greater the size and number of microaggregates.[48,49]

During the first week of storage, the aggregates consist mainly of platelets. Later, the granulocytes lose their cell membranes and adhere to the platelets.[97] Fibrin is then precipitated out of solution onto the pre-existing white cell–platelet aggregates. Even after filtration through a 170 μm filter in a blood giving-set, the presence of up to 100 000 aggregates per millilitre has been demonstrated using a Coulter counter.[40,117]

Various filters have been devised,[39,41,43,128,150,151] but that designed by Swank, using a Dacron wool filter, has gained widespread acceptance.

Care of the patient with severe haemorrhage during surgery

It is, of course, impossible to reproduce those conditions in man that can be observed in the experimental animal; but examination of physiological changes in man described on page 191 indicate that a patient undergoing surgery with positive pressure ventilation must be treated differently during haemorrhagic shock from patients undergoing surgery where blood loss is not a prominent factor. We have seen how a relatively small fall in blood volume is of great importance during positive pressure ventilation, whereas a relatively large volume of blood loss can be tolerated when a patient is breathing spontaneously. This intolerance to blood loss during positive pressure ventilation results in a much more marked change in the body biochemistry. In the first place it is necessary to increase ventilation and the oxygen tensions of the anaesthetic gases.

The lungs should be ventilated in such a way that there is the minimum impairment of capillary blood flow and the inflation pressure must therefore be kept as low as possible, while maintaining adequate alveolar ventilation. This may be achieved by inflating the lungs by hand instead of with an automatic ventilator and following a similar pattern of tidal volume to that occurring in spontaneous ventilation. For example, the compression of the rebreathing bag can be performed so that one in five compressions supplies a large tidal volume and the lungs are fully expanded and this is followed by four rapid compressions of the rebreathing bag so that a small tidal volume of low inflation pressure is supplied to the patient.

During a surgical procedure, blood replacement must keep pace with blood loss as any tendency to fall behind will rapidly produce the very changes that lead to the onset of irreversible shock and tissue damage. Furthermore, during prolonged and continuous blood loss, the changes in body biochemistry should be corrected before they become detectable by blood analysis. The metabolic acidosis requires correction from an early stage if impairment of cardiac output is to be prevented. Adequate amounts of Ca^{++} must also be given in the form of calcium gluconate or calcium chloride. It is necessary to give 5 ml of the 10% solution for every unit of blood transfused. It is also essential to raise the osmolality of the ECF and expand the volume of this compartment. If problems arising from this cause are to be avoided, either hypertonic sodium bicarbonate or hypertonic sodium chloride should be infused from the moment that severe blood loss is detected. Following the operation when the incisions are closed and the anaesthetic is terminated, the results of prolonged tissue anoxia may once again become manifest as equilibration of the intracellular products with the ECF takes place. When there is a major biochemical change in the body as a whole so that many aspects are altered, even a moderate deficit of base may have profound physiological effects. This can result in inadequate ventilation and hypotension. The arterial oxygen saturation then falls and the PCO_2 rises. This has been referred to as secondary CO_2 retention.[26] It is then necessary to infuse hypertonic sodium bicarbonate solution in order to revert the condition of apparent neostigmine-resistant curarization. Although sodium bicarbonate solution having twice the osmolality of plasma (2.74 or 2.8% $NaHCO_3$) is suitable for this purpose, solutions of greater tonicity are also effective; however expansion of the ECF with water is not then as readily available as when the more dilute solutions are used. In practice, however, at this stage of the operation when adequate volumes of fluid have been infused and there is a large volume of water available from the ACD solution of stored blood, this factor is of relatively less importance, and 4.2% or 8.4% $NaHCO_3$ should be given.

Case history. A 36-year-old male patient, weighing 77 kg, underwent a thoracotomy for exploration of the thoracic aorta. He was grossly hypertensive prior to surgery, and had undergone unilateral nephrectomy at the age of 10 for parasitic infiltration of one kidney.

An aneurysmal dilatation of part of a thoracic aorta was found on the posterior aspect of the vessel. The aneurysm was filled with clot but had been leaking slowly in one part. It was therefore decided to plicate the aneurysmal sac so as to prevent rupture at a later date. Although this was performed successfully the vessel was entered at one point with consequent major blood loss which was replaced as quickly as possible. For a short period of time, however, it was impossible to maintain a normal blood volume. In addition to 5 ml calcium gluconate given with every unit of blood, 1 unit (540 ml) of 2.74% sodium bicarbonate solution was infused. During part of this time the blood pressure was unrecordable. At the end of the operation when the patient was slightly hypotensive and failed to breathe spontaneously, demonstrating the syndrome described on page 137, a further 200 ml of 2.74% sodium bicarbonate was infused with good effect so that spontaneous ventilation returned and the blood

pressure rose. The patient was returned to bed and the blood analysis at that time showed the following:

Na^+	129 mmol/l (mEq/l)
K^+	4.7 mmol/l (mEq/l)
pH	7.27
$[HCO_3^-]$	21.1 mmol/l (mEq/l)
and PCO_2	47 mmHg

The patient was breathing spontaneously.

The blood sugar was 6.7 mmol/l (120 mg%). During the subsequent days the patient became extremely jaundiced and produced a dilute urine, specific gravity 1.009, the volume approximately 500–600 ml. The blood urea, therefore, rose. During the next 3 days the jaundice deepened and a more profuse urine of low specific gravity (1.010) containing large quantities of sodium and potassium was passed. This low specific gravity urine represented the diuretic phase of acute renal failure (see p. 110). The bicarbonate ion concentration of the plasma also fell and this was an additional indication of acute or parenchymatous liver damage. The diagnosis of hepatorenal syndrome was therefore made. Although this is a condition of very poor prognosis, it was decided to infuse hypertonic solutions, so that the potential electrolyte deficiencies arising from renal loss were made good, the osmolality of the ECF was raised and the deficit of HCO_3^- was repaired. In order to assist in the maintenance of liver function and reduce the blood urea concentration, hypertonic glucose (dextrose) and fructose (laevulose) were also infused. A regimen for the treatment of anuria similar to that described on page 107 was instituted. The solutions used were 2.74% $NaHCO_3$ with the addition of KCl, 20% dextrose and 20% laevulose. After a period of 3 weeks the jaundice had disappeared and the kidneys began to concentrate so that the specific gravity of the urine rose and the blood urea which had already fallen during the diuretic phase more nearly approached normal values. The patient then made a successful recovery.

This patient illustrates a case in which the replacement of hypertonic solutions during the operative procedure was insufficient to compensate for the fall in osmolality that was produced. In this case only a small rise of blood sugar occurred so that the temporary benefit which a rise in blood sugar concentration affords during haemorrhage was not available. The maintenance of a hypertonic regimen in a potentially lethal condition, together with correction of the acidosis and treatment of the renal failure, appeared to be of benefit. One can speculate that the onset of jaundice resulting from parenchymatous liver damage acquired as a result of blood loss during surgery may also result because of the influence that a fall in the osmolality of the ECF may have upon the cells of the liver. Further work, however, is required to establish this point.

Stress Ulceration

Probably the most common cause of stress ulceration today is prolonged artificial ventilation of the lungs, but historically it is associated with burns. Stress ulceration is known to follow all forms of trauma and major surgery, especially when recovery from the condition is slow. Successful surgical procedures are frequently vitiated by uncontrollable haemorrhage from the gastro-intestinal tract.[62] It is a common cause of sudden hypovolaemic shock.

Although acute gastro-intestinal ulceration was documented in 1842 by Curling, who described a discrete ulcer on the anterior wall of the duodenum, which could perforate in addition to causing haemorrhage, we now know that ulceration can occur almost anywhere in the gut.[45,130,139] It is almost always associated with profound pathophysiological changes in the patient prior to the onset.[100]

Stress ulceration, therefore, is associated with a number of different conditions which include burns, trauma, surgery, respiratory failure, central nervous system abnormalities, sepsis, myocardial failure, jaundice and poliomyelitis.[62,82,110,137]

Curling's publication reported ulceration occurring in four people from a series of 10 who had suffered burns. In 1969, a syndrome of respiratory failure, hypotension, sepsis and jaundice, which was associated with lethal haemorrhage from acute gastro-intestinal ulceration, was reported by Skillman et al.[143] Since that time, however, clinicians have become aware, when they have treated a large number of patients in intensive care wards who have developed respiratory failure (often following open-heart surgery), that stress ulceration can develop when the only pathology present is failure of gas exchange in the lungs.[22,23] In the past this has sometimes led to total gastrectomy, but the association of widespread sepsis and jaundice is not an essential concomitant of this condition.

Stress ulceration is associated with a high mortality. A review of the published reports of

Curling's ulcer in 1938 by Harkins,[82] indicated that out of 107 patients, 94 had died and only 13 had recovered. He was able to correlate the severity of the burn and the association of sepsis with the severity and degree of ulceration.

The aetiology of the condition, however, has not been firmly established with regard to all the conditions producing it.

Because of the frequency of stress ulceration in battle casualties who were severely injured, the committee on trauma of the National Research Council held a conference on the subject.[57] There was little agreement regarding the incidence of stress ulceration following trauma and the incidence in the Navy appeared to differ from that in the Army. Army casualties in Vietnam were usually evacuated after 3 or 4 days to a base hospital. This modified the significance of the assessment of an incidence of only 1.4% because stress ulceration has its highest incidence during the sixth to fourteenth days following surgery or trauma. The incidence in the Navy was only 0.4% among 5350 casualties. The actual incidence from all the published figures was difficult to assess, but it is generally accepted that when there is prolonged recovery from surgery and a high incidence of sepsis, the probability of developing stress ulceration increases.

During this meeting it emerged that there was marked disagreement as to the location of the ulceration, the importance of steroids and the influence of gastric acidity. All these factors have been considered by numerous investigators.[50,51,144] It is evident from the published work that severe stress ulceration can develop in the absence of free hydrochloric acid (HCl) in the stomach, and a low acidity, and therefore a high pH, of gastric fluid is a common finding.[22,31,51,143] The blood cortisol level following the administration of high doses of steroids (e.g. following heart transplant), does not appear to cause stress ulceration.

The pH of the nasogastric fluid was investigated in a number of patients following surgery.[22] It was found that in some patients—who, because of cardiac failure, respiratory failure or cerebrovascular accident, required prolonged artificial ventilation of the lungs and had a prolonged recovery period—the pH of the nasogastric drainage rose to a relatively high value, for example 5.6 or 6.0. Some of these patients had no free hydrochloric acid (HCl) present in their gastric secretions. It was found that when the pH rose to 4.0 or more, the growth of bacteria in the nasogastric fluid was possible. The organisms identified were E. coli, Klebsiella, Proteus sp. and a number of non-pathogenic organisms. When the nasogastric fluid had a pH of 2.0 or more, it remained sterile so that no growth of organisms of any kind could be found after many hours of incubation, even when the fluid had been left in an open container below the patient's bed for 5 hours or longer.

Before these observations had been made, a continuous alkaline ($NaHCO_3$) milk drip down the nasogastric tube was given to one patient who developed severe haemorrhage, but this had no effect upon the blood loss and indeed an exacerbation of the condition occurred so that a partial gastrectomy had to be performed.

In all patients who developed bleeding from stress ulceration, the pH of the fluid was 3.5 or higher. Whenever the nasogastric drainage has been examined, bacteria have been present. Examples of these bacteria are listed in Table 6.5.

The administration of alkali was discontinued, although it is recognized that when given continuously in high concentration it has some bactericidal effect. Appropriate non-absorbable antibiotics were inserted into the stomach in saline via the nasogastric tube in some patients. In other patients dilute HCl was given at intervals.

Table 6.5 pH of nasogastric fluid and types of bacterial growth in fluid of postsurgical patients with stress ulceration

Patient	pH of nasogastric fluid	Organism identified
E.K.	5.0	Pseudomonas Klebsiella
E.D.	4.6	Pseudomonas
K.D.	4.5	Eschericia coli Klebsiella
M.H.	3.5	Eschericia coli Pseudomonas
M.C.	4.0	Eschericia coli Streptococcus Pseudomonas
H.L.	4.6	Eschericia coli Klebsiella
D.J.	6.0	Eschericia coli Pseudomonas

The observation that organisms are present in the stomach following achlorhydria is not new. It has been reported in association with carcinoma. Lactic and pyruvic acids have been found to be present which contribute to the varying pH of the fluid in the stomach.

Another important implication of the achlorhydric stomach acting as a reservoir for organisms is that when the tracheal aspirate was cultured, having been sucked into a sterile trap through a sterile catheter, organisms identical to those in the stomach were found in the lungs, Brooks (1972, 1978).[22,23,24] Because these organisms are motile, prolongation of the respiratory failure is inevitable. When bacteria are present in the stomach, following achlorhydria, the cycle of respiratory failure followed by stress ulceration is self potentiating until the cycle is broken by eliminating the bacteria, from both sites, and positive pressure ventilation ceases.

When stress ulceration occurs the methods of treatment commonly used are irrigation of the stomach with iced saline using a nasogastric tube, partial gastrectomy and cannulation of the superior mesenteric artery via the femoral artery for the constant infusion of Pitressin. In the author's experience the latter method can be very effective.

Intra-arterial infusion of Pitressin (vasopressin)

Pitressin is infused into the superior mesenteric artery in doses of 0.2 units/minute by means of a constant infusion pump; this can be increased to 0.4 units/minute if bleeding does not stop.[5] It is indicated that between 40% and 70% of patients benefit from this treatment, in that bleeding is either reduced or stopped completely. Conn *et al.* (1975)[38] found the treatment more effective when the bleeding did not originate from oesophageal varices. The author's own experience with two patients suffering from acute gastric erosion has indicated that this can be a valuable form of treatment when other methods fail.

Intravenous somatostatin

Somatostatin is also effective in controlling acute haemorrhage from peptic ulcers. A bolus intravenous injection of 250 µg of somatostatin, followed by a continuous intravenous infusion of 250 µg/ hour for 20–67 hours was found to control bleeding ulcers in 5 out of 9 patients (Limberg and Kommerell, 1979).[101] A controlled trial in which somatostatin was compared with ranitidine was performed by Coraggio and his colleagues in 1984.[42] The dose of somatostatin given was the same as that above. They found that intravenous somatostatin was superior to intravenous ranitidine given in doses of 50 mg every 4 hours. Other workers (Somerville *et al.*, 1985)[147] were unsure about the long-term benefits and mortality when somatostatin was used. It was conceded that this form of treatment may be suitable in some patients.

Cimetidine

More than 100 publications are available regarding the use of the H_2 receptor blocking agent cimetidine (Tagamet) in the presence of upper intestinal tract bleeding.[17] These reports indicate that cimetidine is of little value in the treatment of stress ulceration. We have used dilute HCl, given down the nasogastric tube, as reported on page 149 (Brooks, 1978).[23] Antibiotics are also of value.

Expansion of the Vascular Space

Several solutions are available for the treatment of hypovolaemic shock.

Electrolyte solutions

For many years it has been recognized that the blood pressure rises following the infusion of saline, but it required the work of Shires et al.[141] to popularize the use of electrolyte solutions as the primary treatment of shock. They preferred to use Ringer's solution with added lactate which they called 'balanced salt solution'. However, there seems to be little advantage in using Ringer's solution rather than isotonic saline. It was then demonstrated that the osmolality of the circulating plasma fell as haemorrhage progressed and that hypertonic solutions had a protective effect on the tissues that were damaged by hypovolaemic shock in animals; there was some evidence that this applied to man.[27]

Hyperosmotic solutions

A controlled study of the incidence of acute renal failure (ARF) in man is not possible, but the routine use of markedly hypertonic solutions in a number of varying conditions does allow some conclusions to be drawn. For example, ARF is rare in patients surviving cardiac arrest even when resuscitation is prolonged. In the patient suffering from severe diabetic ketosis, hypotension lasting for considerable periods does not appear to give rise to ARF. The hyperosmotic nature of diabetes would appear to be protective. In the experiments performed by Brooks et al. in 1963[27] it was found that the protective effect of hypertonic solutions was independent of acid–base changes, and that hypertonic saline was as protective against tissue damage as sodium bicarbonate. Hypertonic glucose solutions also afforded some protection. The infusion of hypertonic sodium bicarbonate, usually

2.74% but frequently 8.4%, has been used almost routinely in the author's department in cases of hypovolaemic shock. The infusion of 100 ml of 8.4% $NaHCO_3$ raises the total body water [HCO_3^-], of the average adult, by only 2 mmol/l, even if no HCO_3^- is excreted. Initial blood concentrations of HCO_3^-, however, are considerably higher until equilibration with the other body fluid compartments has occurred. Other authors have advocated the use of hypertonic solutions in the treatment of shock.[60,156,158]

Small quantities of very concentrated NaCl, for example 10–20 ml of 23.4% (4 mmol/ml), given into a large vessel will raise the blood pressure in man when all other methods have failed, assuming that there is no major metabolic acidosis present and the rectal temperature is not greatly reduced.[25]

Dextran (Dextraven, Gentran, Lomodex, Macrodex)

Dextran is a polysaccharide of bacterial origin. Until recently, it was the most widely used plasma expander in many centres, especially in solution in isotonic saline. It is also produced as a sodium-free solution in which the tonicity is maintained with isotonic glucose. It is available in various concentrations of dextran with different molecular weights; the period of time that dextran is retained within the circulation varies with the molecular weight of the substance used.

Dextran 70. The most commonly used solution contains 6% dextran which has a molecular weight of 65 000–70 000. (It is to be noted that albumin has a molecular weight of 65 000.) In a 0.9% solution of saline, therefore, the solution is hypertonic. This solution is normally retained in the plasma for 4–6 hours, but this time will vary with the condition of the patient, whether blood loss is continuous, renal function and permeability of the capillary bed. The larger particles of dextran are stored temporarily in the reticuloendothelial system of the liver and are released when the concentration of dextran in the blood decreases. A small part of the dextran is metabolized.

Dextran 110. This has an average molecular weight of 110 000. It has been used in the 6% solution in the treatment of burns, severe haemorrhage and gut obstruction. It remains within the circulation for a longer period of time than dextran 70.

Dextran 40. This is commonly referred to as low molecular weight dextran; the average molecular weight is in the region of 40 000. In the 10% solution there are a greater number of particles than in either dextran 110 or dextran 70. Following infusion of dextran 40, therefore, water is drawn into the vascular space from the extravascular compartments. Marked haemodilution therefore occurs and there is a decrease in both the packed cell volume (PCV) and the plasma protein concentration. It thus improves blood flow and decreases blood viscosity and is indicated where there are abnormalities of blood perfusion.[116] It is used in polycythaemia especially prior to surgery, vascular surgery following cerebral thrombi, burns and frostbite.

The dextrans do, however, have certain side-effects which must be considered. They have an anticoagulant effect and therefore should not be used in the presence of a bleeding diathesis or thrombocytopenia. Severe allergic reactions have been reported, although sensitivity to the drug is uncommon. These reactions occur shortly after starting the dextran infusion.[134]

When the sensitivity reaction occurs there is a *fall* in blood pressure, flushing of the skin, nausea, pain in the lumber region and an increase in heart rate. This condition is best treated with corticosteroids (e.g. hydrocortisone, 1 g i.v. or methylprednisolone, 80 mg i.v.).

Degraded gelatin solution, polygelline (Haemaccel)
The synthetic colloidal solution Haemaccel consists of 3.5% degraded gelatin which can be kept unrefrigerated on the shelf until it is required. In addition to its colloidal content, it contains 145 mmol/l (mEq/l) of Na^+, 5.1 mmol/l (mEq/l) of K^+ and 12.5 mmol/l (mEq/l) of Ca^{++}. Haemaccel has been used in the various forms of hypovolaemic shock, for example following haemorrhage, burns, peritonitis, pancreatitis and in extracorporeal perfusions. It has also been used in isolated organ perfusion, indicating its low incidence of complications. At room temperature it is said to be stable for at least 8 years, and under tropical conditions it is stable for at least 5 years. It can be mixed with other solutions including saline, dextrose and Ringer's solution. It is a very effective plasma expander, and is free from the hepatitis virus. The degraded gelatin that the solution contains has a molecular weight ranging between 5000 and 50 000; the mean molecular weight is approximately 35 000, and is equivalent to 3.15 g of nitrogen. The pH of Haemaccel is 7.25 so that, like blood, no immediate benefit to the acid–base state will be produced. It can be infused rapidly in cases of haemorrhagic shock and at least 2 litres can be given for volume replacement without ill-effects. It is recommended, however, when more than 2 litres are administered, alternate treatment of 500 ml of solution and 1 unit of whole blood should be given. Haemaccel should not be mixed with citrated blood because the relatively high concentration of Ca^{++} in the solution may allow coagulation to occur. Transfusion of blood should therefore be performed using a separate intravenous infusion set into a different vein. Blood can also be transfused directly following an infusion of Haemaccel. Haemaccel can be warmed to body temperature before use when this is indicated.

In the absence of plasma and in the early treatment of burns, Haemaccel will replace blood volume very satisfactorily.

Human plasma protein fraction (PPF)
This preparation of fractionated human albumin can be stored at room temperature for at least 3 years or in a cold room above 2°C for longer periods. It is heat treated and, therefore, unlike plasma, does not contain the active hepatitis virus. It contains 17–19 g of protein per unit (400 ml), and Na^+ 140–160 mmol/l (mEq/l) and K^+ 2 mmol/l (mEq/l).

Because human PPF is readily available and has a long shelf life and has no effects on blood coagulation and renal function, it is a valuable solution to have when expansion of the blood and plasma volume is indicated. Also, it is free from the hepatitis virus and can therefore be given in relatively large quantities.

Although it is highly effective in the treatment of burns, it does not appear to be retained within the circulation for as long a period as plasma, which is preferred by some workers in this field.

Summary of the Management of Hypovolaemic Shock

When confronted with a patient suffering from hypovolaemic shock, blood transfusion is contraindicated when the hypovolaemia is caused by loss of plasma (as a result of gut obstruction, peritonitis, paralytic ileus, anaphylactoid reactions or burns) or loss of water. Blood transfusion is *also* contraindicated in haemorrhagic shock before correction of the metabolic acidosis has been at least partially achieved and rehydration has been established.

There is, therefore, a growing opinion that the immediate transfusion of large volumes of stored blood is undesirable because of the acidosis, high

[K$^+$] and other metabolic consequences that develop from or are caused by storage. The following protocol has been shown to be effective.

1. Infuse saline, Ringer's solution or Ringer Lactate (Hartmann's solution) together with 2.74% or 8.4% NaHCO$_3$. Not more than 200 mmol (mEq) of NaHCO$_3$ should be administered without estimating blood-gas levels.

Try to establish that water depletion is not a factor as none of the above solutions provides electrolyte-free water, but the plasma osmolality must be maintained during hypotension.

2. If hypovolaemia is the result of plasma loss into the gut or peritoneal cavity and the haemoglobin concentration and haematocrit are high, PPF (purified protein fraction, fractionated human albumin) or plasma should be administered in preference to other fluids,* although Haemaccel can be used if these are not available. Isotonic saline is effective as an initial treatment.

3. In the case of sudden haemorrhage which is continuing, a plasma expander such as PPF, Haemaccel or dextran 70 can be infused, bearing in mind the anticoagulant effects that dextrans may have. Remember, blood and Haemaccel cannot be mixed because of the high [Ca^{++}] of Haemaccel.

4. When large volumes of blood have to be infused (e.g. 4 or 5 units in 30 minutes), 10 ml of 10% calcium gluconate or calcium chloride should be given intravenously following each litre of blood given subsequently.

5. One unit of fresh frozen plasma (FFP) should be given following transfusion of the first 6 units of stored blood, and after every 4 units of stored blood transfused subsequently. Remember, the effects of FFP may be lost if a 'normal' bicarbonate

*Take note that only PPF is hepatitis and probably AIDS free.

concentration is not maintained. The FFP should be from group AB donors and cross-matching with the patient's blood group should be performed. FFP should therefore be obtained as soon as its use is considered necessary.

6. A central venous pressure (CVP) measurement is essential following severe haemorrhage because metabolic changes may reduce cardiac output so that a low blood pressure and raised CVP can be observed before the correction of the blood volume has been achieved.

7. Insert a Swank blood transfusion filter between the transfusion set and the patient.

8. Make sure that hypothermia has not developed by recording the rectal temperature. Hypothermia will contribute to a low blood pressure.

9. If the blood pressure fails to rise, take into account that blood may be present in the stomach, lumen of the bowel, thorax, abdomen, areas of bruising and fracture sites. In these circumstances the CVP is low and the oxygen saturation of blood obtained from the femoral vein is below 50% and further expansion of the blood volume is necessary. Correct the metabolic acidosis and confirm that the ventilation of the lungs is adequate. When these are abnormal and the blood volume is adequate, the CVP is usually raised.

10. Confirm that lung pathology has not given rise to anoxia. It may be necessary to give oxygen by mask or tent or to assist ventilation. Remember that cyanosis is a physical sign with a double aetiology. It is produced not only by desaturation of the arterial blood (anoxic anoxia) but also by desaturation of the venous blood caused by inadequate tissue perfusion (low cardiac output). Only volume replacement and increased cardiac output will correct the latter.

11. If hypotension persists, hydrocortisone in doses of 1–2 g should be given intravenously.

12. Relieve pain with analgesics.

SEPTIC SHOCK

This is a condition which has an extremely high mortality. It is most commonly seen after surgical intervention or severe trauma. Patients are more prone to develop septic shock when they have some intercurrent disease process such as diabetes, liver disease, malnutrition and vitamin deficiency, anaemia or carcinoma.

Hypotension results from the presence of circulating toxins arising from a bacteraemia. The Gram-negative organisms that most commonly cause septic shock are *Escherichia coli*, *Proteus* and *Pseudomonas*. Gram-positive organisms also produce this condition, staphylococcus being most common, but cases of streptococcal infections also occur. The gas-forming organisms also constitute an important group which may produce a profound form of septic shock. An endotoxin is produced by Gram-negative organisms and an exotoxin is produced by Gram-positive organisms.

Septic shock is commonly seen in clinical practice following operations upon the gastro-intestinal tract, the genitourinary tract, especially in the presence of existing infections, following septic abortions, endoscopy and quite commonly following the incising of abscess cavities. This last procedure is very rarely seen in modern surgical practice because of the recognition of its attendant dangers. Septic shock can also occur following the transfusion of infected blood or infusion fluid.

The author experienced more than 20 instances of septic shock in Houston, Texas, USA, three episodes occurring in one patient, when a batch of infusion fluids was contaminated with bacteria during manufacture. Injection via the open end of a CVP manometer was suspected and a carrier was sought, but this proved to be wrong. Rapid recognition and prompt treatment with high doses of steroids, antibiotics and $NaHCO_3$ resulted in complete recovery in all cases. Some systemic infections give rise to septic shock, these being typhoid, amoebic dysentery and cholera. Intermittent loss of recordable blood pressure associated with intermittent loss of vision occurred in one patient, and blood culture proved that this was due to the tubercle baccillus emanating from a lung cavity. In this condition, as on many other occasions, early treatment and correction of the acid–base state were important in the maintenance of cardiac output and blood pressure.

Clinical Picture of Septic Shock

Those workers who have taken an interest in this field are able to define clearly two forms of septic shock. These have distinct features and are probably separated only by the degree of toxicity or the intrinsic resistance of the patient to the toxic stimulus.

The first sign of a bacteraemia which may produce the condition of toxic or septic shock is usually a severe rigor accompanied by a sudden rise in body temperature reaching 40–41.1°C (104–106°F) or more. The patient feels cold and severely ill and is unable to control the muscular movements no matter how hard he tries. He may, however, be unaware of any fall of blood pressure

and may wonder why such active measures are being taken and why the foot of the bed is being raised. Profound hypotension may accompany the first rigor, but quite commonly there is a time interval of up to 24 hours. It cannot be stressed too strongly that a rigor occurring after an accident, trauma or surgery should be treated from its first appearance, the patient should be examined for a source of infection and blood must be taken for culture of the organisms. Quite frequently the rigor or hypotension is preceded by a feeling of being very unwell, influenza-like pains and aches in the muscles, a sudden rise in erythrocyte sedimentation rate (ESR), a marked leucocytosis in the region of 15 000–20 000 cells per mm^3. Sometimes patients are aware that all is not well and have been known to complain of a 'feeling of impending doom' or have made a similar observation before the onset of hypotension or the appearance of a rigor. They may complain of transitory loss of vision.

The less severe form of toxic shock that is recognizable is that in which the skin is warm and generalized, peripheral vascular dilatation has occurred, the patient is conscious, talkative, intelligent and alert and sometimes excitable, has an adequate urinary output of reduced specific gravity (1.010–1.018) and relatively moderate hypotension. The systolic blood pressure is in the region of 80–70 mmHg and the diastolic pressure is approximately 40 mmHg. Blood for analysis can be taken without difficulty from the veins on the back of the hand and the AV difference is so small under these conditions that the oxygen saturation is high and the acid–base results similar to those of the arterial blood. This is not unlike the situation in which the hand has been artificially warmed for the purposes of the arterialization of the venous blood.[29] This situation may continue for many days before this 'warm hypotension' is relieved. During this time, if normal hydration and electrolyte balance are maintained, the biochemical alterations in the patient as measured in the blood are relatively unimportant. The venous haematocrit does not alter very much, in the absence of blood or plasma loss, ventilation is unimpaired and the metabolic component of acid–base balance remains at near-normal values. Although the urine-concentrating power is impaired, the plasma sodium level does not fall appreciably unless loss of sodium through sweat and urine is not replaced or if excessive hydration is allowed in the presence of a reduced response to a water load (see p. 26). While the prognosis in this form of 'warm hypotension' is therefore relatively good, great care must be taken to maintain a normal metabolic state in addition to treating the basic infection with appropriate antibiotics.

Another form of 'warm hypotension' is that which occurs with marked plasma loss into the lumen of the gut and fluid loss from the extracellular fluid (ECF). The loss of fluid from the interstitial compartment may in fact be only a manifestation of plasma loss, but may also occur independently. It is most commonly seen with infections involving Gram-negative organisms, such as *E. coli*, and follows surgical procedures within the abdominal cavity, such as resection of part of the alimentary canal or large blood vessel replacement in which the arterial tree supplying the gut has been altered in such a way that it becomes ischaemic. Operations performed upon the intestine when the primary condition has already caused localized or generalized peritonitis not infrequently give rise to this form of toxic shock. Distension of the bowel because of paralytic ileus occurs sometimes with radiographical and clinical signs of obstruction. If the abdomen is opened because mechanical obstruction is feared, it is possible to remove more than 4 litres of fluid from the lumen of the gut without difficulty. Even when this is done it is well recognized that much more fluid is left behind. This volume of fluid represents approximately one tenth of the total body water and more than one third of the volume of the ECF. It may contain as much as 7 g% of protein, 120 mmol/l (mEq/l) of sodium and 14 mmol/l (mEq/l) of potassium. As this is removed from the effectively active circulating body fluids, it represents a major loss and replacement must be made good. In contrast to warm toxic hypotension without plasma loss, the CVP falls as depletion of body fluids progresses. The low arterial blood pressure falls further when these losses are not replaced with plasma and electrolyte-containing fluids. Under these circumstances the arteriovenous oxygen and acid–base differences increase as during haemorrhagic shock, and the blood packed cell volume (PCV) rises as haemoconcentration occurs. This form of toxic hypotension gradually evolves into one in which hypovolaemic hypotension is superimposed upon the underlying toxic condition and death rapidly follows even when there is no increase in the severity of the infection.

The clinical condition that begins as 'warm septic hypotension' gradually changes to that of 'cold septic hypotension' when the infusion of electrolyte and plasma is inadequate. Peripheral vasoconstriction and cyanosis together with coldness of the extremities can then be observed.

The management of this condition is made difficult because of the magnitude of the protein, fluid and electrolyte loss and the rapid onset of hypotension resulting from hypovolaemia. On examination the patient may be found to be comatose but in the early stages is sometimes conscious or even alert, though feeling extremely ill. The hypovolaemia is indicated by an extremely rapid tachycardia and by the fact that frequently the thorax and abdomen are warm while the arms and legs are cold and vasoconstricted. Blood volume determinations with albumin labelled with ^{131}I are of no value because of the loss of this material into depots of fluid such as the protein-containing liquid of the gut. A better measurement of blood volume is with ^{51}Cr, although this is of limited value in a situation which may alter from minute to minute. A much more useful guide to blood volume is the measurement of central venous pressure (CVP) with its limitations kept in mind (see p. 179). It is essential that, if it is to be measured properly, it should be done by means of direct manometry through a catheter passed into the inferior vena cava and kept open with an intravenous drip. It is true that patients have recovered when rapid infusions of plasma and, electrolyte-containing solutions have been instituted 'until the veins are full'. This is, however, a very crude method and open to error. When possible, the simple procedure of inserting a cannula into the SVC should always be performed because, in addition to the measurement of the CVP, the cannula is an avenue for rapid infusion should the necessity arise.

Case history. A 47-year-old man underwent a resection of bowel for Crohn's disease. Ten hours after the operation he had a markedly distended bowel and signs of obstruction on X-ray. No bowel sounds were present and no flatus had been passed. A quantity of fluid, which was bile stained, had been aspirated from the stomach. The patient was returned to theatre and the abdomen was re-opened because it was felt that mechanical obstruction of the bowel had been produced. This was not confirmed at the second operation and 4 litres of fluid were aspirated from the lumen of the bowel. During the anaesthetic, the blood pressure fell to below a systolic value of 65 mmHg as registered by means of a sphygmomanometer cuff. The rates of infusion of plasma, hypertonic saline and hypertonic sodium bicarbonate were increased and the blood pressure rose to 85 mmHg. Throughout the night the patient breathed spontaneously and was given oxygen intermittently. Intravenous hydrocortisone was given in doses of 300 mg at intervals of 4 hours. After each injection a moderate rise in systolic blood pressure to 90 mmHg followed after a period of 20–30 minutes. In all, during the next 12 hours, 9 litres of fluid were infused, these being composed of 1 litre of 1.8% NaCl, 1 litre of 2.8% $NaHCO_3$ and 7 litres of pooled plasma. The rate of infusion of all these fluids was maintained by careful monitoring of the CVP, which fluctuated widely between 2 and 15 cmH_2O, tending to fall when the rate of infusion was slowed. Intravenous tetracycline was given in each bottle of electrolyte solution so that in all 1 g of this substance was infused over this period.

After 12 hours the rate of infusion that was required to maintain an adequate CVP could be reduced so that in the next 12 hours only 3 litres of plasma and 1 litre of 1.8% NaCl needed to be given. Acid–base investigations demonstrated a moderate alkalosis, so that no more sodium bicarbonate was infused that day. Urine output during the 24 hours was approximately 900 ml, with a specific gravity of 1.017, containing 23 mEq/l (mmol/l) of Na^+ and 48 mEq/l (mmol/l) of K^+. In the next 24 hours the blood pressure was maintained in the region of 85–90 mmHg systolic, and fluid replacement presented no difficulty. Twenty-four hours later the blood pressure was still maintained in the region of 85 mmHg, urine output was similar to that of the previous 24 hours and because of a moderate hypernatraemia, the plasma sodium being 147 mmol/l (mEq/l), the patient was given 2 litres of fluid, half of which was 0.9% NaCl and the other half being 1 litre of 5% glucose. This regimen was continued until the sixth day when the blood pressure rose to 100/80 mmHg, the urine output increased to 1200 ml, the urine having a specific gravity of 1.020, and the bowel sounds began to return. On the ninth day flatus was passed and the patient progressed to a normal recovery. During the whole period of time renal function caused no concern, but without a proper CVP measurement it is almost certain that fluid replacement would have been inadequate at a time when it was most needed.

Although there is some experimental evidence that shock produced by intravenous *E. Coli* endotoxin does not alter the blood volume,[79] the clinical circumstances that are present in a patient as in the one described above, are such that major blood volume changes must take place, because of the loss and sequestration of fluid. This loss is distributed through all the body fluid compartments, but has its most profound effect in the early stages upon the vascular compartment of the ECF.

The second form of toxic shock is often referred to as 'cold hypotension'. Unlike the previous cases described above, the patient on examination has a cold skin over virtually the whole of the body surface. The vessels are universally reduced in calibre and venepuncture is difficult. Profuse sweating often accompanies the hypotension and may be a major source of fluid loss. Although some patients are capable of understanding the situation lucidly, others are either comatose or have impaired cerebration. The urine output is markedly diminished and the hypotension often results in the onset of acute renal failure. In this form of shock there may be only a small loss of fluid from the body. In the early stages, especially before the effects of sweating appear, fluid replacement may play only a small part in the treatment of some patients. In others the venous haematocrit may later rise to high levels and fluid replacement becomes necessary. The arteriovenous oxygen difference widens and tissue anoxia itself may be a factor in producing a rise in the venous haematocrit by causing fluid to pass into the cells.

The prime causes for the fall in blood pressure in this form of toxic shock, which become manifest just before, during or just after a severe rigor, appear to be the result of the action of toxins upon the myocardium and the loss of circulating blood volume as fluid is lost from the extracellular fluid space into the cells. The difference in oxygen content between the arterial and mixed venous blood is increased greatly because the venous oxygen saturation falls with little or no change in the arterial blood oxygen saturation. There may be a rise in CVP initially and this can be followed by a fall when the blood packed cell volume (PCV) increases, and fluid leaves the vascular compartment and enters the intracellular fluid compartment (ICF).* The volume of fluid that must be infused can be regulated by monitoring the CVP and by calculating the fluid deficit from serial estimations of PCV.

A small excess of fluid replacement may give rise to a raised CVP because of cardiac failure. A further factor which can contribute to the severity of the hypotension is the rapid onset of a metabolic acidosis. The effects of bacterial toxins upon the patient appear to become more severe as the metabolic acidosis progresses. It has as yet not been possible to elucidate whether this is because

---

*This movement of fluid should not be confused with the clinical condition where fluid, similar in composition to plasma, is lost into the lumen of the gut when the bowel is obstructed.

of the increased numbers of bacteria within the bloodstream or because of an increase in the concentration of toxins or because in the presence of a metabolic acidosis toxins have a greater effect upon the metabolism. It is possible that the reticuloendothelial system functions less well in the presence of a metabolic acidosis, for many workers, notably Fine,[61] consider that removal of endotoxin is one of the functions of the spleen. There is, however, no doubt that in some patients correction of the acidosis causes a marked clinical improvement both with Gram-negative and Gram-positive organisms.

Toxins appear to have two distinct modes of action and therefore can be divided into: (a) toxins acting upon the myocardium, and (b) toxins acting upon the blood vessels. However, other important aspects of toxic shock require further subdivision if the best care of the patient is to be obtained. Therefore, the simple classification of cold and warm toxic shock is unsatisfactory with regard to both treatment and diagnosis.

Clinical experience allows us to identify four main types of toxic shock. These can be summarized as follows.

Type 1: toxins acting primarily on the myocardium
This develops suddenly, often following a rigor. The pulse is impalpable, the blood pressure unobtainable, and, although a rapid tachycardia usually develops, the heart rate is commonly below 100/minute.

The extremities are cold and, while the oxygen saturation (and PO_2) of the arterial blood may be normal, peripheral cyanosis is seen, including the tongue, and this results from a fall in cardiac output.

There are also large arteriovenous differences of pH and PCO_2. Blood analysis reveals a marked metabolic acidosis, a fall in plasma [Na$^+$] and a rise in plasma [K$^+$], PCV and plasma protein concentration. Oliguria with urine of low osmolality develops. The CVP is raised above normal.

Parker et al. (1984)[127] found that severe myocardial depression, with a reduction in stroke volume, occurred during toxic shock. Simultaneous radionuclide cineangiographic studies and haemodynamic evaluation demonstrated a marked reduction in cardiac index which was reversible in some of the patients in their series.

Even when fluid is infused until the CVP is raised to 15 or 20 mmHg and the metabolic acidosis is corrected, the blood pressure may not rise and vasopressors that induce vasoconstriction remain largely ineffective.

Rapid intravenous digitalization sometimes improves myocardial function, but the inotropic action of isoprenaline infusions (2–5 mg/litre at approximately 10 drops/minute) dramatically raises the blood pressure, lowers the CVP, and increases the urine output. Dopamine infusions are also sometimes of value, but a vasoconstricting vasopressor may also need to be given.

Type 2 (a and b): toxins producing generalized vasodilatation
Type 2a Usually no rigors are present and generalized vasodilatation develops. The blood pressure is in the region of 80 mmHg. The CVP is normal or only slightly raised. A metabolic acidosis does not develop and the arteriovenous oxygen difference is normal. The patient's skin is pink and warm. Urine of low osmolality is excreted in adequate quantities. Isoprenaline is ineffective unless the mixed venous oxygen tension falls below 30 mmHg (saturation below 50%). If a normal fluid balance is maintained, the condition may continue for 3 weeks or longer. A water deficit of more than 8 litres can develop in 24 hours, so that hypovolaemia exacerbates the degree of shock. Urine excretion then ceases and the extremities become cold and cyanosed. Clinically, the condition becomes similar to Type 1, *but the CVP is low*.

Type 2b When a severe metabolic acidosis develops during Type 2 shock, hypotension, resistant to vasopressors, increases. The CVP rises and the extremities become cold and blue. The condition is indistinguishable from Type 1 until adequate volumes of hypertonic NaHCO$_3$ have been infused.

Type 3: septic shock associated with loss of protein-rich fluid
Septic shock associated with loss of large volumes of fluid into the gut lumen or peritoneal cavity develops from obstruction or perforation of the bowel and peritonitis. The protein concentration of the fluid may be similar to that of plasma. Before the condition can be recognized as Type 1 or Type 2 shock, plasma must be infused and the acid–base state corrected. The infusion of 1 litre of plasma or PPF hourly during the first 12 hours (controlled by the CVP) may be necessary. The patient described on page 208 would be a typical example, but in this case toxic shock developed after repair of the hypovolaemia.

Type 4: irreversible septic shock
Initially, the condition is similar to Type 1 shock, but a relatively slow intravenous infusion can

cause the CVP to rise above 20 mmHg and the patient to hyperventilate for 3 or 4 minutes after the infusion is stopped. The urine excreted is of small volume and dilute. No rise in blood pressure follows when isoprenaline and other vasopressors are given. As time passes, the CVP gradually rises further, even when fluids are withheld. Any significant reduction in blood volume is followed immediately by a further fall in blood pressure. Correction of the metabolic acidosis produces no significant clinical improvement. It is not possible to maintain a normal $[HCO_3^-]$ by infusions of $NaHCO_3$ solutions except for a very short period of time. Injections of cortisol and digitalis are also ineffective. Jaundice is often present. Death occurs after a variable period of intractable hypotension.

Only haemodialysis and hyperbaric oxygen (which is effective when toxicity is due to *Clostridia*) afford any hope of recovery.

Coagulopathies occasionally develop in Type 4 toxic shock, but these can be delayed (and prevented in other types of toxic shock) by correction of the acid–base state.

Case history. A 24-year-old male patient was admitted via the accident and emergency department with a history of vomiting, constipation and intermittent abdominal pain. On examination, he was grossly dehydrated, had marked abdominal distension with hypersensitive bowel sounds. X-ray of the abdomen revealed multiple fluid levels and possibly a faecolith in the appendiceal area. Blood analysis at this time is shown in Table 6.6 and designated A.

Rectal examination revealed a mass in the pouch of Douglas. At laparotomy it was found that the patient had a dense adherent small bowel which was grossly dilated. A periappendiceal abscess was found which was obstructing loops of small bowel in the pouch of Douglas. A faecolith was found in the appendix and 4.5 litres of foul-smelling pus was aspirated from the abdominal cavity. A small perforation was found following excision of the appendix. The abdominal cavity was irrigated with a 2.5% solution of the antibacterial and antifungal agent noxythiolin (Noxyflex), and then closed; a tube drain was inserted into the pelvic cavity. The pus was subsequently found to contain *E. Coli* and *Bacteroides* sp. During the anaesthetic, the patient was infused with 1 litre of normal saline, 500 ml of plasma, 500 ml of dextran '70' and 500 ml of dextrose/saline. Two units of blood were also transfused. Following the operation, 1 litre of saline was given over 2 hours together with 1 unit of blood during a period of 3 hours.

At 11 a.m. the following morning, having progressed well during the night, the patient was found suddenly to be markedly vasoconstricted and diaphoretic. The pulse was 160/minute and the blood pressure could not be measured using a sphygmomanometer. It was observed that he was not bleeding from the drains and that the urinary output up to the time hypotension had developed had been satisfactory,* and had a specific gravity of 1.025. A diagnosis of toxic shock was made and a CVP cannula was inserted into the SVC. The CVP was found to be 18 cmH₂O measured from the midaxillary line. Hydrocortisone, 2 g, i.v. and methylprednisolone (Solu-medrone) 250 mg 6-hourly i.v. were given. Sodium bicarbonate 180 mmol i.v. was infused. Four antibiotics were given as described on page 000. Blood analysis at this time is shown in Table 6.6 and designated B.

The rate of infusion of fluid had been

*Greater than 30 ml/hour.

Table 6.6 Changes in some of the blood components, electrolytes, biochemical content of the blood and plasma of a 24-year-old man suffering from peritonitis and toxic (septic) shock

	WBC (× 1000)	PCV (%)	Hb (g%)	[Na⁺] (mmol/l)	[K⁺] (mmol/l)	Urea (mg%)	TCO₂ (mmol/l)	Glucose (mg%)
A 26.9	19.6	53	17.5	130	4.0	55		
B 27.9 (9 a.m.)	11.9	56	17.7	136	3.7	63	36	
C 27.9 (4 p.m.)		47	15.3	132	4.1			250 (14)
D 28.9			11.6	139	4.2		25	120 (6.7)
E 30.9	13.7		11.1	137	3.8	57	27	115 (6.4)

WBC, white blood cell count; PCV, packed cell volume; Hb, haemoglobin; [Na⁺], plasma [Na⁺]; [K⁺], plasma [K⁺]; urea, blood urea; TCO₂, plasma total CO₂; glucose, blood glucose concentration (figures in parentheses are mmol/l values).

increased but was reduced following the measurement of CVP and a small dose of fruse-mide (Lasix)—20 mg—was given intravenously.

Approximately 6 hours later the patient was much improved. The systolic blood pressure fluctuated a little but was in the region of 90–100 mmHg, and a urinary output of approximately 150 ml/hour was recorded. The urine pH was 7.0 and contained 30 mg protein/100 ml. The specific gravity of urine had fallen to 1.016. The results of blood analysis at this time are shown in Table 6.6 and designated C.

The following day the blood pressure was 120/70 mmHg, stable and not fluctuating significantly. The heart rate was between 80 and 100 beats/minute. The CVP remained at 16 cmH$_2$O. The biochemical findings at this time are shown in Table 6.6 and designated D.

The dose of methylprednisolone was reduced to 125 mg every 6 hours. The improvement in the patient's clinical condition was such that he was able to sit up in bed and talk at great length in an apparently untiring manner to his relatives. Two days later he sat out of bed. The abdominal drains were shortened, although pus was still being discharged from the orifice. The dose of methylprednisolone was reduced to 62.5 mg every 6 hours. The results of blood analysis at this time are shown in Table 6.6 and designated E.

Three days later the patient became apyrexial, his pulse rate fell to 60/minute and his blood pressure was 100/60 mmHg. The CVP was 4.5 cmH$_2$O. It was noted that bowel sounds were present. The white cell count fell gradually to normal levels and the patient's subsequent progress was uneventful, so that a complete recovery was made and he was discharged 29 days after surgery.

It can be commented that this patient is very interesting in that he illustrates some important factors in management. When he first entered hospital he was in danger of developing hypovolaemic shock, but this was prevented by adequate fluid replacement. He later developed normovolaemic shock due to bacterial toxins (toxic shock).

Initially, the patient was volume depleted and dehydrated. The degree of haemoconcentration was indicated by a packed cell volume (PCV) of 56% and Hb of 17.7 g%. In addition to an inadequate H$_2$O intake, movement of electrolyte- and protein-containing fluid occurred.

Although a raised plasma [Na$^+$] is associated with dehydration, this patient's plasma [Na$^+$] was low because of the loss of Na$^+$ and protein into the peritoneal cavity and into the lumen of the gut.

Dilution had occurred when he drank water to replace his fluid loss. In his case, therefore, the plasma [Na$^+$], if considered alone, would have been misleading with regard to the degree of volume depletion that was present. He corresponded to toxic shock Type 3.

When the following morning the blood pressure fell so that the pulse and blood pressure were unrecordable, it might well have been considered that he had bled into the abdominal cavity and was suffering from hypovolaemic shock had it not been for the CVP reading which indicated that transfusion had probably expanded the blood volume more than required, blood loss having been minimal at surgery. In this patient's case, correct management would not have been possible without a CVP measurement. Treatment with four antibiotics was necessary and these were given before identification of the organisms causing the bacteraemia could be established. The mortality from toxic shock is so high that it was not possible to wait for bacteriological results to be obtained. High doses of steroids, which were rapidly reduced as clinical improvement progressed and appeared to be effective in reducing the effects of toxic shock, may have been instrumental in an early return to bowel sounds and the cessation of paralytic ileus. When high doses of steroids are given for a short period of time, slow curtailment of therapy is not necessary.

Tissue damage and disseminated intravascular coagulation (DIC)

Bacterial toxins, particularly endotoxins, induce tissue damage not only by their vasoconstrictor action but also by their ability to damage the vascular endothelium. This can in turn induce disseminated intravascular coagulation (DIC). This ability is frequently recognized as being the result of a Schwartzmann reaction and tissue manifestations of this are considered to be cortical necrosis of the kidney and shock lung. Endotoxins are known to play a procoagulant role in that they also damage platelets and activate factor XII. Toxins have a number of other effects including damage to the Kupffer cells of the liver. It is recognized, however, that platelet aggregation and the formation of thrombi are more likely to occur when there is a slow, stagnant circulation, as in severe hypotension, a metabolic acidosis or a depressed reticuloendothelial cell function;[52] the last of these occurs following surgery, in association with jaundice and sometimes when very large doses of corticosteroids are given.

Carbohydrate metabolism

In clinical practice, disturbances have to be assessed by the blood-glucose concentration and insulin level. These vary according to the severity of the endotoxin effects, the phase of the attack and the length of time that hypotension has been present.[37] Impaired production of glucose can occur because of liver damage and when gluconeogenesis is prevented.[123]

Plasma osmolality

A fall in the plasma osmolality which results from a decrease in the plasma [Na⁺] without any concomitant rise in the plasma glucose level is a common finding in 'cold septic shock'. It can readily be appreciated that if there is a continuous infusion of glucose solution which supplies a large volume of electrolyte-free water in the presence of reduced renal function, further dilution of the body fluids will take place. When haemoconcentration develops and the packed cell volume (PCV) rises, an increase in the plasma osmolality is sometimes found, especially in the early stages of septic shock. It is also essential to maintain a high plasma osmolality in order that some degree of renal function continues in the presence of toxaemia. The patient is, therefore, more likely to recover when only relatively small volumes of non-electrolyte-containing fluid are infused. When a low plasma sodium concentration is detected it is preferable to infuse solutions having twice the osmolality of plasma (e.g. 1.8% NaCl or 2.74% NaHCO₃) as a continuous intravenous drip, until the plasma concentrations are corrected.

Vaginal tampons as a cause of toxic shock (staphylococcal Toxic Shock Syndrome—TSS)*

A number of cases of toxic shock have been reported associated with the use of vaginal tampons when staphylococci have been present in the vagina.[58,153,155] Hypocalcaemia has been reported to occur during this condition.[153] Both the total and ionized calcium levels are reduced in patients with severe sepsis, and relatively low parathyroid hormone levels have been found to be present. It has been reported by Wagner *et al.* (1981)[157] that in nine patients with the 'toxic shock syndrome' caused by *Staphylococcus aureus* toxins, low serum calcium and phosphate concentrations and calcitonin levels are founded. Only one patient demonstrated clinical evidence of tetany. Low parathyroid hormome levels were also present.

*A symposium on TSS (1985) Edited by R. Goulding has been published. *Postgrad. med. J.*, **61** Suppl. I.

Profound erythema followed by desquamation is a feature of the condition. Muscle pain with subsequent rhabdomyolysis has also been observed.

Toxic shock has also been found in association with the use of contraceptive diaphragms.[90,106] The treatment is the same as in other forms of toxic shock, although more attention is required with regard to eliminating staphylococci from the vagina and skin surface.

Treatment of Septic Shock

The forms of 'cold toxic shock' (Types 1, 2b, 3 and 4) can present as exacerbations of other conditions, especially 'warm septic shock' (Types 2a and 3). Cold toxic shock may, however, develop suddenly with no or few prodromal manifestations. When it occurs there should be no delay in instituting active treatment and this should be directed towards correcting the underlying physiological and biochemical changes while counteracting the bacterial infection. The mortality of this condition is extremely high, and therefore every effort must be made to restore a normal blood pressure.

General measures

In order to assist the venous return, the foot of the bed and elevation of the legs should be maintained during the period of hypotension. This sometimes is beneficial in raising the blood pressure. During the periods when hypotension is less marked and when a relatively satisfactory blood pressure is recorded, the patient may be moved to a more comfortable position, or even allowed to sit up.

Because of the myocardial failure produced by the toxaemia, routine digitalization is usually of benefit. Rapid digitalization with ouabain (see page 367) may initially be preferable to the more slow action of digoxin.

Antibiotics

When blood has been obtained for culture of the organisms and a swab taken of any infective discharge (i.e. from an abscess cavity, vagina, rectum, etc) antibiotic therapy should be started as quickly as possible, preferably by the intravenous route.

When the causative organism is not known, a combination of antibiotics that will probably completely span the spectrum of sensitivities of both Gram-positive and Gram-negative organisms must be used. The patient almost certainly will be unable to take oral medication, so that intravenous medication is essential. A combination of ampicillin, flucloxacillin and gentamicin together with metronidazole or lincomycin is an effective form of treatment. Ampicillin can be replaced with amoxycillin.

In the majority of cases, a bacteraemia causes impaired opsonization because of the lack of type-specific antibody,[163] thus reducing the defence mechanisms against endotoxic shock.* This is most marked when *Pseudomonas* organisms are present. *Bacteroides* organisms are anaerobic and are abundant in the bowel. They cause disseminated intravascular coagulation (DIC).[162] It is important, therefore, that antibiotics, such as clindamycin phosphate (Dalacin C), 300 mg 6-hourly diluted in 100 ml of fluid and given over 30 minutes, or intravenous metronidazole (Flagyl), 100 ml by intravenous infusion 8-hourly of the 0.5% solution in the adult, are administered.

Clavulanic acid has been found to inhibit the β-lactamases that are present on the surface of Gram-positive organisms and within the cytoplasm of Gram-negative organisms. Included amongst the β-lactamases are the penicillinase and cephalosporinase groups of enzymes. Gram-negative organisms, when they are present in the bladder for example, destroy amoxycillin so that no trace of the antibiotic is found in the urine. Clavulanic acid inhibits lactamase activity and thus, when added to amoxycillin (Augmentin), provides a much broader spectrum of antibacterial action. An intravenous form of clavulanic acid with amoxycillin is available from Beecham Laboratories Ltd, UK.

Naloxone in septic shock

It has been demonstrated[131] that naloxone can effectively treat the hypotension of septic shock. Eight patients who had not received corticosteroids had a 45% increase in their systolic blood pressure after being given 0.4–1.2 mg of naloxone. The increase in blood pressure was maintained for 45 minutes or longer. Two patients given a further dose after recurrence of the hypotension had a further increase in blood pressure. Four patients who had hypo-adreno-corticotropism did not respond to intravenous naloxone, and it was therefore concluded that endorphins may contribute to the hypotension of septic shock.

*It has been noted that antibiotics may increase the level of circulating endotoxins when these are released from the dead bacteria and thus increase the degree of endotoxic shock. This has been reviewed in an Editorial (1985) A nasty shock from antibiotics. *Lancet*, **ii**, 594.

Plasma

The presence of a toxaemia often gives rise to a lowering of the plasma protein concentration, either by the effect it has on the metabolism of the body or by causing it to be lost through the kidneys or into the lumen of the gut. If the renal output is low and the patient is already overhydrated, the danger of causing pulmonary oedema by the infusion of plasma is extremely great. Plasma should therefore be given in quantities that do not cause the central venous pressure (CVP) to rise above normal. If severe hypoproteinemia occurs in the absence of overhydration, it produces peripheral oedema in the same way that it is produced during prolonged starvation (ansarca). This brings in its train numerous metabolic problems and its correction by the slow infusion of hypertonic fractionated human albumin or triple strength plasma is of benefit. Because of the strain imposed upon the cardiovascular system, the infusions should be given with caution and a careful watch should be maintained on the respiratory rate and CVP. It is well known that during toxic shock acute dilatation of the stomach and paralytic ileus are commonly present. While paralytic ileus may be detected because of the absence of bowel sounds and the passing of flatus, acute dilatation of the stomach is often not suspected. It is wise, therefore, to pass a Ryles tube to determine whether there is a large accumulation of fluid, which requires replacement by infusion, within this viscus. Because cardiac failure tends to raise the CVP, the loss of a large volume of fluid from the circulation may result initially in a measured venous pressure that is within normal limits.

Vasopressors

It is extremely rare for any patient to survive a long period of 'cold septic shock' with an unrecordable blood pressure, associated with marked peripheral vasoconstriction. It is sometimes considered that, because vasoconstriction is already present, vasopressors may have no effect either on raising the blood pressure or on the outcome of the disease. This is by no means so, because lack of perfusion of the coronary vessels exacerbates the cardiac failure produced by the circulating bacterial toxins and this leads to death. The blood pressure therefore must be raised. The most easily controllable substance that can be used is *l*-noradrenaline (Levophed). It may be given in any normally infused intravenous solution in concentrations of up to 72 mg/l. In this way, overloading the circulation with an excess of fluid is avoided. It is best administered into a large vein so that intense constriction of the vessel does not occur. Although there is a danger that skin necrosis may be produced when there is prolonged administration of highly concentrated solutions, this may be avoided by the injection of phentolamine (Rogitine) around the site of the infusion. Alternatively, 5 mg of phentolamine may be added to each litre of solution infused without affecting the vasopressor effect, but avoiding the danger of necrosis. Other pressor drugs (see p. 226) are often not as effective, but they may be used either alone or to assist the action of *l*-noradrenaline. It is well recognized that these substances have their own side-effects which may tend to produce tissue damage. Their action upon both the heart itself and the gut is questionable, and ischaemia of tissues, caused by the unnatural degree of vasoconstriction, is a possibility that must be borne in mind. It may be advisable, therefore, if hypotension is prolonged, to give vasoconstrictor agents intermittently even if a brief period of hypotension is unavoidable. It is possible, for example, to maintain an adequate blood pressure in the region of a systolic value of 80–90 mmHg with *l*-noradrenaline for 30 minutes and then to stop the infusion for 3–5 minutes so that perfusion of the bowel through the mesenteric vessels is temporarily restored. In this way the effectiveness of these substances may be prolonged in the presence of fewer side-effects.

A slow intravenous infusion of isoprenaline (isoproterenol) may be given when the toxin is acting mainly on the myocardium and the CVP is raised. It is administered as described on page 228. It is frequently highly effective in raising the blood pressure.

Other vasopressors include dopamine, which like isoprenaline, acts directly upon the myocardium;[13,76,86,88,105] its actions are discussed on page 229. It is infused in concentrations of 40–100 mg/l and given at a rate which is sufficient to maintain the systolic blood pressure at 90 mmHg.[73–75]

Dobutamine also acts directly on the myocardium and has less β_2-receptor activity than isoprenaline. It is effective in toxic shock as well as cardiogenic shock,[72,75,88,95] although like dopamine it may be more beneficial in raising the blood pressure when it is used in combination with another vasopressor agent, such as metaraminol[148] (see page 230) which is given as a separate infusion at a different rate when necessary.

In 1967, Loeb *et al.*[104] investigated the effects of different forms of medication in 21 patients suffering from toxic shock. The cardiac output was measured in conjunction with blood pressure,

central venous pressure (CVP) and other parameters. The patients were given methoxamine 0.5 μg/ml, noradrenaline (norepinephrine) 16 μg/ml, isoprenaline 2 μg/ml, low molecular weight dextran (40 000 molecular weight) in volumes of 500–1000 ml, digitalis glycosides in the form of lanatoside C (1.2 mg) or strophanthin (0.5 mg), chlorpromazine, 10 mg followed by a further 5 or 10 mg after a period of 30 minutes, and hydrocortisone 2.0 g, all given intravenously. They found that the various forms of therapy had varying haemodynamic effects. The most positive haemodynamic effect appeared to occur in those patients who survived and who had the greatest response to volume loading, isoprenaline and digitalis.

Isoprenaline was infused at a rate that was sufficient to raise the arterial systolic pressure to 100 mmHg. Strophanthin was given to two patients and lanatoside C to nine patients. Cardiac output increased in eight patients and remained unchanged in two patients. Chlorpromazine was given to seven patients, all of whom had received low molecular weight dextran. Chlorpromazine was useful, as the author can confirm, in reducing the CVP by vasodilatation, thereby reducing the systemic vascular resistance. Even in small amounts, chlorpromazine is an effective vasodilator.[98]

It is well recognized that vasopressor agents become ineffective in the presence of a gross metabolic acidosis. It is, therefore, essential from this point of view alone, as well as the possibly beneficial effect a normal acid–base state may have on the toxic condition, that any fall in the bicarbonate ion content of the ECF should be corrected with sodium bicarbonate solution. Because it is necessary to avoid overloading the body with fluid and at the same time raising the osmolality of the ECF, hypertonic solutions should be used. In general the most concentrated solution available should be injected at intervals at a slow rate. Excess administration of alkali and the overcorrection of a metabolic acidosis are preferable to inadequate treatment. Some degree of metabolic alkalosis is desirable during septic shock, although it is rarely achieved. If there is any doubt as to the acid–base state, routine administration of 200 mmol (mEq/l) of alkali in hypertonic solution should be administered every 24 hours. If highly concentrated solutions are not available, this should not preclude its administration. In general, sodium lactate should not be administered as a raised blood lactate level is already present. Tris hydroxymethyl aminomethane (THAM) may be of value and may help to produce an osmotic diuresis.[122]

Corticosteroids

The intravenous administration of hydrocortisone has been frequently noted to produce a marked rise in blood pressure when it is injected in doses of 1 or 2 g. Smaller doses appear to be of relatively little benefit in many cases. A gradual rise of blood pressure over a period of 10–30 minutes occurs. Like vasopressors such as l-noradrenaline, it is less likely to be effective in the presence of a gross metabolic acidosis.

Experience has shown that the intravenous administration of methylprednisolone (Solu-Medrone) in doses that are used during the initial phases of cardiac transplantation, 250 mg i.v. 3-hourly, has a markedly beneficial effect in many forms of toxic shock. A rise in blood pressure occurs, the peripheral constriction decreases and may disappear entirely, and the recovery of the patient is enhanced. The author's impression is that there is an increase in the rate at which paralytic ileus is cured. It should not be continued in this very high dosage for more than 2–3 days, but when confined to this period a rapid decrease in dosage can be achieved and, in many cases corticosteroid therapy can be stopped after 5 days. The intravenous administration of much larger doses appears to have no greater beneficial effect and may be implicated in coagulation problems that can arise. Also, very large single doses may suppress the lymphocyte responses to such a degree that the immunological responses of the body to bacteria are also suppressed, so that the body defences are weakened rather than enhanced. Certainly the above regimen appears to be effective.

Alcohol

The infusion of alcohol intravenously sometimes appears to be of benefit—50 ml of sterile absolute alcohol may be added to a litre of solution. Alcohol may be beneficial because it is a readily metabolizable material releasing energy so that the defence mechanisms of the body may become more active. It has also the effect of inhibiting ADH and tends to produce vasodilation. In the early stages of 'cold septic shock', however, vasoconstriction predominates over the vasodilator effect of alcohol.

Intravenous vitamins

These do not appear to be of any value in the treatment of septic shock and may in fact be contraindicated as they tend to enhance the proliferation of bacteria. In the early stages of the condition they should, therefore, be withheld.

Summary of the Management of Septic Shock

1. The presence of a severe rigor following trauma or surgical intervention should always be considered as a prodromal sign of septic shock, and a blood culture should be taken, preferably at the height of the pyrexia. Arterial blood-gas and acid–base analysis should be made.

2. In the presence of hypotension (which commonly follows a rigor), general measures such as raising the foot of the bed, possibly digitalization and setting up of an intravenous infusion should be instituted immediately; thus valuable time is not lost.

3. Set up central venous pressure (CVP) measurement. When possible, insert a Swan–Ganz catheter for the measurement of left atrial pressure, and measure the arterial pressure directly by means of an electrical transducer; the pressure is displayed on a cathode-ray oscilloscope (CRO).

4. When there is a marked loss of fluid into the lumen of the gut or peritoneal cavity, replacement with plasma should be started; the volume of fluid infused is controlled by measuring the CVP.

5. Corticosteroids, hydrocortisone in doses of 1 or 2 g i.v., should be followed immediately by methylprednisolone 250 mg i.v., and repeated every 3 hours.

6. Apply antibiotic therapy as if every organism possible was causing the toxic shock. For example, a combination such as:

ampicillin	500 mg i.v. 4-hourly
flucloxacillin	500 mg i.v. 4-hourly
gentamicin	80 mg i.v. 8-hourly
metronidazole	400 mg i.v. 8-hourly

This should be continued for 48 hours before re-assessing the condition and the results from the blood cultures are known.

7. A careful measurement of fluid losses should be maintained when this is possible. In order to assess renal function, care must be taken to make sure that the volume, the specific gravity and osmolality of urine passed are known (see p. 130). The amount of fluid infused is maintained at that volume which will keep a normal fluid balance while permitting the infusion of vasopressor agents when this is necessary. The fluid should, in general, contain a sufficient concentration of electrolyte to maintain the osmolality of the body fluids.

8. The metabolic acidosis should be corrected by infusions of hypertonic sodium bicarbonate solution as early as possible. Frequent blood-gas

estimations are required. The infusion of 100 mmol/l (mEq/l) of $NaHCO_3$ can be given prophylactically.

9. When hypotension does not respond to fluid replacement, antibiotics, digitalization and hydrocortisone, the vasopressors should be used. The most effective vasopressors are isoprenaline (isoproterenol, Isuprel, Suscardia), dopamine (Intropin), metaraminol (Aramine) and *l*-noradrenaline (norepinephrine, Levophed).

10. Maintain the blood pressure, if possible, above 90 mmHg systolic, by means of vasopressors if necessary, after correction of blood volume and acid–base disturbances.

11. Substances such as alcohol (50 ml absolute sterile ethanol, 1 litre of isotonic saline) may be tried when other measures prove to be ineffective.

HYDATID DISEASE (ECHINOCCUS)

Another cause of profound and sometimes unexplained shock is hydatid disease. It is most commonly seen in sheep-rearing areas such as those in New Zealand and Australia and in the Middle and Far East. It is transmitted to man via the dog.

When the ova have been ingested, the hexacanth embryo hatches in the upper part of the alimentary canal and makes its way to the liver via the tributaries of the portal vein and then forms a hydatid follicle. Mononuclear and eosinophil leucocytes accumulate around the parasite. The follicle becomes vesicular by the end of 2 or 3 weeks as fluid is formed within a laminated wall. At first the surrounding tissue reaction is highly cellular, but this later becomes replaced by concentrically arranged fibroblasts. As the cyst grows, a slow pressure necrosis of the surrounding tissue occurs and more fibrous tissue is laid down. The outer layers of the laminated hyaline capsule rupture as these become more stretched than the inner lamination. The outer laminations possess a greater degree of elasticity than the inner laminations and thus if splitting of the capsule occurs, eversion of the cyst is produced, emptying the contents completely. The cyst most commonly bursts when it is situated close to a serous cavity such as the thoracic or peritoneal cavity, or when it is adjacent to a hollow viscus. The contents therefore tend to empty into the bile ducts, the bronchi, the alimentary canal or the urinary tract.[47] Rupture can also occur into the ventricles of the brain or the spinal theca, or into a myocardial cavity. Life, however, is usually short when the cysts are primarily deposited either in the myocardium or the brain because of the profound effect on the function of these organs. In other sites, however, the cysts may remain undetected for years.

The fluid contained within the cyst may produce an anaphylactoid reaction when it is dispersed within the body. It is used in small quantities to detect the presence of hydatid disease in man. This is known as the Casoni test, but all too often this test is negative when hydatid disease is present.

A positive reaction is identified when a weal develops within 15 minutes of the intradermal injection of sterile standard hydatid fluid. It has also been found to be positive in 75% of people with hydatid disease.[9] Eosinophilia is seen in approximately 30% of patients.[102] The complement fixation test is positive in approximately 80% of patients. Haemagglutination and latex glutination tests are also used. The principle of the haemagglutination test is that hydatid antigen is absorbed onto tanned erythrocytes and agglutination occurs when specific antibodies are added. The latex test is similar except that latex particles are used in place of erythrocytes.[115] Other means of identification include radioisotope scanning, ultrasound and intravenous viscerography.[77] Computerized axial tomography (CAT scan) is now being used increasingly.[140]

Anaphylactoid Shock

It must be presumed that the anaphylactoid reaction follows leakage of hydatid fluid into the systemic circulation. Sensitivity to hydatid fluid can vary from a mild reaction of a feeling of being unwell to a profound shock-like state which may result in death. In its mildest form it is associated with a moderate pyrexia, pruritus, a generalized or a localized erythematous reaction which may develop into an urticarial rash, weals, or bullae. A more severe manifestation of this condition may have visual disturbances, a feeling of faintness, delirium, abdominal pain and vomiting. When the complete picture of hydatid anaphylaxis develops the blood pressure falls so that it becomes un-recordable and the pulse impalpable. The patient is unconscious, but may remember conversations that have taken place during this period and the methods and attempts that are made to resuscitate him. Cyanosis is present and breathing is stertorous and laboured and associated with high-pitched inspiratory and expiratory rhonchi resulting from narrowing of the bronchial tree. Vomiting almost invariably occurs. The pupils are sometimes dilated. The reaction of the individual to leakage of hydatid fluid is extremely variable. It commonly occurs spontaneously and is often seen following surgery in which attempts have been made to remove hydatid cysts. The sensitivity reaction, however, does not necessarily accompany the loss of fluid into the abdominal cavity when a hydatid cyst bursts. Bursting the cyst should be avoided, how-ever, because of the secondary spread of the para-site. Profound hypotension and other manifesta-tions of the anaphylactoid reaction may be delayed postoperatively for 24–48 hours or may never occur at all.

The treatment of anaphylactoid shock due to hydatid disease

The shock that occurs when some of the hydatid fluid leaks into the systemic circulation must be considered as one of the manifestations of normo-volaemic shock. Although death does sometimes result from this condition, full recovery almost always occurs. Even after a very low blood pressure has resulted from the anaphylactoid reaction, acute renal failure does not commonly develop.

Any vasopressor will be effective in raising the blood pressure when this is found to be necessary. The intravenous injection of hydrocortisone hemi-succinate is found to be an effective form of therapy. This treatment should be tried in the first instance. Hydrocortisone should be given intravenously in doses of 100 mg and repeated every 10 minutes until an effective return of blood pressure occurs. It may be necessary in the large heavy individual to give larger doses (e.g. as much as 300 mg i.v. in the first instance). Adrenaline given as a 1–1000 solu-tion subcutaneously at the rate of 0.1 ml/minute as for asthma, is also an effective method of treatment in many cases.

It is important to maintain adequate ventilation and it is highly probable that when death has occurred, respiratory failure has contributed as much as cardiac failure. Artificial ventilation, if possible with oxygen, should be given whenever necessary.

When excessive sweating has occurred resulting in a marked loss of fluid from the body, replace-ment with the appropriate solution should be insti-tuted. The following case history illustrates some of the difficulties in diagnosis and treatment.

Case history. A soldier was moving house in the Far East and while carrying some heavy cases he suddenly began to feel unwell. He noticed that his hands and arms and legs were red in colour. He also experienced paraesthesia in the hands and fingers and itching in other parts of the body. He felt sufficiently unwell to go to bed and stayed there until the following day. He then got up and moved about the room, but suddenly collapsed, hitting his fore-head on a piece of furniture and cutting it. He remained unconscious and when the medical attendant arrived a few minutes later it was noticed that the soldier was cyanosed, especially peripherally at the finger tips, that his breathing was noisy and laboured that he was sweating profusely so that his clothes were wet. His pupils were dilated and his blood pressure was unrecordable. He was given intravenous hydro-cortisone 100 mg and, within half an hour, his blood pressure had returned to 90/50 mmHg. It was not known at that time that he was suffer-ing from hydatid disease and, although an electrocardiogram showed no gross deviation from normality, it was considered that he was suffering from a coronary occlusion. When, therefore, his blood pressure had returned to normal values some hours later, he was placed on anticoagulants. One week later he had a mild attack of asthma and a marked haemop-tysis. He was returned to England and a chest X-ray (Fig. 6.7) demonstrated mediastinal lymphadenopathy and discrete rounded shadows in both lungs. In spite of the fact that he had already experienced at least two major anaphylactoid reactions, the Casoni test was negative. A large hard mass was palpable abdominally attached to the liver. During laparotomy it was found that the mass was a multilocular hydatid cyst, but this burst before excision could be performed. The hydatid fluid was under high pressure and spread through-out the abdominal cavity even though the major part of it was directed away from the operation site. No marked fall in blood pressure occurred, but the patient developed paralytic ileus which

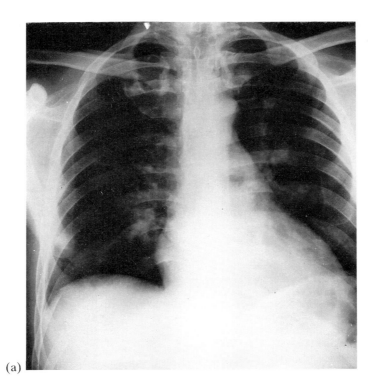

(a)

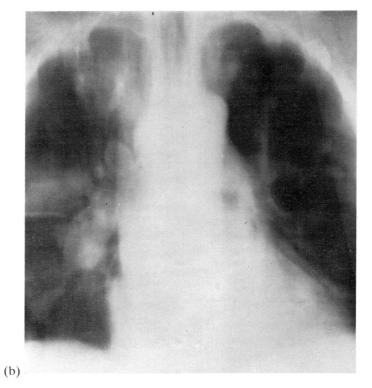

(b)

responded to conservative treatment over a period of 3 weeks. During this time he became hyponatraemic from sodium depletion so that intravenous replacement with hypertonic saline was necessary. He also developed a low serum albumin. Renal disease and dilution by excessive fluid administration were absent and the low serum albumin was partially corrected by infusions of fractionated human albumin until normal values in the plasma returned after a period of 3 weeks.

At a later date he was operated upon in an effort to remove some of the cysts, but because many of these were in the lumen of the pulmonary vessels, postoperative respiratory failure developed.

Treatment of Hydatid Disease

Although there have been advances in medication for this disease, surgery is still considered to be the treatment of choice. When possible, the cyst is removed *in toto* so that the scolices contained within are not set free to be available for secondary infection. Multilocular cysts are more difficult to remove, but those contained within the lung can sometimes be extruded by increasing the inflation pressure when the compressed overlying tissue has been incised. When the surrounding tissue has been damaged or destroyed, or in the lung has given rise to bronchiectasis, partial excision of the area is necessary. Another mode of treatment that has been advocated is the injection of 10% formalin into the cyst. This method of treatment can be used when excision is considered to be either impossible or undesirable.

Medical treatment

Bekhti *et al.*[12] gave mebendazole to four patients with hydatid disease of the liver who were considered unsuitable for surgery. The hydatid cysts regressed, as demonstrated by ultrasound, within 4–13 months. Clinical improvement was observed and specific IgE levels fell. It was later found that doses of 50 mg/kg per day were more effective.[11] The effectiveness of this treatment was also demonstrated by Wilson *et al.*[160] Complications have been found to be associated with this treatment, these include liver dysfunction, glomerulonephritis, gastric irritation, pyrexia, pruritis and leukopenia.[120] Poor absorption of mebendazole was found by Osborne in 1980.[126] Flubendazole has also been used to treat hydatid disease.

Generalized Anaphylactoid Shock

This is a frightening condition which usually occurs when it is least expected. It has, however, been observed following injection with penicillin and other substances and sometimes following the ingestion of various medications. It is associated with generalized cardiovascular collapse and respiratory dysfunction. The author induced anaphylaxis in a patient, who had received a heart transplant some 3 months earlier, following an intravenous injection of antilymphocytic globulin (ALG).

Case history. The patient was a 54-year-old male who had received a transplanted heart for severe myocardial ishaemia. Three months later, having received azathioprine (Imuran), methylprednisolone and ALG, the ALG in doses of 2 ml/day i.m., changes in the electrocardiogram were noted. These were thought to be due to rejection of the myocardium and it was decided that the patient should receive 5 ml of ALG intravenously. No reaction of any kind had been noted following the intramuscular injection of the ALG.

Antilymphocytic globulin 3 ml was given intravenously over a period of 5 minutes and no changes occurred. The remaining 2 ml were then given over a period of 3 minutes. Approximately 5 minutes after the completion of the injection, the patient became extremely dyspnoeic, was grossly cyanosed and had loud inspiratory and expiratory rhonchi which were audible without a stethoscope. The patient also became comatose, had a rapid tachycardia and his blood pressure was difficult to measure by means of a sphygmomanometer cuff but the systolic pressure was found by palpation to be in the region of 50–60 mmHg. All the patient's veins were engorged, indicating a high CVP, although this was not measured. An intravenous infusion of isoprenaline (isoproterenol, Suscardia) 5 mg in 1 litre of 5% dextrose was begun and administered at 10–20 drops/minute. A rapid improvement took place:

Fig. 6.7 (a) Chest X-ray of patient with hydatid disease. (b) Tomogram of the chest of the same patient demonstrating the hydatid cysts in the lungs with greater clarity.

the blood pressure rose immediately, the respiration improved within a very short time and the rhonchi disappeared. The patient coughed and expectorated pure white plugs of mucus. These were smooth and approximately 1 cm in diameter and just over 1 cm in length. The venous distention disappeared with the improvement in cardiac output. Continued complete recovery was made with no apparent ill-effects. No further ALG was given, either intramuscularly or intravenously.

Although the accepted treatment for anaphylactoid shock is considered to be subcutaneous adrenaline, in this instance, because of the nature of the patient's condition, a more controlled form of medication appeared to be indicated, although it is probable that adrenaline would have worked equally well. The venous engorgement facilitated the establishment of an intravenous infusion.

Metabolic Causes of Hypotension

Reduction in blood pressure due to a low plasma bicarbonate concentration has been discussed elsewhere (see p. 142). This may be seen following haemorrhage, cardiogenic shock or trauma which causes bruised, ischaemic muscles, and following release of the clamps after the insertion of a prosthetic abdominal aorta (Dacron graft). A 'washout acidosis' develops when high concentrations of lactate which have accumulated in the ischaemic tissues are released into the circulation. This is seen in patients presenting with peritonitis or acute obstruction of the gut.

Hypotension in diabetic ketosis and in nonketotic 'hyperosmolar' diabetes caused by the acidosis alone can be observed. In the former, hypotension is due to a combination of ketoacids and lactic acid, and in the latter it is due to lactic acid alone. A contribution to the accumulation of lactate in both forms of hyperglycaemia may be made by the presence of hypothermia.

Hypermagnesaemia also induces hypotension either by direct administration or by perforation of the gut allowing faeces to enter the peritoneal cavity and absorption to occur from the peritoneal surface. Magnesium-containing enemas have also produced hypotension.

Hypophosphataemia is now recognized as a cause of hypotension. It is seen in the malnourished, the elderly and in those suffering from chronic diseases. A low plasma phosphate induces a fall in cardiac output (see page 55).

Neurogenic Shock

In addition to direct damage to the vasomotor centre or head injury, which may cause a most profound degree of hypotension, injury to the upper part of the spinal cord causes a loss of vasomotor tone, vasodilatation and a fall in arterial blood pressure, and the peripheral resistance. The blood pressure rises following the administration of a vasopressor such as noradrenaline (norepinephrine), methoxamine or phenylephrine (Neosynephrine) or metaraminol (Aramine).

Drug-induced Hypotension

There are many substances in general use which may produce a marked fall in blood pressure because of their action on the myocardium, the vascular system, or the suprarenal gland and its secretions. They include morphine, pethidine, chlorpromazine and promethazine. The effects of morphine and pethidine may be corrected by naloxone HCl (Narcan) or by nalorphine (N-allylnorephine, Lethidrone). Naloxone (Narcan) is available in ampoules of 0.4 mg in 1 ml and is given initially in doses of 0.1–0.2 mg. It is also available for neonates in a concentration of 0.02 mg/ml in 2-ml ampoules. It is given in doses of 5–10 μg/kg body weight. It can be given intravenously, intramuscularly or subcutaneously. Nalorphine (Lethidrone) is available for intravenous use as a solution containing 10 mg/ml for adults and 1 mg/ml for neonates.

General Principles in the Treatment of Normovolaemic Shock

1. A central venous pressure (CVP) measurement or a pulmonary wedge pressure measurement is essential for management of the patient and avoidance of overtransfusion.

2. Vasopressors are indicated when the cause is toxic, metabolic or neurogenic and may be indicated when the cause is cardiogenic.

3. Correction of metabolic abnormalities is essential when these are acid–base, abnormal $[K^+]$, $[Na^+]$, $[Mg^{++}]$ and $[PO_4^-]$.

4. When in doubt, a broad-spectrum antibiotic regimen should be instituted.

5. Steroids in high doses are indicated in the early treatment of cardiogenic, toxic, anaphylactic and many forms of metabolic hypotension and some forms of neurogenic shock.

6. A close observation of the physiological changes is essential from the moment the patient is admitted. The parameters which should be watched include respiratory rate, heart rate, blood pressure and urine output. Urine output should be maintained at a minimum of 30 ml/hour.

PATHOLOGICAL FIBRINOLYSIS

The fibrinolytic mechanism in the blood is a natural one, which is maintained to remove fibrin from blood vessels and body tissues. The exact pathway through which it works is not known with certainty, but the concentration of the active proteolytic enzyme (plasmin) may be increased in the circulating blood by many factors, such as violent exercise, emotional states, the injection of adrenaline and the presence in the body of necrotic tissue. It is well known that an increase in the concentration of fibrinolytic activator (which results in an increase in concentration of plasmin) occurs following acute traumatic episodes which cause profuse haemorrhage and obstruction to the flow of blood to large area of muscle tissue. It can also develop after the sudden onset of a severe infection.

When pathological fibrinolysis occurs after trauma not only does the fibrinolytic bleeding develop because of clot dissolution, but there is also destruction of many of the essential plasma proteins involved in blood coagulation, such as fibrinogen antihaemophilic globulin (Factor VIII) and Factor V.

Pathological fibrinolysis can therefore occur in two ways. First, the plasma proteins essential to blood coagulation are destroyed at a faster rate than they can be replaced and the normal process of blood coagulation is either impaired or completely destroyed. Second, it is possible that the changes in the body biochemistry may be so altered that the production of these plasma proteins is reduced to such an extent that there is an insufficient quantity present in the circulation for normal blood coagulation to take place, although initially some of these factors are increased. As continuous blood loss progresses, these alterations in the body biochemistry are increased and replacement becomes more difficult.

It is well recognized that pathological fibrinolysis frequently appears after spontaneous attempts have been made at clotting. It is not surprising, therefore, that it is sometimes seen following vascular surgery in which large areas of ischaemic tissue join the general circulation following emergency vessel grafting operations or endarterectomy and are suddenly perfused with blood after many hours of anoxia. These operations are often associated with major blood loss and the replacement of a large volume of stored blood. Blood transfusion is a further factor in the production of pathological fibrinolysis because the condition also follows the transfusion of incompatible blood and may be produced either by the lysing of cells or by intravascular clotting which stimulates fibrinolysis. It also occurs after obstetrical conditions such as concealed accidental antepartum haemorrhage, criminal abortion or postpartum haemorrhage; it is commonly seen after open-heart surgery using an extracorporeal circulation and perhaps is more commonly observed when a pump oxygenator is used in association with a heat exchanger in order to produce hypothermia. Abnormal fibrinolytic activity has also been measured during profound hypothermia using autogenous lung perfusion.[91] An abnormal biochemistry, especially a metabolic acidosis, may be a predisposing condition towards the inadequate production of plasma protein involved in the coagulation of blood. Certainly, there is evidence that a metabolic acidosis is a contributory cause of consumption coagulopathy and fibrinolysis.

In the experiments performed by Kenyon et al.,[94] when a pumpoxygenator and heat exchanger were used to produce deep hypothermia with circulatory arrest, the infusion of sodium bicarbonate from the beginning of the procedure prevented pathological fibrinolysis.[19] If the sodium bicarbonate was infused after the period of circulatory arrest, although many of the physiological abnormalities such as hypotension and respiratory failure were prevented, fibrinolysis still occurred.

Cirrhosis of the liver is a well-recognized cause of increased fibrinolytic activity and may give rise to spontaneous bleeding. Other conditions which may give rise to spontaneous blood loss are leukaemia in which both fibrinolysis and defibrination may develop in the later stages, carcinoma of the prostate and other malignant conditions.

Treatment of Pathological Fibrinolysis

1. *Blood transfusion*. In practice, the replacement of whole blood has little effect upon the reversal of the condition of pathological fibrinolysis in the majority of cases.

It is obviously necessary to replace the red blood cells when they are lost, and the transfusion of fresh blood taken into plastic containers is preferable to that of ordinary stored blood. The fresh blood taken into and transfused from plastic containers helps to correct the thrombocytopenia which often develops during this condition, and when the platelet count is very low (less than 30 000/mm^3) transfusion of platelets may be necessary.

2. *Concentrated fibrinogen*. The infusion of concentrated fibrinogen is the best and easiest method of restoring low fibrinogen levels and it can be given at the rate of 6 g of fibrinogen every 15 minutes until normal values are obtained; 3 g of fibrinogen are contained in 1 litre of fresh or frozen plasma (FFP) and this may be given over a period of 30–60 minutes. Complement components and antithrombin III are also present in FFP, but FFP carries a risk of the transmission of hepatitis. If FFP is not from group AB donors, matching with the patient's ABO group is necessary.[7]

Although these substitutes for concentrated fibrinogen can be used with benefit, they are less effective than the concentrated preparation. Frozen plasma has the advantages, however, of containing antihaemophilic globulin and Factor V which, with other factors important in blood coagulation, are, as we have seen, frequently destroyed by the proteolytic fibrinolysin. If the fibrinolytic activity is intense, all the coagulation factors may be destroyed immediately following infusion. All preparations, including fresh frozen plasma, are then relatively ineffective.

3. *Specific antifibrinolytic therapy*. The most commonly used and undoubtedly most effective substance for reversing the fibrinolytic process is epsilon-aminocaproic acid (EACA). There is no doubt as to its effectiveness in many cases, but Naeye (1962) has reported widespread intravascular thrombosis after its use.[121] Such occurrences, however, are rare. It should, however, be used with caution and administered very slowly. Intravenous injection as a 'bolus' should be avoided, as it has been incriminated in acute renal failure.[35] Renal function abnormalities have been observed on numerous occasions by the author, when moderately large doses of Σ-aminocaproic acid have been given following open-heart surgery.

Intravenous *heparin* is also used in reversing pathological fibrinolysis.

Prevention of Fibrinolysis

We have already seen that fibrinolysis was prevented during an extracorporeal circulation in dogs for the production of profound hypothermia when alkali was infused at the earliest possible moment after the induction of anaesthesia. There is also much evidence that this is true in man. It might be argued, therefore, that after trauma and haemorrhagic shock, the infusion of hypertonic solutions of sodium bicarbonate might play a part in the prevention of the fibrinolytic mechanism of pathological proportions if infused into the patient in the first instance, even before the infusion of blood. Stored bank ACD blood is extremely acidotic and contributes to the metabolic acidosis already produced by the trauma and haemorrhage. In other words, it makes the abnormal biochemical condition already present very much worse. The author has had experience of both types of patients: those who have been treated with sodium bicarbonate in the very first instance and then later transfused with more than 24 units of blood (11 litres) and have not produced fibrinolytic bleeding, and those who have in a similar manner been transfused with stored (ACD) blood and have not been given alkali until later when a metabolic acidosis has been detected by blood analysis and who have developed a lethal form of generalized bleeding. The initial infusion of hypertonic sodium bicarbonate does no harm, but whether it has any pronounced benefit in preventing pathological fibrinolysis still requires further investigation.

A very good review of blood coagulation in the critically ill patient has been written by Bain.[7]

References

Shock

1. Allardyce, D. B., Yoshida, S. H. and Ashmore, P. G. (1966). The importance of microembolism in the pathogenesis of organ dysfunction caused by prolonged use of the pump oxygenator. *J. Thorac. Cardiovasc. Surg.*, **52**, 706.

2. Arrington, P. and McNamara, J. J. (1974). Mechanism of microaggregate formation in stored blood. *Ann. Surg.*, **179**, 146.

3. Arrington, P. J. and McNamara, J. J. (1975). Effect of agitation on platelet aggregation and microaggregate formation in banked blood. *Ann. Surg.*, **181**, 243.

4. Ashmore, P. G., Svitel, V. and Ambrose, P. (1968). Incidence and effects of particulate aggregation and microembolization in pump oxygenator systems. *J. Thorac. Cardiovasc. Surg.*, **55**, 691.

5. Athanasoulis, C. A. (1980). Therapeutic applications of angiography. *N. Eng. of med.*, **302**, 1117.

6. Aub, J. C. and Wu, H. (1920). Studies in experimental traumatic shock. III. Chemical changes in blood. *Amer. J. Physiol.*, **54**, 416.

7. Bain, B. (1982). Coagulopathies. In *Intensive Care.* Edited by E. Sherwood-Jones. Lancaster, England: MTP Press.

8. Barrett, J., Dawidson, I., Dhurandhar, H. N., Miller, E. and Litwin, M. S. (1975). Pulmonary microembolism associated with massive transfusion. 11. The basic pathophysiology of its pulmonary effects. *Ann. Surg.*, **182**, 56.

9. Barros, J. L. (1978). Hydatid disease of the liver. *Amer. J. Surg.*, **135**, 597.

10. Beecher, H. K., Simeone, F. A., Burnett, C. H., Shapiro, S. L., Sullivan, E. R. and Mallory, T. B. (1947). The internal state of the severely wounded man on entry to the most forward hospital. *Surgery*, **22**, 672.

11. Bekhti, A., Nizet, M., Capron, M., Dessaint, J. P., Santoro, F. and Capron, A. (1980). Chemotherapy of human hydatid disease with mebendazole. Follow up of 16 cases. *Acta Gastroenterologica, Belgica*, **43**, 48.

12. Bekhti, A., Schaaps, J-P., Capron, M., Dessaint, J. P., Santoro, F., Capron, A. (1977). Treatment of hepatic hydatid disease with mebendazole: preliminary results in four cases. *Brit. med. J.*, **II**, 1047.

13. Beregovich, J., Bianchi, C., Rubler, S., Lemnitz, E., Cagin, N. and Levitt, B. (1974). Dose-related hemodynamic and renal effects of dopamine in congestive heart failure. *Amer. Heart J.*, **87**, 550.

14. Bernard, C. (1877). *Leçons sur le diabète et la glycogénèse animale.* p. 120. Paris: Baillière.

15. Blaisdell, F. W., Lim, R. C., Amberg, J. R., Choy, S. H., Hall, A. D. and Thomas, A. N. (1966). Pulmonary microembolism—a cause of death and morbidity after major vascular surgery. *Arch. Surg.*, **93**, 776.

16. Brennan, R. N., Patterson, R. H. and Kessler, J. (1971). Cerebral blood flow and metabolism during cardiopulmonary bypass: evidence of microembolic encephalopathy. *Neurology*, **21**, 665.

17. British Medical Journal (1980). Editorial: Prevention or cure for stress-induced gastrointestinal bleeding? *Brit. med. J.*, **281**, 631.

18. Brooks, D. K. (1964). Osmolar, electrolyte and respiratory changes in hemorrhagic shock. *Amer. Heart J.*, **68**, 574.

19. Brooks, D. K. (1965). Physiological responses produced by changes in acid-base equilibrium following profound hypothermia. *Anaesthesia*, **20**, 173.

20. Brooks, D. K. (1967). The mechanism of shock. *Brit. J. Surg.*, Lister Centenary No. 441.

21. Brooks, D. K. (1967). *Resuscitation*, 1st edn. London: Edward Arnold.

22. Brooks, D. K. (1972). Organ failure following surgery. Advances in Surg., **6**, 289.

23. Brooks, D. K. (1978). Gastrointestinal bleeding in acute respiratory failure. *Brit. med. J.*, **1**, 922.

24. Brooks, D. K. (1978). Stomach as a reservoir for respiratory pathogens. *Lancet*, **ii**, 1147.

25. Brooks, D. K. (1980). Treatment of refractory hypovolaemic shock. *Lancet*, **i**, 1256.

26. Brooks, D. K. and Feldman, S. A. (1962). Metabolic acidosis; a new approach to 'neostigmine resistant curarisation'. *Anaesthesia*, **17**, 161.

27. Brooks, D. K., Williams, W. G., Manley, R. W. and Whiteman, P. (1963). Osmolar and electrolyte changes in haemorrhagic shock; hypertonic solutions in the prevention of tissue damage. *Lancet*, **i**, 521.

28. Brooks, D. K., Williams, W. G., Manley, R. W. and Whiteman, P. (1963). Respiratory changes in haemorrhagic shock. The association of respiratory failure with gross changes in biochemistry and osmolarity. *Anasthesia*, **18**, 363.

29. Brooks, D. K. and Wynn, V. (1959). Use of venous blood for pH and carbon-dioxide studies, especially in respiratory failure and during anaesthesia. *Lancet*, **i**, 227.

30. Brown, C., Dhurandhar, H. N., Barrett, J. and Litwin, M. S. (1977). Progression and resolution of changes in pulmonary function and structure due to pulmonary microembolism and blood transfusion. *Ann. Surg.*, **185**, 92.

31. Bryant, L. R. and Griffin, W. O. (1966). Vagotomy and pyloroplasty: an inadequate operation for stress ulcers? *Arch. Surg.*, **93**, 161.

32. Cannon, W. B. (1918). A consideration of the nature

of wound shock. *J. Amer. med. Ass.*, **70**, 611.

33. Cannon, W. B. (1923). *Traumatic shock*. New York: Appleton.

34. Cannon, W. B., Fraser, J. and Cowell, E. M. (1918). The preventive treatment of wound shock. *J. Amer. med. Ass.*, **70**, 618.

35. Charytan, C. and Purtilo, D. (1969). Glomerular capillary thrombosis and acute renal failure after epsilon-amino caproic acid therapy. *N. Engl. J. of Med.*, **280**, 1102.

36. Clowes, G. H., Farrington, G. H., Zuschneid, W., Cossette, G. R. and Saravis, C. (1970). Circulating factors in the etiology of pulmonary insufficiency and right heart failure accompanying severe sepsis (peritonitis). *Ann. Surg.*, **171**, 663.

37. Clowes, G. H. A., O'Donnell, T. F., Ryan, N. T. and Blackburn, G. L. (1974). Energy metabolism in sepsis: treatment based on different patterns in shock and high out put stage. *Ann. Surg.*, **179**, 684.

38. Conn, H. O., Ramson, G. R., Storer, E. H., Mutchnick, M. G., Joshi, P. H., Phillips, M. M., Cohen, G. A., Fields, G. N. and Petroski, D. (1975). Intraarterial vasopressin in treatment of upper gastrointestinal hemorrhage: a prospective controlled clinical trial. *Gastroenterology*, **68**, 211.

39. Connell, R. S., Page, U. S., Bartley, T. D., Bigelow, J. C. and Webb, N. C. (1973). The effects of pulmonary ultrastructure of dacron wool filtration during cardiopulmonary bypass. *Ann. Thorac. Surg.*, **15**, 217.

40. Connell, R. S. and Webb, M. C. (1975). Filtration characteristics of three new in-line blood transfusion filters. *Ann. Surg.*, **181**, 273.

41. Cooksey, W. B. and Puschelberg, G. C. (1948). Disposable fine mesh filter for blood and plasma. *J. Amer. med. Assoc.*, **137**, 788.

42. Coraggio, F., Scarpato, P., Spina, M. and Lombardi, S. (1984). Somatostatin and ranitine in the control of iatrogenic haemorrhage of the upper gastrointestinal tract. *Brit. med. J.*, **289**, 224.

43. Creighton, B. W. and Solis, R. T. (1973). Microaggregation in canine autotransfusion. *Amer. J. Surg.*, **126**, 25.

44. Crenshaw, C. A., Canizaro, P. C., Shires, G. T. and Allsman, A. (1962). Changes in extracellular fluid during acute hemorrhagic shock in man. *Surg. Forum*, **13**, 6.

45. Cushing, H. (1932). Peptic ulcers and the intestines. *Surg., Gynecol. & Obst.*, **551**, 1.

46. DeGowin, E. L. (1949). Transfusion equipment. In *Blood Transfusion*. p. 515. Edited by E. L. DeGowin, R. C. Hardin and J. B. Alsever. Philadelphia: Saunders.

47. Dew, H. (1930). Some complications of hydatid disease. *Brit. J. Surg.*, **18**, 275.

48. Dhall, D. P., Engeset, J., McKenzie, F. N. and Matheson, N. A. (1969). Screen filtration pressure of blood—an evaluation. *Cardiovasc. Res.*, **3**, 147.

49. Dhall, D. P. and Matheson, N. A. (1969). Platelet aggregation filtration pressure—a method of measuring platelet aggregation in whole blood. *Cardiovasc. Res.*, **3**, 155.

50. Douglas, H. O. and LeVeen, H. H. (1970). Stress ulcers—a clinical and experimental study showing the roles of mucosal susceptibility and hypersecretion. *Arch. Surg.*, **100**, 178.

51. Dragstedt, L. R., Ragins, H., Dragstedt, L. R., II and Evans, S. (1956). Stress and duodenal ulcer. *Amer. Surgeon.*, **144**, 450.

52. Drivas, G., Pullan, L., Uldall, P. R. and Wardle, E. N. (1976). Altered reticuloendothelial function in long term allograft recipients. *Arch. Surg.*, **111**, 1368.

53. de Duve, C. (1959). Lysosomes: a new group of cytoplasmic particles. In *Subcellular Particles*. New York: Ronald Press Company.

54. Egeblad, K., Osborn, J. J., Burns, W., Hill, J. D. and Gerbode, F. (1972). Blood filtration during cardiopulmonary bypass. *J. Thorac. Cardiovasc. Surg.*, **63**, 384.

55. Ehrenhaft, J. L. and Clasman, M. A. (1961). Cerebral complications of open heart surgery. *J. Thorac. Cardiovasc. Surg.*, **41**, 503.

56. Ehrenhaft, J. L., Clasman, M. A., Layton, J. M. and Zimmerman, G. R. (1961). Cerebral complications of open heart surgery: further observations. *J. Thorac. Cardiovasc. Surg.*, **42**, 514.

57. Eiseman, B. and Heyman, R. L. (1970). Medical intelligence. *N. Eng. J. of Med.*, **282**, 372.

58. Epidemiologic notes and reports (1980). Follow-up on toxic shock syndrome. *Morbid Mortal Weekly Rep.*, **29**, 441.

59. Evans, E. I. and Butterfield, W. J. H. (1951). The stress response in the severely burned: an interim report. *Ann. Surg.*, **134**, 588.

60. de Felippe, J.Jr., Timoner, J., Velasco, I. T., Lopes, O. U. and Rocha-e-Silva, M.Jr. (1980). Treatment of refractory hypovolaemic shock by 7.5% sodium chloride injections. *Lancet*, **ii**, 1002.

61. Fine, J. (1954). *The bacterial factor in traumatic shock*. p. 43. Springfield, Ill.: Charles C Thomas.

62. Fletcher, D. G. and Hoskins, H. N. (1954). Acute peptic ulcer as a complication of major surgery stress or trauma. *Surgery*, **36**, 212.

63. Freeman, J. and Nunn, J. F. (1963). Ventilation-perfusion relationships after haemorrhage. *Clin. Sci.*, **24**, 135.

64. Fulton, R. L. (1970). The absorption of sodium and water by collagen during hemorrhagic shock. *Ann. Surg.*, **172**, 861.

65. Fulton, R. L. and Fischer, R. P. (1974). Pulmonary changes due to hemorrhagic shock resuscitation with isotonic and hypertonic saline. *Surgery*, **75**, 881.

66. Fulton, R. L. and Jones, C. (1975). The cause of post-traumatic pulmonary insufficiency in man. *Surg. Gynecol. & Obstet.*, **140**, 179.

67. Fulton, R. L. and Peter, E. T. (1974). Metabolic and physiologic effects of sodium in the treatment of hemorrhagic shock. *Amer. Surg.*, **40**, 152.

68. Gaisford, W. D., Pandey, N. and Jensen, C. G. (1972). Pulmonary changes in treated hemorrhagic shock. II. Ringer's lactate solution versus colloid solution. *Amer. J. Surg.*, **124**, 738.

69. Gerst, P. H., Rattenborg, G. and Holaday, D. A. (1959). The effects of hemorrhage on pulmonary circulation and respiratory gas exchange. *J. clin. Invest.*, **38**, 524.

70. Gervin, A. S., Mason, K. G. and Wright, C. B. (1974). Microaggregate volumes in stored human blood. *Surg. Gynecol. & Obstet.*, **139**, 519.

71. Gervin, A. S., Mason, K. G. and Wright, C. B. (1974). Source of microaggregates in aged human blood anticoagulated in CPD. *Clin. Res.*, **22**, 177.

72. Gillespie, T. A., Ambos, H. D., Sobel, B. E. and Roberts, R. (1977). Effects of dobutamine in patients with acute myocardial infarction. *Amer. J. Cardiol.*, **39**, 588.

73. Goldberg, L. (1972). Cardiovascular and renal actions of dopamine: potential clinical applications. *Pharmacol. Rev.*, **24**, 1.

74. Goldberg, L. I. (1975). The dopamine vascular receptor. *Biochem. Pharmacol.*, **24**, 651.

75. Goldberg, L. I., Hsieh, Y. and Resnekov, L. (1977). Newer catecholamines for treatment of heart failure and shock: an update on dopamine and a first look at dobutamine. *Prog. Cardiovasc. Dis.*, **19**, 327.

76. Goldberg, L. I., McDonald, R. H. and Zimmerman, A. M. (1963). Sodium diuresis produced by dopamine in patients with congestive heart failure. *N. Engl. J. of Med.*, **269**, 1060.

77. Gonzales, L. R., Marcos, J., Illanas, M., Hernandez-Mora, M., Pena, M. D., Picouto, J. P., Cienfuegos, J. A. and Alvarez, J. L. R. (1979). Radiologic aspects of hepatic echinococcosis. *Radiology*, **130**, 21.

78. Goolden, R. H. (1854). On diabetes and its relation to brain affections. *Lancet*, **i**, 656.

79. Grable, E., Israel, J., Williams, J. and Fine, J. (1963). Blood volume in experimental endotoxic and hemorrhagic shock. *Ann. Surg.*, **157**, 361.

80. Grant, R. T. and Reeve, E. B. (1951). Observations on the general effects of injury in man with special reference to wound shock. *Spec. Rep. Ser. med. Res. Coun. (Lond.)*, **No. 277**.

81. Greenall, M. J., Blewitt, R. W. and McMahon, M. J. (1975). Cardiac tamponade and central venous catheters. *Brit. med. J.*, **2**, 595.

82. Harkins, H. N. (1938). Acute ulcer of the duodenum (Curling's ulcer) as a complication of burns. *Surgery*, **3**, 608.

83. Hill, J. D., Aguilar, M. J., Baranco, A., DeLanerolle, P. and Gerbode, F. (1969). Neuropathological manifestations of cardiac surgery. *Ann. Thorac. Surg.*, **7**, 409.

84. Hill, J. D., Osborn, J. J., Swank, R. L., Aguilar, M. J., Primal de Lanerolle, and Gerbode, F. (1970). Experience using a new dacron wool filter during extracorporeal circulation. *Arch. Surg.*, **101**, 649.

85. Hirsch, H., Swank, R. L., Brever, M. and Hissen, N. (1964). Screen filtration pressure of homologous and heterologous blood and electroencephalogram. *Amer. J. Physiol.*, **206**, 811.

86. Holloway, E. L., Stinson, E. B., Derby, G. C. and Harrison, D. C. (1975). Action of drugs in patients early after cardiac surgery. I. Comparison of isoproterenol and dopamine. *J. Amer. med. Assc.*, **35**, 656.

87. Horovitz, J. M., Carrico, C. J. and Shires, G. T. (1974). Pulmonary response to major surgery. *Arch. Surg.*, **108**, 349.

88. Horwitz, D., Fox, S. M. and Goldberg, L. I. (1962). Effects of dopamine in man. *Circ. Res.*, **10**, 237.

89. Howard, J. M. (1955). Studies of the absorption and metabolism of glucose following injury. *Ann. Surg.*, **141**, 321.

90. Jaffe, R. (1981). Toxic-shock syndrome associated with diaphragm use. *N. Engl. J. of Med.*, **305**, 1585.

91. James, D. C. O. (1966). Private communication.

92. Janoff, A., Weissmann, G., Zweifach, B. W. and Thomas, L. (1962). Pathogenesis of experimental shock. IV. Studies on lysosomes in normal and tolerant animals subjected to lethal trauma and endotoxemia. *J. Exper. Med.*, **116**, 451.

93. Jenkins, M. R., Jones, R. F., Wilson, B. and Moyer, C. A. (1950). Congestive atelectasis: a complication of intravenous infusion of fluids. *Ann. Surg.*, **132**, 327.

94. Kenyon, J. R., Ludbrook, J., Downs, A. R., Tait, I. B., Brooks, D. K. and Pryczkowski, J. (1959). Experimental deep hypothermia. *Lancet*, **ii**, 41.

95. Kersting, F., Follath, F., Moulds, R., Mucklow, J., McCloy, R., Sheares, J. and Dollery, C. (1976). A comparison of cardiovascular effects of dobutamine and isoprenaline after open heart surgery. *Brit. Heart J.*, **38**, 622.

96. Kim, S. I. and Shoemaker, W. C. (1973). Role of acidosis in the development of increased pulmonary vascular resistance and shock lung in experimental hemorrhagic shock. *Surgery*, **73**, 723.

97. Kolmer, J. A. (1940). Studies on the preservation of human blood. *Amer. J. med. Sci.*, **200**, 311.

98. Lancet (1955). Editorial: Pharmacology of chlorpromazine. *Lancet*, **i**, 337.

99. Landis, E. M. and Hortenstine, J. C. (1950). Functional significance of venous blood pressure. *Physiol. Rev.*, **30**, 1.

100. Lillehei, C. W., Roth, R. E. and Wangensteen, O. H. (1952). The role of stress in the etiology of peptic ulcer. *S. Forum*, **2**, 43.

101. Limberg, B. and Kommerell, B. (1979). Somatostatin after failure of cimetidine for acute bleeding ulcers. *Lancet*, **ii**, 1361.

102. Little, J. M. (1976). Hydatid disease at Royal Prince Alfred Hospital 1964–1974. *Med. J. Australia*, **1**, 903.

103. Litwin, M. S. and Hurley, M. J. (1978). The filtration of blood. *Surgery Annual*, **10**, 105.

104. Loeb, H. S., Cruz, A., Teng, C. Y., Boswell, J., Iietras, R. J., Tobin, J. R. and Gunnar, R. M. (1967).

Haemodynamic studies in shock associated with infection. *Brit. Heart J.*, **29**, 883.

105. Loeb, H. S, Winslow, E. B. J., Rahimtoola, S. H., Rosen, K. M. & Gunnar, R. M. (1971). Acute hemodynamic effects of dopamine in patients with shock. *Circulation*, **44**, 163.

106. Loomis, L. and Feder, H. M. Jr. (1981). Toxic-shock syndrome associated with diaphragm use. *N. Engl. J. of Med.*, **305**, 1585.

107. Lowrey, B. D. and Sugg, J. M. (1972). Pulmonary dysfunction after shock and trauma. *Adv. Exp. Med. Biol.*, **23**, 415.

108. Ludbrook, J. and Wynn, V. (1958). Citrate intoxication: a clinical and experimental study. *Brit. med. J.*, **2**, 523.

109. McNamara, J. J. (1973). Microaggregates in stored blood—physiologic significance. In *Preservation of Red Blood Cells*. p. 336. Edited by H. Chaplin. Washington DC: National Academy of Sciences.

110. McNamara, J. J. and Austen, W. G. (1955). Gastrointestinal bleeding occurring in patients with acquired valvula heart disease. *Arch. Surg.*, **97**, 538.

111. McNamara, J. J., Boatright, D., Burran, E. L., Molot, M. D., Summers, E. and Stremple, J. F. (1971). Changes in some physical properties of stored blood. *Ann. Surg.*, **174**, 58.

112. McNamara, J. J., Molot, M. D. and Stremple, J. F. (1970). Screen filtration pressure in combat casualties. *Ann. Surg.*, **172**, 334.

113. Marston, A. (1964). Patterns of intestinal ischaemia. *Ann. Roy. Coll. Surg. Engl.*, **35**, 151.

114. Martin, A. M., Simmons, R. L. and Heisterkamp, C. A. (1969). Respiratory insufficiency in combat casualties—pathogenic changes in the lungs of patients dying of wounds. *Ann. Surg.*, **170**, 30.

115. Matossian, R. M. (1977). The immunological diagnosis of human hydatid disease. *Transactions of the Roy. Soc. of Trop. Med. and Hygiene*, **71**, 101.

116. Matsuda, H. and Shoemaker, W. C. (1975). Cardiorespiratory responses to Dextran 40. *Arch. Surg.*, **110**, 296.

117. Maycock, W. D. A. and Mollison, P. L. (1960). A note in testing filters in blood transfusion sets. *Vox Sang.*, **5**, 157.

118. Mollison, P. L. (1980). *Blood Transfusion in Clinical Medicine*. London: Blackwell Scientific Publications.

119. Moore, F. D., Lyons, J. H. and Pierce, E. C. (1969). *Post-traumatic pulmonary insufficiency*. Philadelphia: W. B. Saunders.

120. Murray-Lyon, I. M. and Reynolds, K. W. (1979). Complication of mebendazole treatment for hydatid disease. *Brit. med. J.*, **II**, 1111.

121. Naeye, R. L. (1962). Thrombotic state after a hemorrhagic diathesis, a possible complication of therapy with epsilon-aminocaproic acid. *Blood*, **19**, 694.

122. Nahas, G. G., Manger, W. M., Mittleman, A. and Ultmann, J. E. (1961). The use of 2-amino-2-hydroxymethyl-1,3-propanediol in the correction of addition acidosis and its effect on sympathetic adrenal activity. *Ann. N.Y. Acad. Sci.*, **92**, 596.

123. Nolan, J. P. (1975). The role of Endotoxin in liver injury. *Gastroenterology*, **69**, 1346.

124. Nusbaum, M., Baum, S. and Blakemore, W. S. (1969) Clinical experience with the diagnosis and management of gastrointestinal haemorrhage by selective mesenteric catheterization. *Ann. Surg.*, **170**, 506.

125. Osborn, J. J., Swank, R. L., Hill, J. D., Aquilar, M. J. and Gerbode, F. (1970). Clinical use of a dacron wool filter during perfusion for open heart surgery. *J. Thorac. Cardiovasc. Surg.*, **60**, 575.

126. Osborne, D. R. (1980). Mebendazole and hydatid disease. *Brit. med. J.*, **280**, 183.

127. Parker, M. M., Shelhamer, J. H., Bacharach, S. L., Green, M. V., Natanson, C., Frederick, T. M., Damske, B. A. and Parrillo, J. E. (1984). Profound but reversible myocardial depression in patients with septic shock. *Ann. Int. Med.*, **100**, 483.

128. Patterson, R. H. and Twichell, J. B. (1971). Disposable filter for microemboli. *J. Amer. med. Assoc.*, **215**, 76.

129. Patterson, R. H., Wasser, J. S. and Porro, R. S. (1974). The effect of various filters on microembolic cerebrovascular blockade following cardiopulmonary bypass. *Ann. Thorac. Surg.*, **17**, 464.

130. Penner, A. and Bernheim, A. I. (1959). Acute postoperative esophageal, gastric and duodenal ulceration. *Arch. Path.*, **28**, 129.

131. Peters, W. P., Friedman, P. A., Johnson, M. W. and Mitch, W. E. (1981). Pressor effect of naloxone in septic shock. *Lancet*, **i**, 529.

132. Reul, G. J., Greenberg, S. D., Lefrak, E. A., McCollum, W. B., Beall, A. C. and Jordan, G. L. (1973). Prevention of post-traumatic pulmonary insufficiency. *Arch. Surg.*, **106**, 386.

133. Ruckley, C. V. (1985). Ruptured aortic aneurysm: an avoidable disaster. *Brit. med. J.*, **290**, 179.

134. Rudowski, W. and Kostrzewska, E. (1976). Aspects of treatment. Blood substitutes. *Ann. roy. Col. Surg.*, **58**, 115.

135. Rushmer, R. F. (1961). *Cardiovascular dynamics*. p. 53. 2nd edn. Philadelphia: Saunders.

136. Sarnoff, S. J. (1955). Myocardial contractility as described by ventricular function curves; observations on Starling's law of the heart. *Physiol. Rev.*, **35**, 107.

137. Schaberg, A., Hildes, J. A. and Alcock, A. J. W. (1954). Upper gastrointestinal lesions in acute bulbar poliomyelitis. *Gastroenterology*, **27**, 828.

138. Schweizer, O. and Howland, W. S. (1962). Potassium levels, acid-base balance and massive blood replacement. *Anesthesiology*, **23**, 735.

139. Sevitt, S. (1957). *Burns: Pathology and Therapeutic Applications*. London: Butterworth.

140. Sherer, U., Weinzierl, M., Sturm, R., Schildberg, F. W., Zrenner, M. and Lissner, J. (1978). Computed tomography in hydatid disease of the liver: a report on 13 cases. *Journal of Computer Assisted Tomography*, **2**, 612.

141. Shires, T., Brown, F. T., Canizaro, P. C. and Somerville, N. (1960). Distributional changes in extracellular fluid during acute hemorrhaghic shock. *Surg. Forum*, **11**, 115.

142. Shires, T., Williams, J. and Brown, F. (1960). Simultaneous measurement of plasma volume, extracellular fluid volume, and red blood cell mass in man utilizing I^{131}, S^{35}, O_4 and Cr^{51}. *J. Lab. clin. Med.*, **55**, 776.

143. Skillman, J. J., Bushnell, L. S. and Goldman, H. (1969). Respiratory failure, hypotension, sepsis and jaundice: a clinical syndrome associated with lethal hemorrhage from acute stress ulceration of the stomach. *Amer. J. Surg.*, **117**, 523.

144. Smith, G. P. and Brooks, F. P. (1967). Hypothalamic control of gastric secretions. *Gastroenterology*, **52**, 727.

145. Solis, R. T., Goldfinger, D., Gibbs, M. B. and Zeller, J. A. (1974). Physical characteristics of microaggregates in stored blood. *Transfusion*, **14**, 538.

146. Solis, R. T., Noon, G. P., Beall, A. C. and DeBakey, M. E. (1974). Particulate microembolism during cardiac operation. *Ann. Thorac. Surg.*, **17**, 332.

147. Somerville, K. W., Henry, D. A., Davies, J. G., Hine, K. R., Hawkey, C. J. and Langman, M. J. S. (1985). Somatostatin in treatment of haematemisis and melaena. *Lancet*, **i**, 130.

148. Spink, W. W. and Vick, J. (1961). Evaluation of plasma metaraminol, and hydrocortisone in experimental endotoxin shock. *Circ. Res.*, **9**, 184.

149. Swank, R. L. (1961). Alteration of blood on storage: measurement of adhesiveness of "aging" platelets and leucocytes and their removal by filtration. *N. Engl. J. of Med.*, **265**, 728.

150. Swank, R. L. (1968). Platelet aggregation: its role and cause in surgical shock. *J. Trauma*, **8**, 872.

151. Swank, R. L. and Porter, G. A. (1963). Disappearance of microbemboli transfused into patients during cardiopulmonary bypass. *Transfusion*, **3**, 192.

152. Swank, R. L., Ruth, J. C. and Jansen, J. (1964). Screen filtration pressure method and adhesiveness and aggregation of blood cells. *J. appl. Physiol.*, **19**, 340.

153. Taylor, B., Sibbald, W., Edmonds, H., Holliday, R. and Williams, C. (1978). Ionized hypocalcemia in critically ill patients with sepsis. *Canad. J. Surg.*, **21**, 429.

154. Thomsen, V. (1938). Studies of trauma and carbohydrate metabolism with special reference to the existence of traumatic diabetes. *Acta. med. scand.*, **91** (Suppl).

155. Todd, J., Fishaut, M., Kapral, E. and Welch, T. (1978). Toxic shock syndrome association with phage-group-1 staphylococci. *Lancet*, **ii**, 1116.

156. Tristani, F. E. and Cohn, J. N. (1970). Studies in clinical shock and hypotension. VII. Renal hemodynamics before and during treatment. *Circulation*, **42**, 839.

157. Wagner, M. A, Batts, D. H., Colville, J. M. and Lauter, C. B. (1981). Hypocalcaemia and toxic shock syndrome. *Lancet*, **i**, 1208.

158. Walker, J. B. (1936). Intravenous injection of hypertonic sodium chloride solution in the treatment of some conditions of low blood-pressure. *Brit. J. Surg.*, **24**, 105.

159. Weissman, G. and Thomas, L. (1962). Studies on lysosomes: I. Effects of endotoxin, endotoxin tolerance, and cortisone on the release of acid hydrolases from a granular fraction of rabbit liver. *J. Exper. Med.*, **116**, 433.

160. Wilson, J. F., Davidson, M., Rausch, R. I. (1978). A clinical trial of mebendazole in the treatment of alveolar hydatid disease. *Amer. Rev. Resp. Dis.*, **118**, 747.

161. Wilson, J. N., Grow, J. B., Demong, C. V., Prevedel, A. E. and Owens, J. C. (1962). Central venous pressure in optimal blood volume maintenance. *Arch. Surg.*, **85**, 563.

162. Yoshikawa, T. T., Chow, A. W., Guze, L. B. (1974). Bacteroidaceae bacteremia with disseminated intravascular coagulation. *Amer. J. Med.*, **56**, 725.

163. Young, L. S. (1977). Gram-negative rod bacteremia: microbiologic, immunologic and therapeutic considerations. *Ann. Int. Med.*, **86**, 456.

164. Zeller, J. A., Gerard, J. D., Gibbs, M. B. and Solis, T. (1972). An electron microscopic study of microaggregates in ACD stored blood. *Abstracts of the 111 Congress on Thrombosis and Haemostasis*. Washington, DC, p. 264.

Further Reading

Bamber, M. G. and Welsby, P. D. (1985). Toxic Shock: Clinical presentation and management I. *Postgrad. med. J.*, **61** (Suppl. 1), 25.

de Saxe, M. J., Hawtin, P. and Wieneke, A. (1985). Toxic Shock Syndrome in Britain—epidemiology and microbiology. *Postgrad. med. J.*, **61** (Suppl. 1), 5.

Fox, H. (1985). The pathology of tampon usage and of the Toxic Shock Syndrome. *Postgrad. med. J.*, **61** (Suppl. 1), 31.

Howorth, P. J. N. (1985). The role of isotonic and hypertonic solutions in the resuscitation of shocked patients. *J. R. Med. Corps.*, **131**, 100.

Shires, G. T. (Editor) (1984). *Shock and Related Problems*. Edinburgh: Churchill Livingstone.

PRESSOR DRUGS

Although pressor drugs should always be used as a last resort, they are in fact a valuable form of treatment when all else fails, and on occasions when they cease to act or produce undesirable side-effects, it is quite often because other biochemical and physiological factors have been neglected. For example, the presence of a gross metabolic acidosis quite commonly produces a lack of response to pressor amines or allows only a transitory, weak response even when large doses are given.[4,28] On the other hand, all pressor drugs work at reduced body temperatures and, in the author's own experiments, they were effective in the dog when the oesophageal temperature was below 17°C. They have been observed to be effective in man at 28°C in the oesophagus. Although the treatment of haemorrhagic shock is by blood replacement and the infusion of isotonic or hypertonic electrolyte solutions, it is quite common for blood loss to be associated with pain, toxicity and biochemical disorders related to a specific disease process. Under these circumstances, when an acute emergency presents in a situation removed from formal medical care and delay in treatment is unavoidable, it would be unrealistic to withhold pressor amines until a more correct form of therapy is available. It is, therefore, necessary to deal with the more common pressor amines that are commercially available so that we are familiar with their prime mode of action.

The majority of pressor agents are derivatives of adrenaline, and differences in their potency and predominant mode of action, their stability in the presence of amine oxidase which destroys adrenaline, and whether they have a stimulant effect upon the central nervous system are determined either by substitution of the OH groups of the benzene ring or upon the composition of the side chain (Fig. 6.8). In a similar manner, the molecular structure of a substance determines whether its action is one that is primarily vasconstrictor or one that causes it to act directly upon the heart muscle. Let us, therefore, deal with the two naturally occurring vasopressors first.

Adrenaline (epinephrine)

This sympathomimetic amine stimulates some nerve endings while inhibiting others. It is, there-

PRESSOR DRUGS

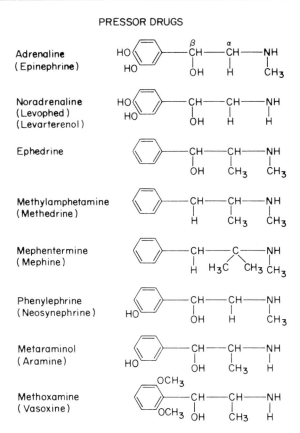

Fig. 6.8 The molecular structures of the most commonly used catecholamines.

fore, considered that there are two kinds of receptors at sympathetic nerve endings, called alpha-receptors and beta-receptors. The α-receptors deal with excitatory effects which are peripheral vasoconstriction, dilatation of the pupils, inhibition of gut movements and the mobilization of glucose from liver glycogen. The β-receptors are mainly concerned in inhibition so that they produce the effects of vasodilatation of blood vessels which supply skeletal muscle, reduction of tone of the smooth muscle supplying the bronchial tree, relaxation of the uterus, increase in the rate of beating of the heart, together with an increase in cardiac output. Adrenaline, therefore, acts on both α- and β-receptors. (For a more detailed account see p. 375–378.)

Adrenaline is not usually given for raising the blood pressure but it may be used in bronchial asthma or in restarting the heart after cardiac arrest when it is injected into the right ventricle as a 1–10 000 solution of the acid tartrate preparation. Even in normal therapeutic doses injected subcutaneously, adrenaline may have unpleasant side-effects such as anxiety, headache, palpitations and tremor. If the dose of adrenaline is too large, it will cause cardiac arrhythmias and even ventricular fibrillation. Adrenaline should therefore not be given when there are underlying disease processes such as hyperthyroidism or a history of cardiac disease giving rise to the acute onset of a tachycardia. It should, of course, not be withheld following cardiac arrest when there is asystole or ventricular fibrillation which is so inactive that electrical countershock will not produce a contracting myocardium.

When given intravenously as a bolus injection, adrenaline (epinephrine) is probably the most powerful vasopressor available. It raises the blood pressure; its effect is most marked on the systolic pressure. The pulse pressure therefore increases. The effect is *dose* related. When adrenaline is given in this way the rise in blood pressure is due to: (a) increased force of myocardial contraction, (b) rise in heart rate, and (c) vasoconstriction.

When adrenaline is given slowly intravenously or subcutaneously in therapeutic doses, the effect is very different. The β_2-receptor agonist actions allow vasodilatation to occur, and minute doses, 0.1 μg/kg, may cause a fall in blood pressure in man. When infused intravenously at a rate of 10–30 μg/minute, there is usually a moderate increase in systolic pressure (largely induced by an increase in cardiac output), a fall in diastolic pressure, an increase in pulse pressure and a fall in peripheral resistance. This is largely due to the effect on the β_2-receptor sites present in the blood vessels of skeletal muscle.

Noradrenaline (norepinephrine, Levophed, Adrenor)

This hormone is liberated at the terminations of the post-ganglionic adrenergic nerve fibres. It is also present in the adrenal glands and in chromaffin tissue scattered throughout the body. It is released from these tissues with adrenaline. It acts on the α-receptors to produce vasoconstriction, an increase in the size of the pupil and a rise in the blood glucose level by liberating glucose from the liver. It causes an increase in coronary flow and may produce slowing of the heart through reflex vagal inhibition as the blood pressure rises.

It is used to treat peripheral vasomotor failure in such conditions as the postoperative period of removal of a phaeochromocytoma, after acute myocardial infarction and during postoperative hypotension of unknown aetiology. Noradrenaline is administered by means of an intravenous infusion at a rate which is sufficient to raise the blood pressure to its desired level. Because it produces a marked constriction of the vessels to the gut in addition to reducing motility, its infusion should be discontinued periodically to allow a few minutes during which the abdominal organs can be perfused with blood.

The β-receptors, unlike the α-receptors, are not blocked by the adrenergic blocking agents, phentolamine (Rogitine), phenoxybenzamine (Dibenzyline) or tolazoline (Priscol, Priscoline), and thus when the occasion and need arises it is possible to infuse, for example, *l*-noradrenaline with phentolamine.

Pressor Amines which are mainly Vasoconstrictor

Noradrenaline
Phenylephrine—no chronotropic or positive inotropic effect.
Methoxamine—no chronotropic action.*
Metaraminol—some positive inotropic effect.

The substances listed above act mainly on the α-receptors. In addition to producing vasoconstriction of peripheral vessels, they also act upon the hepatic and splanchnic vascular systems and upon the renal vessels. The pulmonary artery pressure often rises after their use, but there is some evidence that this is because of a redistribution of blood and a rise in the systemic arterial blood pressure. With the exception of metaraminol, they do not appreciably increase the force of contraction of the heart. There is much evidence that coronary blood flow may increase with their use, but this may be said of all drugs that increase the arterial blood pressure and may reflect only this function. In general, cerebral vasoconstriction may reduce cerebral blood flow in the non-hypotensive patient but, because of the redistribution

*Does not increase heart rate in patients with heart block.

of blood, vasopressors may increase cerebral blood flow when hypotension is present. This action is separate from any stimulating effect that these substances may have upon the central nervous system.

Metaraminol is commonly used for its pressor effect following myocardial infarction and open-heart surgery. When given during heart–lung by-pass operations, the perfusion pressure rises and there is sometimes a dramatic increase in blood pressure, which is sustained in patients suffering from cardiogenic shock.

Pressor Amines acting mainly upon the Heart and Causing Vasodilatation

Adrenaline (epinephrine)
Isoprenaline
Dopamine
Dobutamine
Ephedrine
Methamphetamine
Mephentermine

The overall action of adrenaline (epinephrine) is to produce vasodilatation in those organs which are essential for survival. We therefore find that the vessels of the brain and muscles dilate so that the blood flow through these organs is increased. On the other hand, there is constriction of the veins, the renal arteries and the arteries of the mesentery. The overall effect is to increase the perfusion of essential tissues and to increase the venous return to the heart so that the cardiac output is improved while conserving fluid and minimizing blood loss in structures which are unprotected.

Isoprenaline (isoproterenol, isopropyl-noradrenaline Suscardia)

Isoprenaline (isoproterenol), a synthetic derivative of noradrenaline (isopropyl-noradrenaline, Neo-Epinine), is infrequently administered parenterally in some centres because its action on the heart is considered to produce arrhythmias. Its action is almost entirely upon the β-receptors producing marked vasodilatation, tachycardia and marked bronchial dilatation. It is used mainly in asthma, during septic shock, for increasing the rate of contraction of the heart in the presence of heart block and after cardiac arrest.

Isoprenaline has been used successfully in cardiogenic shock following myocardial infarction.[9,15,26,36] It acts on the β_1- and β_2-adrenergic receptors and has no significant activity on the α-receptors, and therefore produces vasodilatation and sometimes a fall in blood pressure. It causes little change in renal blood flow.[31] Not all clinicians have found it to be of value.[21,35,33] The author's own experience has confirmed these diverging views—isoprenaline (isoproterenol, Suscardia) being readily effective in some patients and unpredictably ineffective in others. As experienced by other workers,[36] a combination of dopamine (Intropin) and isoprenaline (isoproterenol, Suscardia) has succeeded in raising the blood pressure when neither agent alone has been effective. (The molecular structures of these substances are shown in Figs. 6.8 and 6.9.)

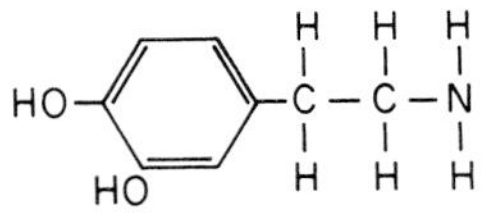

Dopamine (Intropin)

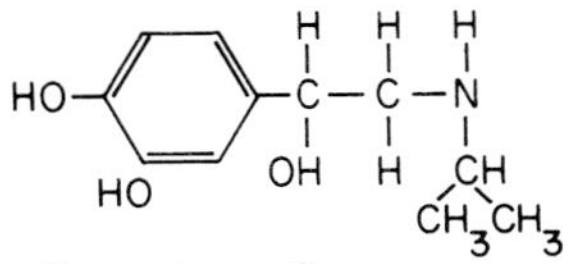

Isoprenaline (Isoproterenol)

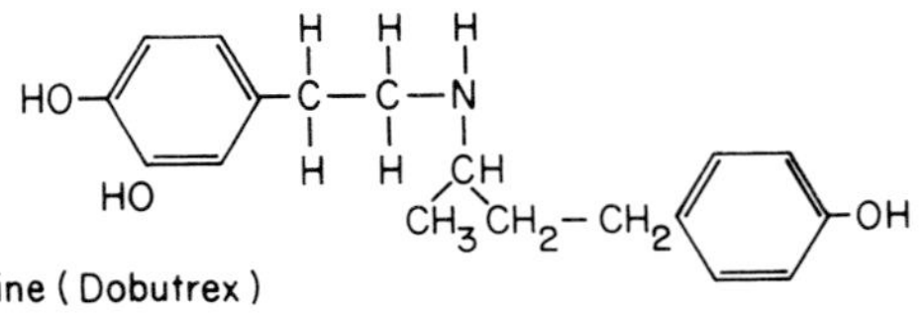

Dobutamine (Dobutrex)

Fig. 6.9   The molecular structure of dopamine, isoprenaline, and dobutamine. Note that dopamine has a basic molecular structure while dobutamine has the most complex structure. Both isoprenaline and dobutamine are synthetic and, unlike dopamine, they do not occur naturally.

Isoprenaline is infused in 5% glucose or 0.9% NaCl; 5 mg of the substance is added to 1 litre of solution and the rate of infusion is controlled so that a rapid tachycardia does not result and the blood pressure is maintained at a systolic value of 90 mmHg or more. When isoprenaline is given in the presence of complete heart block, it is very effective in reversing bradycardic shock.

Dopamine (Intropin)

This substance (3,4 dihydroxy phenylethylamine) is a precursor of noradrenaline (norepinephrine) (Blaschko, 1959).[2] It is therefore a naturally occurring catecholamine. As described in this chapter, a number of sympathomimetic amines have been found to raise the blood pressure and to increase the contractility of the heart. Because of vasoconstriction in vital organs, including the coronary and renal vessels, the use of these agents has been widely questioned, and even vasodilatation has been advocated.[30] Until dopamine became available for general clinical use, isoprenaline (isoproterenol) was usually used in the many forms of normovolaemic shock or when shock was unresponsive to volume expansion.[15,26,36]

The vasoactive pressor amines of most value in clinical practice have both α- and β-receptor activity so that vasoconstriction occurs in some organs, vasodilatation occurs in some vital organs, and myocardial output and contractility are improved.

The benefits of infusion of dopamine are well illustrated (Goldberg, 1972)[16] when it is noted that even small quantities of adrenaline (epinephrine) reduce renal blood flow by α-adrenergic vasoconstriction.[29]

Although the positive inotropic effect upon the heart has been found to be due to stimulation of the β-adrenergic receptors,[24] the vasodilator activity was found to be of non-adrenergic origin, as this manifestation was not blocked by either α- or β-receptor antagonists.[14,27] The ability of dopamine to cause vasodilatation in the renal and mesenteric vessels is, however, blocked by haloperidol.[39] The presence of specific dopamine receptors has been suggested (Yeh et al., 1969 and Goldberg, 1975).[17,39]

Dopamine is added to physiological solutions of saline or glucose in doses of 40–100 mg/l and infused at a rate which raises the systolic blood pressure to 90 mmHg.

When dopamine is given rapidly in high concentration, the α-adrenergic receptor response predominates and vasoconstriction occurs.[1] In therapeutic doses in man, however, cardiac output and stroke volume increase with little or no change in heart rate. Also urine flow, Na^+ excretion[18,19] and creatinine clearance increase (McDonald et al., 1962),[25] and vascular resistance is decreased. Dopamine is commonly used in conjunction with another vasopressor (e.g. metaraminol or isoprenaline).

Dobutamine HCl (Dobutrex)

This inotropic agent has no action on dopamine receptors. It acts directly and almost exclusively on the β_1-receptors, thus increasing myocardial contractility and cardiac output.[37] It is less active on the β_2- and α-adrenergic receptor sites than either noradrenaline (norepinephrine) or isoprenaline (isoproterenol). It has been used during toxic and cardiogenic shock.[22] The effective infusion rate is 2.5–10 μg/kg/minute.

Ephedrine

Ephedrine has a stimulatory effect upon both the α- and β-receptors and, when administered therapeutically, its action at these sites is of value.

In its overall action within the body, ephedrine has a vasoconstrictor effect. It causes the vessels of the skin, the splanchnic area and kidneys to contract. The vessels to the brain, the muscles and the coronary arteries all undergo vasodilatation. (The pressor effect of ephedrine is therefore largely due to increased cardiac output with some vasoconstrictor action).

The two derivatives, methamphetamine and mephentermine, tend to produce peripheral vasodilatation rather than vasoconstriction and this is sometimes more noticeable with mephentermine. They increase blood flow through the limbs and, unlike adrenaline, through the kidneys. Their pressor effect is considered to be mainly by action upon the myocardium; although constriction of the skin vessels may also occur, they have little direct action on the veins. In some cases methamphetamine has a vasodilator effect which does not involve the receptor sites.[8] Both these substances produce marked cerebral stimulation and their effect on the central nervous system may be an important part of their action in producing reflex vasoconstriction in other parts of the body when it has previously been absent. Both these substances are particularly useful for raising the blood pressure during hypothermia and, like metaraminol, they increase urine output when given during hypothermic heart–lung bypass operations.

Mode of Action of Pressor Drugs on Small Vessels

The mechanism by which these drugs act has been a subject of considerable interest. In 1958 and 1959[5-7] Burn and his co-workers put forward the suggestion that the response of a vessel was dependent upon the store of noradrenaline that was contained within the muscle wall. This store was being continually diminished and in this way the vessels could respond to noradrenaline which was present in the blood. If, therefore, there was a continuously large concentration of noradrenaline in the circulation, the receptors in the vessel wall would become saturated and thus the response of the vessel would be diminished. This would be similar to the situation which occurs during the continuous infusion of noradrenaline when resistance appears. Conversely, if the stores within the walls of the vessel were decreased, such as following treatment with reserpine (Serpasil), the response to *l*-noradrenaline would be increased. Since this fact has been shown, Burn has divided the pressor amines into three groups.

Group 1: *l*-noradrenaline (norepinephrine), adrenaline (epinephrine), and phenylephrine. Pressor action is powerfully maintained following treatment with reserpine, but a reduced response occurs after infusions of *l*-noradrenaline.

Group 2: metaraminol and methoxamine. This intermediate group has a reduced response following noradrenaline (epinephrine) infusions, but a moderately good pressor response following previous treatment with reserpine.

Group 3: methamphetamine, mephentermine and ephedrine. These substances are unable to act if noradrenaline (epinephrine) is absent from the blood vessel walls and have little action following treatment with reserpine. This group, in addition to giving some indication as to the mode of action of these substances, also helps in the treatment of prolonged shock when one or more of these substances has been used but a poor response obtained. It also indicates that, in addition to the action of reserpine, other substances may modify their action. For example, it has been shown that drugs of the phenothiazine group, while not affecting the pressor action of *l*-noradrenaline, may act on other pressor amines. Chlorpromazine (Largactil) reduces the pressor action of adrenaline, methoxamine and phenylephrine while promethazine (Phenergan) acts similarly on the latter two substances.

Clinical applications

Generally, the measures outlined previously should first be taken to resuscitate a patient suffering from haemorrhage or toxic shock. This should be done to increase the effectiveness of the pressor drugs and, therefore, reduce the amount that is required for achieving a therapeutic effect. However, in certain circumstances, predominantly those of toxicity induced by infections, or hypotension induced by other drugs, vasopressors may sometimes be the treatment of choice.

Anaesthetic Hypotension

When analgesia is induced by the injection of local anaesthetics into the subarachnoid or epidural spaces, a profound fall of blood pressure sometimes results. It occasionally occurs when continuous analgesia is being maintained and the rate of infusion inadvertently becomes too great. Stopping the infusion altogether does not always result in a rise of blood pressure.

It was shown some time ago that the intravenous injection of hypertonic sodium chloride would often be effective in returning the blood pressure to normal.[38] The infusion of 10–20 ml of a 23.4% solution of NaCl (4 mmol/ml) into a large vein or intra-arterially will raise the blood pressure when other agents have failed, and this may prevent renal and other tissue damage.

When hypotension is caused by vasodilator action of the anaesthetic agent, the use of a substance which produces vasoconstriction is indicated. Phenylephrine, methoxamine or metaraminol would on theoretical grounds appear ideal. In practice, however, other substances such as ephedrine and methylamphetamine have been used with success,[11,13,23] although ephedrine is rarely used today.

Compensatory mechanisms to changes in blood pressure are impaired during anaesthesia. If a pressor drug is given in the absence of hypotension, it may lead to gross hypertension resulting in cerebrovascular accidents.[10,20] Pressor drugs should therefore never be given prophylactically.

Other substances used primarily for anaesthesia, such as thiopentone and *d*-tubocurarine, can lead to a profound fall of blood pressure. *D*-tubocurarine can give rise to the release of histamine. Thiopentone itself has a depressing effect on myocardial action, and the hypotension resulting from *d*-tubocurarine may also be caused by myocardial insufficiency. Although other vasopressors are effective in reversing hypotension form both these causes, methamphetamine appears to be most effective.

Removal of Phaeochromocytoma and Adrenalectomy

There are two dangers associated with removal of a phaeochromocytoma: (a) gross hypertension during manipulation of the abnormal gland because of the excessive release of noradrenaline (norepinephrine) and (b) postoperative hypotension when the abnormally high concentrations of circulating noradrenaline are no longer present.[12,32,34] The first danger is largely overcome by the injection of phentolamine (Rogitine, Regitine) and care in handling of the tumour during surgery. The postoperative hypotension is usually controlled by maintaining a continuous *l*-noradrenaline infusion, the rate of administration of which can be varied according to the patient's needs. In some cases, however, the hypotension fails to respond adequately to *l*-noradrenaline infusions, even in high concentrations, and this may well be because of the saturation of the receptors when it was previously present in excessive quantities. This situation coincides well with the suggestions put forward by Burn[5] and substances such as methamphetamine or mephentermine are then indicated. Such a case has been reported in which resistance to noradrenaline was present, but a rise in blood pressure followed the injection of 10 mg of methamphetamine.[3] The tachycardia can be controlled with phentolamine and inderal.

Hypotension resulting from Cardiac Insufficiency

In this condition it is essential to try to improve the heart action before resorting to vasopressors. Attention, therefore, must be directed initially to the rapid digitalization of the patient (see p. 367), the acid–base state (especially the correction of a metabolic acidosis), the potassium concentration of the plasma, and the correction of disorders of hydration and blood volume. Because anoxia is a potent cause of cardiac failure, oxygen therapy by mask, tent or, if possible, by hyperbaric oxygen bed should never be neglected. On theoretical grounds it could be advocated that pressor amines which improve the heart beat (ejection fraction) without causing vasoconstriction would be those of choice. These would be methamphetamine (Desoxin, Fetamin) and mephentermine (Wyamine, Mephine). It is often necessary, however, to avoid increasing the irritability of the myocardium which would make ventricular fibrillation more probable. This is especially so in cases of myocardial infarction. For this reason noradrenaline is commonly used in cardiac shock produced by coronary occlusion. There is no doubt, however, that its action could be reinforced with very small doses of methamphetamine, methoxamine or phenylephrine.

There is no doubt that prolonged hypotension resulting from myocardial disease has a poor prognosis and the use of vasopressors in this condition may be beneficial when other measures are to no avail.

Hypotension resulting from Decreased Blood Volume

It must be remembered that a great degree of reduction in circulating blood volume can occur before there is any measurable change in the systemic arterial blood pressure. This is not so, however, of the venous pressure. The vasoconstrictor mechanisms that are normally functioning when the circumstances arise are maintained for a considerable period of time, and during disease processes may suddenly become exhausted so that there is an abrupt fall of blood pressure of sudden onset to very low levels. Before this occurs there are usually physical signs which reflect increased sympathetic activity, such as profuse sweating, marked tachycardia, vasoconstriction of the skin vessels, an anxious appearance, hyperventilation and restlessness.

This appearance is produced by haemorrhagic shock and also sometimes occurs in severe dehydration and electrolyte abnormalities such as gross sodium depletion. It is therefore necessary to correct these factors before using a pressor amine if the situation and time allow. Sometimes, however, the disease has progressed to a point at which immediate treatment is essential and under these circumstances a pressor amine is sometimes lifesaving and provides sufficient time for the correct forms of therapy to be applied. In this sort of situation, methamphetamine, phenylephrine or noradrenaline infusions can prevent circulatory failure.

Hypotension resulting from Pulmonary Embolus

Although nearly all the vasopressors have been used at some time for the treatment of this condition, and because of the doubt that surrounds the effect of these substances on the pulmonary blood flow and, therefore, their effect upon the pulmonary resistance and resulting strain on the right heart, it is probable that those that are least likely to cause constriction of the pulmonary vessels are to be advocated. Thus methamphetamine, methoxamine and mephentermine can be recommended; *l*-noradrenaline has also been used successfully.

General Measures during use of Pressor Drugs

1. It is essential that the blood pressure is measured repeatedly during use of pressor drugs.
2. A large vein should always be chosen for the injection of vasopressors, and continuous infusions of substances like noradrenaline should preferably be given through a catheter into the inferior vena cava. If any of the material leaks backwards along the catheter, the tissue should be injected with phentolamine (Rogitine); 5 mg of phentolamine may be added to each litre of solution containing noradrenaline without affecting its pressor qualities, but avoiding local tissue necrosis.

3. Withdrawal of vasopressors such as noradrenaline may be accompanied by a profound fall of blood pressure, so that gradual withdrawal is preferable. Because of the marked vasoconstrictor affect of noradrenaline in the splanchnic area, withdrawal of the infusion for 2–3 minutes every hour is to be recommended, even though it results in a short period of hypotension.

4. Doses of vasopressors should be kept to a minimum and this is assisted by combining a vasopressor, which produces vasodilatation but increases output, with a pure vasoconstrictor. Their action is also assisted by the administration of intravenous hydrocortisone and the correction of metabolic acidosis.

References

Pressor drugs

1. Beregovich, J., Bianchi, C., Rubler, S. Lomnitz, E., Cagin, N. and Levitt, B. (1974). Dose-related effects of dopamine in congestive heart failure. *Amer. Heart J.*, **87**, 550.
2. Blaschko, H. (1959). Development of current concepts of catecholamine formation. *Pharmacol. Rev.*, **11**, 307.
3. Bromage, P. R. (1960). Vasopressors. *Canad. Anaesth. Soc. J.*, **7**, 310.
4. Brooks, D. K. (1965). Physiological responses produced by changes in acid–base equilibrium following profound hypothermia. *Anaesthesia*, **20**, 173.
5. Burn, J. H. (1958). Reserpine and vascular tone. *Brit. J. Anaesth.*, **30**, 351.
6. Burn, J. H. and Rand, M. J. (1959). Sympathetic postganglionic mechanism. *Nature*, **184**, 163.
7. Burn, J. H. and Walker, J. M. (1959). The action of sympathomimetic amines on the heart rate. *J. Physiol.*, **145**, 10P.
8. Caldwell, R. W. and Goldberg, L. I. (1970). An evaluaion of the vasodilation produced by mephentermine and certain other sympathomimetic amines. *J. Pharmacol. Exp. Ther.*, **172**, 297.
9. Carey, J. S., Brown, R. S., Mohr, P. A., Monson, D. O., Yao, S. T. and Shoemaker, W. C. (1967). Cardiovascular function in shock: responses to volume loading and isoproterenol infusion. *Circulation*, **35**, 327.
10. Casady, G. N., Moore, D. C. and Bridenbaugh, L. D. (1960). Postpartum hypertension after use of vasoconstrictor and oxytocic drugs; etiology, incidence, complications and treatment. *J. Amer. med. Ass.*, **172**, 1011.
11. Coleman, D. J. (1959). Mephentermine: its value as a pressor agent in anaesthesia. *Anaesthesia*, **14**, 240.
12. Cooperman, L. H., Engelman, K. and Mann, P. E. G. (1967). Anaesthetic management of phaeochromocytoma employing halothane and beta-adrenergic blockade. *Anesthesiology*, **18**, 575.
13. Dripps, R. D. and Deming, M. van N. (1946). An evaluation of certain drugs used to maintain blood pressure during spinal anesthesia: comparison of ephedrine, paredrine, pitressin-ephedrine and methedrine in 2500 cases. *Surg. Gynecol. & Obstet.*, **83**, 312.
14. Eble, J. N. (1964). Proposed mechanism for depressor

effect of dopamine in anesthetized dog. *J. Pharmacol. Exp. Therap.*, **145**, 64.

15. Eichna, L. W. (1967). Treatment of cardiogenic shock III. Use of isoproterenol in cardiogenic shock. *Amer. Heart J.*, **74**, 848.

16. Goldberg, L. I. (1972). Cardiovascular and renal actions of dopamine: potential clinical applications. *Pharmacol. Rev.*, **24**, 1.

17. Goldberg, L. I. (1975). The dopamine vascular receptor. *Biochem. Pharmacol.*, **24**, 651.

18. Goldberg, L. I., Hsieh, Y. Y. and Resnekov, L. (1977). New catecholamines for treatment of heart failure and shock: an update on dopamine and a first look at dobutamine. *Prog. Cardiovasc. Dis.*, **19 (4)**, 327.

19. Goldberg, L. I., McDonald, R. H. and Zimmerman, A. M. (1963). Sodium diuresis produced by dopamine in patients with congestive heart failure. *N. Eng. J. Med.*, **269**, 1060.

20. Greene, B. A. and Barcham, J. (1949). Cerebral complications resulting from hypertension caused by vasopressor drugs in obstetrics. *N.Y. St. J. Med.*, **49**, 1424.

21. Gunnar, R. M., Loeb, H., Pietras, R. J. and Tobin, J. R. (1967). Ineffectiveness of isoproterenol in shock due to acute myocardial infarction. *J. Amer. med. Assoc.*, **202**, 1124.

22. Kersting, F., Follath, F., Moulds, R., Mucklow, J., McCloy, R., Sheares, J. and Dollery, C. (1976). A comparison of cardiovascular effects of dobutamine and isoprenaline after open heart surgery. *Brit. Heart J.*, **38**, 622.

23. King, B. D. and Dripps, R. D. (1950). The use of methoxamine for maintenance of the circulation during spinal anesthesia. *Surg. Gynecol. & Obstet.*, **90**, 659.

24. McDonald, R. H. and Goldberg, L. I. (1963). Analysis of cardiovascular effects of dopamine in dog. *J. Pharmacol. Exp. Ther.*, **140**, 60.

25. McDonald, R. H., Goldberg, L. I. and Tuttle, E. P. (1962). Saluretic effect of dopamine in patients with congestive heart failure. *Clin. Res.*, **10**, 19.

26. McLean, L. D., Duff, J. H., Scott, H. M. and Peretz, D. I. (1965). Treatment of shock in man based on hemodynamic diagnosis. *Surg. Gynecol. & Obstet.*, **120**, 1.

27. McNay, J. L. and Goldberg, L. I. (1966). Comparison of effect of dopamine, isoproterenol, nor-epinephrine and bradykinin on canine renal and femoral blood flow. *J. Pharmacol. Exp. Ther.*, **151**, 23.

28. Nahas, G. G., Manger, W. M., Mittelman, A. and Ultmann, J. E. (1961). The use of 2-amino-2-hydroxy-methyl-1,3-propanediol in the correction of addition acidosis and its effect on sympathetic adrenal activity. *Ann. N.Y. Acad. Sci.*, **92**, 596.

29. Nickel, J. F., Smythe, C. M., Papper, E. M. and Bradley, S. E. (1954). Study of mode of action of adrenal medullary hormones on sodium, potassium and water excretion in man. *J. Clin. Invest.*, **33**, 1687.

30. Nickerson, M. (1964). Vasoconstriction and vasodilation in shock. In *Shock*, p. 227. Edited by S. G. Hershey. Boston: Little Brown.

31. Rosenblum, R., Berkowitz, W. D. and Lawson, D. (1968). Effect of acute intravenous administration of isoproterenol on cardiorenal hemodynamics in man. *Circulation*, **38**, 158.

32. Ross, E. J., Pritchard, B. N. C., Kaufman, L., Robertson, A. I. G. and Harries, B. J. (1967). Preoperative and operative management of patients with phaeochromocytoma. *Brit. med. J.*, **I**, 191.

33. Sandler, H., Dodge, M. T. & Murdaugh, H. V. (1961). Effects of isoproterenol on cardiac output and renal function in congestive heart failure. *Amer. Heart J.*, **62**, 643.

34. Sheps, S. G. and Maher, F. T. (1967). Comparison of glucagon and histamine tests in diagnosis of pheochromocytoma. *Circulation*, **36**, 236.

35. Smith, H. C., Oriol, A., March, J. and McGregor, M. (1967). Hemodynamic studies in cardiogenic shock. Treatment with isoproterenal and metaraminol. *Circulation*, **35**, 1084.

36. Talley, R. C., Goldberg, L. I., Johnson, C. E. and McNay, S. L. (1969). A hemodynamic comparison of dopamine and isoproterenol in patients in shock. *Circulation*, **39**, 361.

37. Tuttle, R. R. and Mills, J. (1975). Dobutamine: development of a new catecholamine to selectively increased cardiac contractility. *Circ. Res.*, **36**, 185.

38. Walker, J. B. (1936). Intravenous injection of hypertonic sodium chloride solution in the treatment of some conditions of low blood-pressure. *Brit. J. Surg.*, **24**, 105.

39. Yeh, B. K., McNay, J. L. and Goldberg, L. I. (1969). Attenuation of dopamine renal and mesenteric vasodilation by haloperidol: evidence for a specific dopamine receptor. *J. Pharmacol. Exp. Ther.*, **168**, 303.

PANCREATITIS

It is readily apparent, when treating patients suffering from pancreatitis, that there are at least two separate forms of the disease, though the condition is of apparently acute onset. One form of acute pancreatitis has a high mortality rate[11,45,57] and causes severe shock even when haemorrhagic complications do not occur. The other form is recurrent, episodic, relatively mild and benign in its manifestation, and is associated with a relatively low mortality.[44,57]

Unfortunately sometimes the clinician has no way of knowing in the very early stages of the disease when the patient presents with symptoms which include abdominal pain, pyrexia and constipation, whether it is an acute attack, whether it is the mild episodic form and has occurred before and has been dismissed as of no consequence, or whether the attack will continue to progress to the more severe form of the disease. The patient may present with misleading physical signs, for example, a discoloured lump in the groin (Dennison and Royle, 1984).[16] Precautions, therefore, have to be taken in the full knowledge that there are limitations to the degree of help that can be obtained from the clinical laboratory. The serum amylase concentration is raised for a notoriously short time and, in both the normal and abnormal circumstances, appears to circulate in the blood only to be excreted in the urine or destroyed at some, as yet unidentified, site. As demonstrated below, both the serum and urine amylase levels may be above normal in a large number of widely differing conditions unrelated to pancreatitis.

patients in this study the diagnosis was made only following an autopsy. When Trapnell and Duncan[57] reviewed the incidence and mortality of acute pancreatitis in 1975, they concluded that the overall incidence of the disease in Great Britain was not known and that the overall mortality rate in the Bristol area of the UK was approximately 17%. They reviewed other mortality rates, some of which were considerably lower.

In Bourke's series,[6] when the diagnosis was made during life, the mortality was just over 10%. The wisdom of treating the patient for hypovolaemia and correcting the severe metabolic and toxic changes before the correct diagnosis of the condition is established, is therefore well illustrated.

The MRC multicentre study in 1977[44] confirmed that the mortality rate (in 257 patients) was approximately 11%.[13] Other authors[29] gave similar figures for patients treated after the condition had been diagnosed.

When Glazer and Dudley reviewed acute pancreatitis in 1977,[23] they noted that there were regional variations in mortality, and these variations could be partly explained by the number of patients who developed fulminant haemorrhagic or necrotizing pancreatitis or pancreatitis associated with severe biliary sepsis. In this particular type of subdivision, which varies between 10% and 25% of any series, the mortality is approximately 40–70%.[3]

It is apparent that early diagnosis of acute pancreatitis increases the possibility of a successful outcome, and that mortality varies from one centre to another.

Incidence and Mortality of Acute Pancreatitis

Both the incidence and mortality of acute pancreatitis are very difficult to assess. Unfortunately in many cases the diagnosis is not made until necropsy. This is because in a large number of patients it is not possible to arrive at a correct diagnosis. In Pollock's series of 100 patients with acute pancreatitis,[53] nine were incorrectly diagnosed and the true nature of their condition was only revealed at necropsy. The overall mortality of the series was 25%. In another series,[56] the mortality was more than 20% of 590 patients; in 6% of the

Aetiology of Pancreatitis

A number of drugs have been implicated as causative factors in pancreatitis, but because many of these preparations are used routinely, it is sometimes difficult to designate an individual drug as a definite cause. In 1977, Nakashima and Howard[46] reviewed the English, German and Japanese literature with regard to drugs in the aetiology of the disease. Since then, other drugs have been added to the list.[42] Treatment with corticosteroids appeared to be a predominant factor in 51 out of the 112 patients studied by Mallory and Kern (1980).[42] The underlying disease which necessitated the corticosteroid treatment did not appear to be a contributory cause; the conditions for which these patients were receiving corticosteroids included asthma, nephrotic syndrome and disseminated lupus erythematosus. The contraceptive pill was found to be a cause of pancreatitis and has been implicated on several occasions. It is also known to induce gall-stones in a number of women taking the drug.

The diuretic frusemide (Lasix, Dryptal) was implicated by Jones and Oelbaum[35] in a clearly recorded case in which the serum amylase rose during therapy with this preparation, fell when the frusemide was withdrawn, and rose again when it was reintroduced as a part of therapy. As frusemide is used in the treatment of many conditions, frequently in large doses, this drug and other diuretics have to be borne in mind as a possible cause of pancreatitis.

Acute haemorrhagic pancreatitis has been reported in patients treated with both chlorothiazide and hydrochlorothiazide.[33,60] Chlorthalidone has also been implicated in the onset of acute pancreatitis.[34]

In a further review,[45] the antibiotic rifampicin (Rimactane) appeared to be responsible for pancreatitis in 20 patients. Phenformin has been implicated directly as causing acute pancreatitis by Goodley et al.,[24] Levitan,[40] and Wilde,[62] and a number of other authors. In 1976, Graeber et al.[25] described two patients, one developed lactic acidosis and recovered, and the other, aged 85 years developed acute pancreatitis, following treatment for her phenformin-induced lactacidosis. The diagnosis was confirmed at surgery and artificial ventilation was given. Certainly, this account clearly demonstrates the success of skilled treatment and clinical management. Paracetamol poisoning can result in acute pancreatitis.[12,21] Cimetidine (Tagamet) has also been reported as causing the disease;[2] in this case, however, the patient was also receiving frusemide (Lasix), although this did not appear to be a contributing factor. Mumps, Coxsackie B viruses and gall-bladder disease were excluded. The patient recovered following withdrawal of the cimetidine. In animal experiments, Joffe and Lee[32] found that acute pancreatitis could be induced by cimetidine in rats, and it is apparent that the H_2-receptor inhibitor may induce cellular damage if large doses are given to some species of animals.

Acute pancreatitis has been reported to occur after an excessive intake of phenolphthalein which is widely used for its cathartic effect (Lambrianides and Rosin, 1984).[37]

Respiratory Failure During Acute Pancreatitis

The changes in the lung are commonly associated with a radiological appearance of pulmonary oedema. However, clinically the disease is quite different. Warshaw et al.,[58] when reviewing a series of patients from the Massachussets General Hospital, stated that as many as 30% of patients suffering from acute pancreatitis developed some form of respiratory insufficiency. They quoted a number of authors who have considered iatrogenic fluid overload to be the cause. In the absence of a central venous pressure (CVP) or pulmonary wedge pressure measurement, this possibility is apparent. Myocardial insufficiency as a result of metabolic changes and circulating toxins also appears to contribute to the respiratory insufficiency.

There is, however, much evidence that the changes in the lung are the result of what Warshaw and his colleagues describe as an 'alveolar-capillary leak syndrome'. Certainly, the author has noted a decrease in the lung compliance prior to the onset of either radiological changes or marked alterations in the blood-gas tensions, although reduced arterial oxygen tensions have been observed shortly after the onset of the disease. Controlled ventilation, especially with prolonged positive-end-expiratory pressure (PEEP), produces an improvement in blood-gas tension, but, as noted elsewhere (see p. 132), it may reduce the cardiac output. In these circumstances, the administration of high concentrations of humidified O_2 are preferable to PEEP. The similarity between the changes that occur in acute pancreatitis and fat embolus are so great that damage to the alveolar-capillary wall can be postulated to be caused by some, as yet unidentified, factor. It may also be noted that the high incidence of hyperlipidaemia in this condition may indicate a similarity of aetiology.

Cardiogenic Factor in Acute Pancreatitis

Some investigators have identified a myocardial depressant factor during acute pancreatitis.[38] Certainly, low cardiac output contributes to the hypotension that is observed in some patients. The contribution made by the cardiovascular system is usually difficult to define when large volumes of plasma and electrolyte-containing fluid are being continuously lost into the abdominal cavity and lumen of the gut over several days. A metabolic acidosis can cause cardiac insufficiency. Circulating vasoactive substances have been identified, for example kinins[48] and prostaglandins.[22]

It can be seen that measurement of the CVP or the pulmonary artery pressure (PAP) by means of a Swan–Ganz catheter is essential in this condition, in which restoration of the blood volume, while avoiding overloading the circulation, is of primary importance. It would appear that in some cases the cardiogenic factor is a manifestation of toxic shock.

Case history. A 24-year-old man, who was not an alcoholic, had no significant previous medical history and who was subsequently shown not to be suffering from gall-stones or gall-bladder disease, presented at the hospital with abdominal pain. The pain was fairly generalized over the abdomen and had lasted for 1 or 2 hours on two previous occasions when it appeared, subjectively, to have been worse in the upper part of the abdomen radiating into the back. He had a feeling of nausea but had not vomited on either of the two previous occasions. Although the pain had not dis-

appeared, he had gained some relief from lying in bed in the prone position. Both the attacks had occurred during the previous 4–6 weeks. He had not had diarrhoea, but he appeared to have gained some relief from a large, bulky bowel movement.

Because of the severity of the pain and its continuous character, the patient decided to seek medical attention. The abdominal pain, although generalized, appeared to be most severe in the epigastrium and radiated into the back. He had vomited earlier that morning and had a feeling of nausea. He had not had a bowel movement, although he had a desire to do so. He had taken no medication of any kind.

On examination, the patient was slightly toxic and dehydrated in appearance. The only positive physical findings were a heart rate of 92 beats/minute and marked lower right quadrant tenderness. There was minimal rebound tenderness and the bowel sounds were normal. The serum amylase was slightly raised, being 460 units. The white cell count was 8600/mm^3. An X-ray of the abdomen revealed no abnormality and an upright film showed that no gas was present under the diaphragm. (See Table 6.7 for blood and biochemical changes.)

Table 6.7   The blood and biochemical changes which occurred in a 24-year-old man who was suffering from acute pancreatitis

	Hb g%	PCV %	WBC mm^3	Serum amylase	[Na$^+$] mmol/l	[K$^+$] mmol/l	Albumin g%	[Ca^{++}] mmol/l (mg%)	[HCO$_3^-$] mmol/l	PO$_2$ mmHg
	15.5	45	8600	460	138	4.7		2.1 (8.4)	22	94
	16.1	47	13 800	1325	127	5.8	3.3			
	12.4	32	14 700	3600	138	4.6			21	86
1st Post-op. day	13.7	36	12 200	280	140	4.7	2.9	2.0 (8.0)	18	65
2nd Post-op. day	14.0	38	10 900	273	136	3.7	2.7	1.9 (7.6)	20	285
4th Post-op. day	14.5	37	11 200	190	137	3.5			22	78
7th Post-op. day	15.1	40	7300		142	3.4	4.9	2.3 (9.3)	28	92

Hb = Haemoglobin g%
PCV = Packed cell volume
WBC = White blood cell count per mm^3
Serum amylase = Total serum amylase in international units
[Na$^+$] = Plasma [Na$^+$] mmol/l (mEq/l)
[K$^+$] = Plasma [K$^+$] mmol/l (mEq/l)
Albumin = Plasma albumin
[Ca^{++}] = Plasma [Ca^{++}] mmol/l (mg%)
[HCO$_3^-$] = Bicarbonate ion concentration mmol/l
PO$_2$ = Partial pressure in O$_2$ in mmHg

Six hours later the patient's blood pressure was found to have fallen to 80/60 mmHg. The abdomen was distended. There was marked rebound tenderness and a further X-ray of the abdomen revealed distended loops of bowel and, again, the absence of air under the diaphragm. It was, nevertheless, decided to perform a laparotomy and, before the patient was taken to the operating room, further blood samples were obtained for analysis. These results are shown in Table 6.7. The operation revealed an inflamed pancreas with areas of fat necrosis within the peritoneal cavity. The gall bladder and ducts were normal and no stones were found.

The blood samples demonstrated a raised serum amylase of 1325 units. The packed cell volume (PCV) was 47%; a low plasma [K^+], a raised plasma [Na^+] a fall in the plasma albumin concentration and [Ca^{++}] were present. A metabolic acidosis had also developed. During the anaesthetic, infusions of saline and plasma produced a rise in the blood pressure and a central venous pressure line was placed in the superior vena cava (SVC). During surgery, 110 mmol/l (mEq/l) of sodium bicarbonate were given intravenously. The blood glucose concentration prior to surgery was 350 mg% (19.4 mmol/l).

The patient was returned to the ward with a haemoglobin of 12.4 g% and a PCV of 32%. The CVP was 6 cmH$_2$O. Postoperative estimations of the acid–base state and plasma protein concentrations and electrolytes demonstrated 'normal' sodium and potassium concentrations, a continued low albumin concentration and a moderate degree of metabolic acidosis, in spite of the infusion of bicarbonate during surgery. The blood pressure was 105/70 mmHg when the patient was first returned to the ward. The arterial blood oxygen tension was also reduced, and the patient was ventilated with 100% oxygen which was well humidified and positive pressure ventilation was continued with a patient-triggered, pressure-cycled (Bird) ventilator. High values of PO_2 (Table 6.7) and low values of PCO_2 were therefore recorded.

Ventilation of the lungs was continued overnight and during that period the patient received 2 litres of saline, 4 units of plasma, 2 units of blood and 180 mmol/l (mEq/l) (180 ml of 8.4% solution) of sodium bicarbonate. A blood sugar measurement taken during the night revealed a glucose concentration of 480 mg% (26.6 mmol/l), and 20 units of soluble insulin were therefore given intramuscularly at approximately 3 a.m. Blood-glucose estimations were then made at 6-hourly intervals and treatment was maintained with intravenous soluble insulin. During the first 48 hours following surgery, the blood pressure was approximately 125/75 mmHg and the CVP was 9–11 cmH$_2$O. Instructions were given that infusions of saline and plasma should proceed at such a rate that the CVP did not fall below 8 cmH$_2$O. Urine output was well maintained with the specific gravity lying between 1.007 and 1.017. The plasma amylase fell to within normal limits (280 units). The urinary amylase, however, was found to be high. The acid–base state demonstrated a moderate metabolic acidosis which was corrected with two infusions of sodium bicarbonate solution which amounted to 220 mmol (mEq) (220 ml of 8.4% NaHCO$_3$) on the first postoperative day. No further rise in serum amylase was noted, although the urinary amylase level remained high for 4 days following surgery. The plasma [Ca^{++}], although low post-operatively, rose as the plasma protein concentration increased and, by the seventh postoperative day, when the patient was well on the way to recovery, a metabolic alkalosis was noted and the lowest plasma [K^+] was recorded. The hyperglycaemia which was present both pre- and postoperatively disappeared by the fifth postoperative day and insulin was no longer required after that period Carbohydrate intake was restricted.

The patient was removed from the respirator after 48 hours and the PO_2, although lower than normal following the discontinuation of positive pressure ventilation, gradually climbed to normal levels and oxygen therapy was also discontinued. By the twelfth day, the patient had made an uneventful recovery and antibiotic therapy was ceased. The patient was walking well and regaining strength, although he felt very weak. When the patient was followed up 1 year later, no recurrence of pancreatitis had occurred.

The author has observed and treated acute pancreatitis following a number of different conditions including mitral valve replacement, surgery for the implantation of an abdominal aortic prosthesis, and major trauma. He has also treated patients in whom the aetiology could not be identified, as in the case described above. The hypocalcaemia, as recorded in the first edition of this book (Brooks, 1967),[8] was associated with hypoalbuminaemia and is in keeping with the findings of Imrie et al. (1976)[30] and Imrie (1976)[28] and other workers in this field. Much assistance can now be obtained by the differentiation of amylasaemia into different fractions (especially the salivary fraction and the pancreatic fraction) when a diagnosis has to be made.[49] In the case described above, pancreatitis was confirmed at surgery, but it should be noted that an increased amylase activity in the plasma is found not only in patients with diseases of the salivary glands, but also in cases of lung cancer, perforation of the gut, pneumonia, diabetic coma, diseases of the fallopian tube and following surgery. The hyperamylasaemia in these conditions is due to the salivary fraction.[1,19,27,50–52]

Clinical Presentation of Acute Pancreatitis

There appear to be three *types* of *acute* pancreatitis that are clinically identifiable and superimposed upon the two forms described on page 234. Type 2, however, could be divided into two subgroups: (a) that in which toxaemia is absent, and (b) that in which there is a toxic element in the condition, or a 'cardiodepressant' factor is present in the circulatory blood.

Type 1

The patient presents with a history of intermittent, acute abdominal pain, severe in nature, relieved in part by bedrest, sometimes by lying in the prone position on the abdomen, and sometimes by a bowel movement. Bending forwards at the trunk, approximating the shoulders to the knees, also appears to give relief of pain. The serum amylase is moderately raised above normal values if a blood sample is obtained during the acute attack. Body temperature is sometimes raised to a moderate degree, especially in the early morning. The patient occasionally feels cold but tends not to have a rigor and his condition appears to be improved by a broad-spectrum antibiotic such as oxytetracycline (Terramycin). Even when no treatment is given, the patient appears to improve and may not have a second attack. This type of acute pancreatitis may be associated with drug therapy, and a vast number of drugs have been implicated in its initiation, although it is difficult to draw conclusions as most patients who receive these preparations experience no problems.

Type 2

The patient may be admitted to hospital with acute abdominal pain and is investigated for this condition. The onset of the manifestation of acute

pancreatitis may be either rapid, developing over a period of 6–8 hours, or relatively slow, taking 2–3 days to develop fully.

The patient may be hyper- or hypopyrexial. The blood pressure falls and the patient's urinary output decreases or ceases altogether; acute renal failure may be suspected and sometimes develops. The low urine output, however, is initially due to hypovolaemia. Toxic shock sometimes appears to be a significant factor. The patient looks pale, is peripherally cyanosed, he has a haggard, dehydrated appearance and cold peripheries. The packed cell volume (PCV, haematocrit) is raised as plasma is lost into the abdominal cavity, and a paralytic ileus may manifest itself at a very early stage. Protein-rich fluid is then lost into the lumen of the gut, this is in addition to that lost into the peritoneal cavity. There is a fall in the plasma protein concentration, largely confined to the albumin fraction, and an associated fall in the serum $[Ca^{++}]$. As the condition progresses and the volume of protein-rich fluid in the peritoneal cavity increases, the CVP falls, and the signs of shock become more pronounced. It is at this stage that early, rapid intervention with fluid, plasma and electrolyte replacement probably affects mortality and, in any case, is essential if success is to be achieved.

Toxic shock, however, can be superimposed upon the hypovolaemia caused by the loss of fluid and plasma into the abdominal cavity, and a complicated clinical presentation develops. Toxic shock causes the CVP to rise. When an adequate blood volume has been restored by the infusion of saline and PPF or plasma, the CVP rises above 15 cmH$_2$O measured from the mid-axillary line. When a normal CVP is measured the replacement of fluid and repair of the blood volume are inadequate. This makes the control of fluid replacement difficult so that the rate of infusion of fluid requires constant attention, experience and skill.

As a result of either the hypotension or of the low blood volume and resulting poor tissue perfusion, there is a fall in the plasma bicarbonate concentration. Although this fall is not as pronounced as that seen in haemorrhagic pancreatitis low levels of bicarbonate, approximately 10 mmol/l (mEq/l), are sometimes seen. The early correction of the fluid volume, infusions of sodium bicarbonate and broad-spectrum antibiotics administered intravenously are necessary in this condition.

The patient sometimes recovers rapidly, especially when there has been a sudden rise followed by a rapid fall in blood-glucose concentration. Forty-eight hours after the onset of the condition the patient may be recovering well. Nevertheless, the treatment of this condition requires knowledge of its pathophysiology, skill, and experience in treating the acutely ill. Hypothermia can develop insidiously. Occasionally, the sudden onset of ventricular fibrillation occurs and, even if it is possible to restore sinus rhythm on one or more occasion, subsequent episodes of ventricular fibrillation are sometimes impossible to treat successfully even in well-equipped and experienced units, and in spite of every effort complete asystole develops. Brain death also appears to the author to have a relatively early onset.

A controlled clinical trial to determine whether peritoneal lavage produced an improvement in mortality has been performed by Mayer et al. (1985).[43] These workers concluded, however, that this procedure did not have any significant influence on the outcome of the condition.

Type 3 (haemorrhagic pancreatitis)

A third form of pancreatitis is that which may present with relatively mild symptoms and signs in its initial stages and rapidly progresses so that the condition of the patient quickly deteriorates, culminating often in death. As necrosis of the pancreas takes place, due to overwhelming inflammatory changes, both plasma and blood are lost in the peritoneal cavity. A rapid fall in blood pressure occurs and hypoxaemia is sometimes present, even though there is no clinical or X-ray evidence of pulmonary disease.[54] As in other cases of acute pancreatitis, pleural effusions are sometimes present as well as atelectasis, but this may also be seen in other abdominal conditions such as perforation of the gut.

SERUM AMYLASE

The amylases are a group of enzymes that hydrolyse starch glycogen. They are divided into two groups—alpha- and beta-amylases. The alpha-amylases appear in numerous but different animal tissues and convert starch into alpha-maltose and short-chain polysaccharides called dextrins. The beta-amylases also hydrolyse starches, but they yield a higher percentage of maltose at the end of the reaction. The presence of the amylases in both the sera and urine is used for diagnostic purposes.

The amylases are stored within the cells in the zymogen granules. Secretion of pancreatic juice is regulated by two hormones, *secretin* and *pancreozymin*. The parasympathetic nervous system also has a controlling influence. Secretin controls water and bicarbonate production, while pancreozymin and the parasympathetic nervous system govern the secretion of the enzyme.

In normal individuals the serum amylase may vary by as much as 200% on different days. The normal serum concentration of amylase lies between 80 and 150 Somogyi units.

The excretion of amylase in the urine in the normal individual remains uniform in spite of changes in urine volume and output.

In man the highest concentration of amylase is found in the pancreatic and salivary gland tissues. The liver, fallopian tubes, striated muscle and adipose tissue also contain amylase in significant quantities. Experimentally, pancreatectomy in some animals produces only minor changes in the concentration of amylase in the plasma.

In a review of this subject, Janowitz and Dreilig[31] concluded that the amount of amylase from the pancreas and salivary glands was less than that which had been previously accepted, while the contribution from the liver in normal subjects was more significant than that which had previously been assumed. In normal subjects, Dreiling et al.[17] demonstrated that amylase migrated with both the albumin and gamma globulin fractions. However, when serum from patients with acute pancreatitis was examined, the major part of the amylase migrated with the gamma-globulin fraction. They also observed that in normal subjects the sum of the amylase activity of the electrophoretically determined amylase fractions was greater than the total serum amylase activity. In patients suffering from pancreatitis this difference could not be established. It was demonstrated by Berk et al.[4,5] that the pattern of migration of amylase derived from pancreatic tissue was different from that of amylase derived from the salivary gland.

It is therefore not surprising, from the above that different clinical conditions can produce variable amylase activities, and that some confusion still exists with regard to interpretation of amylase levels.

Delcourt and Wettendorff[15] found the urinary amylase clearance in normal subjects to be reasonably constant at 148 ml/hour. Patients suffering from pancreatitis or carcinoma had values greater than 200 ml/hour. The upper limit of amylase excretion in the urine in normal people was found to be 300 units/hour. The mean 1-hour excretion rate in 37 people was 119 Somogyi units. Variations from hour to hour were found in patients suffering from acute pancreatitis.[10]

Hyperamylasaemia

Although the serum amylase activity is commonly regarded as an indication of disturbances of the pancreas, hyperamylasaemia does occur in a number of conditions where primary pancreatic disease is not present and primary pancreatic function has not changed.

Pancreatic disease

Although it is recognized that at the onset of acute pancreatitis many patients have a raised serum amylase activity, as the disease progresses, serum amylase activity returns to normal and urine amylase determinations are considered to be more reliable.[20]

Perforation and obstruction of the gastro-intestinal tract

High serum amylase activity is associated with many cases of perforation of the gut. This causes difficulties in diagnosis, especially when the abdominal pain is not localized and rebound tenderness is present. It is possible that the serum amylase value reflects the amount of gastro-intestinal content that has entered the peritoneal cavity.[9] The condition is quite commonly associated with marked hyperamylasaemia.[9] When the bowel is obstructed, it has been postulated that amylase in the lumen of the bowel in high concentration can penetrate the bowel wall and enter the circulating blood.[7]

Renal disease

Patients suffering from both acute and chronic renal failure demonstrate hyperamylasaemia, and there is considered to be a correlation between the retention of nitrogenous products and the degree of serum amylase activity.[26]

Ectopic pregnancy

The fallopian tubes appear to contain high concentrations of amylase. It is therefore logical that high serum and urinary amylase levels reaching 1600 Somogyi units can be found in the presence of a ruptured ectopic pregnancy.[36]

Trauma and surgery

Patients who have received a severe blow to the abdomen, such as those involved in road traffic accidents, demonstrate hyperamylasaemia. Traumatic rupture or haemorrhage into the bowel also causes a marked rise in serum amylase concentration.[61] Injuries to the brain are associated with hyperamylasaemia; the values sometimes reach 1400 Somogyi units.[18]

Abdominal surgery frequently gives rise to hyperamylasaemia. For example, it has been noted that hyperamylasaemia occurs in association with gastrectomy.[41]

Carcinoma

Very high levels of serum amylase are sometimes found in patients suffering from neoplasia which does not involve the pancreatic gland.[18]

Disease of the liver and biliary tract

In a number of cases, post-mortem studies on patients with cirrhosis of the liver have revealed inflammatory changes of the pancreas.[63]

It is also found that patients suffering from hepatitis exhibit a moderate degree of hyperamylasaemia.[14]

Mumps

This viral infection, which is generalized in nature, and is by no means isolated to the parotid glands, although it is referred to as epidemic parotitis, frequently gives rise to hyperamylasaemia.[47] It is well recognized that mumps may give rise to complications such as pancreatitis and meningo-encephalitis and orchitis. It is therefore logical that in some patients the hyperamylasaemia persists for a considerable period of time after the inflammation of the salivary glands has subsided.

Hypoamylasaemia

Low serum amylase values are seen in a number of conditions in which there is destruction of the pancreatic gland. This occurs following acute exacerbations of chronic pancreatitis and during recovery from the disease.[55,59]

Very low values of amylase are also found in the protein deficiency disease, present in Central Africa, which causes abnormality of liver function and is known as kwashiorkor.[39] It seems that the degenerative processes in this condition are not confined to the liver but also involve the pancreatic gland.

References

Pancreatitis and serum amylase

1. Ammann, R. W., Berk, J. E., Fridhandler, L., Ueda, M. and Wegmann, W. (1973). Hyperamylasaemia with carcinoma of the lung. *Ann. int. Med.*, **78**, 521.
2. Arnold, F., Doyle, P. J. and Dell, G. (1978). Acute pancreatitis in a patient treated with cimetidine. *Lancet*, **i**, 382.
3. Barraclough, B. H. and Coupland, G. A. E. (1972). Acute pancreatitis: a review. *Aus. & N.Z. J. Surg.*, **41**, 211.
4. Berk, J. E. (1967). Serum amylase and lipase. *J. Amer. med. Ass.*, **199**, 98.
5. Berk, J. E., Searcy, R. L., Hayashi, S. and Ujihira, I. (1965). Distribution of serum amylase in man and animals. Electrophoretic and chromatographic studies *J. Amer. med. Ass.*, **192**, 389.
6. Bourke, J. B. (1977). Incidence and mortality of acute pancreatitis. *Brit. med. J.*, **II**, 1668.
7. Boyd, T. F., Perez, J. L. and Byrne, J. J. (1961). Serum amylase levels in experimental intestinal obstruction: does small bowel necrosis cause a rise in serum amylase? *Ann. Surg.*, **154**, 85.
8. Brooks, D. K. (1967). *Resuscitation*, 1st edn. London: Edward Arnold.
9. Burnett, W. and Ness, T. D. (1955). Serum amylase and acute abdominal disease. *Brit. med. J.*, **II**, 770.
10. Calkins, W. G. (1966). A study of urinary amylase excretion in normal persons. *Amer. J. Gastroent.*, **46**, 407.
11. Condon, J. R., Knight, M. and Day, J. L. (1973). Glucagon therapy in acute pancreatitis. *Brit. J. Surg.*, **60**, 509.
12. Coward, R. A. (1977). Paracetamol-induced acute pancreatitis. *Brit. med. J.*, **I**, 1086.
13. Cox, A. G. (1977). Death from acute pancreatitis. *Lancet*, **ii**, 632.
14. Cummins, A. J. and Backus, H. L. (1951). Abnormal serum pancreatic enzyme values in liver disease. *Gastroenterology*, **18**, 518.
15. Delcourt, A. and Wettendorff, P. (1964). Renal amylase clearance in the normal state during the course of pancreatic disorders. *Acta clin. Belg.*, **19**, 265.
16. Dennison, A. R. and Royle, G. T. (1984). Acute pancreatitis—presentation as a discoloured lump in the groin. *Postgrad. med. J.*, **60**, 374.
17. Dreiling, D. A., Janowitz, H. D. and Josephberg, L. J. (1963). Serum isoamylases: an electrophoretic study of the blood amylase and the patterns observed in pancreatic disease. *Ann. int. Med.*, **58**, 235.
18. Edmondson, H. A., Berne, C. J., Homann, R. E. and Wertman, M. (1952). Calcium, potassium, magnesium and amylase disturbances in acute pancreatitis. *Amer. J. Med.*, **12**, 34.
19. Fridhandler, L., Berk, J. E. and Ueda, M. (1972). Isolation and measurement of pancreatic amylase in human serum and urine. *Clin. Chem.*, **18**, 1493.
20. Gambill, E. C. and Mason, H. L. (1963). One-hour value for urinary amylase in 96 patients with pancreatitis. *J. Amer. med. Assoc.*, **186**, 24.
21. Gilmore, I. T. and Tourvas, E. (1977). Paracetamol-induced acute pancreatitis. *Brit. med. J.*, **I**, 753.
22. Glazer, G. and Bennett, A. (1976). Prostaglandin release in canine acute haemorrhagic pancreatitis. *Gut*, **17**, 22.
23. Glazer, G. and Dudley, H. (1977). Acute pancreatitis. In *Recent advances in intensive therapy*, p. 77. Edited by I. McA. Ledingham. London: Churchill Livingstone.
24. Goodley, E., Derasse, J. and Carver, J. (1973). Phenformin and pancreatitis. *Ann. int. Med.*, **28**, 307.
25. Graeber, G. M., Marmor, B. M., Hendel, R. C. and Gregg, R. O. (1976). Pancreatitis and severe metabolic abnormalities due to phenformin therapy. *Arch. Surg.*, **111**, 1014.
26. Gross, J. B., Parkin, T. W., Maher, F. T. and Power, M. H. (1960). Serum amylase and lipase values in renal and extrarenal azotemia. *Gastroenterology*, **39**, 76.
27. Harada, K., Kitamura, M. and Ikenaga, T. (1974). Isoamylase study of postoperative transient hyperamylasemia. *Amer. J. Gastroent.*, **61**, 212.
28. Imrie, C. W. (1976). Proceedings: hypocalcaemia of acute pancreatitis. The effect of hypoalbuminaemia. *Brit. J. Surg.*, **63**, 662.
29. Imrie, C. W., Goldring, J., Pollock, J. G. and Watt, J. K. (1977). Acute pancreatitis after translumbar aortography. *Brit. med. J.*, **2**, 681.
30. Imrie, C. W., Murphy, D., Ferguson, J. C. and Blumgart, L. H. (1976). Arterial hypoxia in acute pancreatitis. *Ann. Roy Coll. Surg. Engl.*, **58**, 322.

31. Janowitz, H. and Dreiling, D. (1959). The plasma amylase: source, regulation and diagnositic significance. *Amer. J. Med.*, **27**, 924.

32. Joffe, S. M. and Lee, F. D. (1978). Acute pancreatitis after cimetidine administration in experimental duodenal ulcers. *Lancet*, **i**, 383.

33. Johnston, D. H. and Cornish, A. L. (1959). Acute pancreatitis in patients receiving chlorothiazide. *J. Amer. med. Ass.*, **170**, 2054.

34. Jones, M. F. and Caldwell, J. R. (1962). Acute haemorrhagic pancreatitis associated with administration of chlorthalidone; report of a case. *N. Engl. J. Med.*, **267**, 1029.

35. Jones, P. E. and Oelbaum, M. H. (1975). Frusemide-induced pancreatitis. *Brit. med. J.*, **1**, 133.

36. Kelly, M. L. (1957). Elevated serum amylase level associated with ruptured ectopic pregnancy. *J. Amer. med. Ass.*, **164**, 406.

37. Lambrianides, A. L. and Rosin, R. D. (1984). Acute pancreatitis complicating excessive intake of phenolphthalein. *Postgrad. med. J.*, **60**, 491.

38. Lefer, A. M., Glenn, T. M., O'Neill, T. J., Lovett, W. L., Geissinger, W. T. and Wangensteen, S. L. (1971). Inotropic influence of endogenous peptides in experimental haemorrhagic pancreatitis. *Surgery*, **69**, 220.

39. Lehndorff, H. (1961). Kwashiorkor ... present problems. *Arch. Pediat.*, **78**, 293.

40. Levitan, A. A. (1973). Phenformin and pancreatitis. *Ann. int. Med.*, **78**, 306.

41. McGowan, G. K. and Willis, M. R. (1964). Diagnostic value of plasma amylase, especially after gastrectomy. *Brit. med. J.*, **1**, 160.

42. Mallory, A. and Kern, F. (1980). Drug-induced pancreatitis: a critical review. *Gastroenterology*, **78**, 813.

43. Mayer, A. D., McMahon, M. J., Corfield, A. P., Cooper, M. J., Williamson, R. C. N., Dickson, A. P., Shearer, M. G. and Imrie, C. W. (1985). Controlled clinical trial of peritoneal lavage for the treatment of severe acute pancreatitis. *N. Engl. J. of Med.*, **312**, 399.

44. MRC Multicentre trial of glucagon and aproprotin (1977). Death from acute pancreatitis. *Lancet*, **ii**, 632.

45. Myren, J. (1977). Acute pancreatitis: pathogenic factors as a basis for treatment. *Scand. J. Gastroent.*, **12**, 513.

46. Nakashima, Y. and Howard, J. M. (1977). Drug-induced acute pancreatitis. *Surg. Gynecol. & Obs.*, **145**, 105.

47. Nakoo, T., Gotooda, T. and Tohoku, J. (1962). Pancreatic ferments in the duodenal fluids in mumps. Subclinical pancreopathy in mumps. *J. exp. Med.*, **78**, 249.

48. Ofstad, E. (1970). Formation and destruction of plasma kinine during experimental acute haemorrhagic pancreatitis in dogs. *Scand. J. Gastroent.*, **5**, 9.

49. Otsuki, M., Saeki, S. and Yuu, H. (1975). Electrophoretic studies on human urinary amylase isoenzymes by using a simple thin layer of polyacrylamide gel electrophoresis. *Physico-Chem. Biol.*, **19**, 139.

50. Otsuki, M., Saeki, S., Yuu, H. and Baba, S. (1975). Amylase and the lung. *Excerpta. Med. Int. Congr. Ser.*, **369**, 67.

51. Otsuki, M., Saeki, S., Yuu, H., Baba, F. and Kondo, T. (1975). Reassessment of clinical significance of amylase isoenzymes. *Clin. Chem.*, **21**, 948.

52. Otsuki, M., Saeki, S., Yuu, H., Maeda, M. and Bana, S. (1976). Electrophoretic pattern of amylase isoenzymes in serum and urine of normal persons. *Clin. Chem.*, **22**, 439.

53. Pollock, A. V. (1959). Acute pancreatitis: analysis of 100 patients. *Brit. med. J.*, **I**, 6.

54. Ranson, J., Roses, D. F. and Fink, S. D. (1973). Early respiratory insufficiency in acute pancreatitis. *Ann. Surg.*, **178**, 75.

55. Smith, E. K. and Allbright, E. C. (1952). Carcinoma of the body and tail of the pancreas. Report of 37 cases studied at the State of Wisconsin Gen. Hospital from 1925–50. *Ann. int. Med.*, **36**, 90.

56. Trapnell, J. E. (1972). The natural history and management of acute pancreatitis. *Clinics in Gastroenterology*, **1**, 147.

57. Trapnell, J. E. and Duncan, E. H. L. (1975). Patterns of incidence in acute pancreatitis. *Brit. med. J.*, **2**, 179.

58. Warshaw, A. L., Lesser, P. B., Rie, M. and Cullen, D. J. (1975). The pathogenesis of pulmonary edema in acute pancreatitis. *Ann. Surg.*, **182**, 505.

59. Webster, P. E. and Zieve, L. (1962). Alterations in serum content of pancreatic enzymes. *N. Engl. J. of Med.*, **267**, 604.

60. Wenger, J. and Gross, P. R. (1964). Acute pancreatitis related to hydrochlorothiazide therapy. *Gastroenterology*, **46**, 778.

61. Wharton, G. K. and Sloan, L. E. (1953). Pancreatitis. *Amer. J. Gastroent.*, **29**, 445.

62. Wilde, H. (1972). Pancreatitis and phenformin. *Ann. int. Med.*, **77**, 324.

63. Woldman, E. E., Fishman, D. and Segal, A. J. (1958). Relation of fibrosis of the pancreas to fatty liver and/or cirrhosis: an analysis of one thousand autopsies. *J. Amer. med. Ass.*, **169**, 1281.

TREATMENT OF BURN SHOCK

With the increasing understanding of the problems in general body metabolism and physiology that are associated with the burning of large areas of tissue, the mortality rate has fallen. Since 1948, however, Phillips and Cope[52] have demonstrated that a more scientific approach has increased the survival time which follows severe burning, but has not very greatly influenced its final fatal outcome. There is, therefore, still scope for more investigation and improved forms of therapy. One of the notable improvements, especially, since 1948, is a decrease in the mortality of treated patients during the shock phase. This has been halved. When people who had been burnt over more than 90% of the body surface were excluded from their series, the mortality within the first 48 hours fell to only 18%. The importance of the early correction of metabolic and fluid volume abnormalities becomes apparent. In the first 24 hours, shock is the prime cause of death. It was shown that the degree of shock was related to the area of burning and age of the patient;[16] this view has not changed.[58] Other factors are damage to the respiratory tract, renal failure, infection, toxaemia, hypoproteinaemia and disturbances of hydration and electrolytes.

Degrees of Burns

Essentially, there are only two degrees of burns: (a) partial skin thickness burning, and (b) full thickness burning, which removes every epidermal cell. It is not always possible in the early stages to know with certainty whether every epidermal cell has been removed, or killed. The treatment of the burn must, therefore, be directed towards preventing the conversion of a partial thickness burn, which may have a layer of epidermis only one cell thick, into a full thickness lesion. It is for this reason that forms of treatment which involve the application of astringent substances or scrubbing the burnt areas under a general anaesthetic have been abandoned. Exposure to air is a form of treatment which is now advocated by many centres.

Because the appearance of the surface of the burnt area is so deceptive, a reliable assessment as to whether a burn is of partial thickness or not is

very difficult. Methods such as sensitivity to pinprick,[37,38] the use of intravenous dyes and fluorescein have been suggested.[34] Partial thickness burns tend to blister and heal without scarring, while full thickness burns always scar and require the application of skin grafts. It is true that there is an intermediate stage in which some regeneration of skin may take place from the sweat glands and from the hair follicles which lie at a deeper level, and partial, patchy scarring which may have a profound effect on function may result. This aspect of the subdivision of burns into various degrees has been emphasized by Clarkson.[19] There is also little doubt that the depth of burn influences the volume of fluid loss and haemodynamic disturbances and therefore the degree of shock.

In general, three degrees of burns are usually recognized in present-day clinical practice.

Grade 1. Erythema of the skin without blistering.
Grade 2. Partial thickness burning of the skin with blistering (vesication).
Grade 3. Full thickness burning of the skin so that blistering cannot occur.

There is initially loss of fluid into and from the burned area. In a grade 3 burn a crust (or eschar) is formed later which sloughs off leaving a granulating ulcer that heals by fibrosis, contraction and much scarring. This area, therefore, has to be grafted with skin.

Changes in Fluid Volume

Although haemoconcentration due to fluid loss had been recognized and described very clearly in 1881,[66] Underhill in 1923[68] was the first to demonstrate the rise in haemoglobin concentration and the benefit of giving intravenous saline solution for the treatment of burns. The changes in fluid volume were quantitatively studied in the experiments of Blalock (1931)[9] who recognized the importance these played in the genesis of shock. He compared the weights of two halves of a burnt animal and demonstrated that the average weight difference of a sagittal section was 3% of the total weight of the dog. In his experiments upon 18 dogs this represented a loss of over half of the plasma volume. It was demonstrated by Harkins (1934)[35] that a fluid shift occurred very shortly after burning. He balanced anaesthetized animals so that the centre of gravity moved towards the burnt side and the board upon which they were placed tilted. A movement of fluid from the extracellular fluid (ECF) space into the intracellular fluid (ICF) space was demonstrated by Fox and Baer.[29] Bull and England[14] concluded from their investigations that the changes in the fluid and salt metabolism that occurred after the age of 55 years were similar to those that were produced in younger age-groups who were more severely burnt.

It is obvious from this work therefore, that changes in water metabolism play an important part in the treatment of the severely burnt patient. Also, it is not suprising that more recent work has shown a decrease in mortality when active fluid therapy has been instituted. It must be remembered, however, that as plasma is lost, a fall in the protein concentration must automatically follow and that there is therefore a reduction in the colloid osmotic activity of the plasma and this has to be restored.

Changes in Serum Proteins

It was very readily established in the early investigations of the changes that occurred in burns that the fluid contained within a bulla was very similar to plasma because of its electrolyte and protein content. It is predictable that the smaller molecules of albumin would be lost more readily than the larger molecules of globulin, and in 1927 Davidson[22] demonstrated a lowering of the total plasma protein with a fall in the serum albumin and a rise in the serum globulin. In 1930, Underhill[69] showed that there was a loss of plasma into the area of burning. Since then, many investigations have been performed on plasma protein concentration including that of the electrophoretic pattern.[44,51,56] It has been suggested[56] that the gamma-globulin concentration was a good indication of the severity of the burn. The infusion of plasma albumin which has been fractionated or of plasma substitutes, such as dextran, has been advocated.

Changes in Na+ Metabolism

The fall in sodium ion concentration in the plasma was demonstrated by Underhill, who advocated large infusions of NaCl solution. Fox (1945) demonstrated the loss of Na^+ from the plasma in the burnt area by means of labelled Na^+.[29,30] The marked improvement in mortality and the clinical improvement of shock state associated with burns that have accompanied the use of large volumes of saline solution have demonstrated that this is an essential part of burn therapy. This is so whether additional colloid in the form of plasma protein or plasma substitute is given or not. The kidneys retain Na^+ immediately following burning, so that if normal ordinary water losses are replaced with NaCl, then hypernatremia will result. It is not uncommon, therefore, for an elevated plasma $[Na^+]$ to be found 3 or 4 days after an extensive burn. Replacement of water is the only method by which this condition can be reversed, but it must be borne in mind that if renal function is depressed and fluid is being retained, the infusion of large volumes of water will result in expansion of the ECF and lead to pulmonary oedema.

Plasma K+ Metabolism

A rise in the serum $[K^+]$ after burns was demonstrated in 1921 by Kramer and Tisdall[41] and this rise has since been considered to be of some importance.[60] Nevertheless, other workers in the field have not placed much stress on this aspect of metabolism. Unlike Na^+, large quantities of K^+ are excreted in the first few days by the kidneys so that in certain circumstances a low plasma $[K^+]$ may sometimes be found.[19] If renal failure develops, a rise in plasma $[K^+]$ automatically follows and it is under these circumstances that a raised plasma level becomes of greatest importance.

Destruction of Erythrocytes and Anaemia

When a burn extends over more than 10–15% of the body surface, anaemia usually develops. Where there is a large deep burn, immediate red cell destruction occurs and during the following 2 or 3 weeks the average loss may amount to 45% of the patient's red cells.[23,67] When estimates of red cell loss were made by Muir[49] using ^{32}P and ^{51}Cr, it was found that 0.5–1% of the circulating cells were lost for each 1% of deep burn during the first

3 days. A moderate degree of hyperplasia of the bone marrow has been demonstrated by Sevitt,[62] but he believed that this was insufficient to compensate fully for the loss of erythrocytes. Damage to the red cell membrane occurs as blood perfuses burnt areas so that erythrocyte fragility increases.[50]

Hyperglycaemia

In common with other forms of acute change in body function, such as haemorrhagic shock and acute myocardial infarction, the blood sugar in the burnt patient is commonly raised and glucose is often found in the urine for a short period. Sometimes the situation may give rise to a more prolonged and more greatly raised concentration of blood sugar so that it may be considered to be a form of 'pseudo-diabetes'.[3,27] In addition to hyperglycaemia, the degree of glycosuria produces an osmotic diuresis so that dehydration can become more marked. The specific gravity of the urine is raised because of the presence of sugar and, therefore, may be misleading if it is considered to be a sign of the ability of the kidneys to concentrate. Throughout the period of glycosuria ketone bodies are absent.

Renal Function

Immediately following burning there is a decrease in the renal excretion of both sodium and water and an increase in the excretion of potassium and nitrogen. Retention of fluid by the kidneys when severe burns have been treated with adequate volumes of fluid so that the oligaemia and hypotension are not severe, lasts for 2–3 days. Two forms of renal failure which may develop have been described by Sevitt.[61,62] One form follows the course of acute tubular necrosis (see p. 110) and in the other form there is a high blood urea with only moderate oliguria and this form is associated with passing a urine of low specific gravity. The importance of adequate therapy following burn trauma in preventing renal damage has been stressed by Artz and Reiss.[5]

Changes in the Endocrine System

Elevation of the urinary catecholamines occurs for several days after a severe burn.[32] When serial specimens of urine were examined it was found that adrenaline (epinephrine) and noradrenaline (norepinephrine, levarterenol) were present in their highest concentrations within the first 8 hours. Because there is sodium retention, increased potassium excretion, increased urinary nitrogen concentration, elevation of the blood sugar, an increase in the urinary 17-ketosteroids and corticosteroids and a fall in the number of circulating eosinophils, the similarity between the effects of treatment with ACTH and the endocrine changes and metabolic effects that follow burns has been noted.[27] The correlation between increased adrenocortical function and protein breakdown has been demonstrated.[63] It was found that the rate of excretion of 17-hydroxycorticoids was greatest during the catabolic phase which occurs in the days following recovery from the initial burning episode.

Curling's Ulcers

Damage to the gut is present in most cases of fatal burns. This is generally superficial and may occur in various parts of the gut.[62] The ulcer described by Curling[21] was approximately 5.1 cm (2 inches) long and situated on the anterior wall of the duodenum. Ulceration of the gut had previously been reported by others.[24,45,65] The ulceration may give rise to perforation or melaena.[4] A young child reported by Clarkson[19] survived a major blood loss from bloody melaena which was associated with a reduction in urine output, the urine also contained blood. The importance of this complication in causing death after burning has also been demonstrated by Choudhury,[18] who has reported two children, one aged 12 years and the other 2 years, in whom ulceration gave rise to melaena, perforation and peritonitis.

Stress ulceration following burns and other conditions, such as respiratory failure, is discussed elsewhere (see p. 199). While bacterial erosion appears to play a part in the aetiology of stress ulceration when burns are not the precipitating cause, and low concentrations of HCl or complete achlorhydria are found,[11] other factors may give rise to Curling's ulcers.

Damage to the Lungs and Respiratory Tract

The importance of damage to the respiratory tract has been emphasized by Phillips and Cope,[53,55] although the seriousness of these burns has been noted by others.[6,7,15] The inhalation of toxic gases which are at a high temperature is one of the main causes of death following the burning episode. This becomes especially important when there are burns in the region of the mouth and face.[54] Damage to the respiratory tract gives rise to dyspnoea, stridor, cyanosis associated with râles and rhonchi. The sputum is blood-stained and may contain bronchial casts. An X-ray of the chest may reveal increased areas of density caused by inhalation of smoke and other vapours, patchy atelectasis or lobar collapse. Lobar collapse is caused by plugs of necrotic material occluding bronchioles. Damage to the respiratory tract is very largely avoided if it is possible to place a wet pad across the mouth and to breathe through this while in the area of the fire.

Fortunately, the specific heat of gas is so low that only the upper respiratory tract is usually damaged by heat.[36] Since the first edition of this book was published in 1967, however, polyurethane and other plastics have been used increasingly in furniture manufacture. When polyvinyl chloride is burnt it can give rise to phosgene gas. Thus respiratory damage occurs in modern fires with much greater frequency, and death from asphyxiation at the time of the fire is a common occurrence. However, those people who survive the fire present with respiratory failure in the emergency department of the hospital as much as 8–24 hours later.

When heat damages the oral cavity and pharynx, oedema of the posterior pharyngeal wall develops and early tracheal intubation or tracheostomy under general anaesthesia is indicated. When left too late because of a reluctance to perform a tracheotomy, on understandable humanitarian grounds, tragedy due to obstructed airway can follow.

Because of the consequences of lung damage from inhaled chemicals and gases, even when obstruction of the airway is absent, many centres give a single dose of corticosteroids,[36] for example methylprednisolone 250 mg i.v., sometimes repeated twice at 8-hourly intervals. Continued use of steroids, except when there is a direct indication, is usually not advocated because of the increased risks of infection.

An early fall in arterial PCO_2 is often the first indication of impending respiratory damage. The PCO_2 and pH will vary with the degree of ventilation of the lungs.

During the Vietnam War, a large number of burns were treated, most of which had resulted from flame-throwing weapons, napalm, bombs and petrol. There was a high mortality. When death occurred from respiratory failure during the first 48 hours of treatment for burns, the major cause was overhydration and overloading with infused fluid in the presence of renal failure.

Infection also played an important role, particularly with *Pseudomonas aeruginosa*,[39,40] which, as demonstrated, can grow freely in the stomach.[11,12] Inhalation pneumonitis (see p. 122) has also been identified as a cause of respiratory failure, even in those patients who are receiving nasogastric suction.

Burn Encephalopathy

The onset of convulsions, hyperpyrexia and coma has been observed following burns. This is sometimes preceded by cerebral irritability, paraesthesia, muscle cramps or twitching, vomiting and nausea. Burn encephalopathy is probably a manifestation of cerebral oedema as seen in other conditions when large volumes of fluid are infused at a rapid rate, as in diabetic ketosis and the non-ketotic (hyperosmolar) form of the disease.

Convulsions can also occur, as in an 11-year-old child who was treated by the author and in whom excessive volumes of glucose/saline had been infused; the patient's plasma $[Na^+]$ fell to 126 mmol/l (mEq/l). This was really a manifestation of water intoxication, as described on page 26.

Shock

In every patient, burn shock remains the greatest danger during the first few hours. As well as being the prime cause of death within the first 3 days, it also results in additional damage to tissues that is not a direct result of burning, such as acute renal failure and possibly ulceration of the bowel.

It arises because there is a loss of fluid from the circulation resulting in hypovolaemia. This occurs in the following ways.

There is a movement of fluid from the ECF into the ICF and there is a movement of fluid into the tissues which surround and are involved in the burn; also fluid passes from the burnt area into blisters or drains from the burnt surface. In addition there is a loss of red cells by haemolytic processes. In this way more than *half* the effective blood volume may be lost within the first 2–3 hours of the burning episode when there is a 50% burn of the skin surface.

We have seen how this loss of fluid also produces hypoproteinaemia because of the high protein content of the fluid that is lost. Because of this, a deep burn covering a large area is associated with such a large depletion of osmotically active colloid that the correction of the oligaemia may be insufficient if replacement of fluid loss is made by infusions of saline or solutions such as that of Ringer or Hartmann alone. For this reason it has been the practice in many centres to infuse plasma, human albumin or dextran. The effects of loss of fluid from the circulation are not immediately apparent from the clinical appearance of the patient. Although there is a tachycardia, the blood pressure may remain high for some time. The patient, however, is almost invariably thirsty, has an anxious appearance and is restless and may have beads of sweat on the unburnt areas of skin. Peripheral cyanosis caused by hypovolaemia will be present, especially at the extremities such as the ear lobes, the nose, fingernail beds and finger tips. The tongue is pale and may also have a cyanotic appearance, even when the arterial blood has a normal oxygen tension.

It is therefore, essential, that the infusion of electrolyte-containing fluid should begin immediately after the burning episode and be continued in adequate volumes until the initial danger period of 3 days is passed. Increased capillary permeability in the burn areas continues for approximately 48 hours and after this time major fluid losses usually cease unless there is gross hyperventilation or diarrhoea. It may be necessary to continue large volume fluid therapy for a longer period than this if a fluid deficit has accrued and if there are associated complications, such as acute dilatation of the stomach.

Infection

The problem of infection of the burn surface is always present and there seems to be little doubt that in almost all cases infection is the result of contamination either from the surroundings or from the medical attendants.[62] Almost any organism may invade the burnt area, although those most feared are *Pseudomonas*, pyocyaneus and tetanus. However, in the experience of the Birmingham Burns Unit, infection with tetanus spores is uncommon.[62] The toxicity of infective processes is one of the major dangers of burns, and it is now quite common for the burst surface to be gently cleaned with a mild antiseptic detergent, such as 1% Savlon applied before the method of exposure is used.[70] In this way the dried eschar acts as a barrier to infective processes and the circumstances that least favour the growth of bacteria— coolness and dryness—are established.[71] Hyperbaric oxygen treatment may assist in inhibiting bacterial growth.

For the immediate treatment of burns, one should refer to an up-to-date reference work on the subject.[58]

Much progress has been made in the prevention of *Pseudomonas* infections with the use of a polyvalent vaccine. For example it is well recognized that *Pseudomonas aeruginosa* can give rise to bacteraemia and therefore to toxic shock. It has been found that patients vaccinated with the polyvalent vaccine have not developed a generalized infection. No *Pseudomonas* organisms were found when blood cultures were obtained in all cases, and raised titres of circulating protective antibody were present.

Alterations in the body's immunity to infection and immune responsiveness have been documented and the possibility of 'burn induced immuno-deficiency syndrome' has been postulated (Antonacci *et al.*, 1984).[2]

Choice of Solution for Infusion in Burn shock

There are certain experiments that have tended to show that the level of plasma protein does not play an important part in the maintenance of the circulation.[1,73] It was found that when the blood was removed and the plasma separated and the red cells returned with saline, twice the blood volume could be removed in one day and the plasma protein concentrations reduced to 1 g% without any evidence of circulatory failure or causing death.

In clinical practice, a low plasma protein concentration in the sick patient commonly complicates treatment, causing oedema, oliguria, circulatory insufficiency and hypotension. In the burned patient, unless an adequate volume of fluid is infused within an hour of suffering burn trauma, profound shock may develop.[38,43]

Haemaccel (see p. 202) has been used during the treatment of burns and will reverse the hypovolaemic shock that develops.[31,59] It can be given in volumes based upon 1 ml of Haemaccel per percentage of skin area burnt, per kilogram body weight. The colloid particles have a molecular weight of between 5000 and 50 000, (mean 35 000), and are contained in isotonic saline. One possible advantage of using Haemaccel is that the solution induces a diuresis.

Particular care must be taken to avoid overloading children with excess fluid.[17]

From a knowledge of the basic physiological changes, it can therefore be seen that an adequate volume of fluid must be infused as soon after the burning episode as possible and that this fluid must contain a high concentration of electrolyte. NaCl or a mixture of NaCl and $NaHCO_3$ is suitable in the early stages, and it is now generally believed that additional colloid in the form of plasma or plasma substitute must also be given. Squire et al.[64] found that when they performed a controlled trial, dextran was associated with a slightly, but not significantly, greater mortality than plasma. Although they considered the great fall in plasma protein concentration a disadvantage, the use of this plasma substitute is free from the dangers of homologous serum jaundice, now known as hepatitis B, which is a complication found by Sevitt[62] to be associated with 0.16% of patients who have received blood transfusions.

Plasma is now being discarded by many countries and is being replaced by purified protein fraction (PPF), also known as fractionated human albumin. It is heat-treated during manufacture (page 202) and is therefore free from the hepatitis viruses and probably the acquired immune deficiency syndrome (AIDS) agent.

The presence of colloid in the infusion solution does not appear to be essential. In 1968 Baxter and Shires demonstrated that fluid losses associated with large areas of burns could be replaced with 'balanced electrolyte solution', which was lactated Ringer's solution, also known as Hartmann's solution.[8] In 1973 Monafo and his co-workers used hypertonic saline solutions and, although this sometimes leads to hypernatraemia, they have proved to be successful.[46] Indeed hypernatraemia, sometimes of a very severe degree, is seen when isotonic solutions are used and an inadequate

volume of electrolyte-free water is either infused or taken orally. If 5% Dextrose is infused to provide free water, care must be taken that hyperglycaemia does not develop even in the non-diabetic patient. The use of various solutions has been reviewed by Pruitt (1981) and Goodwin (1984).[33,57]

It is important to avoid over infusion, which produces respiratory insufficiency and hypoxia, while maintaining an adequate blood volume and therefore blood pressure and circulatory response.

A guide to adequate hydration is the urine output; this should not fall below 30 ml/hour in the adult or 1 ml/kg body weight in a child weighing 30 kg or less.

A further indication to the adequacy of volume replacement is heart rate. There is always a tachycardia unless some cardiac or other abnormality prevents an increase in heart rate. A persistent very fast tachycardia may indicate hypovolaemia. A central venous pressure (CVP) measurement may be essential.

Volume of Fluid Required

When the burnt area is greater than 15% of the body surface in the adult or 10% in the child, the infusion of electrolyte–colloid solutions is essential. Various formulae have been devised for the calculation of the patient's fluid requirements.[13,20,25,26] These are based upon age of the patient and the area burnt.

The percentage of the surface area burnt can be assessed for clinical purposes from the 'Rule of 9', (see Fig. 6.10).[72]

An example of a formula for fluid replacement which has been used successfully is that reported by Evans in 1963.[25]

Adults. The total quantity of fluid infused in the first 48 hours is calculated as follows: 120 ml dextran is infused for each 1% of the body surface area burnt up to a maximum volume of 6 litres. Half of this volume is given in the first 8 hours following burning. One-quarter of the volume is given in the following 16 hours. The remaining quarter is given in the final 24 hours. In addition, approximately 50 ml/kg of water are given orally every 24 hours for normal fluid balance. In the presence of deep burns, up to one-third of the total calculated volume of dextran is replaced with acid-citrate-dextrose (ACD) blood.

Children.* When burns are less than 30% of the body surface area, the volume of dextran is calculated as follows:

Age	Dextran (ml)
0–3 months	15
3–6 months	21
6–9 months	24
9–12 months	27
1–2 yr	30
2–3 yr	42
3–4 yr	48
4–5 yr	54
5–6 yr	63
6–7 yr	69
7–8 yr	81
8–9 yr	87
9–10 yr	93
10–11 yr	102
11–12 yr	111

The figure under dextran is multiplied by the per cent surface area burnt to give the volume of dextran saline to be infused during the 48 hours which follow burning. As in the adult, half is infused in the first 8 hours, a quarter in the next 16 hours and a quarter in the remaining 24 hours.

When burns are greater than 30% of the surface area, 10% of the body weight of dextran is infused (1 kg = 1 litre) and the same proportion of fluid is given during the same time period. In the presence of deep burns, up to a quarter of the volume is given as ACD blood. In addition all fluids are given at the following rates:

0–2 yr	160 ml/kg
2–5 yr	100 ml/kg
5–8 yr	80 ml/kg
8–12 yr	50 ml/kg

All formulae are only rough guides as to the requirements of individual patients and it will be obvious that the volume and rate and nature of the fluid infused will have to be modified in many cases. The physical signs such as the presence or absence of peripheral vasoconstriction, pulse rate, ventilation, blood pressure, and serial estimations of packed cell volume (PCV) will determine the precise nature of the treatment given. Even when the eschar is formed, there is a marked loss of fluid from the surface of the burn; it has been shown that it is 75 times faster than that of normal skin.[10,28]

*The formula for children is based on the charts of Kyle and Wallace.[42]

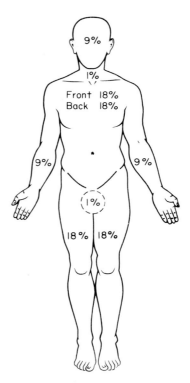

Fig. 6.10 The 'rule of 9' for assessing the area burnt in percentage of body surface. (Reproduced from the *Lancet*, Wallace, 1951.)[71]

Head and face	9%
Neck	1%
Trunk	18% front
Trunk	18% back
Arms	9% each
Genital areas	1%
Legs	18% each

One of the aspects associated with the irrigation of burnt areas with normal saline is the transfer of Na^+ and Cl^- back across the burnt area into the circulation,[47] together with water contributing to the blood volume.

If the plasma [Na^+] did not vary, the formula given on page 000 would be satisfactory, but in practice it is not found to be of very great value in the early stages following burns. A better formula based on estimated blood volume and PCV is:

$$\text{plasma deficit} = \text{blood volume (ml)} - \frac{\text{blood volume} \times \text{normal PCV\%}}{\text{observed PCV\%}}$$

For example, if in an adult male the normal blood volume is 5000 ml and the PCV is 55%, the plasma deficit is:

$$5000 - \frac{5000 \times 45}{55} = 909 \text{ ml.}$$

If the calculation is made every hour, some indication of the rate of fluid loss can be obtained even if the absolute values are inaccurate. However, as we have seen, changes in the PCV can occur. Care must be taken that reliance is not placed too firmly on any formula so that over-expansion of the vascular space or, conversely, hypovolaemic shock does not develop.

The formula recommended for the first 4 hours by Muir (1981)[48] is:

ml of fluid required =

$$\frac{\text{total area of burn} (\%) \times \text{wt (kg)}}{2}$$

Muir noted that intravenous fluid therapy may not begin until 2 hours after the burn has occurred. The volume of plasma required is therefore transfused over a period of 2 hours. At the end of the first 4 hours the patient's condition, packed cell volume (PCV) and urine output are assessed and the same volume as calculated may need to be transfused during the next 4 hours making 8 hours altogether. Subsequently, further transfusions are based on very careful assessment of the patient and the medical attendant should not hesitate to change either the rate of infusion or the regimen that is followed.

Based upon the experience at Mount Vernon Hospital, a scheme for fluid replacement in which there are two further successive periods of 6 hours followed by 12 hours has been produced. During these periods the same volume of fluid is used. However, frequent checks as to the suitability of these volumes have to be made according to the physiological responses of the patient.

During the first 48 hours, very careful clinical attention is necessary and constant observations by the nursing and medical staff are essential. The assistance of the pathology department is an important aspect when success is achieved.

Sedation

It is important on both clinical and humanitarian gounds to decrease the amount of pain that is suffered by the patient and to blunt the unpleasant aspects of the experience.

Morphine
This should be given intravenously in doses of 0.1–0.2 mg/kg body weight. This can be achieved by diluting 10 mg of morphine sulphate in isotonic saline in a 10-ml syringe.

Diazepam (Valium)
Intravenous administration of 5–10 mg of this substance to an adult produces a satisfactory sedation and sometimes complete amnesia with regard to the starting of infusions and other procedures. When morphine has been administered, the smaller dose of diazepam should be given.

Chlorpromazine
All substances in the phenothiazine group potentiate the action of morphine, so that the lower doses of both drugs should be given. Chlorpromazine, however, has a number of advantages. It relieves nausea and vomiting and has a vaso-dilatory action. It can be administered at 6-hourly intervals so that the patient remains asleep for a long period of the time. It should be given in doses of 0.5 mg/kg body weight; 50 mg of the substance can be diluted in a suitable solution in a 10-ml syringe so that each millilitre contains 5 mg. When given in these doses chlorpromazine does not appear to increase the dangers of respiratory depression that can be induced by morphine.

References

Burn shock

1. Abou, I. A., Reinhardt, W. O. and Tarver, H. (1952). Plasma protein. III. The equilibrium between blood and lymph protein. *J. biol. Chem.*, **194**, 15.
2. Antonacci, A. C., Reaves, L. E., Calvano, S. E., Amand, R., De Riesthal, H. F. and Shires, T. (1984). Flow cytometric analysis of lymphocyte subpopulations after thermal injury in human beings. *Surg. Gynecol. & Obs.*, **159**, 1.
3. Arney, G. K., Pearson, E. and Sutherland, A. B. (1960). Burn stress pseudodiabetes. *Ann. Surg.*, **152**, 77.
4. Artz, C. P. (1954). *Curling's ulcers*. Ann. Rept. Surg. Res. Unit, Brooke Army Medical Center, Texas.
5. Artz, C. P. and Reiss, E. (1957). *The treatment of burns*. Philadelphia: Saunders.
6. Aub, J. C., Pittman, H. and Brues, A. M. (1943).

Management of the Cocoanut Grove burns at the Massachusetts General Hospital. The pulmonary complications: a clinical description. *Ann. Surg.*, **117**, 834.

7. Baker, R. D., Grinvalsky, H. T., Hicks, S. P., Liebow, A. A., Madden, S. C., Moore, R. A., Moritz, A. R., Ross, O. A., Smith, E. B., Warren, S. and Waterman, W. B. (1950–53). Forty-one fatal burn injuries. In *Adhoc Panel Report to National Research Council*, p. 3. Washington.

8. Baxter, C. R. and Shires, G. T. (1968). Physiological response to crystalloid resuscitation of severe burns. *Ann. of N.Y. Acad. Sci.*, **150**, 874.

9. Blalock, A. (1931). Experimental shock. VII. The importance of the local loss of fluid in the production of the low blood pressure after burns. *Arch. Surg.*, **22**, 610.

10. British Medical Journal (1964). Leading Article: Loss and gain in burns. *Brit. med. J.*, **2**, 1090.

11. Brooks, D. K. (1972). Organ failure following surgery. *Advances in Surgery*, **6**, 289.

12. Brooks, D. K. (1978). Gastrointestinal bleeding in acute respiratory failure. *Brit. med. J.*, **i**, 922.

13. Bull, J. P. (1954). Shock caused by burns and its treatment. *Brit. med. Bull.*, **10**, 9.

14. Bull, J. P. and England, N. W. J. (1954). Fluid and electrolyte exchange in patients with burns. *Lancet*, **ii**, 9.

15. Bull, J. P. and Fisher, A. J. (1954). A study of mortality in a Burns Unit: a revised estimate. *Ann. Surg.*, **139**, 269.

16. Bull, J. P. and Squire, J. R. (1949). A study of mortality in a Burns Unit; standards for the evaluation of alternative methods of treatment. *Ann. Surg.*, **130**, 160.

17. Carvajal, H. F. (1980). A physiologic approach to fluid therapy in severely burned children. *Surg. Gynecol. & Obstet.*, **150**, 379.

18. Choudhury, M. (1963). Two further cases of Curling's ulcer in major burns in children. *Brit. med. J.*, **1**, 448.

19. Clarkson, P. (1963). Burns: Critical review. *Brit. J. Surg.*, **50**, 457.

20. Cope, O. and Moore, F. D. (1947). The redistribution of body water and the fluid therapy of the burned patient. *Ann. Surg.*, **126**, 1010.

21. Curling, T. B. (1842). On acute ulceration of the duodenum in cases of burn. *Med.-Chir. Trans.*, **25**, 260.

22. Davidson, E. C. and Matthew, C. W. (1927). Plasma proteins in cutaneous burns. *Arch. Surg.*, **15**, 265.

23. Davies, J. W. L. and Topley, E. (1956). The disappearance of red cells in patients with burns. *Clin. Sci.*, **15**, 135.

24. Dupuytren, G. (1832). Des brulures. De leurs Causes, de leurs divers Degrés, de leurs complications, de leurs caractères anatomiques et de leur traitement. In *Leçons orales de clinique chirurgicale*, Vol. 1, pp. 413–516. Paris: Ballière.

25. Evans, A. J. (1963). The treatment of burns. In *Recent advances in the surgery of trauma*, **1**, p. 76. Edited by D. N. Matthews. London: Churchill.

26. Evans, E. I. (1951). Treatment of high intensity burns. *Arch. Surg.*, **62**, 335.

27. Evans, E. I. and Butterfield, W. J. H. (1951). The stress response in the severely burned: an interim report. *Ann. Surg.*, **134**, 588.

28. Fallon, R. H. and Moyer, C. A. (1963). Rates of insensible perspiration through normal, burned, tape stripped, and epidermally denuded living human skin. *Ann. Surg.*, **158**, 915.

29. Fox, C. L. and Baer, H. (1947). Redistribution of potassium, sodium and water in burns and trauma, and its relation to the phenomena of shock. *Amer. J. Physiol.*, **151**, 155.

30. Fox, C. L. and Ketson, A. S. (1945). The mechanism of shock from burns and trauma traced with radio-sodium. *Surg. Gynecol. & Obstet.*, **80**, 561.

31. Froeschlin, W. (1962). The treatment of shock with Haemaccel® a new plasma volume expander. *Dtsch. med. Wschr.*, **87**, 811.

32. Goodall, McC., Stone, C. and Haynes, B. W. (1957). Urinary output of adrenaline and noradrenaline in severe thermal burns. *Ann. Surg.*, **145**, 479.

33. Goodwin, C. (1984). Burn Shock. In *Shock and Related Problems*, p. 70. Edited by G. T. Shires. London: Churchill Livingstone.

34. Goulian, D. (1961). Early differentiation between necrotic and viable tissue in burns: a review of the problem and development of a new clinical approach. *Plast. reconstr. Surg.*, **27**, 359.

35. Harkins, H. N. (1934). Shift of body fluids in severe burns. *Proc. Soc. exp. Biol. (N.Y.)*, **31**, 994.

36. Head, J. M. (1980). Inhalation injury in burns. *Amer. J. Surg.*, **139**, 508.

37. Jackson, D. MacG. (1953). The treatment of burns: an exercise in emergency surgery. *Ann. roy. Coll. Surg. Engl.*, **13**, 236.

38. Jackson, D. MacG. (1959). Diagnosis in the management of burns. *Brit. med. J.*, **1**, 1263.

39. Jones, R. J., Roe, E. A. and Gupta, J. L. (1978). Low mortality in burned patients in a pseudomonas vaccine trial. *Lancet*, **ii**, 401.

40. Jones, R. J., Roe, E. A. and Gupta, J. L. (1979). Controlled trials of a polyvalent pseudomonas vaccine in burns. *Lancet*, **ii**, 977.

41. Kramer, B. and Tisdall, F. F. (1921). A clinical method for the quantitative determination of potassium in small amounts of serum. *J. biol. Chem.*, **46**, 339.

42. Kyle, M. J. and Wallace, A. B. (1950). The exposure method of treatment of burns. *Brit. J. plast. Surg.*, **3**, 144.

43. Kyle, M. J. and Wallace, A. B. (1950). Fluid replacement in burnt children. *Brit. J. plast. Surg.*, **3**, 194.

44. Lanchantin, G. F. and Deadrick, R. E. (1957). Serum protein changes in thermal trauma. I. Electrophoretic analysis at pH 8.6 and pH 4.5. *Brooke Army Medical*

Center. *Surgical Research Unit. Research Report* No. 1–57. Project No. 6-59-12-028. Jan.

45. Long, J. (1840). On the postmortem appearances found after burns. *Lond. med. Gaz.*, **25**, 743.

46. Monafo, W. W., Chuntrasakul, C. and Ayvazian, V. H. (1973). Hypertonic sodium solutions in the treatment of burn shock. *Amer. J. Surg.*, **126**, 778.

47. Moser, M. H., Robinson, D. W. and Schloerb, P. R. (1964). Transfer of water and electrolytes across granulation tissue in patients following burns. *Surg. Gynecol. & Obstet.*, **118**, 984.

48. Muir, I. (1981). The use of the Mount Vernon formula in the treatment of burn shock. *Intensive care med.*, **7**, 49.

49. Muir, I. F. K. (1960). Red cell destruction in burns. In *Transactions second congress of the International society of Plastic Surgeons, London 1959*, p. 481. Edited by A. B. Wallace. Edinburgh: Livingstone.

50. Muir, I. F. K. and Barclay, T. L. (1974). *Burns and their treatment*. London: Lloyd-Luke.

51. Perlmann, G. E., Glenn, W. W. L. and Kaufman, D. (1943). Changes in the electrophoretic pattern in lymph and serum in experimental burns. *J. clin. Invest.*, **22**, 627.

52. Phillips, A. W. and Cope, O. (1960). Burn therapy: I. Concealed progress due to a shifting battlefront. *Ann. Surg.*, **152**, 767.

53. Phillips, A. W. and Cope, O. (1962). Burn therapy: II. The revelation of respiratory tract damage as a principal killer of the burned patient. *Ann. Surg.*, **155**, 1.

54. Phillips, A. W. and Cope, O. (1962). Burn therapy: III. Beware the facial burn. *Ann. Surg.*, **156**, 759.

55. Phillips, A. W., Tanner, J. W. and Cope, O. (1963). Burn therapy: IV. Respiratory tract damage (an account of the clinical, X-ray and post-mortem findings) and the meaning of restlessness. *Ann. Surg.*, **158**, 799.

56. Prendergast, J. J., Fenichel, R. L. and Daly, B. M. (1952). Albumin and globulin changes in burns as demonstrated by electrophoresis. *Arch. Surg.*, **64**, 733.

57. Pruitt, B. A. (1981). Fluid resuscitation for extensively burned patients. *Journal of Trauma*, **21** (Suppl.), 690.

58. Quinby, W. C. (1983). Burns. In *Modern Emergency*

Department Practice, p. 288. Edited by D. K. Brooks and A. J. Harrold. London: Edward Arnold.

59. Schäfer, H. (1969). Results of treatment with gelatin plasma substitutes in accident surgery. Modified gelatins as plasma substitutes. *Bibl. Haemat. (Basel)*, **33**, 518.

60. Scudder, J. (1940). *Shock; blood studies as a guide to therapy*. Philadelphia: Lippincott.

61. Sevitt, S. (1956). Distal tubular necrosis with little or no oliguria. *J. clin. Path.*, **9**, 12.

62. Sevitt, S. (1957). *Burns: pathology and therapeutic applications*. London: Butterworth.

63. Soroff, H. S., Pearson, E. and Artz, C. P. (1961). An estimation of the nitrogen requirements for equilibrium in burned patients. *Surg. Gynecol. & Obstet.*, **112**, 159.

64. Squire, J. R., Bull, J. P., Maycock, W. d'A. and Ricketts, C. R. (1955). *Dextran: its properties and use in medicine*. Oxford: Blackwell.

65. Swan, J. (1823). Practical observations; case of a severe burn. *Edinb. med. surg. J.*, **19**, 344.

66. Tappeiner (1881). Ueber Veränderungen des Blutes und der Muskeln nach ausgedehnten Hautverbrennungen. *Zbl. med. Wiss.*, **19**, 385; 401.

67. Topley, E. and Jackson, D. MacG. (1957). The clinical control of red cell loss in burns. *J. clin. Path.*, **10**, 1.

68. Underhill, F. P., Carrington, G. L., Kapsinow, R. and Pack, G. T. (1923). Blood concentration changes in extensive superficial burns and their significance for systemic treatment. *Arch. Int. Med.*, **32**, 31.

69. Underhill, F. P., Fisk, M. E. and Kapsinow, R. (1930). Studies on the mechanism of water exchange in the animal organism. III. The extent of edema fluid formation induced by a superficial burn. *Amer. J. Physiol.*, **95**, 325.

70. Wallace, A. B. (1949). Treatment of burns; a return to basic principles. *Brit. J. plast. Surg.*, **1**, 232.

71. Wallace, A. B. (1951). Treatment of burns. *Med. Press.*, **225**, 191.

72. Wallace, A. B. (1951). The exposure treatment of burns. *Lancet*, **i**, 501.

73. Whipple, G. H., Smith, H. P. and Belt, A. E. (1920). Shock as a manifestation of tissue injury following rapid plasma protein depletion. The stabilizing value of plasma proteins. *Amer. J. Physiol.*, **52**, 72.

Chapter 7
Hypothermia and Hyperthermia

HYPOTHERMIA

The normal body temperature is 37°C (98.4°F) when measured in the mouth. Temperatures in the rectum are usually 0.5°C higher than those in the mouth. Skin temperatures vary enormously and depend in part upon the temperature of the environment. They vary with exercise and the degree of peripheral vasoconstriction and are therefore dependent upon the peripheral circulation, which is itself altered by endocrine, myocardial, haemodynamic and body temperature changes. Therefore, the two commonly taken temperatures that show most variation are those of the skin of the axilla and the mucous membranes of the mouth. The latter alters with the degree of 'mouth breathing' and the ingestion of hot or cold substances. The rectal temperature may also vary if a sufficient amount is eaten or drunk. It is therefore possible to lower the body temperature by drinking a large volume of iced liquid, and in a tropical region this may be sufficiently effective to make life more comfortable for a very short period of time (e.g. sweating may cease for a few minutes). On the other hand, drinking warm soup in a temperate climate can raise the body temperature and produce sweating.

The behaviour of the homoiothermic* organism is quite different from that of the poikilothermic† organism. The hibernating homoiothermic animal also behaves quite differently from the non-hibernating one. The hearts of poikilothermic and hibernating homoiothermic animals continue to beat at very low temperatures. The human heart and that of other non-hibernating homoiothermic

organisms will, in general, not tolerate temperatures much below 28°C because, below this temperature, ventricular fibrillation commonly occurs. It was shown, however, that rats and hamsters could be frozen and supercooled and would readily survive if certain precautions were taken to maintain body temperature after rewarming.[6,7,89,90] These impressive series of experiments by Andjus and Smith indicated the viability of living tissue after cooling to extremely low temperatures. After investigating total body cooling in dogs, Bigelow et al.[12] were able to suggest that it would be possible to perform open-heart surgery under these conditions. The elective reduction of the body temperature to 30°–28°C is now common clinical practice and is also used routinely for open-heart operations and when occlusion of major vessels, supplying vital organs such as the brain, is necessary during surgery.

Total body cooling was produced by means of an extracorporeal circulation using a heart–lung machine and heat exchanger by Gollan.[55] Kenyon et al.,[64] using a pump-oxygenator and Drew et al.,[38,39] using autogenous lung perfusion, cooled the body and produced total circulatory arrest. In these latter procedures very low temperatures, for example 12°C in the nasopharynx and 9° or 10°C in the oesophagus, may be reached. The circulation can then be stopped for various periods of up to one hour or more; the patient recovers when rewarming has been completed. In some patients the heart continues to beat during the assisted circulation to very low temperatures (e.g. 10°C in the oesophagus).

Because hypothermia can be used with safety for clinical purposes, it is often asked why people die when they are accidentally exposed to cold environments for such lengths of time that their tissue temperatures are reduced to low levels. We must look initially at the physiological and biochemical changes that occur when the body of the homoiothermic animal is cooled. We will then be

* Homoiothermic organisms are 'warm blooded'. Body temperature is maintained at a 'constant' level above that of the surroundings and, except in extreme conditions, does not normally vary greatly with changes in ambient temperature.
† Poikilothermic organisms are 'cold blooded'. Body temperature changes with the environment, usually being a little higher than ambient temperature.

able to observe how these differ from those occurring in the naturally hibernating animal and the poikilothermic animal and why the organism that is not naturally able to survive cooling can, only under special circumstances, withstand very low body temperatures.

Respiration

As cooling proceeds the respiratory rate becomes slower, and breathing becomes more shallow and finally often ceases altogether between 27° and 24°C. Although cooling reduces the oxygen requirements of the body tissues, we shall see later how as soon as oxygen supply to a cooled animal is no longer available, the blood rapidly becomes desaturated and gross anoxia supervenes within a very few minutes. Respiration is maintained only under special circumstances and these do not apply to the homoiothermic organism under normal conditions. The naturally hibernating animal can maintain a slow respiratory rate of 4 or 5 breaths/minute throughout the whole period of cooling. It is for this reason that during clinical hypothermia (i.e. hypothermia electively induced for surgery) an adequate alveolar ventilation has to be maintained throughout the whole procedure. In man alcohol in high concentration may assist in maintaining respiration at lower temperatures, but this is not found consistently in experimental animals.[25]

Heart beat

The heart beat gradually slows as cooling proceeds so that an intense bradycardia occurs when temperatures in the region of 20°C are reached. Except in exceptional circumstances, temperatures as low as this cannot be used either in man or the majority of animals because the ventricular fibrillation which usually occurs cannot, in most cases, be reverted to a normal rhythm by means of internal or external electrical countershock. When lower temperatures are reached in some animals and in humans accidentally exposed to a cold environment, the blood pressure falls and the arterial and mixed venous difference in oxygen tension and saturation *increases*. When the mixed venous oxygen saturation falls below 40%, or the PO_2 falls below 20 mmHg, it indicates that the cardiac output is inadequate for the needs of the tissues.

Case history. A 75-year-old woman living in an old people's home was given her 2.5-mg tablet of diazepam (Valium) when she went to have her bath before going to bed. She apparently fell asleep in the bath and she was not found until the following morning, when her rectal temperature was that of room temperature, 24.4°C.

No 'afterdrop' (further fall in rectal temperature) occurred when she was transferred to the relatively warm surroundings of the accident and emergency department of the hospital.

Her respiratory rate was 11/minute, she was unconscious and no pulse could be detected or blood pressure obtained. An electrocardiogram (Fig. 7.1) revealed a marked bradycardia with typical Osborn or 'J' waves. Blood gases revealed a marked metabolic acidosis, the plasma $[HCO_3^-]$ was approximately 10 mmol/l. An endotracheal tube was inserted and the patient was ventilated manually with 100% oxygen at a rate of approximately 10 breaths/minute using the lowest possible inflation pressure. An infusion of 8.4% $NaHCO_3$ solution was begun and the patient was covered with an electric blanket.

The rectal temperature was continuously monitored by an electric rectal probe which was connected to a digital display, and a rise in temperature of just 1°C per hour was noted. When the rectal temperature had increased to 29°C, vigorous spontaneous respiration returned and the carotid and femoral pulses could be palpated, but the blood pressure could not be obtained by means of a sphygmomanometer cuff. At this time just over 100 mmol of $NaHCO_3$ had been infused; the rate of infusion of $NaHCO_3$ was increased and an immediate rise in blood pressure occurred; blood pressure was found to be 110/60 10 minutes later. When the rectal temperature had increased to 33.8°C, the patient was moved to the intensive care ward; warming by the use of the electric blanket was discontinued when the rectal temperature reached 36.5°C.

The venous pressure in these circumstances often rises, but because of movements of fluid into the cells a marked rise of venous pressure is sometimes delayed. The failing heart, which worsens as lower temperatures are reached, is therefore one of the major causes of death during exposure to cold. It is possible that cardiac failure may be linked with respiratory failure, because when the flow of blood to the brain becomes inadequate, the function of the respiratory centre becomes even more depressed. We have already mentioned how the heart of man and other homoiothermic organisms differs from the heart of the naturally hibernating and poikilothermic organisms,

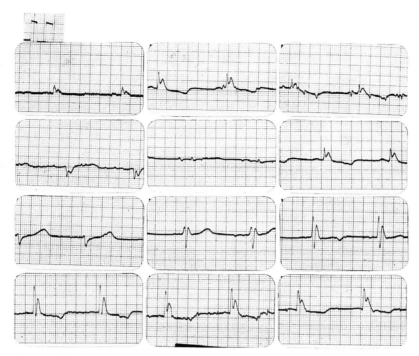

Fig. 7.1 Electrocardiogram of a 75-year-old woman who had fallen asleep in the bath after taking a tablet of diazepam (Valium) and was found the following morning. Her rectal temperature was 24.4°C when she was found and 24.9°C when this recording was taken. 110 ml of 8.4% sodium bicarbonate (110 mmol NaHCO₃) had been given.

which can withstand cooling to lower temperatures. They have this in common, however, that, when in isolated circumstances, cooling in man proceeds in an uneventful manner, gradual slowing of the myocardium occurs until the heart beats at only 10 beats/minute or less.

The onset of ventricular fibrillation is usually abrupt and sudden. Reversion to a normal rhythm at low temperatures, by means of electrical counter-shock, is often very difficult and sometimes the re-establishment of a normal heart beat is impossible.

Electrocardiogram changes with hypothermia

There is commonly early prolongation of the P–R interval and, later, prolongation of the Q–T interval. As the body temperature falls, the heart rate slows so that a severe bradycardia is present. Widening of the QRS complex develops and, at temperatures below 26°C in the rectum, the P wave usually disappears and a biventricular type of QRS complex is seen and an 'Osborn' or 'J' wave is present.[76] This secondary wave represents the widened extrinsicoid deflection of the QRS complex and appears to be related to temperature

alone and not to changes in the plasma [K⁺] or [HCO₃⁻]. Although it is possible for patients to be rewarmed from these temperatures, there is great danger of ventricular fibrillation following the appearance of the 'Osborn' wave. Similar findings have been reported by Emslie-Smith.[43,44]

Central nervous system

Gradual central nervous system depression develops as cooling proceeds. Consciousness is lost somewhere below 30°C; in most homoiothermic animals consciousness is lost completely at 27°C. Muscle reflexes (e.g. the knee jerk) are, however, retained to much lower temperatures, and the eyelid reflex may not be abolished until the temperature falls below 23°C. The pupil gradually dilates as cooling proceeds and the fundus may be inspected without difficulty. On rewarming, gradual contraction of the pupil occurs and when there is a constant blood flow, as may occur when hypothermia is induced by means of an extra-corporeal circulation, the pupil size reflects the rise in temperature. At temperatures below 17°C the pupils are almost completely fully dilated and there is almost complete muscle flaccidity. Response to painful stimuli disappears at relatively high temperatures, for example, in most animals in the region of 30°C. This is usually referred to as cold narcosis. The electroencephalogram (EEG) demonstrates waves of decreasing frequency which become slower as the temperature falls until finally, at very low temperatures, an isoelectric recording is obtained. Transection of the spinal cord produces an inability to vasoconstrict and, because of lack of continuity between the hypothalamus and autonomic system, shivering does not occur below the transection and is not possible because of interruption of the motor pathways.[78]

Endocrine gland function

In common with other metabolizing tissues, secretions of essential substances from the endocrine glands are reduced. It is well recognized that a malfunctioning endocrine gland may give rise to a so-called accidental hypothermia. This condition may arise from myxoedema, from Simmonds disease and from Addisons's disease. In the hypothermic animal the administration of adrenaline and hydrocortisone appears to have a thermogenic effect.[25,28,46,47] The substances also have a marked effect on the regulation of the heart beat and the maintenance of blood pressure.

Biochemical effects of hypothermia

Changes in the body biochemistry are of major importance to the homoiothermic animal. Naturally hibernating and poikilothermic animals are able to keep the same concentrations of electrolytes and the same acid–base state that they have at normal body temperatures. The non-hibernating mammal is at a great disadvantage in that the moment cooling begins, abnormal biochemical changes can be detected when the blood is analysed. When cooling is of a moderate degree and other parameters such as respiration and gas exchange in the lungs and maintenance of adequate cardiac output are kept close to normal, these abnormal changes in biochemistry do not reach significant proportions. It is when cooling is permitted to proceed below the normally acceptable safe temperatures that larger changes in the concentrations of electrolytes and a rise in the blood lactate concentration occur.

Some of the changes are common to all animals and are of a beneficial nature, such as the increase in oxygen content of the blood carried through the body; this is of benefit, however, only if the circulation (i.e. the cardiac output) is maintained. The increased capacity of the circulating blood for oxygen, because more is dissolved, and the decreased oxygen requirements of the tissues assist in maintaining a normal metabolism.

Blood oxygen content

As cooling proceeds, the oxygen requirements of the body are decreased. Bigelow et al.[12] found that the decrease in oxygen consumption was almost linear, so that at 10°C it fell almost to zero. It has been noted, however, that the oxygen consumption of individual tissues is still high at relatively low temperatures, and in the collected data of Fuhrman,[51] for example, muscle is still using 25% of its oxygen requirements at normal temperatures when the temperature of the muscle is at 15°C. Experiments in the author's laboratory confirmed that a surprisingly high quantity of oxygen is required when the tissue temperatures are low. For example, when the ventilation is stopped at an oesophageal temperature of 17°C in the dog and the muscle temperatures are very low (e.g. in the region of 11°C to 21°C), and an adequate circulation is maintained by the heart so that the blood pressure is 100/70 mmHg, then complete desaturation of the blood occurs within 5 minutes. However, while the increase in the dissolved oxygen content of the plasma and body water assists in the maintenance of an adequate oxygen supply, because the dissolved oxygen content of the plasma is 20% greater at 20°C than at 37°C, the oxygen saturation curve for haemoglobin moves to the left during cooling so that full saturation of the blood occurs at a much lower oxygen tension. Also, less oxygen is readily available to be taken up by the tissues when they are cold. It has therefore been suggested that the CO_2 tension of the blood which tends to reverse this change should be kept at a high level. In practice, the quantitative difference made to the oxygen-carrying power of the blood at low temperatures by CO_2 is insignificant. A decreased blood oxygen saturation is an important factor in the causation of ventricular fibrillation when the period of anoxia is prolonged. Anoxia is less likely to have an immediate effect when acid–base abnormalities are corrected or partly corrected by intravenous infusions.

pH at low temperatures

The interpretation of pH at low temperatures is an extremely complicated and involved subject and has been discussed elsewhere.[15, 19, 20, 74] In the hibernating animal or man that has been surface cooled either electively or by exposure where there are small temperature gradients between separate tissues, the pH of blood is best measured at the temperature of the nasopharynx, the oesophagus or the rectum. It is then possible to have some measure of the overall change in the buffer components. However, a low pH reading alone will give no indication as to whether there has been CO_2 retention or whether there is a deficit of plasma bicarbonate ion. A measurement of these acid–base components can be achieved by equilibrating the blood sample at the same temperature (i.e. the temperature of the rectum or elsewhere) with two gases of known CO_2 tension. If this is done, then an assessment of the blood PCO_2 and bicarbonate ion concentration may be obtained. When resuscitating a person, however, it is essential to maintain ventilation and therefore, as most pH meters are maintained at 37°C or 38°C, it may be more convenient to measure the bicarbonate ion concentration alone so that an indication of the degree of metabolic acidosis may be obtained. This can best be done by equilibrating the blood sample, which must be arterial because of the large arteriovenous differences that may occur due to an impaired circulation, in an apparatus such as that designed by Astrup and his colleagues,[9] with two known gas samples. As long as the pH measurements are made at the same temperature as that at which the blood was equilibrated with the gases of known PCO_2 tension, then an accurate estimate of the bicarbonate ion concentration will be obtained. The value for PCO_2, however, is for a normal body temperature, and this value is abnormally high. There remains the problem of pH measurement. When blood is taken from a normal patient and the pH is measured at room temperature (using a pH electrode that has been calibrated with known buffer solutions at room temperature), the pH is found to be approximately 7.7. In order to relate this rise of pH to what are known to be normal values at normal body temperatures, workers in this field have produced conversion factors so that the values obtained may be corrected to 37°C or 38°C.[32,34,69] Until the introduction of more involved correction factors,[53, 81,101] such as those of Severinghaus[83] and Siggaard-Andersen,[86] the most commonly used correction factor was that of Rosenthal (1948)[81]

$$pH_{38} = pH_t - 0.0147 (38 - t), \text{ sometimes written}$$
$$\Delta pH = -0.0147 \times \Delta t$$

where t is the temperature of the blood at which the pH was measured. The formula Rosenthal produced relates the pH of blood measured at room temperature to the pH of blood at body temperature. For every degree below normal body temperature at which the pH of blood was measured, a rise of 0.0147 of a pH unit can be expected. A wide variation of this coefficient is found in the papers quoted above and, for reasons explained below, the coefficient must be dependent upon haemoglobin concentration and PCO_2. Its value is therefore limited to special conditions.

The Rosenthal factor is still of value, even when blood is removed from pump-oxygenators. There are, however, inaccuracies. During total body cooling, the rectal and oesophageal temperatures are measured for t or Δt and, as we have seen, these can be different, especially during rapid cooling. Also, even during accidental hypothermia, there are gradients and differences of temperature between the muscles, organs and available sites of measurement.

The Rosenthal factor also refers to blood that has cooled anaerobically in a syringe before being transferred to the pH meter. This is quite different from the situation present in the cold patient when CO_2 is being lost from the lungs, or CO_2 from a gas cylinder is being added with O_2 to the cold blood circulating in an artificial heart–lung machine.

If a constant ventilation has not been maintained throughout cooling, correction factors are of little value in assessing the actual PCO_2 of the blood at its reduced temperature.[12,18,19]

Care must also be taken when using corrected pH for the calculation of the metabolic component of acid–base $[HCO_3^-]$. For a more detailed account, see Brooks (1964).[22]

Changes in alveolar carbon dioxide tension (PCO_2)

As the body cools and the metabolism is reduced, the production of carbon dioxide falls. This is reflected in low alveolar carbon dioxide tensions. The alveolar PCO_2 level therefore falls but, because in the spontaneously breathing organism ventilation is reduced and the solubility of carbon dioxide in the blood at lower temperatures is increased, the total carbon dioxide content remains very much the same if the metabolic component of the buffer system is not altered. In this way it has been shown that the PCO_2, when measured at these low temperatures in a hibernating animal such as the bat,[5] is 40 mmHg—the same as that at 37°C or 38°C. In the experiments by Andjus and Smith, the animals were placed in closed jars so that PCO_2 rose in this compartment. However, in these experiments no anaesthetic was given and shivering, which has a marked thermogenic effect, had to be eliminated so that cooling would proceed. Many people have been operated upon at very low temperatures using anaesthetic agents and muscle relaxants to control shivering in the early stages when no CO_2 has been given, and alveolar CO_2 tensions have fallen to approximately 15 mmHg. This situation is similar to that of the naturally hibernating animal.[5] It has also been shown, however, that patients who are being artificially ventilated after hypothermia require a PCO_2 close to 40 mmHg in order to avoid impairment of myocardial function and hypotension.[23]

Plasma bicarbonate ion concentration

The naturally hibernating animal does not show a marked increase in fixed acid and therefore the bicarbonate ion concentration does not fall very much in the extracellular fluid (ECF). When the pH is measured at the temperature of hibernation it is in the region of 7.4.[5] When the non-hibernating organism is cooled a metabolic acidosis is gradually produced, and when cooling is extended so that cardiac function is depressed, the $[HCO_3^-]$ of the plasma may fall to very low levels. The non-hibernating, warm-blooded animal lacks the ability to adapt biochemically during cooling for a normal acid–base state to be maintained. The onset of ventricular fibrillation is always hastened when a metabolic acidosis of significant proportions is present. When defibrillation of the heart is attempted by electrical means, correction of the metabolic acidosis by means of infusions of sodium bicarbonate is essential. In an elective procedure the metabolic acidosis is best avoided by slowly infusing small quantities of hypertonic $NaHCO_3$ solution from the beginning of the cooling. Care should be taken that gross hyperventilation is not allowed so that the alveolar PCO_2 is not reduced to below 30 mmHg.[23] A fall in cardiac output causing hypotension and associated with an abnormal electrocardiogram may occur when the alveolar PCO_2 is allowed to fall below 30 mmHg during hypothermia.

A deficiency in the bicarbonate ion concentration in the plasma will itself lead to hypotension, largely because of inadequate myocardial function. The hypotension does not respond to blood transfusions and, when extremely severe, does not respond to adrenaline and noradrenaline.[20] A metabolic acidosis also produces hypothermia and a syndrome in which there is central nervous system depression, so that tendon reflexes are absent and there is continued unconsciousness and failure to breathe.[22,23]

Plasma potassium concentration

As cooling proceeds, the plasma $[K^+]$ falls. When some urine is passed this may well have a very high $[K^+]$, but the quantity excreted is insufficient to account for the fall that occurs in the concentration present in the extracellular fluid (ECF). In the naturally hibernating animal the potassium concentration varies only to a small degree. When the heart is diseased, such as in those patients who are cooled for corrective myocardial surgery by means of an extracorporeal circulation or by surface cooling, then the correction of this decrease in plasma K^+ level may have a beneficial effect upon the myocardium.[22,64] It is usually sufficient to infuse enough KCl during the operation to raise the ECF concentration by 1 mmol (1 mEq).

Packed cell volume

It is often stated that the packed cell volume (PCV) increases with hypothermia. Most of the blood samples in which this has been found have been taken when there has been a marked degree of hypotension or after the onset of ventricular fibrillation. It is stated that the increase in blood viscosity is one of the factors contributing to ventricular fibrillation because the work the heart needs to perform is so much greater. Examination of the PCV in the author's own laboratory indicates that there is no significant rise when the non-hibernating animal, such as the dog, is cooled and the arteriovenous oxygen difference is kept either within the values that are to be expected at normal temperatures or are reduced as metabolism itself is reduced. The moment tissue anoxia is allowed to occur or the heart fails for any reason, so that there is an increase in the arteriovenous oxygen difference, then the haematocrit begins to rise as there is a movement of fluid from the exracellular fluid (ECF) space into the intracellular compartment. This movement of fluid occurs rapidly so that a rise in the PCV is detectable within a minute of the onset of anoxia. It is also reversible so that when the anoxic episode is over, the PCV returns to its previous value. A rise in the viscosity of blood, therefore, as reflected in the concentration of the erythrocytes within the vascular space, is not a factor in hypothermia until anoxia has developed. It is when attempting to resuscitate a patient from exposure to cold, when both ventilation and myocardial output have been impaired that, in addition to maintaining ventilation and rewarming, the infusion of hypertonic sodium salts should be performed as soon as possible so that fluid is available for the expansion of the ECF space and for the dilution of the erythrocytes within the vascular space. Because an acidosis may be corrected at the same time as the changes in volume of the ECF, the infusion of hypertonic $NaHCO_3$ is advocated. It should be noted that the normally hibernating animal tends to maintain both its PCV and the electrolyte content of its body spaces at normal values.

Blood sugar

We have noted that the blood sugar concentration rises during shock. Claude Bernard[11] observed that the rise also occurred during hypothermia. Finney et al., in 1927,[46,47] who also observed the rise in blood sugar, demonstrated that the rise could be inhibited by insulin. Talbott et al., in 1941[94] observed the same in man and suggested that hypoglycaemia would abolish shivering. A rise in blood sugar was also found later during the horrifying experiments performed by Rascher on the Dachau prisoners. Therefore, an increase in the concentration of blood glucose both in man and in non-hibernating mammals is a common association of hypothermia however it is produced. It occurs during cooling, produced by means of an extracorporeal circulation for open-heart surgery.[20] The infusion of ACD (acid-citrate-dextrose) blood, with its high glucose concentration of approximately 600 mg% (33 mmol/l) is a contributory cause of hyperglycaemia during this procedure. Hyperglycaemia is reversed spontaneously during rewarming. The rise in blood glucose concentration contributes to the osmotic activity of the ECF so that the blood volume is maintained even when there is a tendency for it to decrease as the $[Na^+]$ falls. The alteration in plasma electrolytes is caused by the increased concentration of glucose, as discussed by Wynn.[100]

Resuscitation of man from the cold

Man has been interested in this problem from very early times. In 1776, John Hunter[61] gave one of the earliest accounts of electively induced hypothermia. He demonstrated that small animals such as eels could survive cooling to very low temperatures. In 1798, John Currie[35] investigated hypothermia so that sailors who were exposed to cold by shipwreck could be resuscitated. Many animals, both hibernating and non-hibernating, were investigated from very early times.[77,87,88,92,95] In this way a vast quantity of data was collected. In 1902 Simpson was able to anaesthetize monkeys with ether and cool them to below 14°C; two of these monkeys survived. He noted that the respiration ceased before the heart beat and that this

tended to occur at 25°C when the animals were insensitive to pain. In 1930 Britton examined a series of patients who had been exposed to low ambient temperatures in Canada. The lowest rectal temperature of the patients who survived was 24°C. All the survivors had drunk sufficient alcohol to make them completely inebriated at the time of exposure. In the abominable and scientifically unrewarding experiments performed on victims confined within the Dachau concentration camp during the Second World War, the mean rectal temperature at which cardiac arrest was produced was found to be 26.8°C. The unfortunate victims were exposed to an environment of 4°C by immersion in iced water.[1] Attempts were made to suppress the knowledge of these experiments,[4] but they were investigated by Dr Leo Alexander.[3] A chance meeting with a Padre, Lt. Bigelow led indirectly to the documentation being discovered (Fig. 7.2). Some of the prisoners who survived the first experiment were cooled a second time. All the crude physiological changes that were recorded during these human experiments were already known to interested investigators.

A curious coincidence played into my hands. On my way to Goettingen, by way of Hadamar and Dillenburg, on 14 June 1945, while having dinner at the Officers' mess of the 433rd A.A. Bn., then in camp in Rennerod, Westerwald, I happened to meet another casual guest, an army chaplain, Lieut. Bigelow. In the course of our conversation Lt. Bigelow told me and was quite eager to get my ideas about rather cruel experiments on human beings which had been performed at Dachau concentration camp. He had learned of them from a broadcast a few days earlier when ex-prisoners of Dachau had talked about these grim experiences over the Allied radio in Germany. Lt. Bigelow stated that he had been particularly horrified by experiments in which prisoners were placed in tubs of ice water while their sufferings and death throes respectively were recorded by sets of electrical instruments attached to their bodies. The description of the experiments as given by the prisoners and related to me by Lt. Bigelow was strikingly similar to the animal experiments performed by Dr. Weltz and his group. I asked Lt. Bigelow whether any experimentor's name had been mentioned over the radio, and he said yes, but he had forgotten the name.

Dr. Paul Hussarek, philologist from Prague, who has been confined in the concentration camp in Dachau for 5 years because of "literary relations with foreign countries", stated that Dr. Rascher had been arrested sometime in 1944, later escaped with two other prisoners, but was caught again. In April 1945 he was taken to the stronghouse (Bunker) in Dachau, and there he was shot by S.S. executioners, two weeks before the arrival of the Americans, after being stripped of his rank as S.S. Hauptsturmführer. It is likely, but not definitely known, that his wife was shot together with him. His wife, Mrs. Nini Rascher, had assisted him in his experiments. Dr. Hussarek remembers her as a "petite, elegant, lively woman". One of Dr. Rascher's chief helpers was an ex-prisoner named Walter Neff, who later became a policeman; he was last heard of in Munich.

Fig. 7.2 From a personal communication from Dr Leo Alexander. The lieutenant Bigelow mentioned in the text was in no way related to the Dr Bigelow of reference No. 12 (1950) who pioneered hypothermia for heart surgery.

In 1951 Laufman[68] described how a 23-year-old lightly dressed Negro woman, who had been drinking continuously for some hours, was exposed to an ambient temperature of between $-18°C$ and $-24°C$ before she became comatose. While in her drunken stupor, she cooled so that on admission to hospital her rectal temperature was $18°C$. She was successfully resuscitated by means of external heating.

Alcohol in hypothermia

In addition to the series of Britton and the case reported by Laufman, there is further evidence that survival from the reduction of body temperature to low levels by exposure is made more probable by the presence of high alcohol concentrations in the blood. Experiments in the author's own laboratory largely confirm these findings.[25]

The level of blood alcohol required to produce unconsciousness is somewhere between 450 and 550 mg%. It is well known that it may itself give rise to respiratory depression. Loomis[73] found that respiratory depression occurred in dogs at normal body temperature when the blood alcohol level rose to 400 mg%. Death occurred from respiratory failure when it reached 690 mg%. If artificial ventilation was maintained, no change in the heart rate or electrocardiogram occurred until the concentration was 985 mg% or more. Alcohol has a marked thermogenic effect. It is converted into CO_2 and water as it is metabolized and only 2–6% is excreted in the urine unchanged. Each gram provides 7.1 calories. We have observed that when an animal is cooled to low temperatures by being immersed in iced water, having been anaesthetized with ether and ventilation of the lungs is maintained by means of intermittent positive pressure, there is a rise in muscle temperatures following the intravenous infusion of alcohol.[25]

In the inebriated alcoholic, therefore, there seems to be little doubt that the rate of cooling is slowed and, for this reason alone, the onset of ventricular fibrillation must be delayed. There is also some evidence that alcohol may afford some protective influence upon the myocardium, by means of either a nutritional or other metabolic effect, so that lower temperatures may be reached with relative safety. It must be borne in mind, however, that alcohol has a vasodilator action which would increase the heat exchanger effect of the skin in the thinly clad person exposed to low ambient temperature. It would appear, however, that the stimulus of cold causing vasoconstriction, predominates over the vasodilator effect of alcohol.

However, when alcohol is taken in large quantities over a long period of time, it is, as we have seen, commonly associated with profound accidental hypothermia.[68,98]

Other thermogenic substances

In the author's laboratory the correction of an acidosis during hypothermia appears to have a thermogenic effect. A rise in tissue temperatures has been observed in a manner similar to that which occurred during the infusion of alcohol. It must be noted, however, that this is possibly only an apparent thermogenic effect for it has been observed only when positive pressure ventilation has been applied wrongly or there has been some form of lung pathology, such as a basal pneumonia, and desaturation of the arterial blood has been present so that a gross metabolic acidosis has developed. The infusion of alkali has always been associated with a rise in blood pressure on these occasions and, therefore, it must be assumed that improved tissue perfusion and generalized body metabolism have been the prime cause. Adrenaline has also been reported to have an apparent thermogenic effect, but it is highly probable that, in a manner similar to the infusion of sodium bicarbonate, an increased cardiac output (and therefore circulation of blood within the tissues) has been the prime cause for the rise in tissue temperatures.

Glycine has also been observed to possess thermogenic activity and, as this amino acid is rapidly metabolized and is essential for the maintenance of metabolism within the central nervous system, it may possess an intrinsic thermogenic effect similar to that of alcohol.[10]

Process of rewarming

When a living organism is exposed to a cold environment so that surface cooling occurs, temperature gradients are produced so that the limbs may be colder than the oesophagus and the rectum, and the skin and subcutaneous fat are colder than any other part of the body. The bones also, because of their low intrinsic metabolism, cool very rapidly. It is well recognized, by anaesthetists especially, that when surface cooling is produced electively in man in the operating theatre, the patient continues to cool after being removed from the cold environment before the desired temperature in the oesophagus, usually $30°$–$28°C$, is reached. This is because gradients of temperature diminish so that the temperatures of individual tissues within the body become more alike. It is because the skin and subcutaneous fat remain at a lower temperature than the rest of the body for some time after the patient has been removed from the iced water bath and exposed to room temperature that temperatures in other parts of the body, such as the oesophagus and rectum, continue to fall. For this reason most anaesthetists and surgeons prefer to operate on the surface-cooled patient at the time when the process of spontaneous rewarming is just beginning. Thus inadvertent ventricular fibrillation is avoided.

Experiments on animals have shown repeatedly that if cooling is stopped when the oesophageal or rectal temperature is 25°C, a further fall of 5°C or more in these temperatures may occur before any spontaneous rewarming takes place. In the case of animals it is true that, although they are exposed to room temperature in the region of 20°–25°C, the iced water is contained within the fur and is a source of further heat loss. However, removing the fur before the experiment or replacing the iced water with water at or just above room temperature makes little difference to the pronounced further fall of oesophageal and rectal temperatures. These observations are an important aspect of active resuscitation in man.

The dangers associated with continued cooling have been stressed by Burton and Edholm. During the Second World War shipwrecked sailors, who had been exposed for many hours or days, were alive when taken from the water, but died a short while later.[27] The normal practice at that time was to remove the wet clothing, which may have necessitated a certain degree of man-handling and movement, and to wrap the victim in blankets or warm clothing so that a spontaneous rise in body temperature could be assisted. Experience has shown that these measures are insufficient and that further cooling almost certainly occurred in most of these people and that active steps have to be taken to apply external heating in any form available, including numerous hot-water bottles, electric blankets or infra-red lamps, immersion of the limbs or whole body in water at 42–44°C. Warm peritoneal dialysis fluid was successfully used by Lash et al. (1967)[67] to rewarm a patient who had cooled to 21°C after taking barbiturate and meprobamate.

It is important that further cooling should be avoided in all circumstances, not only because there is an increased impairment of myocardial function, but also because respiratory depression is made greater as further falls in body temperature occur. Because ventricular fibrillation will follow respiratory depression and anoxia, this aspect of resuscitation must always be borne in mind. Fortunately, the heart will beat sometimes for many minutes at low temperatures, even in the presence of anoxia, and this period can be extended by the infusion of sodium bicarbonate and alcohol.

Animal experiments have demonstrated repeatedly that the more rapid the rate of rewarming the more likely survival is possible. In the animal that has received infusions of sodium bicarbonate and KCl so that the metabolic acidosis is largely corrected and the plasma potassium concentration is adequate, immersion in a water bath at 45°C will cause a rapid rise in both heart rate and blood pressure. It has been observed that a return to a blood pressure of 120 mmHg has occurred within 2 minutes of the onset of rewarming, when there has been relatively little rise in the temperature of the oesophagus and rectum. There has also been a vigorous spontaneous ventilation which had previously been failing. These animals had been anaesthetized with an ether–air mixture and placed in an iced water bath at 7°C. The blood pressure was recorded electrically by means of a transducer. The electrocardiogram was also recorded. As cooling proceeded the heart rate was reduced, the blood pressure fell and the central venous pressure (CVP) rose. Infusions of bicarbonate and KCl were maintained so that the 'standard bicarbonate' was kept at a relatively normal value. No ill-effects from the procedure could be detected, in spite of prolonged hypotension, and the post-mortem examination revealed no abnormalities when the animal was sacrificed 6 weeks later (Brooks, 1963).[21] Renal function tests have shown normal values. Because of the apparently immediate effect of rapid rewarming upon the myocardium, active measures for rewarming by applying heat in the form of a water bath at 40°–44°C or an electric blanket, or hot-water bottles insulated with blankets should be performed as quickly as possible.

It has been observed in man that a more rapid rewarming after surface cooling can be achieved when a metabolic acidosis is absent, and when the ventilation is maintained at a value that gives an arterial blood PCO_2 close to 40 mmHg at 38°C.

Accidental Hypothermia

We have seen that during hypothermia the respiration becomes depressed, the pulse slows, the blood pressure falls and the pupils dilate. It is not surprising, therefore, that when accidental total body cooling has taken place, especially in the aged, the condition may be mistaken for death. This has lead to mistakes being made; patients have been found to be alive by mortuary attendants, and this has quite understandably, led to graphic newspaper reports. It is essential, therefore, that accidental hypothermia should be recognized when it occurs.

In accidental hypothermia the skin is cold to the touch and the body tissue temperatures are below those which can be measured using a normal clinical thermometer; a low-reading rectal thermometer is therefore required. The patient may be comatose for reasons other than hypothermia, although it is known that a normal conversation can be held with a patient whose temperature is below 29°C.[13] It may be necessary to record an electrocardiogram in order to determine the presence or absence of cardiac activity.

Causes of accidental hypothermia

Cooling of the body will only occur when heat loss exceeds heat production. These circumstances will arise when there is a low ambient temperature, when metabolism is impaired, when muscle tone is lost or when foreign substances enter the circulation and cause depression of the central nervous system control.

Exposure to cold

This factor in accidental hypothermia is most important at the extremes of age. The premature baby has less control than a mature neonate and requires an incubator. Malnutrition is an important factor and is commonly seen in vagrants who during the winter have spent the night in a shop doorway, often close to the hostel which they cannot enter because they have insufficient money. Hypothermia is also seen in old people living alone who have a relatively mild infection, but are unable to care for themselves.

When people are shipwrecked or fall overboard, rapid cooling occurs. In arctic conditions life cannot last for long. Even today with improved communications and the carriage of improved lifesaving apparatus at sea, this form of exposure is a recurrent problem. When the temperature of the water is in the region of 4°C, death usually occurs within 1.5 hours.

Saturation diving in the North Sea can cause a significant fall in body temperature.[63] The temperature of the divers' urine which was passed as soon as they returned to the diving bell was recorded; the lowest temperature found was 34.7°C. The divers had been breathing an oxygen–helium mixture at a depth of 130–145 m where the water temperature is below 10°C. Cooling developed in spite of warm water being pumped into the divers' suits. When cooling occurred, shivering was often absent so that the development of hypothermia was unsuspected by the diver. Experimental investigations in man have shown that unsuspected hypothermia, without shivering, can occur following exposure to circulating water at 29°C and can lead to cardiac arrhythmias.[60] Cooling appears to occur more readily in the patient whose skinfold thickness is small. Nearly six divers die each year in the North Sea, and some divers are known to have had periods of unexplained mental confusion and unconsciousness, yet have survived;[29] undetected hypothermia is one possible cause.

Drugs and anaesthetics

The antihistamine groups of drugs may cause hypothermia when taken in large quantities. Chlorpromazine (Largactil) is sometimes given to reduce the raised body temperature following a cerebrovascular accident or head injury. However, its hypothermic effect may not occur until it is given in doses which also produce hypotension.

Anaesthetics, especially when used in conjunction with muscle relaxants, also produce a fall in body temperature which is most apparent in the old and very young. The temperature of a child below the age of 1 year may fall by 2°C in the oesophagus after 30 minutes of anaesthesia.

Alcohol

Although alcohol delays cooling and may assist in rewarming and is an ideal substance to be taken when exposure to cold is envisaged,* it can, when absorbed in excessive quantities sufficient to cause unconsciousness, produce accidental hypothermia when the ambient temperature is low.[98]

Endocrine disorders

A rise in the temperature may occur in the early stages of an Addisonian crisis; this is followed by an abrupt fall in temperature when peripheral circulatory failure develops.

Hypothermia is a common accompaniment of myxoedema, hypopituitarism and diabetic coma.

In myxoedema coma, cooling to very low levels may occur so that the patient becomes unconscious and the respiration is depressed, causing hyper-

---

*The vasoconstrictor effect of cold appears to predominate over the vasodilator effect of alcohol.

carbia and hypoxia. The heart slows, the pulse becomes imperceptible and the blood pressure unrecordable. The electrocardiogram is of low voltage and the serum cholesterol is high. The hypotension and hypoxia give rise to a metabolic acidosis. Approximately 80% of patients with myxoedema have a reduced body temperature. There is also a correlation between mortality and body temperature.[8,48,85]

The patient may require assisted ventilation. It may be possible to rewarm the patient with external heating, such as an electric blanket. In other cases it may be necessary to correct the metabolic acidosis with sodium bicarbonate solution and to give l-tri-iodothyronine (liothyronine, Cytomel) intravenously. It can be given slowly by means of intravenous drip, 0.05–0.1 mg in 500 ml of solution. Intravenous hydrocortisone 100–300 mg i.v. may also be of benefit.

Hypopituitarism may give rise to a similar clinical condition but in this case, if active thyroid preparations are administered, an acute adreno-cortical insufficiency may be produced. It is therefore essential in this circumstance to give intravenous hydrocortisone before starting other forms of treatment.

When diabetic ketosis is allowed to develop to a serious degree so that the blood pressure falls, hypothermia is almost always present.

Diabetic coma is discussed on page 417. External warming is not often necessary but when the body temperature is raised, glucose is metabolized more readily and it can form an essential part of treatment. A raised blood sugar is a normal occurrence in hypothermia.[45,67,72]

Hypoglycaemic patients develop severe hypothermia, as was observed when psychiatric patients were being treated with 'insulin shock'.[50]

Benign episodic hypothermia occurs when there is impaired development of the corpus callosum and has been described by Shapiro et al.[84] There is also a related disorder in which episodic hypoglycaemia occurs, but no lesion or endocrine abnormality can be found.[40,82]

Disorders of the hypothalamus also predispose to hypothermia, whether these are developmental degenerative disorders, primary tumours, metastatic tumours or trauma.

Myocardial infarction

It has been reported by Doherty et al. (1984)[37] that two patients cooled to 35°C in the rectum following myocardial infarction. Both patients were women and, following an increase in cardiac output achieved by means of intra-aortic balloon pump-ing, the rectal temperature returned to normal. The rise in body temperature followed very closely to the rise in cardiac output. There might have been a number of causes for both the fall in body temperature and the subsequent recovery.

Poisoning

Barbiturate overdose commonly gives rise to accidental hypothermia. If, because of hypoventilation, prolonged anoxia causes brain damage, hyperpyrexia may result. Coal gas and morphine poisoning may also produce hypothermia.

It is well recognized that very low barbiturate concentrations can be found in the blood after death. Large doses of barbiturates kill by causing respiratory depression. Small doses of barbiturates can kill when sleep occurs while the patient is exposed to a low ambient temperature. Cold narcosis replaces and potentiates the effects of the barbiturates as the body temperature falls.

This aspect has been discussed by Edwards et al.,[42] when reporting the resuscitation of a 23-year-old woman exposed to an ambient temperature of 10°C after taking a small amount of barbiturate; her rectal temperature was found to be 26°C. Edwards et al. considered that the early administration of 200 mmol (mEq) of $NaHCO_3$ was a contributory factor in the successful resuscitation of this patient and the absence of cardiac arrhythmias during rewarming.

Head injury and paralysis

If head injury causes brain damage, hyperpyrexia may result, but when there is paralysis of the muscle or simple concussion, accidental hypothermia may gradually develop.

Hypothermia in Hodgkin's Disease

At least seven cases of severe and prolonged hypothermia have been reported; the lowest rectal temperature was 29°C. Hypothermia appears to develop irrespective of whether chemotherapy is being given or not (Jackson et al., 1983; Buccini, 1985).[62,26]

General management

Accidental hypothermia is best avoided by recognizing its existence and potential dangers and supplying external heat, especially in those groups of patients in which it is likely to occur. Even in hospital, the temperature of the patient may be noted regularly during the night with no steps taken to prevent its fall. Abnormal electrolyte concentrations and acid–base equilibrium should be corrected. Resistance to infection is reduced during hypothermia so antibiotics should be given when the condition is prolonged. External heat is essential once hypothermia has been recognized and care must be taken to maintain ventilation of the lungs.

There has been no satisfactory investigation and no satisfactory statistical evidence is available with regard to morbidity or mortality, which allows the clinician to decide whether the best form of treatment is rapid or slow rewarming, following severe accidental hypothermia.

When a patient passes into ventricular fibrillation during rapid rewarming, it is usually impossible to say that the rate of rewarming was the cause. Patients also die when the rate of rewarming is slow. Experimental evidence in the dog indicates that rapid rewarming by means of heat applied to the surface is immediately effective and quickly results in improved spontaneous ventilation of the lungs and a rise in heart rate and blood pressure. Certainly, in the young patient, suffering from a moderate degree of hypothermia (32°C in the rectum), rapid rewarming appears to be both effective and safe. In addition to the author, therefore, rapid rewarming has its advocates.[1,2,54]

At present, treatment is dictated by age, degree of cooling and the cause of the accidental hypothermia. If the cause is endocrine gland dysfunction, it is usual, and safer, to correct the underlying deficiencies before attempting to raise the body temperature by means of external heat. In diabetic ketosis, rehydration, correction of the metabolic acidosis and administration of insulin in small intermittent doses are usually sufficient to raise the body temperature.

The following procedures for rewarming should therefore be followed.

1. Make sure the airway is maintained. If the patient is unconscious, and if respiratory depression is present, an endotracheal tube should be passed. When the cuff is inflated, the inhalation of vomit is prevented. The tube should be connected to an anaesthetic apparatus and 100% O_2 should be administered, preferably through a warm humidifier so that the periodic deflation of the bag during spontaneous respiration can be observed. When the patient is covered with blankets, breathing is often too shallow to be observed by a nurse or clinician, and depression or cessation of respiration, which can occur suddenly, is most readily observed by the expansion and deflation of the bag. The endotracheal tube should *never* be covered by an O_2 *mask*, because when the patient vomits the stomach contents are channelled by the mask down the lumen of the endotracheal tube, even when the cuff is inflated.

2. Begin rewarming immediately by any means available, for example, wrap patient in electric blanket, immerse an arm in water at 45–46°C, immerse the whole body in a water bath at 45°C. Covering the naked body with the metallic surface of a 'space blanket' *increases* body cooling.

For a 'space blanket' to be effective, the patient has to be placed upon it and wrapped tightly (cocooned) within it. Warm blankets then have to be placed over the patient, and under these circumstances spontaneous rewarming, for example from a rectal temperature of 30°C or less, can occur. It is readily apparent that, if very severe hypothermia is present and intravenous infusions are required, wrapping the patient in this way is made more difficult.

3. Monitor the electrocardiogram.

4. Monitor the rectal temperature.

5. Take arterial blood samples to measure pH, $[HCO_3^-]$, PCO_2, full blood count, urea, electrolytes and blood glucose. If indicated, blood should also be taken for the estimation of barbiturate level, amylase activity and thyroxine index.

6. Set up an intravenous infusion of $NaHCO_3$. A metabolic acidosis is almost always present so that a slow infusion (the rate of which can be increased later if necessary) will do no harm and may have an immediate thermogenic effect.

7. If the plasma $[K^+]$ is low and the patient is old, add 200 mmol of KCl to 1 litre of 0.9% saline solution and infuse at 100 ml/hour.

8. If the patient is slow to rewarm and the acid–base state is normal, add 50 ml of absolute alcohol to 1 litre of glucose and infuse at 100 ml/hour.

9. Be prepared for respiratory failure and ventricular fibrillation to occur at any moment, even when the patient is rewarming at a satisfactory rate. The patient should not be removed from the emergency department until the rectal temperature has reached at least 35°C unless there are adequate facilities and staff in the ward.

10. Hydrocortisone in small doses, 100-200 mg i.v., may be given, but this has not been proved to be of consistent benefit.

HYPERTHERMIA

Two main disorders are associated with hyperthermia. One, an increasingly common disorder, is 'heat stroke', and the other is 'malignant hyperthermia'; this develops in members of susceptible families during an anaesthetic.

Heat disorders that result from a high ambient temperature can be divided into three main forms according to severity. These are:

1. heat syncope and muscle cramps,
2. heat exhaustion,
3. heat stroke.

Heat syncope

This rarely leads to a more severe heat disorder. It usually occurs in those people who lead a relatively sedentary life and are not adapted to a hot environment. In special circumstances, for example when standing for long periods of time in a hot uniform, it can also afflict physically fit soldiers on parade, girl guides and boy scouts. Muscle cramps are sometimes associated with heat syncope, but these are probably caused by sodium imbalance. Heat syncope is of a relatively mild nature and not of the severity seen in heat exhaustion or 'miners cramps' which are caused by severe Na^+ depletion and water intoxication. The rectal temperature is normal in heat syncope.

Heat exhaustion

The usual description of heat exhaustion is that of man's inability to continue to work or exercise in a high ambient temperature. This is associated with excessive salt and water loss.[66,70]

The condition commonly presents as a syncopal attack, extreme weakness, tetany, headache, dizziness and cramping of the muscles, both of the abdomen and in the extremities. Frequently, hyperventilation is present and this factor, in addition to those noted above, was first described by Haldane in 1905.[57] He considered that hyperventilation caused the tetany and muscle cramps. The observation that hyperventilation could produce tetany was also reported by Wingfield[99] in men working in intense heat in the Persian Gulf. Gaudio and Abramson[52] found that hyperventilation in response to high ambient temperatures was achieved by an increase in the tidal volume rather than by an increase in respiratory rate (see p. 118). This explains the low PCO_2 found in the arterial blood of patients suffering from heat exhaustion in whom tachypnoea has not been observed.

In 1975, Boyd and Beller[14] investigated 17 patients suffering from heat exhaustion; 11 of these patients presented with syncope, 16 had severe extremity and abdominal muscle cramps, and 9 had obvious tetany with carpopedal spasm. Although the mean respiratory rate on admission was 26 breaths/minute, the arterial PCO_2 was decreased in all patients, the mean value being 23.5 mmHg. The range of PCO_2 was between 14.7 mmHg and 34 mmHg. The arterial pH varied between 7.44 and 7.78. Boyd and Beller stated that, surprisingly, very few (only three) of their patients developed hypernatraemia, which they defined as a serum $[Na^+]$ greater than 148 mmol/l (mEq/l). It is possible, however, that dehydration would have been identified in a greater number of their patients had they accepted the lower figure of 145 mmol/l(mEq/l) as being the upper limit of normal, with the knowledge that a significant number would normally have a plasma $[Na^+]$ of 140 mmol/l(mEq/l) or less. All their patients recovered following rest in an air-conditioned room and the administration of oral fluids.

It should be noted that the aetiology of muscle cramping in heat exhaustion is different from that due to water intoxication and hyponatraemia seen in foundry workers and 'miners cramps' described on page 24–26.

Heat exhaustion occurs insidiously during exposure to heat over a long period of time. The rectal temperature is usually below 40°C, although all the characteristics of heat stroke can be observed at this temperature and below. Unless rehydration and removal to a cool environment is possible immediately, the condition can develop into 'heat stroke'.

Heat stroke

This sometimes develops from heat exhaustion. As stated above, the rectal temperature is usually found to be high, 41°C or more, and 46°C has been recorded. The patient is semiconscious or unconscious, has often ceased to sweat and frequently convulses. Without rapid and effective external cooling, the condition progresses to death.

Before unconsciousness develops, the patients are sometimes aware that they have been exposed to the hot environment for too long, and that steps have to be taken to reverse the situation. Some patients have convulsed and are comatose before being seen or are delirious and violent. Some patients convulse shortly after being admitted to hospital.[31] Hypernatraemia and hypoglycaemia are commonly present. Occasionally, haemolysis occurs and this may be precipitated during a convulsion.

Heat stroke and its treatment were investigated in Saudi Arabia; the patients were people on their annual pilgrimage to Mecca.[65,96] The mean rectal temperature of 18 patients was found to be 42.3°C, ranging from 41.2 to 43.1°C. Glucose 5% in normal saline and 250 ml of 4.2% $NaHCO_3$ solution were administered. Three patients with oliguria were given 500 ml of 10% mannitol and 40 g frusemide (Lasix). The main factor in the successful treatment of the patients was ascribed to blowing *warm* air at 45–48°C and spraying the body with water. This was stated to prevent the skin temperature from falling below 30°C. As a result, vasoconstriction did not occur and rates of cooling of 0.30–0.40°C per minute were achieved. A 2°C fall of rectal temperature was recorded in less than 7 minutes. This rapid rate of cooling was achieved using an apparatus specially designed for this purpose. Investigations confirmed the observation that by wetting the skin and using warm air to induce evaporation, cooling was superior to immersion in iced water.[97]

With the increasing popularity of jogging, marathon and other foot races in the Western world, it has been found that heat stroke can develop, especially in the poorly trained,[75] even when the ambient temperature is ideal, for example 16°C.[93] Air humidity appears to be an important factor. This is in keeping with the observations of Fox et al.,[49] who found that wetting the skin suppressed sweat gland activity. They concluded from their investigations that when acclimatization took place in a hot, wet environment, the time required for suppression of sweat to develop was lengthened. This was not seen in those who had undergone acclimatization in hot, dry conditions. This may be an important factor in man's ability to adapt to a hot environment.

When heat stroke has developed, however, wetting the skin artificially and allowing evaporation to occur is a valuable and effective method of inducing body cooling.

Case history. A fit, healthy, 39-year-old Caucasian male in Texas decided he would re-roof his house using his own skills. The process took rather longer than he expected so that he continued his work into the height of summer and, having once started, was reluctant to abandon

the project. He continued to work in a temperature of 35.5°C (96°F) and suddenly became overcome with exhaustion and a feeling of faintness. He successfully reached the ground floor of his house. He was found by his wife who noticed that he was semiconscious and was 'breathing heavily'. From the state of his clothing and that of the rug upon which he was lying, it is possible that he had convulsed prior to being found, and he had a single grand mal attack in the ambulance. When he arrived at the hospital, it was noted that he was intermittently disorientated, that he had a carpopedal spasm and collapsed veins. His blood pressure was 105/65 mmHg. His rectal temperature was 39.9°C.

Analysis of his blood revealed a pH of 7.60, a PCO_2 of 18.5 mmHg and a $[HCO_3^-]$ of 17.6 mmol/l(mEq/l). The base excess was −1 mmol/l. The PCV (packed cell volume) was 49.5%, the plasma $[Na^+]$ 149 mmol/l(mEq/l), plasma $[K^+]$ 4.5 mmol/l(mEq/l). Plasma $[Ca^{++}]$ was 9.5 mg% (2.4 mmol/l, 4.8 mEq/l). Blood enzyme values were raised, CPK (creatinine phosphokinase) 1475 i.u./l, LDH (lactic-acid dehydrogenase) 1270 i.u./l, alkaline phosphatase 101 i.u./l, SGOT (aspartate transaminase) 1025 i.u./l, SGPT (alanine transaminase) 960 i.u./l.

The patient's clothing was removed and he was placed on a water-cooled blanket and infused with glucose/saline. Two litres were infused over a period of 1½ hours and, when he became less disorientated, he was given water by mouth. The hyperventilation ceased after approximately 3 hours and no further carpopedal spasm occurred. The patient's temperature rapidly fell to normal so that 4 hours later it was 38.2°C. The patient received 3.5 litres of fluid parenterally over a period of 5 hours, and 1.5 litres of water orally over a similar period. The urine specific gravity on admission was 1.025 and had a $[Na^+]$ of 3 mmol/l (mEq/l). Five hours later the urine had a specific gravity of 1.018 and a $[Na^+]$ of 5 mmol/l (mEq/l). Blood taken at that time revealed the following values: PCV 46.5%, $[Na^+]$ 140 mmol/l (mEq/l), $[K^+]$ 3.8 mmol/l (mEq/l), pH 7.42, PCO_2 37 mmHg, $[HCO_3^-]$ 23.8 mmol/l, base excess −1 mmol/l.

The following day the patient was orientated but lethargic, and had to be reminded to take oral fluids. He was unwilling to talk, and although fully conscious, his intellect was blunted and his verbal responses were slow. There was some fear at that time, which was quite unfounded, that some permanent brain damage had occurred. Rectal temperature had been recorded constantly, and when it had fallen to 37.2°C, the cooling blanket had been removed. When blood analysis was performed, the CPK had fallen to 478 i.u./l, but was still raised, as was the SGOT (485 i.u.), SGPT (364 i.u.) and LDH (960 i.u.). Clotting and pro-thrombin times were normal. Although overt haemolysis did not occur, the plasma haemo-globin concentration rose to 58 mg%.

The patient made steady progress, but was slow to eat, complained of muscle pain and feeling unwell for a further 4 days, even though he had no significant clinical signs. His further recovery was uneventful. He showed no signs of bruising and no evidence of renal insufficiency.

Treatment and management of heat stroke

1. The patient should be placed in cool surround-ings and all unnecessary clothing should be removed. Wetting the skin and applying cold, damp cloths are emergency measures of some value. Sprinkling with cold water and keeping the cloths damp until more specific cooling measures can be taken is usually of value. Fanning the body either manually or by means of an electric fan is also effective.

2. Patients with heat stroke tend to hyperven-tilate, but when the patient is unconscious and when convulsions develop, a clear airway must be maintained and care should be taken to avoid respiratory depression. Artificial ventilation of the lungs should be performed if necessary. Pure humidified oxygen should be given.

3. If cooling cannot be achieved by wetting the body and blowing air over the wet surface by means of electric fans, the patient should be immersed in iced cold water as soon as possible. Alternatively, the patient should be covered with ice packs or placed on a cooled water blanket.

4. An intravenous infusion of 5% glucose or glucose/saline should be given immediately, both for the purposes of rehydration and to facilitate the giving of drugs. At the time of setting up the infusion, specimens of blood should be taken for analysis later. A 2.74% solution of $NaHCO_3$ should be infused until 500 ml have been given.

5. If convulsions occur, chlorpromazine 100 mg i.m. should be given and if this is ineffective, paraldehyde 8 ml i.m. may be injected, 4 ml into each thigh. Depression of respiration does not occur with these substances.

Alternative substances are diazepam 10 mg i.v. and chlormethiazole edisylate (Heminevrin). Chlormethiazole is available in solution containing 8 mg/ml and is infused at 10–15 drops/minute.

Haloperidol (Haldol, Serenace) is available in ampoules containing 10 mg/ml. This can be diluted in saline and infused at a rate which is sufficient to control the convulsions. Care must, however, be taken that respiratory depression and a profound fall in blood pressure do not occur. In order to suppress convulsions in an emergency, 10–30 mg can be given either intramuscularly or intra-venously; by either route, the smallest dose should be given.

6. It is important to make repeated estimations of the acid–base state, haemoglobin and plasma haemoglobin, packed cell volume (PCV) and plasma electrolyte concentrations. The blood glucose is also of importance as both hypogly-caemia and hyperglycaemia can develop.

Malignant Hyperpyrexia (Malignant Hyperthermia)

Denborough[36] reported from Australia that the first case that was recognized in the Royal Melbourne Hospital was in 1960. A 21-year-old student was brought to the casualty department with a compound fracture of the right leg. As the patient was concerned about the anaesthetic, 10 of his relatives having died during anaesthesia with ether, halothane was given. Ten minutes after the induction, he was found to be acutely ill and hyperpyrexial. The anaesthetic was stopped and he was packed in ice and survived, the only affected member of his family to do so.

The earliest sign of impending hyperpyrexia is usually muscular contraction after the administra-tion of suxamethonium chloride. The muscle rigidity is often interpreted as being due to an insufficient dose of suxamethonium, and as a result of this a further dose of the relaxant is given. The rigidity of the jaw muscles may be so marked that tracheal intubation is either difficult or impossible. The associated rise in body temperature is, however, frequently not noticed and no early steps for correction are taken.

The development of malignant hyperpyrexia is sometimes slow and insidious, with no muscular rigidity and little warning to the anaesthetist. There would therefore appear to be two forms: (a) those patients who develop muscle rigidity, and (b) those patients in whom muscle rigidity is never present. When muscle rigidity appears shortly after induction of the anaesthetic, the body temperature rises within minutes. Patients who develop the condition later may have no marked rise in temperature for as long as 4 hours after the induction of the anaesthesia. A rise in body temperature to malignant levels can occur occasionally after the anaesthetic has ceased. The rise in body temperature is associated with an increased respiratory rate, this is sometimes noted before the onset of muscle rigidity. Later, rigidity of the respiratory muscles increases and with it the degree of respiratory impairment. The heart rate increases sometimes to over 200 beats/minute. Prior to death, the patient is in a coma with widely dilated, often unequal, pupils.

In reviewing the aetiology and pathophysiology of malignant hyperthermia,[17] it was reported that the most consistent initial observation during the development of the condition was a rapid multifocal ventricular arrhythmia together with an unstable blood pressure. A mottled cyanosis of the skin also develops.[16] Rigidity of the skeletal muscles occurs in about 80% of cases and is almost always observed after the administration of succinylcholine. Following the initial rise in temperature, a rapid increase takes place so that values of 44–46°C are measured.

Hyperkalaemia accompanies the condition but is probably not the cause of ventricular fibrillation when this occurs, because when the heart is examined at *post mortem* it is found to be in a state of contraction. A severe metabolic acidosis is also present. Respiratory failure and impairment of diffusion of respiratory gases lead to hypoxia and hypercarbia. With the raised PCO_2 and low plasma $[HCO_3^-]$, blood pH values as low as 6.6 have been observed. For a more full account see Brooks (1983).[24]

A very lucid account of a successfully treated case of malignant hyperthermia, occurring in a patient suffering from osteogenesis imperfecta, has been reported by Rampton *et al.* (1984).[80] The patient's sister had died from an 'overdose of anaesthetic' at the age of 14 years. Other cases of malignant hyperthermia associated with osteogenesis imperfecta have been reported.[30,33,71]

Dantrolene

The drug dantrolene sodium has been introduced specifically for treating malignant hyperthermia,[58] although it has been used for treating muscle spasticity in children.[41,91]

This substance is a member of a group of new skeletal muscle relaxants which act directly upon the muscle, producing relaxation and reducing contraction, but which do not alter neuromuscular transmission.[56,79] Dantrolene appears to act by diminishing the amount of Ca^{++} available to the sarcoplasmic reticulum.*

Dantrolene sodium was effective when given intravenously in controlling malignant hyperpyrexia in pigs.[59] In the initial treatment in man, dantrolene approximately 2.5 mg/kg body weight has been effective, although as much as 7.5 mg/kg body weight was used during investigation of malignant hyperthermia in pigs.

The substance is obtained in vials containing 20 mg dantrolene, 300 mg mannitol and sodium hydroxide which gives a pH of 9.5 when reconstituted with 60 ml of sterile water.

Treatment of malignant hyperpyrexia (malignant hyperthermia)

1. Terminate the anaesthetic immediately and terminate surgery as quickly as possible.

2. Uncover the patient and begin cooling as rapidly as possible.

3. Increase fluid intake of glucose and water intravenously, preferably using an infusion bottle or bag that has been immersed in ice and cold water. Large volumes of fluid will be needed and 20 g of mannitol should be injected intravenously to encourage an osmotic diuresis.

4. Inject a large dose of corticosteroid intravenously, for example 1 g of 6-methylprednisolone (Solu-Medrone) in the adult over a period of 10 minutes.

5. Maintain artificial ventilation of the lungs by hand using high concentrations of O_2. If muscle spasm prevents adequate ventilation, muscle relaxation may be obtained by administering pancuronium (Pavulon). However, this may not produce any effect as the muscle contracture is the result of the movement of Ca^{++} and is not influenced by blocking the muscle end-plate. Pancuronium is given intramuscularly in doses of 0.03–0.06 mg/kg body weight.

6. An arterial blood sample should be taken for estimation of blood gases and, at the same time, serum electrolytes, CPK and other biochemical parameters. Before the results are known, an infusion of 200 ml of 8.4% $NaHCO_3$ should be started and the dose adjusted according to the measured base deficit—$[HCO_3^-]$.

7. If the plasma $[K^+]$ is found to be high, an infusion of hypertonic glucose and insulin can be

---

*The Ca^{++} channel blocker diltiazem (Cardizem, Tildiem) has also been used.

started: 20% glucose containing 1 unit of soluble insulin per 3 g of glucose can be instituted (33 units of insulin in 500 ml of a 20% solution of glucose). This also helps to reverse the hypoglycaemia that is sometimes present.

8. Begin the infusion of dantrolene sodium with an initial intravenous dose of approximately 1 mg/kg body weight, usually approximately 70–80 mg. This is given by rapid intravenous infusion. Up to 10 mg/kg body weight has been recommended in the acute phase. Dantrolene infusions may need to be repeated three or four times per day in the succeeding days following recovery. Repeated estimations of serum electrolytes, especially $[K^+]$, are required and serial estimations of the blood glucose is also of value. Plasma haemoglobin should also be estimated when this is possible.

9. A catheter should be inserted into the bladder so that the urine output can be measured and the urine osmolality and myoglobin content can be estimated.

10. The patient should be cooled as soon as possible by placing him/her in a bath of iced, cold water. If it is not possible to place the patient in a bath of iced water at 4°C, ice packs should be applied to all parts of the body. Wetting the skin and fanning air over the body are also beneficial.

11. Vasodilatation can be achieved by means of droperidol (Droleptan), which is supplied in 2 ml ampoules containing 5 mg/ml. It is used as an adjunct to anaesthesia and can therefore be administered early when the condition is diagnosed and the formal anaesthetic is stopped. It can be given intravenously in doses of 5–15 mg to the adult (0.2–0.3 mg/kg). Droperidol has an alpha-adrenergic blocking action which causes the vasodilatation, and it may have a beneficial effect in reducing muscle spasm. It should not be given with fentanyl, as the latter induces muscle spasm.

12. The fall in blood pressure that is associated both with the condition itself and with the specific therapy, such as dantrolene sodium and droperidol, can be corrected by administering the vasopressor isoprenaline. This may be infused in solutions containing 4–5 mg of isoprenaline (isoproterenol) at a rate of 10 drops/minute, or at a rate which is sufficient to raise the blood pressure. Cardiac arrhythmias tend to be prevented by dantrolene and verapamil (which has a similar action in that it reduces the transfer of Ca^{++} through the cell wall). If neither of these is effective, a beta-blocker, such as propranolol 1 mg i.v. or practolol 5 mg i.v., should be given slowly.

References

1. Alexander, L. (1946). Combined intelligence objectives Sub-Committee, item 24, file Nos. 26–37.
2. Alexander, L. (1946). The treatment of shock from prolonged exposure to cold, especially in water. Report No. 250. Office of the Publication Board. Department of Commerce, Washington, D. C.
3. Alexander, L. (1949). Medical science under dictatorship. *New Engl. J. Med.*, **241**, 39.
4. Alexander, L. (1966). Limitations in experimental research on human beings. *Lex et Scientia*, **3**, 8.
5. Andersen, O. S. and Egsbaek, W. (1962). Hypotermiens indvirkning på syre-base-status hos hibernerende flagermus. *Ugeskr. Læg.*, **124**, 929.
6. Andjus, R. (1951). Sur la possibilité de reanimer le rat adulte refroidi jusqu'à proximité du point de congélation. *C. R. Acad. Sci. (Paris)*, **232**, 1591.
7. Andjus, R. K. (1955). Suspended animation in cooled, supercooled and frozen rats. *Journal of Physiology*, **128**, 547.
8. Angel, J. H. and Sash, L. (1960). Hypothermic coma in myxoedema. *Brit. med. J.*, **1**, 1855.
9. Astrup, P., Jørgensen, K., Andersen, O. S. and Engel, K. (1960). The acid–base metabolism: a new approach, *Lancet*, **i**, 1035.
10. Beavers, W. R. and Covino, B. G. (1956). Immersion hypothermia: effect of glycine. *Proc. Soc. exp. Biol. (N.Y.)*, **92**, 319.
11. Bernard, C. (1877). *Leçons sur le diabète et la glycogénèse animale*, p. 190. Paris: Baillière.
12. Bigelow, W. G., Lindsay, W. K., Harrison, R. C., Gordon, R. A. and Greenwood, W. F. (1950). Oxygen transport and utilization in dogs at low body temperatures. *Amer. J. Physiol.*, **160**, 125.
13. Bloch, M., Bloom, H. J. G., Penman, J. and Walsh, L. (1961). Irradiation of cerebral astrocytomata under whole-body hypothermia. *Lancet*, **ii**, 906.
14. Boyd, A. E. and Beller, G. A. (1975). Heat exhaustion and respiratory alkalosis. *Ann. int. Med.*, **83**, 835.
15. Brewin, E. G., Gould, R. P., Nashat, F. S. and Neil, E. (1955). An investigation of problems of acid base equilibrium in hypothermia. *Guy's Hosp. Rep.*, **104**, 177.
16. Britt, B. A. (1977). Malignant Hyperthermia. In *Complications in Anesthesiology*. p. 120. Edited by F. K. Orkin and L. H. Cooperman. Philadelphia: Lippincott.
17. Britt, B. A. (1979). Etiology and pathophysiology of malignant hyperthermia. *Fed. Proc.*, **38**, 44.

18. Britton, S. W. (1930). Extreme hypothermia in various animals and in man. *Canad. med. Ass. J.*, **22**, 257.

19. Brooks, D. K. (1962). Acid–base balance in hypothermia. In *Modern Trends in Anaesthesia*, p. 102. Edited by F. T. Evans and T. C. Gray. London: Butterworths.

20. Brooks, D. K. (1962). M.D. Thesis. London University.

21. Brooks, D. K. (1963). Ph.D. Thesis, London University.

22. Brooks, D. K. (1964). The meaning of pH at low temperatures during extracorporeal circulation. *Anaesthesia*, **19**, 337.

23. Brooks, D. K. (1965). Physiological responses produced by changes in acid–base equilibrium following profound hypothermia. *Anaesthesia*, **20**, 173.

24. Brooks, D. K. (1983). Hypothermia and hyperthermia. In *Modern Emergency Department Practice*, p. 343. Edited by D. K. Brooks and A. J. Harrold. London: Edward Arnold.

25. Brooks, D. K. Unpublished data.

26. Buccini, R. V. (1985). Hypothermia in Hodgkin's Disease. *New Engl. J. Med.*, **312**, 244.

27. Burton, A. C. and Edholm, O. G. (1955). *Man in a cold environment*. London: Edward Arnold.

28. Cannon, W. B., Querido, A., Britton, S. W. and Bright, E. M. (1927). Studies on conditions of activity in endocrine glands; role of adrenal secretion in chemical control of body temperature. *Amer. J. Physiol.*, **79**, 466.

29. Childs, C. M. and Norman, J. N. (1978). Unexplained loss of consciousness in divers. *Medécine Subaquatique et Hyperbare*, **17**, 127.

30. Cole, N. L., Goldberg, M. H., Loftus, M. and Kwok, V. (1982). Surgical management of patients with osteogenesis imperfecta. *J. Oral Maxillofac. Surg.*, **40**, 578.

31. Costrini, A. M., Pitt, H. A., Gustafson, A. B. and Uddin, D. E. (1979). Cardiovascular and metabolic manifestations of heat stroke and severe heat exhaustion. *Amer. J. Med.*, **66**, 296.

32. Craig, F. A., Lange, K., Oberman, J. and Carson, S. (1952). A simple, accurate method of blood pH determination for clinical use. *Arch. Biochem.*, **38**, 357.

33. Cropp, J. G. A. and Myers, D. N. (1972). Physiological evidence of hypermetabolism in osteogenesis imperfecta. *Paediatrics*, **49**, 375.

34. Cullen, G. E. (1922). Studies of acidosis. Part 19. The colorimetric determination of the hydrogen ion concentration of blood plasma. *J. Biol. Chem.*, **52**, 501.

35. Currie, J. (1798). *Medical reports on the effects of water, cold and warm, as a remedy in fever; appendix II*. Liverpool: Cadell & Davies.

36. Denborough, M. A. (1977). Malignant hyperpyrexia. *Med. J. Aust.*, **2**, 757.

37. Doherty, N. E., Ades, A., Shah, P. K. and Seegal, R. J. (1984). Hypothermia with acute myocardial infarction. *Ann. Int. Med.*, **101**, 797.

38. Drew, C. E. and Anderson, I. M. (1959). Profound hypothermia in cardiac surgery: report of three cases. *Lancet*, **i**, 748.

39. Drew, C. E., Keen, G. and Benazon, D. B. (1959). Profound hypothermia. *Lancet*, **i**, 745.

40. Duff, D. S., Farrant, P. C., Leveaux, V. M. and Wray, S. M. (1961). Spontaneous period hypothermia. *Quart. J. Med.*, **30**, 329.

41. Dykes, M. H. M. (1975). Evaluation of a muscle relaxant: Dantrolene sodium (Dantrium). *J. Amer. med. Ass.*, **231**, 862.

42. Edwards, H. A., Benstead, J. G., Brown, K., Makary, A. Z. and Menon, N. K. (1970). Apparent death with accidental hypothermia: a case report. *Brit. J. Anaesth.*, **42**, 906.

43. Emslie-Smith, D. (1956). Changes in the electrocardiogram during pre-operative hypothermia in man. *Australasian Ann. Med.*, **5**, 62.

44. Emslie-Smith, D. (1958). Accidental hypothermia:a common condition with a pathognomonic electrocardiogram. *Lancet*, **ii**, 492.

45. Fell, R. H., Gunning, A. J., Bardhan, K. D. and Triger, D. R. (1968). Severe hypothermia as a result of barbiturate overdose complicated by cardiac arrest. *Lancet*, **i**, 392.

46. Finney, W. H. and Dworkin, S. (1927). Artificial hibernation in woodchuck (Arctomys monax). *Amer. J. Physiol.*, **80**, 75.

47. Finney, W. H., Dworkin S. and Cassidy, G. J. (1927). Effects of lowered body temperature and of insulin on respiratory quotients of dogs. *Amer. J. Physiol.*, **80**, 301.

48. Forester, C. F. (1963). Coma in myxoedema. *Arch. Int. Med.*, **111**, 734.

49. Fox, R. H., Goldsmith, R., Hampton, I. F. G. and Hunt, T. J. (1967). Heat acclimatization by controlled hyperthermia in hot–dry and hot–wet climates. *J. appl. Physiol.*, **22**, 39.

50. Freinkel, N., Metzger, B. E., Harris, E., Robinson, S. and Mager, M. (1972). The hypothermia of hypoglycemia. *N. Engl. J. of Med.*, **287**, 841.

51. Fuhrman, F. A. (1956). Oxygen consumption of mammalian tissues at reduced temperatures. In *The physiology of induced hypothermia. Proceedings of a symposium, 28–29 October 1955*, p. 50. Edited by R. Dripps. Washington: National Academy of Sciences—National Research Council.

52. Gaudio, R. and Abramson, N. (1968). Heat-induced hyperventilation. *J. appl. Physiol.*, **25**, 742.

53. Gleichmann, U. and Lübbers, D. W. (1960). Vergleichende Untersuchungen des Kohlensäuredruckes mit der Micro-pH-Methode (Astrup) und der stabilisierten Ganzglas-pCO_2-Elektrode in Normo– und Hypothermie. *Pfluegers Arch.*, **273**, 190.

54. Golden, F. (1973). Recognition and treatment of immersion hypothermia. *Proceedings of the Royal Society of Medicine*, **66**, 1058.

55. Gollan, F. (1954). Cardiac arrest of one hour duration

in dogs during hypothermia of 0°C followed by survival. *Fedn. Proc.*, **13**, 57.

56. Gronert, G. A., Milde, J. H. and Theye, R. A. (1967). Dantrolene in porcine malignant hyperthermia. *Anesthesiology*, **44**, 488.

57. Haldane, J. S. (1905). The influence of high air temperature. *J. Hyg.*, **55**, 495.

58. Hall, G. M. (1980). Dantrolene and the treatment of malignant hyperthermia. *Brit. J. Anaesth.*, **52**, 847.

59. Harrison, G. G. (1975). Control of the malignant hyperpyrexic syndrome in MHS swine by dantrolene sodium. *Brit. J. Anaesth.*, **47**, 62.

60. Hayward, M. G. and Keatinge, W. R. (1979). Progressive symptomless hypothermia in water: possible cause of diving accidents. *Brit med. J.*, **1**, 1182.

61. Hunter, J. (1776). *The works of John Hunter, F.R.S., with notes*, Vol **4**, p. 20. Edited by J. F. Palmer. London: Longman, 1837.

62. Jackson, M. J., Proctor, S. J. and Leonard, R. C. F. (1983). Hypothermia during chemotherapy for Hodgkin's disease. *Brit. med. J.*, **286**, 1183.

63. Keatinge, W. R., Hayward, M. G. and McIver, N. K. (1980). Hypothermia during saturation diving in the North Sea. *Brit. med. J.*, **280**, 291.

64. Kenyon, J. R., Ludbrook, J., Downs, A. R., Tait, I. B., Brooks, D. K. and Pryczkowski, J. (1959). Experimental deep hypothermia. *Lancet*, **ii**, 41.

65. Khogali, M. and Weiner, J. S. (1980). Heat stroke: report on 18 cases. *Lancet*, **ii**, 276.

66. Ladell, W. S. (1957). Disorders due to heat. *Trans. Roy. Soc. Trop. Med. Hyg.*, **51**, 189.

67. Lash, R. F., Burdette, J. A. and Ozdil, T. (1967). Accidental profound hypothermia and barbiturate intoxication. *J. Amer. med. Assoc.*, **201**, 269.

68. Laufman, H. (1951). Profound accidental hypothermia. *J. Amer. med. Assoc.*, **147**, 1201.

69. Laug, E. P. (1930). The application of the quinhydrone electrode to the determination of the pH of serum and plasma. *J. Biol. Chem.*, **88**, 551.

70. Leithhead, C. S. and Lind, A. R. (1964). *Heat Stress and Heat Disorders*, p. 127. Philadelphia: F. A. Davis.

71. Libman, R. M. (1981). Anaesthetic considerations for the patient with osteogenesis imperfecta. *Clin. Orthop.*, **159**, 123.

72. Linton, A. L. and Ledingham, I. McA. (1966). Severe hypothermia with barbiturate intoxication. *Lancet*, **i**, 24.

73. Loomis, T. A. (1952). Effect of alcohol on myocardial and respiratory function. *Quart. J. Stud. Alcohol*, **13**, 561.

74. Neil, E. (1959). Discussion. In *A Symposium on pH and blood gas measurement*, p. 44. Edited by R. F. Woolmer and J. Parkinson. London: Churchill.

75. Nicholson, M. R. and Somerville, K. W. (1978). Heat stroke in a 'run for fun'. *Brit. med. J.*, **1**, 1525.

76. Osborn, J. J. (1953). Experimental hypothermia: respiratory and blood pH changes in relation to cardiac function. *Amer. J. Physiol.*, **175**, 389.

77. Pembrey, M. S. and Hale White, W. (1896). The regulation of temperature in hybernating animals. *J. Physiol.*, **19**, 477.

78. Pledger, H. G. (1962). Disorders of temperature regulation in acute traumatic tetraplegia. *J. Bone Joint Surg.*, **44B**, 110.

79. Putney, J. W. and Bianchi, C. P. (1974). Site of action of dantrolene in frog sartorius muscle. *J. Pharm. Exp. Ther.*, **189**, 202.

80. Rampton, A. J., Kelly, D. A., Shanahan, C. and Ingram, G. S. (1984). Occurrence of malignant hyperpyrexia in a patient with osteogenesis imperfecta. *Brit. J. Anaesth.*, **56**, 1443.

81. Rosenthal, T. B. (1948). The effect of temperature on the pH of blood and plasma *in vitro. J. Biol. Chem.*, **173**, 25.

82. Sadowsky, C. and Reeves, A. G. (1975). Agenesis of the corpus callosum with hypothermia. *Arch. Neurol.*, **32**, 774.

83. Severinghaus, J. W., Stupfel, M. and Bradley, A. F. (1956). Variations of serum carbonic acid pK' with pH and temperature. *J. appl. Physiol.*, **9**, 197.

84. Shapiro, W. R., Williams, G. H. and Plum, F. (1969). Spontaneous recurrent hypothermia accompanying agenesis of the corpus callosum. *Brain*, **92**, 423.

85. Sheehan, H. L. and Summers, V. K. (1952). Treatment of hypopituitary coma. *Brit. med. J.*, **1**, 1214.

86. Siggaard-Andersen, O. and Egsbaek, W. (1962). Hypotermiens indvirkning pa syre–base status hos hibernerende flagermus. (The influence of hypothermia on the acid–base status of hibernating bats) (English summary). *Ugeskr. Laeger*, **124**, 929.

87. Simpson, S. (1902). Some observations on the temperature of the monkey. *J. Physiol.*, **28**, xxi.

88. Simpson, S. (1902). Temperature range in the monkey in ether anaesthesia. *J. Physiol.*, **28**, xxxvii.

89. Smith, A. U. (1959). Viability of supercooled and frozen mammals. *Ann. N. Y. Acad. Sci.*, **80**, 291.

90. Smith, A. U., Lovelock, J. E. and Parkes, A. S. (1954). Resuscitation of hamsters after supercooling or partial crystallization at body temperatures below 0°C. *Nature (Lond.)*, **173**, 1136.

91. Snyder, H. R., Davis, C. S., Bickerton, R. K. and Halliday, R. P. (1967). 1-(5-Arylfurfurylidene amino) hydantoins: a new class of muscle relaxant. *J. med. Chem.*, **10**, 807.

92. Spallanzani, L. (1803). *Tracts on the natural history of animals and vegetables*. 2nd ed. Translated by J. G. Dalyell. Edinburgh: Creech & Constable.

93. Sutton, J. R. and Hughson, R. L. (1979). Heatstroke in road races. *Lancet*, **i**, 983.

94. Talbott, J. H., Consolazio, W. V. and Pecora, L. J. (1941). Hypothermia. *Arch. Int. Med.*, **68**, 1120.

95. Walther, A. (1862). Beiträge zur Lehre von der thierischen Wärme. *Virchows Arch.*, **25**, 414.

96. Weiner, J. S. and Khogali, M. (1979). Heatstroke. *Lancet*, **i**, 1135.

97. Weiner, J. S. and Khogali, M. (1980). A physiological body-cooling unit for treatment of heat stroke. *Lancet*, **i**, 507.
98. Weyman, A. E., Greenbaum, D. M. and Grace, W. J. (1974). Accidental hypothermia in an alcoholic population. *Amer. J. Med.*, **56**, 13.
99. Wingfield, A. (1941). Hyperventilation tetany in tropical climates. *Brit. med. J.*, **1**, 929.
100. Wynn, V. (1954). Electrolyte disturbances associated with failure to metabolise glucose during hypothermia. *Lancet*, **ii**, 575.
101. Yoshimura, H. and Fujimoto, T. (1937). Is the hydrogen gas electrode not applicable to the determination of the pH of oxygenated blood. (Studies on the blood pH estimated by the gas electrode method. VI). *J. Biochem., Tokyo*, **25**, 493.

Further Reading

Editorial (1985). Deaths in winter. *Lancet*, **ii**, 987.

Ilias, W. K., Williams, C. H., Fulfer, R. T. and Dozier, S. E. (1985). Diltiazem inhibits halothane-induced contractions in malignant hyperthermia-susceptible muscles *in vitro*. *Brit. J. Anaesth.*, **57**, 994.

Keatinge, W. R., Coleshaw, S. R. K., Millard, C. E. and Axelsson, J. (1986). Exceptional case of survival in cold water. *Brit. med. J.*, **292**, 171.

Ranklev, E., Monti, M. and Fletcher, R. (1985). Microcalorimetric studies in malignant hyperpyrexia susceptible individuals. *Brit. J. Anaesth.*, **57**, 991.

Chapter 8
Hyperbaric Oxygen

Inspired Oxygen

Oxygen was discovered by Priestley in 1775:[30,31]

> From the greater strength and vivacity of the flame of a candle in this pure air, it may be conjectured, that it might be peculiarly salutary to the lungs in certain morbid cases. . .But, perhaps, we may also infer from these experiments, that though pure dephlogisticated air might be very useful as a medicine, it might not be so proper for us in the usual healthy state of the body: for as a candle burns out much faster in dephlogisticated than in common air, so we might, as may be said, live out too fast, and the animal powers be too soon exhausted in this pure kind of air. A moralist, at least, may say that the air which nature has provided for us is as good as we deserve. . .The feeling of it to my lungs was not sensibly different from that of common air; but I fancied that my breast felt peculiarly light and easy for some time afterwards. Who can tell but that, in time, this pure air may become a fashionable article of luxury. Hitherto, only two mice and myself have had the prividege of breathing it.

Priestley later found that oxygen, even at atmospheric pressure, was toxic to some animals but not to man.

The first review of the effects and physiology of hyperbaric oxygen is that of Bean in 1945.[4] Men have worked in high pressures of air for considerable periods of time during the building of tunnels under rivers and in caissons. Underwater divers are exposed to high pressures but, except in special circumstances, breathe air usually for relatively short periods.

Although we can increase the oxygen tension in the air we breathe by means of an oxygen tent or close-fitting oxygen mask such as used by airmen, so that almost 100% oxygen is inspired, the relative increase in oxygen content of the blood is small. Unless very large flows are used, the concentration of oxygen in the ordinary clinical oxygen tent does not rise very much above 40% and, unless great care is taken in tucking the edges of the tent under the mattress and folding the bedclothes in such a way that no large gaps are left, the oxygen content very often does not rise above 30%. Although oxygen tents are still used in some medical centres, they have largely been discarded in Britain and the USA in favour of nasal catheters attached to 'spectacles' and oxygen masks which can deliver high and low tensions of O_2. Most oxygen masks used in clinical practice do not provide concentrations of oxygen which are appreciably higher than 70%. An exception to this is the demand valve type of oxygen mask.

It has long been considered that the use of hyperbaric oxygen, that is to say oxygen or air under pressure, may be of clinical value.

Terminology

We refer to normal atmospheric pressure as being 1 atmosphere absolute, thus when the pressure is increased by diving below the surface of water or being compressed in a specially designed tank, we refer to the pressure as being 2, 3 or more 'atmospheres absolute'. For many years now, when tunnelling below rivers, men have had to work at pressures in the region of 4–5 atmospheres absolute so that water would not seep from below the river bed into the working area. Men have been successfully exposed to these pressures for 8 hours/day having been compressed in an airlock before entering the working site. They have used heavy manual implements such as pickaxes and hammers for considerable periods of time. There have been indications that this experience may give rise to pathological effects. It has been reported that certain people may undergo necrotic changes of the bones.[12,13] This has been reported also in sailors who underwent rapid decompression when they escaped from a submarine.[22] These changes have, however, all been produced when rapid decompression has occurred after breathing air at very high pressures.

Physiology of Hyperbaric Oxygenation

The blood consists of two oxygen-carrying compartments; one is the red cells and the other is the plasma. The red cells contain haemoglobin which has unique characteristics in that it is specially designed for carrying oxygen in a loose combination, but in very large quantities; 1 g of haemoglobin combines with 1.34 ml of O_2. When blood contains 15 g of haemoglobin it combines with:

$$15 \times 1.34 = 20.1 \text{ ml } O_2$$

We know, however, that this combination depends upon the tension of O_2 in the gas which ventilates the alveoli. An oxygen saturation of 97% represents a PO_2 of 100 mmHg. An oxygen saturation of 93% represents a PO_2 of only just over 70 mmHg. When, however, the oxygen saturation falls to 75% the PO_2 is only 40 mmHg. As desaturation proceeds further there is a less rapid decline in PO_2 but the volume of oxygen available to the tissues is very small. Cyanosis begins to appear when the oxygen saturation of the arterial blood is reduced to below 85%, but it may not become obvious, except in a bright white light, until oxygen saturation falls to 75%. The oxygen dissociation curve for haemoglobin is altered by numerous factors such as temperature and pH. The blood is arterialized when it passes from the right to the left side of the heart and undergoes a change of pH, the shape of this curve is thus altered so that most curves that are published indicate the mean figures obtained, although in practice the difference is very small.

As the partial pressure of oxygen in the alveoli increases, the amount of oxygen dissolved in the plasma also increases. Unlike haemoglobin, however, gases dissolved in plasma obey Henry's Law so that the amount of gas dissolved in the liquid is proportional, at any given temperature, to the tension to which the liquid is exposed. This applies also to CO_2. The solubility of oxygen in plasma and body water is therefore linear. The coefficient of solubility of oxygen is 0.003 ml O_2/100 ml of blood/mmHg PO_2.

If, for example, a patient is placed in an oxygen tent that is so efficient that the PO_2 rises to 700 mmHg, the amount of oxygen dissolved in the plasma will rise from its normal value of 0.30 ml/100 ml to 2.1 ml/100 ml. If the patient is now placed in a tank full of oxygen and the pressure is increased to 30 lb/in^2, so that he is exposed to an atmosphere of 3 atmospheres of oxygen absolute and the PO_2 is approximately 2000 mmHg, the amount of oxygen dissolved in the plasma will be 6 ml O_2/100 ml of blood. It must be remembered, however, that not only the blood is exposed to this tension, but the whole of the body water is exposed, so that the amount of oxygen carried by the ECF and ICF is also greatly increased when sufficient time has passed for equilibration to have occurred. If this is done abruptly, the tension of both the O_2 and the CO_2 is increased.[3,4] In this way it is theoretically possible to impose an uncompensated respiratory acidosis in an abrupt manner so that the pH of the blood is lowered. This would only occur if ventilation was depressed or kept constant by artificial means. In practice a patient placed in an hyperbaric atmosphere spontaneously increases alveolar ventilation so that the alveolar PCO_2 is maintained at a normal value.

We have seen how by increasing the pressure to 3 atmospheres a patient breathing 100% oxygen dissolves 6 ml O_2/100 ml of blood. This is more than equal to the volume of oxygen extracted from the blood of a patient at rest. At this pressure, therefore, the normal arteriovenous difference of oxygen saturation (i.e. that between the right and left atrium) disappears. There is sufficient oxygen dissolved in the plasma to supply all the body's requirements at rest so that the blood returning to the right side of the heart is fully saturated. The importance of the effect of high pressure atmospheres upon CO_2 tension now becomes clear. Haemoglobin has a dual function. Not only does it carry O_2 but it also plays an essential part in CO_2 transport.[17] When it is fully oxygenated and is behaving as a stronger acid, it is unable to carry carbon dioxide efficiently. There is therefore the danger that CO_2 is retained within the tissue when the normal arteriovenous difference of oxygen content is removed. This appears to be one of the causes of oxygen toxicity convulsions.[9,18]

Oxygen Convulsions

These are not seen in man except during exposure to 100% oxygen at 3 atmospheres or more. They begin with minor focal neurological signs such as twitching of the mouth and eyebrows before developing into a violent and prolonged fit. Even when decompression from 3 atmospheres is begun the moment these signs appear, the characteristic epileptiform fit may still develop. Oxygen convulsions may appear even when 100% oxygen has been breathed at 3 atmospheres for only 3 or 4 minutes. Individual susceptibility varies greatly. It is known both from animal experiments and experience in man that the tolerance to hyperbaric oxygen at these pressures is increased by barbiturates and tolerance is decreased as the tension of CO_2 in the atmosphere rises. Conversely, the infusion of $NaHCO_3$ and the buffer tris hydroxymethylamino-methane (THAM)[32] (see p. 92) tends to reverse the incidence of convulsions when the CO_2 tension in the atmosphere is increased.

Blood Flow

It has been demonstrated that vascular resistance in various parts of the body, especially the brain and pulmonary circulation, is increased by hyperbaric oxygen, but because of the increased O_2 content of the circulation the cardiac output is reduced. Following decompression from oxygen at 2 atmospheres to oxygen at 1 atmosphere absolute, it is noticeable that the pale vasoconstricted skin during compression gives way to generalized flushing. This is very similar in appearance to that seen in patients when a continuous intravenous infusion of *l*-noradrenaline is stopped suddenly.

Hyperbaric Oxygen Chambers

Although the use of air at high pressures had been studied in both man and animals for several centuries, the first recorded medical use of a hyperbaric chamber is that by Henshaw in 1662.[33] His was the first recorded attempt to use high atmospheric pressures to treat disease. His chamber, which he called a 'domicilium', had a large pair of organ bellows with a valve arrangement which allowed the pressure inside the chamber to be raised for acute diseases and lowered for chronic diseases. He wrote:

> In time of good health this domicilium is proposed as a good expedient to help digestion,

to promote insensible respiration, to facilitate breathing and expectoration, and consequently, of excellent use for the prevention of most affections of the lungs.

Numerous chambers were then introduced at various times, including one at the Brompton Hospital in 1885. Apart from the work of Churchill-Davidson[10] in relation to cancer therapy, Boerema, in 1956, introduced a high-pressure chamber which was large enough to be used as an operating theatre.[6]

The author's own clinical experience in this field is that associated with the use of the hyperbaric oxygen bed produced by Vickers Company Limited (Fig. 8.1).

When the tank is closed, it is flushed with 100% oxygen at a rate of 180 l/minute. At the end of 2 minutes, by which time the tank has been sealed by turning a handle, oxygen circulates through a CO_2 absorber and an activated carbon black chamber at 100 l/minute. A pressure of between 0 and 16 lb/in^2 can then be selected and the rate of compression determined by adjusting the control mechanism to suit the patient's comfort or clinical condition. When the desired pressure is reached, the patient can be held at that pressure for an indefinite period of time, the oxygen circulating and being lost from the chamber at a rate of 10 l/minute. It is, therefore, economical in its use of oxygen. Decompression can be effected at either a fast or a slow rate; again this depends upon the patient's clinical condition and comfort.

'The Bends'

This is the term given to the painful condition that arises when rapid decompression in air occurs. It was noticed originally in caisson workers and those who were subjected to high atmospheric pressures so that they could tunnel under river beds. It is also seen in divers who, having remained submerged for a sufficient length of time for a large volume of nitrogen to be dissolved in the body fluids, have risen to the surface of the water too rapidly. It is said that the name is derived from the peculiar posture and positions that victims of this condition adopted in order to alleviate the pain in the joints. Nitrogen is the least soluble of the inspired gases and the sudden release of pressure causes it to form bubbles in the tissue fluids. It is therefore obvious that, because of the relatively low solubility of nitrogen, production of

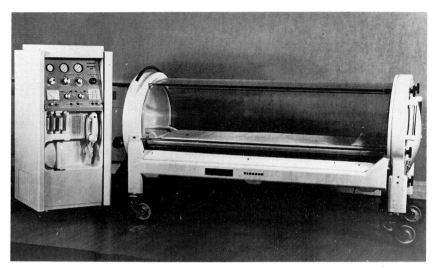

Fig. 8.1 Hyperbaric oxygen bed produced by Vickers Limited, England. The consol to the left of the bed is for regulating pressure up to 3 atmospheres absolute, temperature and humidity. The rate of compression and decompression can be controlled, as can the carbon dioxide content of the atmosphere in the bed. The patient can communicate with the operator, and the patient's blood pressure can be measured when necessary.

the bends is related to the length of time of exposure to air at high pressures and the pressure itself. The shorter the exposure the less probability there is of 'bends' being produced during decompression, and decompression can therefore progress more rapidly. When exposure to high atmospheric pressures in air is prolonged, slow decompression is essential. The treatment of the bends is to recompress the subject as soon as the condition is diagnosed and to maintain the pressure for a time which is relative to the severity of the condition and then to decompress very slowly. A prophylactic measure for the 'bends' is to breathe oxygen during decompression when pressures below 2 atmospheres absolute (plus 15 lb/in^2) are reached. The 'bends' do not occur if, when a patient is subjected to 2 atmospheres absolute in pure oxygen, nitrogen is gradually removed from the body. Because the gas is so soluble and quickly transported, rapid decompression in oxygen can be performed without the danger of 'bends' being caused. If, however, there has been previous exposure to high pressures in air, time is required for the elimination of nitrogen.

Radiotherapy

In 1955 Churchill-Davidson *et al*.[10] introduced the technique of irradiating tumours with the patient

exposed to a pressure of 3 atmospheres in oxygen. Although in a controlled trial it is difficult to establish the benefits of this form of therapy with scientific clarity, the results in difficult cases are so good that it is highly probable that some benefit must be derived. The improved effectiveness of radiotherapy when used at high pressures of O_2, that was found by Churchill-Davidson *et al*. (1957),[11] has been subsequently confirmed by others.[39]

Hyperbaric Oxygen in Resuscitation

The possibility of increasing the oxygen content of the blood offers enormous advantages in many forms of acute disease processes. This is readily apparent when there has been a partial occlusion of the blood supply to a limb or organ after trauma or surgery, following coronary occlusions or ischaemic damage to the brain.

Safety of hyperbaric medicine

The safety of using a hyperbaric chamber in which those inside the chamber breathe air, unless oxygen is specifically administered, was reviewed by Ledingham and Davidson in 1969.[24] Over a period of 3 years, observations were made on 285 patients and 357 staff exposed to air and oxygen at pressures of 1–3 atmospheres absolute (ATA). Decompression sickness had not been observed. Annual radiographs of the skeletal system did not demonstrate a single case of aseptic bone necrosis. Oxygen toxicity had not been observed in any patient. The incidence of barotrauma to the eardrums was 4.7%. It would appear from these figures that, in the hands of knowledgeable physicians, the application of hyperbaric medicine is very safe.[37,38]

Infection

Hyperbaric oxygenation inhibits the growth of bacteria whether they are facultative anaerobes or the more common aerobic pathogens.[26] *Pseudomonas pyocyanea* is inhibited by O_2 at 2 atmospheres absolute. Although the bactericidal qualities of hyperbaric oxygen have still to be investigated fully, it is apparent that its effectiveness in this respect against spore-bearing anaerobes, such as *Clostridium welchii* is incomplete. Because of this, necrotic tissue which may contain anaerobic organisms may still require surgical removal. However, the effect of hyperbaric oxygen on the toxicity of these infections is without doubt.[21] When a patient is exposed to compression to 2 atmospheres absolute of O_2 there is very rapid clinical improvement in that the blood pressure rises, the tachycardia decreases, and the level of consciousness and mental activity markedly improves. Hyperbaric oxygen has been reported to be of benefit in the treatment of tetanus.

A number of other conditions warrant the use of hyperbaric oxygen. It is effective in infections such as gas gangrene. It was noted that, despite the numerous accounts of its dramatic effects on *Clostridium welchii,* there has been a reluctance in Britain to use hyperbaric oxygen instead of the scalpel. At pressures just below 3 atmospheres absolute, organisms are prevented from multiplying and the toxins are inactivated. Ischaemic tissue is also made more viable.

Because of the inhibition of bacterial growth, hyperbaric oxygen has also been used in osteomyelitis[5] and, perhaps not surprisingly, in burns[16] and trauma.[25]

Coronary occlusion

The long-term benefit of treating acute coronary occlusion with hyperbaric oxygen is still unknown. In the acute stage, however, in the presence of cardiac failure giving rise to pulmonary oedema, it appears to produce a remarkable improvement. Improvement in blood pressure that has been reported by Moon et al. (1964),[27] Smith (1964)[34]

and Kioschos et al. (1969)[23] is confirmed in the author's own experience. During compression, however, a bradycardia may develop so that it may be necessary to carry out compression and decompression at a slow rate. However, atropine may be given in small doses (e.g. 0.4–0.8 mg) to increase the heart rate before compression in oxygen is begun.

Although today the conventional treatment for cardiac arrhythmias following acute myocardial infarction involves mainly the use of antiarrhythmic drugs and electrical cardioversion, we know that sometimes this treatment is either unsuccessful or is only sustained for a relatively brief period of time. Hood et al.,[19] however, reported a patient in whom neither procainamide nor quinidine was successful, but in whom hyperbaric oxygen maintained a satisfactory rhythm. Ashfield and Gavey (1969)[1] also found hyperbaric oxygen to be beneficial.

Infarct size

There seems to be some controversy with regard to the effects of hyperbaric oxygen following embolic conditions and myocardial infarction.[8,35] It must be remembered, however, that different chambers have been used. In some cases, oxygen was administered inside an air-containing hyperbaric chamber in which the operators and medical attendants were enclosed, breathing pure oxygen (diluted by water vapour). It is interesting to note that Glauser and Glauser[15] concluded that the improvement in infarct size was dependent upon the radius of the infarct—the smaller the radius, the greater the improvement—and that hyperbaric oxygen was likely to be more beneficial when the blood supply to the infarct was greater.

Coal gas poisoning

Hyperbaric oxygen has been proved to be of value in coal gas poisoning.[36] It is apparent that when the oxygen carrying capacity of the blood is decreased because of the presence of carboxyhaemoglobin, the increased carrying capacity for oxygen of the body fluids at high pressures is of immediate value. It is also highly probable that CO is more rapidly eliminated when the O_2 tension is high. Cerebral complications appear to be fewer when hyperbaric oxygen therapy is used. Because death may occur on the way to hospital, an ambulance containing a perspex (lucite) hyperbaric oxygen chamber has been developed by Vickers Limited and used successfully in Glasgow, UK.

Although coal gas, and therefore CO poisoning, has largely disappeared from Great Britain because of North Sea gas, carbon monoxide poisoning does occur when the exhaust fumes of a motor vehicle are inhaled for a significant period of time. The treatment of this condition is identical to that of coal gas poisoning.[40] The investigations by Ziser et al. (1984)[41] indicated that hyperbaric O_2 should be used following CO poisoning, even when treatment has been delayed.

Respiratory failure

Although anoxia is present during respiratory failure, CO_2 retention also occurs. We have already discussed how this may be a disadvantage during the use of hyperbaric oxygen. This is because compensatory increased ventilation in order to eliminate it in increased quantities may not be possible in this condition. Experience has shown that hyperbaric oxygen may produce unconsciousness and decreased ventilation in the same way that they are produced in patients with uncompensated respiratory acidosis who are placed in an oxygen tent. There is also some evidence that the infective process, far from being inhibited, is exacerbated. It is possible, however, that these difficulties may be overcome.

Resuscitation of the newborn

A neonate may fail to breathe after being born even in the absence of any detectable abnormality and in the presence of a normal circulation and cardiovascular system. Such neonates usually respond to clearing the airway, endotracheal intubation and artificial ventilation with oxygen. This often entails skilled medical attention outside the province of the midwife. Hutchison et al. (1963) have shown that it is possible to resuscitate these babies with a small hyperbaric oxygen chamber.[20] Neonates placed in the tank become pink in colour when completely apnoeic and then begin to breathe after a few minutes. Retrolental fibroplasia does not occur because the exposure to hyperbaric oxygen is limited to only a few minutes. The tank has the advantage that the baby can be placed within it immediately after birth.

Hyperbaric O_2 for multiple sclerosis

Enthusiasm for hyperbaric O_2 treatment for multiple sclerosis continues in the UK, and at least 50 compression chambers have been established privately for treating the condition. Transient improvement was reported by Boschetty and Cernoch (1970)[7] following 10–20 sessions at 2 atmospheres absolute (ATA).

Improvement was also found by Fischer et al. (1983),[14] but a placebo-controlled, double-blind trial performed by Barnes et al. (1985)[2] found that the claims made by others could not be supported except for the fact that bowel and bladder function improved following hyperbaric O_2 therapy. Neubauer (1985),[29] however, could not agree with the findings of the trial performed by Fischer and his co-workers (Neubauer, 1984 and 1985).[28,29] There are widely accepted indications that bladder and bowel function is improved by hyperbaric O_2 therapy, although other methods for achieving this improvement (e.g. oral medication) also exist.

References

1. Ashfield, R. and Gavey, C. J. (1969). Severe acute myocardial infarction treated with hyperbaric oxygen—Report on 40 patients. *Postgrad. med. J.*, **45**, 648.

2. Barnes, M. P., Bates, D., Cartlidge, N. E. F., French, J. M. and Shaw, D. A. (1985). Hyperbaric oxygen and multiple sclerosis: short-term results of a placebo-controlled, double-blind trial. *Lancet*, **i**, 297.

3. Bean, J. W. (1931). Effects of high oxygen pressure on carbon dioxide transport, on blood and tissues acidity, and on oxygen consumption and pulmonary ventilation. *J. Physiol.*, **122**, 27.

4. Bean, J. W. (1945). Effects of oxygen at increased pressure. *Physiol. Rev.*, **25**, 1.

5. Bingham, E. L., Mullen, J. E., Winans, R. G. and Hart, G. B. (1973). The treatment of refractory osteomyelitis with hyperbaric oxygen: a progress report. In *Proceedings of the 5th International Hyperbaric Conference*, p. 264. Edited by W. G. Trapp, E. W. Bannister, A. J. Davison and P. A. Trapp. Burnaby: Simon Fraser University.

6. Boerema, I. (1964). *Clinical Application of Hyperbaric Oxygen*. Edited by I. Boerema, W. H. Brummelkamp and N. G. Meijne. Amsterdam: Elsevier.

7. Boschetty, V. and Cernoch, J. (1970). Aplikace kysliku za pretlaku u nekterych neurologickych anemocneni. *Bratisl Lek Listy*, **53**, 298.

8. *British Medical Journal*. (1978). Editorial. *Brit. med. J.*, **i**, 1012.

9. Case, E. M. and Haldane, J. B. S. (1941). Human physiology under high pressure. *J. Hyg.*, **41**, 225.

10. Churchill-Davidson, I., Sanger, C. and Thomlinson,

R. H. (1955). High-pressure oxygen and radiotherapy. *Lancet*, **i**, 1091.

11. Churchill-Davidson, I., Sanger, C. and Thomlinson, R. H. (1957). Oxygenation in radiotherapy. II. Clinical application. *Brit. J. Radiol.*, **30**, 406.

12. Davidson, J. K. (1964). Pulmonary changes in decompression sickness. Some observations on compressed air workers at the Clyde Tunnel. *Clin. Radiol.*, **15**, 106.

13. Davidson, J. K. (1965). Avascular necrosis of bone. In *Hyperbaric oxygenation. Proceedings of the Second International Congress, Glasgow, September, 1964*, p. 11. Edited by I. McA. Ledingham. Edinburgh: Livingstone.

14. Fischer, B. H., Marks, M. and Reich, T. (1983). Hyperbaric-oxygen treatment of multiple sclerosis: a randomised, placebo-controlled, double blind study. *N. Engl. J. of Med.*, **308**, 181.

15. Glauser, S. C. and Glauser, E. M. (1973). Hyperbaric oxygen therapy: size of infarct determines therapeutic efficacy. *Ann. Int. Med.*, **78**, 77.

16. Grossman, A. A. and Yanda, R. L. (1973). The hyperbaric oxygen treatment of burns. In *Proceedings of the 5th International Hyperbaric Conference*, p. 300. Edited by W. G. Trapp, E. W. Bannister, A. J. Davison and P. A. Trapp. Burnaby: Simon Fraser University.

17. Haldane, J. B. S. (1941). Human life and death at high pressure. *Nature*, **148**, 458.

18. Hill, L. (1933). The influence of carbon dioxide in the production of oxygen poisoning. *Quart. J. Exp. Physiol.*, **23**, 49.

19. Hood, W. B., Yenikomshian, S., Norman, J. C. and Levine, H. D. (1968). Treatment of refractory ventricular tachysystole with hyperbaric oxygenation. *Amer. J. Cardiol.*, **22**, 738.

20. Hutchison, J. H., Kerr, M. M., Williams, K. G. and Hopkinson, W. I. (1963). Hyperbaric oxygen in the resuscitation of the newborn. *Lancet*, **ii**, 1019.

21. Irvin, T. T., Moir, E. R. S. and Smith, G. (1968). Treatment of *Clostridium welchii* infection with hyperbaric oxygen. *Surg. Gynecol. &. Obstet.*, **127**, 1058.

22. James, C. C. M. (1945). Late bone lesions in caisson disease. *Lancet*, **ii**, 6.

23. Kioschos, J. M., Behar, V. S., Saltzman, H. A., Thompson, H. K., Myers, N. E., Smith, W. W. and McIntosh, H. D. (1969). Effect of hyperbaric oxygenation on left ventricular function. *Amer. J. Physiol.*, **216**, 161.

24. Ledingham, I. and Davidson, J. K. (1969). Hazards in hyperbaric medicine. *Brit. med. J.*, **3**, 324.

25. Loder, R. E. (1979). Hyperbaric oxygen treatment in acute trauma. *Ann. Roy. Col. Surg.*, **61**, 472.

26. McAllister, T. A., Stark, J. M., Norman, J. N. and

Ross, R. M. (1965). Hyperbaric oxygen and aerobic micro-organisms. In *Hyperbaric Oxygenation*, p. 250. Edited by I. McA. Ledingham. Edinburgh and London: Churchill Livingstone.

27. Moon, A. J., Williams, K. G. and Hopkinson, W. I. (1964). A patient with coronary thrombosis treated with hyperbaric oxygen. *Lancet*, **i**, 18.

28. Neubauer, R. A. (1984). The effects of hyperbaric oxygen on magnetic resonance imaging in multiple sclerosis. Xth Congress of European Undersea Bio-Medical Society (Marseille, Oct 4, 1984).

29. Neubauer, R. A. (1985). Hyperbaric oxygen for multiple sclerosis. *Lancet*, **i**, 810.

30. Priestley, J. (1772). Observations on different kinds of air. *Philosophical Transactions*, **62**, 147.

31. Priestley, J. (1775–7). *Experiments and observations on different kinds of air*. 3 vols. London: J. Johnson.

32. Sanger, C., Nahas, G. G., Goldberg, A. R. and D'Alessio, G. M. (1961). Effects of 2-amino-2-hydroxymethyl-1,3-propanediol on oxygen toxicity in mice. *Ann. N. Y. Acad. Sci.*, **92**, 710.

33. Simpson, A. (1857). *Compressed air as a therapeutic agent in the treatment of consumption, asthma, chronic bronchitis and other diseases*. Edinburgh: Sutherland & Knox.

34. Smith, G. (1964). Therapeutic applications of oxygen at two atmospheres pressure. *Dis. Chest*, **45**, 15.

35. Smith, G. and Lawson, D. D. (1962). The protective effect of inhalation of oxygen at two atmospheres absolute pressure in acute coronary artery occlusion. *Surg. Gynecol. & Obstet.*, **114**, 320.

36. Smith, G., Ledingham, I. McA., Sharp, G. F., Norman, J. N. and Bates, E. H. (1962). Treatment of coal-gas poisoning with oxygen at 2 atmospheres pressure. *Lancet*, **i**, 816.

37. Thurston, J. G. B. (1969). A controlled trial of hyperbaric oxygen in acute myocardial infarction. *Circulation*, **40**, 203.

38. Thurston, J. G. B. (1970). Hyperbaric oxygen. *Nursing Times*, **66**, 1271.

39. Van den Brenk, H. A. S., Madigan, J. P. and Kerr, R. C. (1964). Experience with megavoltage irradiation of advanced malignant disease using high pressure oxygen. In *Clinical Application of Hyperbaric Oxygen*, p. 144. Edited by I. Boerema, W. H. Brummelkamp and W. G. Meijne. Amsterdam: Elsevier.

40. Winter, A. and Shatin, L. (1970). Hyperbaric oxygen in reversing carbon monoxide coma; Neurologic and psychologic study. *N. Y. State J. Med.*, **70**, 880.

41. Ziser, A., Shupak, A., Halpern, P., Gozal, D. and Melamed, Y. (1984). Delayed hyperbaric oxygen treatment for acute carbon monoxide poisoning. *Brit. med. J.*, **289**, 960.

Further Reading

Mertin, J. and McDonald, W. I. (1984). Regular Review: Hyperbaric oxygen for patients with multiple sclerosis. *Brit. Med. J.*, **288**, 957.

Chapter 9
Cardiac Disease I: practice and theory

Introduction

Although the healthy adult heart has such an enormous reserve that its output can be increased from 5 litres/minute at rest to 30 litres/minute during severe exercise, minor disease processes can severely reduce its function. Minor alterations of rate and rhythm can sometimes have a severe effect on the rest of the body metabolism. Cardiac failure commonly develops postoperatively, especially in the elderly patient, and the treatment of diseases of the myocardium is an important part of resuscitation.

Coronary Occlusion

Although the onset of coronary occlusion is usually sudden, the manner in which it develops can be extremely variable. In many cases there is a premonitory phase which may extend over 1 or 2 days or many weeks. The patient feels unwell or tired, or even exhausted so that slight effort has to be followed by a period of rest. The Oxford Record Linkage Study (Kinlen, 1973)[78] obtained a spontaneous history from relatives that severe tiredness was present in 40% of patients during the weeks or months prior to the death of those who died suddenly. Tiredness was of such a degree, in some cases, that the patient fell asleep at meals. Chest or epigastric pain was a presenting symptom in 82% of patients, while syncope, collapse and the sudden onset of shortness of breath were present in 12%.

The electrocardiogram (ECG) may be normal, even when pains of mild or moderate severity are present which are, in form and position, identical to those of an established coronary occlusion producing infarction of the myocardium. It is now an established practice to treat this phase of the condition in the same way as acute coronary insuf-

ficiency would be treated. The condition, however, may be 'crescendo angina' in which there is usually an intervening period between the onset of chest pain associated with exercise and the development of angina pectoris at rest; this period may be a year or more (sometimes years) following the initial onset of angina. In some patients this intervening period is short (e.g. 6 months or less), and sometimes it is so short that virtually no intervening period is recognized by the patient. Angina at rest, with a normal ECG and normal enzyme studies, can be the *first* indication of heart disease. It is at this stage, before damage to the myocardium has occurred, that aortocoronary by-pass surgery should be performed.

Sometimes there are no premonitory symptoms or physical signs. When coronary occlusion becomes recognizable by such severe pain that the patient repeatedly requests for it to be alleviated, this often indicates impending ventricular fibrillation or cardiac arrest.

The pain is usually substernal, extending across the chest into both arms, up through the neck to the jaw and teeth and backwards to the shoulder blades and spinal column. Not uncommonly, the pain is worse on the left side than the right and pain in the left hand may be present when it is absent in the right. Sometimes the patient will complain of a crushing sensation in the chest and sometimes a burning sensation or a feeling of fullness in the neck. The feeling of fullness is more commonly experienced during the premonitory phase and may be rejected as being of little significance if the history is taken and the examination performed hastily. Even the most severe pain is more intense at certain times than others, waxing and waning for no apparent reason. The pain may be confined to the epigastrium and when accompanied by vomiting may lead to a wrong diagnosis. It may also be confined to the arms, the back, the teeth and neck, the jaw and even the paraumbilical area. The pain is usually accompanied by an increase in the respiratory rate and profuse sweating; the patient looks pale and ill.

Sometimes the pain is absent altogether, this is the so-called silent infarct and the only symptoms are those of tiredness and a mild feeling of being unwell. Sometimes there is a reduced blood pressure or a pulse of irregular volume. This mode of onset is quite commonly associated with sudden death. It is well recognized that the severity of the pain is neither a guide to the seriousness of the condition nor to the degree of infarction.

Fainting sometimes occurs with the onset of coronary occlusion. When an Adams–Stokes attack is caused by asystole, spontaneously reverting ventricular fibrillation or complete heart block, when the heart beat is too slow to maintain cerebral circulation (e.g. 35 beats per minute), then the period of unconsciousness may be associated with convulsions, which are the result of cerebral anoxia.

The usual presentation of acute coronary insufficiency

The patient looks ill, is very pale or grey, sometimes cyanosed, especially peripherally at the finger-tips, nose, cheeks and lips. The skin is cold and clammy and beads of perspiration are seen on the forehead. The patient appears anxious, making restless unnecessary movements and often sighing deeply.

The blood pressure falls to such low levels that it is sometimes unrecordable and it may remain low until death occurs. Although the pulse is usually rapid, in some cases, especially in the presence of cyanosis, a bradycardia develops. Sometimes, even when the infarct is large, the blood pressure may not fall initially and may yet be associated with sudden ventricular fibrillation; therefore, like pain, the blood pressure cannot always be regarded as a guide to the potential danger and severity of the infarction. If cardiac failure has developed by the time the patient is examined, then râles may be heard at the lung bases and the jugular venous pressure (JVP) will be raised. The heart sounds are often faint or 'distant', and when the infarction has occurred some 48 hours before the examination, a pericardial rub may be present which, although transient, lasting perhaps for only an hour or two each time, may recur intermittently for many days.

An S_3* (protodiastolic) gallop is frequently heard and sometimes an S_4 (presystolic) gallop is also present. The pulmonary component of the second sound (S_2) is sometimes accentuated, more

so if there is interstitial oedema of the lungs, associated with cyanosis and a reduced arterial PO_2. Moist râles in the lungs may or may not be present in association with the cyanosis and interstitial pulmonary oedema.

The association of congestive cardiac failure with myocardial infarction has long been recognized as a poor prognostic sign. Although measurements of increase in heart size, stroke volume and left ventricular function demonstrate a close correlation with prognosis, simple clinical signs can be lacking with any degree of conviction. When, however, Harlan et al. (1977)[57] examined two simple criteria—the presence of cardiomegaly and the presence of an S_4 gallop—they found that when these two factors were present, the survival rate at 36 months was approximately 60% compared with 90% when they were absent. There was also a close correlation with a rise in the left ventricular end-diastolic pressure which was invariably greater than 50 mmHg.†

Location of myocardial infarction

Myocardial infarction as a consequence of coronary artery occlusion is confined almost entirely to the left ventricle. In a very small number of cases, however, infarction of the right ventricle occurs. Identification of right ventricular infarction was investigated by Isner and Roberts (1978),[69] and in all cases it was found to be associated with infarction of the posterior wall of the left ventricle; it was not seen in association with infarction of the anterior wall. In addition, the infarction had to be transmural. The vessel involved depended upon the dominant artery supplying the posterior wall of the left ventricle and, as is well recognized from angiographic studies, this can be either the *right* or *left* coronary artery.

---

* There are four heart sounds: S_1 formed by the closure of the mitral and tricuspid valves; S_2 formed by the closure of the aortic (A_2 sound) and pulmonary (P_2 sound) valves; an S_3 sound produced by the ventricles, and an S_4 sound produced by the atria, these are visible on the phonocardiogram. The S_3 and S_4 sounds can be heard normally in the early months of life, puberty and other times, but in the absence of disease they are usually not audible.

† In the absence of disease the end-diastolic pressure in the left ventricle is 2–12 mmHg.

Three types of infarct, related to position, can be identified as occurring in the left ventricle. These are 'anterior', 'inferior' or 'diaphragmatic', and the less common 'true posterior' infarct. The true posterior infarct is referred to as 'true' because the older term 'posterior' infarct has now been largely discarded in favour of the more correct 'inferior or diaphragmatic myocardial infarction'.

The ECG in acute myocardial infarction is characterized by changes that are easily recognizable. When an anterior infarction is present one finds a raised ST segment in leads I, AVL and in the precordial leads (Fig. 9.1). When a full-thickness infarct has occurred, these leads also show Q waves. The T wave is inverted. In leads III and AVF the ST segment is depressed reciprocally. When an inferior infarct is present the ST segment is raised in leads II, III and AVF (Fig 9.2). The precordial leads and lead I show ST depression. Put simply, if the characteristic signs of myocardial infarction (i.e. deep Q waves, elevated upwardly convex ST segment and inverted T wave) are seen

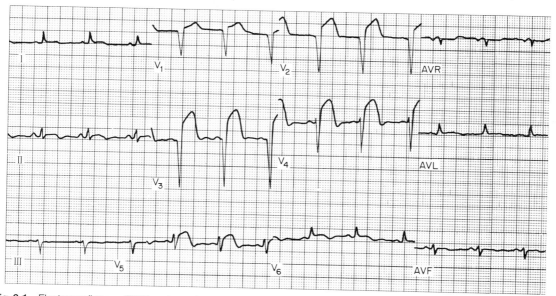

Fig. 9.1 Electrocardiogram (ECG) and anterior myocardial infarction. Note the salient changes are in lead I and AVL. These are exaggerated in the chest leads. There is also poor progression of the R waves. The QRS complex should be upright by V_4 but is still negative by V_5. This is characteristic of an anterior myocardial infarction.

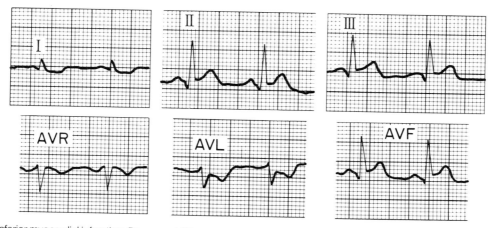

Fig. 9.2 Inferior myocardial infarction. Depressed ST segment in lead I and AVL with reciprocal elevation of the ST segment in leads II, III and AVF.

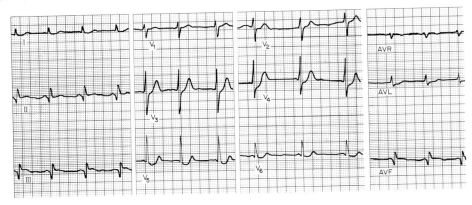

Fig. 9.3 Inferior myocardial infarction showing changes less clearly. Note that the V leads exaggerate the changes in lead I.

in lead I, the diagnosis is anterior infarction, and if these signs are seen in lead III, the diagnosis is inferior infarction (Figs. 9.2 and 9.3).

In 'true posterior infarction', the ECG changes that occur can be observed clearly only in an oesophageal lead. They can be seen as reciprocal changes in the anterior chest leads. The significant ECG changes are an increase in the height of the R waves in the right precordial leads V_{3R}, V_1, V_2, and V_3. There is no Q wave preceding the R wave but the width of the R wave may be increased to 0.14 seconds or more in V_1 and V_2.

Diagnostic tests

The presence of myocardial infarction may be confirmed in difficult cases by the use of biochemical investigations, although in the case of a moderate or minor degree of myocardial damage, the values may be normal.

The serum glutamic oxalo-acetic transaminase (SGOT) level rises above the normal value of 40 units after the first 24 hours and returns to normal 5–6 days later.

The lactic dehydrogenase (LDH) level may be raised 48 hours after the onset of coronary occlusion and may remain raised for 10–12 days. Its normal value is 350–400 units, and after coronary occlusion it often rises above 600 units.

It is now clear that LDH is formed from at least five components called isoenzymes which may themselves be specific for a number of different organs or tissues. The isoenzymes act on the same substrata and act in an identical manner but have different physicochemical characteristics, and can therefore be distinguished.

The hydroxybutyrate dehydrogenase fraction (HBD) is increased in myocardial infarction to a similar degree to the rise of SGOT, and the increased concentration persists for a longer period of time.

Creatine phosphokinase (CPK) is an enzyme which rises in concentration* soon after myocardial infarction[157] and is of value especially when hepatic dysfunction is suspected and the rise in SGOT may be from that cause.

On the second or third day there is a neutrophil leucocytosis and a raised erythrocyte sedimentation rate (ESR) which remains raised for 6 weeks or more and is a guide to the progress made in healing.

Treatment

In the acute stage of myocardial infarction, the main concern should be to relieve the pain, to oxygenate the blood, to counteract the shock that may be present, to protect against the development of arrhythmias and to relieve the psychological and physical stress so that the effects of the coronary occlusion upon the myocardium are not increased.[40] There is increasing evidence that we can add the limitation of infarct size to this list.

Relief of pain

In Europe many clinicians believe that the analgesic of choice is diacetyl-morphine (heroin) given intramuscularly in doses of 10 mg i.m. every

---

* The brain contains the largest amount of CPK in the body; there are also large amounts in skeletal muscle. Following trauma or cerebrovascular accident, misleading values may be obtained. Erythrocytes contain large quantities of LDH; haemolysis therefore results in high blood concentrations of this enzyme.

4 hours. An alternative is morphine sulphate. If the pain is severe, 5–10 mg morphine sulphate should be given intravenously at a very slow rate. If the pain is less severe, 15 mg of morphine sulphate can be given intramuscularly or subcutaneously. Alternative analgesics are pethidine HCl (meperidine, Demerol, Dolantin) 100 mg and papaveretum (Omnopon) 22 mg. If these preparations cause nausea or vomiting, an antihistamine, such as promethazine HCl (Phenergan) 25 mg, will help to counteract it and assist in sedation. Alternative preparations are promethazine theoclate (Avomine) 25 mg by mouth, and dimenhydrinate (Dramamine) 50 mg p.o. or i.m. While perphenazine (Fentazin, Trilafon) 5 mg i.m. or 2–8 mg p.o. may be equally effective, chlorpromazine (Thorazine, Largactil) should be avoided because, in addition to causing jaundice, it may produce hypotension.

Promazine HCl (Sparine) is also a useful method of suppressing nausea and vomiting, but it is *contraindicated* in coronary artery disease, and when given intramuscularly, it can also produce hypotension. Diazepam (Valium) 5–10 mg can be given either intravenously or intramuscularly to relieve both nausea and anxiety; a smaller dose of analgesic is then sometimes required. Metoclopramide HCl (Maxolon) 10–15 mg is also effective.

Oxygen

Following myocardial infarction, almost all patients are found to have a reduced arterial PO_2. Because of hyperventilation and the greater diffusability of CO_2, the carbon dioxide tension (PCO_2) is low and does not rise unless severe pulmonary oedema develops. For this reason, high concentrations of O_2 (e.g. 100%) can be given at high flow rates.

When oxygen is given, the relief of pain is sometimes marked. This can be observed when oxygen is administered through nasal tubes and mask. Another form of administering oxygen is by means of a high-pressure tank (see p. 277). Oxygen administration also assists in the relief of dyspnoea, which is sometimes also relieved by the intravenous injection of theophylline–ethylenediamine (aminophylline, Cardophyllin, Euphyllin) 0.5–1.0 g given very slowly. It may also sometimes relieve pain.

Protection against arrhythmias and sudden death

Approximately 60% of those patients who die do so before they reach hospital and 50% die before receiving medical attention. Almost 80% of the deaths in the Oxford study occurred before 8 hours had passed following the onset of symptoms.[78] We

are therefore looking at a selected group, and the sooner treatment is initiated the better.

One general practitioner study developed a protocol which included:

injection of morphine, 7.5 mg i.v.,
injection of atropine, 0.6 mg, if the pulse was less than 60/minute,
injection of lignocaine (lidocaine, xylocaine) 100 mg i.v. and 200 mg i.m.

For patients under 70 years of age, a marked reduction in the expected death rate was achieved without the use of a Pantridge-type (Pantridge and Geddes, 1967)[112] resuscitation ambulance which has proved to be effective. Of the 115 patients seen within 1 hour of the onset of acute myocardial infarction, only two developed ventricular fibrillation and neither of those had the antiarrhythmic medication described above. The plasma concentration of lignocaine (lidocaine) following an intravenous dose of 100 mg and an intramuscular dose of 200 mg, given into the deltoid, was investigated by Barber *et al.* (1977).[4] They found that the plasma concentrations of lignocaine that resulted from this regimen were maintained at therapeutic levels which were sufficient to provide protection from ventricular arrhythmias for a sufficient length of time to allow transit to hospital. An infusion of lignocaine (see p. 310) can also be given following 100–200 mg i.v. (5–10 ml of the 2% solution).

Nifedipine

Nifedipine (Adalat) is a Ca^{++} antagonist acting on phase 2 of the action potential (see p. 30). It also relieves coronary artery spasm (Richmond, 1980),[118] is effective in the treatment for angina, and may be of value in the treatment and relief of myocardial infarction (British Medical Journal, 1979).[15] It has been found that, experimentally, both nifedipine and verapamil (Cordilox) have a protective effect following myocardial infarction. Nifedipine HCl is available in capsules containing 5 or 10 mg. When a rapid effect is required, the capsule can be bitten and the solution is first held in the mouth and then swallowed.

Improved haemodynamic effects were found (Matsumoto *et al.*, 1980)[100] following a single sublingual dose of 20 mg of nifedipine in patients suffering from congestive cardiac failure. Cardiac output (index) increased and systemic vascular resistance decreased.

Although nifedipine was widely used in the treatment of angina pectoris (Opie, 1980),[109] there is the danger that it may give rise to hyperglycaemia. Severe diabetes of maturity onset type has been reported by Charles et al. (1981).[20] Nifedipine-induced impairment of insulin secretion has been reported by Giugliano et al. (1980).[51] Hepatotoxicity has also been reported (Brodsky et al., 1981).[16]

Although nifedipine causes effective vasodilation unlike verapamil and diltiazem (see p. 332), nifedipine has little or no effect on the SA and AV nodes, and is therefore largely ineffective as an antiarrhythmic agent under these circumstances.

Amiodarone

Amiodarone (see p. 332), which does not have a negative inotropic effect and therefore does not contribute to cardiogenic shock, may be an effective antiarrhythmic agent following myocardial infarction.

Flecainide acetate (Tambocor)

This antiarrhythmic agent can be given orally in doses of 200–400 mg/day. It can also be given by intravenous injection very slowly in doses of 2 mg/kg body weight following dilution, preferably by a constant infusion pump.

Flecainide acetate is used for controlling ventricular arrhythmias and, because it can be given orally, is an extremely useful therapeutic agent. The main effects of flecainide are on the His–Purkinje and intraventricular conduction systems of the myocardium.[61] The effect upon the atrioventricular (AV) node is less pronounced and it seems to have virtually no effect on the sinoatrial (SA) node in the healthy heart. Its effect on the SA node in the condition known as sick sinus syndrome is less predictable.

It has a marked effect on conduction through accessory pathways and therefore upon re-entry arrhythmias in general. It has been demonstrated to have an ability to suppress retrograde conduction through accessory pathways (Hellestrand, 1981).[61] Abitbol et al. (1983)[1] found it to be a very valuable agent when given intravenously for the suppression of ventricular extrasystoles. When taken orally over a long period of time it may give rise to maniacal paranoia.

Tocainide

This agent also can be used for controlling ventricular arrhythmias (see p. 289). This agent should be used to treat life threatening arrhythmias only because of its tendency to produce neutropenia, agranulocytosis, thrombocytopenia, and aplastic anaemia.

Myocardial infarction in the younger patient

When acute myocardial infarction occurs in the third and fourth decade, a frequent cause is familial hyperlipidaemia. There is usually a history of early death occurring in the father and uncles of the patient, and routine screening would permit treatment and diet to at least delay, and sometimes avoid, an early demise.

There is not, however, always a typical family history. In one case of a young naval officer who died in his early thirties (triple vessel disease was found at post mortem), his grandfather (an admiral) was then aged 90 years and his father who suffered from angina, was aged 67 years. It was essential to investigate the naval officer's older brother, with regard to his lipid profile. He was found also to have hyperlipidaemia, but with diet and treatment he has survived and was alive 10 years later.

Myocardial infarction and sudden death do occur as a result of congenital abnormalities in the coronary vessels. Adulthood can be reached and athletic prowess can be demonstrated, but myocardial infarction occurs during a long run or other forms of intense physical effort.

Other causes of myocardial infarction in the young include inborn errors of metabolism. One condition which leads to myocardial infarction in the 20–30-year age-group is Fabry's disease, an inherited disorder of glycolipid metabolism.[165] The deficit is a deficiency of ceramide trihexosidase which is confined to the lysozyme. This particular sphingolipid is found in high concentrations in the arterial walls, red cell membranes and peripheral nerves. It is not found in central nervous tissue, so that when, because of the enzyme deficiency, lysozymal (ceramide trihexosidase) storage disease develops, mental retardation is not a feature, nor is splenomegaly or hepatomegaly. There is saccular dilatation of blood vessels. Angiokeratomata are found around the eyes, periumbilical and scrotal areas, skin of the chest and abdominal walls. In some areas it is not uncommon: in Houston, Texas, USA there are approximately 20 cases of Fabry's disease in a population of 1.2 million (Zeluff et al., 1978).[165]

When Underwood et al. (1985)[144] examined coronary artery disease in 88 men and 13 women below the age of 30 years, the obstructive coronary artery disease having been proven angiographically, they were able to identify clear risk factors. Cigarette smoking was one risk factor, family history of coronary artery disease was another. Serum cholesterol values were significantly higher in the group of patients with coronary artery disease. The 5 year mortality was 20%.

Right Ventricular Infarction

Although isolated infarction of the right ventricle is relatively rare, it occurs in 2.5% (Wartman and Hellerstein, 1948)[150] to 4.6% (Yater *et al.*, 1948) of the population.[164] Involvement of the right ventricular muscle in association with left ventricular infarction is found with much greater frequency. Right myocardial infarction was found to be present in 34% of post-mortems by Rotman *et al.* (1974)[123] and in 43% by Erhardt (1974).[41] The development of radionuclide imaging of infarcts using m99-technicium pyrophosphate has indicated that 37.5% of patients who have suffered inferior left ventricular infarction have right ventricular involvement (Wackers *et al.*, 1978).[149] The view has therefore been expressed that at least one-third of patients who have had an inferior myocardial infarction also have infarction of the right ventricle (Braunwald, 1980).[14]

Blood supply of the right ventricle

This has been studied in detail by Farrer-Brown (1968)[44] in both normal and infarcted hearts. The major part of the free wall of the right ventricle is supplied by the right coronary artery. The anterior portion of the free wall is supplied by the anterior descending branch of the left coronary artery, which also contributes to the blood supply of the anterior papillary muscle of the tricuspid valve.

In the majority (85%) of patients, the infero-posterior wall of the right ventricle receives a more tenuous blood supply from the posterior descending branch of the right coronary artery. In approximately 15% of patients a contribution to the supply of this area of muscle arises from the circumflex branch of the left coronary artery.

It is therefore the infero-posterior wall of the right ventricle that is most vulnerable when there is partial occlusion of the right coronary vessel along its length and there is no added supply from the circumflex branch of the left coronary artery.

Physical signs and diagnosis of right ventricular myocardial infarction

The characteristic ischaemic pain and rise in blood enzyme activities, hypotension, cold peripheries and tachycardia are present. There is a right ventricular 3rd heart sound. Kussmaul's sign* and

---

* Kussmaul's sign is an *increase* in peripheral venous distension and pressure occurring during *inspiration*. This is a truly paradoxical sign and can also be seen during cardiac tamponade.

pulsus paradoxus may be present. The ECG changes are those of inferior myocardial infarction.

The jugular venous pressure (JVP) is significantly raised but pulmonary oedema is absent. Chest X-ray can be used to confirm that the lung fields are clear and free from congestion.

Some clinicians have placed emphasis upon a right precordial lead placed in the 5th intercostal space in the mid-clavicular line demonstrating ST elevation.[42] Others have placed more emphasis on non-invasive, radionuclide investigations or direct right heart catheterization comparing pulmonary artery pressure, which is raised, with pulmonary artery wedge pressure, which is normal. A thermo-dilatation probe can confirm the low cardiac output.

It is necessary, however, to differentiate right ventricular infarction from two other conditions. The three cardinal signs, low cardiac output, a raised CVP (and JVP) and the conspicuous absence of pulmonary oedema, also occur in cardiac tamponade and constrictive pericarditis. Flow-directed right heart catheterization, combined if necessary with angiography, is probably the only certain method of making the differentiation.

Treatment of Arrhythmias Following Myocardial Infarction

Sinus tachycardia

This arrhythmia, although perhaps benign in its appearance, commonly has a serious prognosis. In the very early stages it should be determined that extracardiac causes, such as anoxia, anaemia, hyperthyroidism, pain and anxiety, can be excluded. It is important to establish that hypovolaemia is not present and that congestive cardiac failure is not developing. Most of these factors can be differentiated by means of a central pressure line. Treatment with a beta-blocker, such as propranolol (Inderal) given in doses of 10 mg t.d.s. p.o. in the initial phases, usually effectively decreases the tachycardia; it has a prophylactic effect with regard to the development of arrhythmias, and in this dose usually does not produce marked vasoconstriction and cold peripheries. An initial loading dose of 20 mg is sometimes advisable. Digitalization can also be used if necessary.

Sinus bradycardia

This arrhythmia occurs most commonly following diaphragmatic or inferior wall myocardial infarction. In a number of cases the bradycardia is transient; sometimes it lasts for only a few minutes. However, the bradycardia is sometimes persistent and associated with severe hypotension. Because a severe bradycardia may be associated with decreased flow in the non-occluded coronary vessels, even in the absence of bradycardic shock, early treatment of the arrhythmia should be instituted. An intravenous injection of 0.6 mg of atropine will usually increase the heart rate and raise the blood pressure. If this dose is ineffective, it can be repeated immediately and a further 1 mg can be given after 10 minutes. If treatment with atropine is totally ineffective, an intravenous infusion of isoprenaline (isoproterenol), 5 mg in 1 litre of 5% glucose, or the insertion of a temporary pacemaker becomes essential.

Atrial arrhythmias

If the ventricular rate produced by the atrial arrhythmia is rapid, for example 140 beats/minute or more, it is frequently associated with hypotension. If the degree of hypotension is severe, synchronized electric cardioversion becomes necessary (see p. 403).

If cardioversion is not possible and if the ventricular rate is less than 140 beats/minute and the patient is not hypotensive or haemodynamically unstable, relatively slow intravenous digitalization can be commenced. In the digitalized patient, the original oral dose is given in such a way that toxicity is not produced, and the amount given will depend upon the dosage prior to the onset of myocardial infarction.

In the non-digitalized patient, an initial dose of 0.5 mg of digoxin can be given intravenously with additional doses of 0.25 mg every 2–4 hours until a ventricular response of less than 90 beats/minute has been achieved. Slowing of the heart rate can be assisted by the administration of a beta-blocker, for example propranolol, in the doses recommended above. If atrial flutter is present, cardioversion is probably the treatment of choice. However, this arrhythmia usually responds to an electrical charge of less than 100 joules (watt-seconds), for example 25 joules.

Ventricular arrhythmias

The danger of a ventricular extrasystole falling at the vulnerable part of the cardiac cycle, the downstroke of the T-wave (see p. 313), makes the early treatment with antiarrhythmic agents essential. If, however, numerous ventricular extrasystoles have developed, lignocaine should be given intra-venously in doses of 100–200 mg. This should be followed by an intravenous infusion so that lignocaine is infused at a rate of 2–4 mg/minute. The above regimen may be reinforced from time to time by an intravenous injection of lignocaine if 'R on T' is threatened.

In addition to propranolol, phenytoin (diphenylhydantoin, Dilantin) may be of value, and it is given orally in doses of 100 mg. The sodium salt of diphenylhydantoin (phenytoin sodium, Epanutin, Dilantin) can be given parenterally in doses of 100 mg.

Procainamide (Pronestyl) has been successfully used both orally and intravenously for the treatment of arrhythmias and for prophylaxis. It can be given in doses of 250 mg every 4–6 hours. It can also be given intramuscularly in doses of 100–250 mg every 4–6 hours. To be effective, a plasma concentration of 4–8 μg/ml should be maintained so that the heavier the person, the larger the dose given and the more frequently the dose is given.

The adrenergic beta-blocking drugs have been shown to reduce mortality in the presence of severe myocardial ischaemia. Propranolol (Inderal) given orally immediately following myocardial infarction in a dose of 20 mg and followed by 10 mg t.d.s. or q.d.s. tends to reduce the attacks of pain and has a prophylactic effect. Propranolol should not be given intravenously in a dose which is greater than 1 mg. Practolol, which has been withdrawn for prolonged oral use, is effective in doses of 5 mg.

Disopyramide phosphate (Norpace) has also been used prophylactically against arrhythmias, it was given orally, initially 300 mg and followed by 1.5 mg q.d.s. It should be discontinued in cases of partial or complete heart block.

Mexiletine (Mexitil), which should be given orally except when a close and careful control can be maintained, when it can be given intravenously. It has been shown to prevent ventricular arrhythmias (Achuff *et al.*, 1975)[2] and is active when lignocaine is ineffective. An initial dose of 400 mg is given, followed by 250 mg every 8 hours. When given intravenously at a rate which is too rapid, mexiletine may produce convulsions.

Bretylium tosylate (Bretylate) may prove to be of value in the avoidance of ventricular arrhythmia following myocardial infarction because it is known to convert arrhythmias which are resistant to other forms of treatment (see p. 333). It can be given intramuscularly in doses of 5 mg/kg body weight, so that a 70-kg man would require 350 mg i.m., but it has been given successfully intravenously in doses of 500 mg at a very slow rate.

Tocainide is an antiarrhythmic agent that is structurally related to lignocaine (lidocaine, Xylocaine), and it is active when taken orally. The substance was found to abolish ventricular ectopic complexes produced in the dog by ouabain when the tocainide plasma level was greater than 11.7 μg/ml (Moore *et al.*, 1978).[107] Tocainide was also found to increase the ventricular fibrillation threshold when the plasma level was 48 μg/ml, and it depressed AV nodal conduction. However, it produced no change in His–Purkinje or ventricular muscle conduction. Ligation of the coronary arteries in the dog also demonstrated its antiarrhythmic activity and it was found to decrease the duration of action potential and the effective refractory period. Other workers have also found that tocainide is an active oral antiarrhythmic agent (Lalka *et al.*, 1976; Winkle *et al.*, 1976; Coltart *et al.*, 1974).[22,82,160] Tocainide does, however, produce several side-effects in sensitive patients. An interstitial pneumonitis can develop for example, over a relatively short period of time (Perlow *et al.*, 1981).[113] It has been demonstrated that blood dyscrasias also develop, including aplastic anaemia. Its use should therefore be confined to life threatening arrhythmias.

Amiodarone (see p. 332) is also an effective agent for the treatment of ventricular arrhythmias and is being used with increasing frequency.

Flecainide and encainide have also been used to control ventricular arrhythmias.

Digitalis glycosides

Digitalis is not normally given at the onset of myocardial infarction. It is not always necessary to give digitalis even after cardiac arrest, for often a satisfactory blood pressure and normal cardiac rhythm can be maintained after cardiac arrest, open chest cardiac massage and a difficult resuscitative period. If good progress is being made, administration of digitalis is therefore unnecessary. Intravenous digoxin can, however, have a profound effect on cardiogenic shock in man (Cronin *et al.* 1965)[24] and this is supported by experimental evidence (Cronin and Zsotér, 1965).[25] Digitalis is therefore given when it is necessary to treat heart failure, to improve myocardial contraction and to treat arrhythmias. It is only during the past decade that digitalis has been demonstrated to have a positive inotropic effect when the heart is in sinus rhythm.

Except when digitalis or one of its preparations has been given during the previous 5–6 weeks, intravenous digitalization may be indicated in profound cardiogenic shock. Acute coronary insufficiency may, however, give rise to a sinus bradycardia (e.g. of 45 beats/minute) and further slowing of the heart may follow digitalization. If the bradycardia does not respond to atropine 1.2 mg i.v., digitalis should be withheld.

The preparation that has a most rapid action intravenously, but is too unreliable to administer orally, is ouabain. The digitalizing dose of this substance is 0.25–0.75 mg. It is prepared in ampoules containing 0.25 mg. It should never be used for maintaining digitalization orally because its absorption from the gut is so unpredictable. The next most effective preparation given intravenously is digoxin (Lanoxin), dose 0.75–1 mg; ampoules are prepared containing 0.25 or 0.5 mg. Digoxin is rapidly absorbed from the gut and like digitoxin it is suitable for oral administration for maintenance purposes; digitoxin is less likely to cause vomiting when this is a problem. For each patient the maintenance doses of these substances must be discovered by trial and error, partly because of the rate of elimination and also because of some variance in the degree of absorption from the gut. Digitoxin is almost completely absorbed. The maintenance doses are digoxin 0.25–0.75 mg/day and digitoxin 0.05–0.2 mg/day. Other preparations that may be used are lanatoside C (Deslanoside, Cedilanid), digitalizing dose 6–8 mg, maintenance dose 0.5–0.75 mg every 24 hours.

The action of digitalis is potentiated by calcium ions. Injections of calcium gluconate or calcium chloride during profound cardiogenic shock may have a most dramatic effect on relieving this condition. The rapid injection of either of these compounds, especially in the acidotic patient, is not without its dangers, for it may in its own right give rise to ventricular fibrillation or arrest. On the other hand, it is well recognized that a spontaneous reversion to a normal rhythm has followed the use of calcium salts, especially when the salts are injected directly into the fibrillating heart. The rule, therefore, in cardiogenic shock should be to inject slowly intravenously, the 10% solution of the calcium salt. A fall in the potassium concentration of the plasma results in increased sensitivity to digitalis and this factor must be remembered if the total body potassium has been reduced by malnutrition or prolonged diuretic therapy.

Amrinone

Because digitalis has such a weak inotropic action and because its therapeutic levels in the body are so close to its toxic levels, an alternative substance with a positive inotropic effect has been sought and a number of agents are now being evaluated. Amrinone, which is one of these, does not act in the same way as the glycosides of digitalis, nor does it act by stimulating the beta adrenergic receptors; it appears to act primarily as an inhibitor of phosphodiesterase. When given intravenously, either as a bolus, 2 mg/kg or by an infusion over 12 hours of 2 μg/kg per minute, it has been found to be of benefit in cardiogenic shock and congestive cardiac failure. It has also been given in the treatment of left ventricular failure following myocardial infarction. It may be of value therefore when it is indicated that digitalis should not be used because of its propensity to generate arrhythmias. A review of a Symposium on Amrinone has been published.*

A small number of patients have been noted to develop thrombocytopenia, and other complications include pyrexia, gastro-intestinal discomfort and changes in liver enzymes.

Anticoagulants

Intravenous heparin is given during the first 24–72 hours in doses which summate to 20 000 units/day. Heparin is best administered in a small-volume intravenous drip or by means of a constant infusion pump.

Anticoagulation can be begun with phenindione, 75 mg b.d., and later the dosage, usually 50 mg b.d., is controlled by the laboratory estimation of prothrombin time. The prothrombin time should be two to two-and-a-half times the normal value.

Phenindione is begun 24 hours before stopping treatment with heparin.

The other two anticoagulants which are commonly used are bishydroxycoumarin (Dicumarol) and warfarin (Coumadin). The action of bishydroxycoumarin usually reaches its peak 36–48 hours after beginning treatment. It is supplied in tablets and capsules containing 25, 50 and 100 mg. The maintenance dose is usually between 37.5 mg and 75 mg daily, given in the afternoon following measurement of the prothrombin time. Warfarin reaches its peak 24–36 hours after administration. It is supplied in tablets ranging from 2 mg to 25 mg. The maintenance dose lies between 2 mg and 15 mg daily. In the author's opinion, control is more

easily obtained with warfarin, and this substance has the added advantage that it can be given intravenously or intramuscularly, usually in the same dosage. Unfortunately, there is a rare complication associated with warfarin. This results in thrombosis over a relatively large area (the size of a hand or more) of the vessels in the superficial layers of the skin. When seen it is quite dramatic, with black necrotic areas on the thighs, arms and elsewhere. Immediate withdrawal of warfarin usually results in complete recovery. Numerous other reactions occur including pyrexia, jaundice, leucopenia, thrombocytopenia, nausea, vomiting and diarrhoea, but these are not common.

Antidotes

The antidote for heparin is protamine, which is given intravenously, diluted so that the solution contains 2 mg/ml. It is given in a dose that is equivalent to 50% of the last dose of heparin. A maximum dose of 100 mg is given because in excessive doses protamine itself can act as an anticoagulant. When a continuous infusion of heparin has been used, small doses, for example 5–10 mg, are given and the prothrombin time is measured.

The antidote for the coumarin derivatives is vitamin K_1 (phytomenadione). It can be given orally, but when parenteral administration is required it is given intramuscularly in doses of 10–20 mg. When it is essential to administer the preparation intravenously, it is given slowly over 10–15 minutes in doses of 10–25 mg, preferably diluted. Even with a very slow infusion, rigors, pyrexia, sweating and discomfort in the chest may not be avoided. Very rarely, hypotension and convulsions occur. The effect is not rapid, and 4 hours or longer are required before a significant reversal of the anticoagulant is obtained.

Treatment of shock

The patient is restless, cold to the touch and has a clammy skin and a low or unrecordable blood pressure. The pulse is rapid and may be impalpable at the wrist. Without special treatment severe shock is almost always fatal. Therefore, pressor agents in some form are advisable and enthusiastically advocated by some clinicians. Of those pressor agents listed on page 226 it is possible to suggest methylamphetamine, mephentermine, phenylephrine, methoxamine, metaraminol be used in order of preference. If these preparations are ineffective, intravenous drip of *l*-noradrenaline

* Braunwald, E. (1985). A Symposium: Amrinone. *Amer. J. Cardiol.*, **56**, 1B.

should be tried. The positive inotropic agent amrinone (see page 289) has also been used intravenously in cardiogenic shock.

l-Noradrenaline (*l*-norepinephrine, Levophed)

This solution can be infused in strengths varying from 8 to 72 mg/l. The ampoules of *l*-noradrenaline are usually supplied so that they can contain 2 mg/ml, and each ampoule contains 4 ml of solution. It is usual to dilute 3–4 ampoules in a litre of normal (0.9%) saline, so that in most cases the drip can be run at a slow rate and therefore not overload the body with a large volume of fluid. This is especially important when oliguria follows profound hypotension. The solution should be given at the rate of 10–30 drops/minute and, because intense venospasm may occur if the solution is given into a small peripheral vein, it should ideally be administered through a long polythene catheter, if necessary into the inferior vena cava. To avoid clotting within the catheter when the drip is being run slowly, 1 ml of heparin (1000 units/ml) can be added to the 0.9% saline solution. Extravasation of *l*-noradrenaline around the vein can cause sloughing of the skin. Damage to the skin can be avoided by injecting subcutaneously phentolamine hydrochloride (Rogitine) 5–10 mg in 10–20 ml of normal saline, together with 3–4 ml of procaine HCl 1% around the site.

Angiotensin is an alternative vasopressor, but there is conflicting evidence about its possible vasoconstrictor effects upon the pulmonary circulation. It is added to physiological saline or glucose solutions in doses of 1–2 mg/l and infused at a rate such that it maintains the systolic blood pressure above 90 mmHg.

Isoprenaline (isoproterenol, Suscardia, Saventrine) has been used successfully in cardiogenic shock following myocardial infarction (MacLean et al., 1965; Eichna, 1967; Carey et al., 1967; Talley et al., 1969).[19,32,96,139] It acts on the beta₁- and beta₂-adrenergic receptors and therefore produces vasodilatation and sometimes a fall in blood pressure. It causes little change in renal blood flow (Rosenblum et al., 1968).[120] Not all clinicians have found it to be of value (Gunnar et al., 1967; Smith et al., 1967).[54,133] The author's own experience has confirmed these diverging views that isoprenaline (isoproterenol, Suscardia, Saventrine) is readily effective in some patients and unpredictably ineffective in others. As reported by other workers (Talley et al., 1969),[139] a combination of dopamine (Intropin) and isoprenaline has succeeded in raising the blood pressure when neither agent used alone has been effective.

Dopamine (Intropin), however, is a vasopressor agent that is being used successfully and has a vasodilatory effect on the pulmonary, renal and mesenteric vascular bed.[119,121,127] It was observed by Horwitz et al. (1962)[67] that this catecholamine produced an increase in cardiac output in normal subjects without increasing either the heart rate or the peripheral resistance. It has been used successfully in cardiogenic shock (Holzer et al., 1973).[65] It is added to physiological glucose or saline solutions in doses of 40–80 mg/l and infused at a rate which raises the blood pressure, usually between 4 and 60 µg/kg body weight. At the higher rate of infusion, some vasoconstriction may be produced.

Dobutamine is another inotropic agent that acts directly on the beta₁-adrenergic receptors producing an increase in cardiac output. The beta₂- and alpha-adrenergic actions are markedly less than those of either noradrenaline (norepinephrine) or isoprenaline (isoproterenol) and have no direct action on dopamine receptors. It has been found that following myocardial infarction (Gillespie et al., 1977)[50] there was an increase in cardiac output with no significant increase in heart rate. Dobutamine is infused at a rate of 2.5–10 µg/kg per minute and has been used successfully after open heart surgery (Sakamoto and Yomada, 1977).[125]

Glucagon, which is also used in the treatment of hypoglycaemic coma, has been known for many years to have a positive inotropic effect. It appears to act via the beta-adrenergic receptors and augments the action of both beta-receptor agonists and digoxin. It is active on the denervated heart following cardiac transplant, having both a positive inotropic and chronotropic effect. It appears to have little action on the vascular bed. Following myocardial infarction glucagon has a prolonged action upon the heart, largely improving the force of contraction (Gunnar and Loeb, 1972; Berk, 1975).[9,53] It is infused at the rate of 3–5 mg/hour. A single injection of 10 mg i.v. is sometimes effective in raising the blood pressure.

Corticosteroids

Intravenous hydrocortisone in large doses may have a profound effect on hypotension resulting from myocardial insufficiency following infarction; it often potentiates the action of pressor agents. If corticosteroids have been administered to the patient during the past 2 years, intravenous hydrocortisone should be given routinely. Initially, 100 mg i.v. should be given and doses of this size repeated at 10-minute intervals until 300 mg have been given; 100 mg i.v. can then be given every 2 hours for a further four or five doses.

Corticosteroids have been used prophylactically in patients who have received earlier corticosteroid treatment; a positive inotropic effect, possibly mediated by catecholamines, has also been reported. Peripheral vasodilatation has been considered a more important factor in the beneficial effect of corticosteroids than the stabilization of the cell membranes and the protection of the mitochondria, although they do afford some protection to the mitochondria (Altura and Altura, 1974; Haglund, 1974; Spath *et al.*, 1974).[3,55,136] Some experimental work has indicated that corticosteroids are of benefit only if administered within 24 hours of the onset of myocardial infarction and the development of hypotension and may limit the size of the infarct (Maley *et al.*, 1966)[97] and reduce mortality (Barzilai *et al.*, 1972).[5] The author's own experience suggests that corticosteroids can sometimes have a dramatically beneficial effect in some patients, when given in large doses.

Hyperbaric oxygen in cardiogenic shock

Smith (1964)[132] has reported a case of shock resulting from myocardial infarction which improved markedly when exposed to air compressed at 2 atmospheres absolute,* breathing oxygen through a mask. The author's own experience with a Vicker's research model hyperbaric oxygen bed confirms the beneficial effects of this form of treatment reported by Moon *et al.* (1964).[106]

The patient is placed in the bed without myringotomy being performed, and the pressure is increased slowly using pure oxygen; the CO_2 evolved is absorbed. After cardiac infarction, bradycardia may occur if the pressure of oxygen is increased too rapidly, but this phenomenon usually disappears when the patient has been exposed to the raised pressure more than once or twice. It is highly effective in the presence of pulmonary oedema and makes the management of this type of case very much easier.

The bradycardia, when observed before the patient is placed in the hyperbaric oxygen tank, can be treated with atropine 0.4–1.2 mg i.v. When bradycardia develops after compression has taken place, no special treatment is usually necessary.

While today the conventional treatment for cardiac arrhythmias following acute myocardial

infarction is composed largely of anti-arrhythmic drugs and electrical cardioversion, we know that sometimes this is either unsuccessful or is not sustained except for a relatively short time. However, Hood *et al.* (1968)[66] reported a patient in whom neither procainamide nor quinidine was successful, but in whom hyperbaric oxygen maintained a satisfactory rhythm. This is similar to the author's experience and that of Thurston *et al.* (1973).[142]

Limitation of infarct size

Despite the long-standing use of nitroglycerin in the treatment of angina pectoris, there has been the view that this preparation should not be used to treat the ischaemic pain caused by myocardial infarction. This approach has been based on the belief that cardiac arrhythmias are more likely to occur following the use of nitroglycerin when myocardial damage is present than when only localized ischaemia has developed.

Furthermore, the reduction in arterial blood pressure and the associated reflex increase in heart rate which can exacerbate the degree of ischaemia have been frequently taken into consideration. These observations in man have been supported by experimental investigations which have shown that when hypotension was induced by haemorrhage following myocardial infarction (Smith *et al.*, 1973)[131] (for reflex stimulation of the carotid baroceptors, Thibault *et al.*, 1973),[141] the area of myocardial damage was increased. A simple increase in heart rate also occurs and is considered to be important in determining the extent to which myocardial ischaemia develops.

It is, however, significant that, more recently, the concept that nitroglycerin is contraindicated following acute myocardial infarction, has been challenged by the finding that the degree of myocardial damage and the intensity of the myocardial ischaemia are reduced when it is used (Smith *et al.*, 1973; Hirschfeld *et al.*, 1973).[62,131]

Kent *et al.* (1973)[77] infused nitroglycerin intravenously following occlusion of the left anterior descending coronary artery, approximately 2 cm from its origin. They found that the threshold for ventricular fibrillation was reduced by nitroglycerin and that it was further reduced when the blood pressure was maintained by infusions of either methoxamine or phenylephrine (see p. 227). They concluded that not only did nitroglycerin reduce the area of infarction, but it also enhanced the electrical stability of the heart during myocardial ischaemia, raising the threshold at which ventricular fibrillation developed.

---

* One atmosphere above the normal atmospheric pressure.

Puri (1974)[116] obtained similar findings in dogs. He came to the conclusion that both isoprenaline (isoproterenol) and methoxamine could increase the area of myocardial ischaemia but that nor-adrenaline (norepinephrine) and ouabain did not appear to induce this change. Isoprenaline in the early stages of the infusion appeared to have a beneficial effect when the contractility of the inter-mediate zone of the myocardial infarction was observed. In the later stages of the infusion, isoprenaline appeared to diminish contractility.

Sayen et al. (1960)[126] also observed that nor-adrenaline had a beneficial effect on the ischaemic area of the infarct. It must be remembered, how-ever, that all vasopressor agents and drugs that stimulate the myocardium can increase the size and extent of ischaemic injury by increasing myocardial oxygen consumption (Maroko et al., 1971).[98]

It would appear, however, that the combination of nitroglycerin and an alpha-adrenergic agonist may be of value in diminishing the area of myocardial ischaemia.

The investigations into timolol (Blocadren) indicate that this should be given as a drug of choice in the treatment of acute myocardial infarc-tion and in prophylaxis against the development of a fatal arrhythmia.

In 1971 Mather and his co-workers[99] compared the progress of two groups of patients; one group was treated at home and the other group was treated in hospital. There appeared to be no sig-nificant difference, in the results of treatment, between the two groups. There seems, therefore, to be no set pattern for treating the patient who has an uncomplicated myocardial infarction and, in Scotland, UK, it has been demonstrated that wide variations in the practice of individual clini-cians occur (Heaseman and Carstairs, 1971).[60] The period of immobilization is becoming progressively shorter. In many instances patients with uncom-plicated myocardial infarction can be allowed up and out of bed after 48 hours have elapsed from the time of onset, and therefore the management of the acute myocardial infarction may be advanc-ing so that it is less expensive and very much easier. This is perhaps more possible since the introduction of the antiarrhythmic drugs such as the beta-adrenergic blocking agents that can be used prophylactically.

Mobilization following myocardial infarction

As time has progressed, changing views have developed with regard to bed-rest following myocardial infarction. There is a much greater tendency towards early mobilization and a reduc-tion of the period of bed-rest to 1 or 2 days. This obviously applies to patients who have suffered an uncomplicated myocardial infarct, and not to those patients suffering from cardiogenic shock or from severe cardiac arrhythmias at the time of being seen. Nevertheless, this changing pattern of care must have some bearing on the approach to limiting exercise once the acute stage of myocardial infarction is over, even in those patients who have been severely affected.

In 1952, Levine and Lown reported the progress of 73 patients who had suffered myocardial infarc-tion and were mainly treated in armchairs with no ill-effects.[90] Duke (1971) reviewed the approach of different centres over the years, indicating the increasing brevity of the period of immobilization (Table 9.1).[31]

Prognostic factors

The Framingham studies, in which individuals have been investigated over a considerable period of time, have indicated that the lower the blood pressure (even within the 'normal' range), the lower the incidence of heart disease. This was indicated in its 18th year of continuous study (McGee and Gordon, 1976),[102] and has been con-firmed by further publications since that time.

A highly significant investigation can now be used for the prediction of coronary heart disease. Miller (1975) established that there was a correla-tion between the concentration of high-density lipoproteins and ischaemic heart disease.[103] This view was expanded in 1977 by Miller et al.,[104] and other studies, such as that of Rhoads et al. (1976)[117] and Stanhope et al. (1977),[138] have confirmed these findings. It would appear that the higher the concentration of high-density lipoproteins in the blood, the smaller the tendency to deposit atheroma and develop atherosclerotic heart disease (Miller and Miller, 1975).[103]

A number of prognostic indices have been produced which may be of some value in predict-ing the chances of recovery of an individual patient who has suffered myocardial infarction, but these are not reviewed specifically in this chapter.

The severity of hyponatraemia was found to be of value in predicting the severity of the infarction when 235 consecutive patients were investigated by Flear and Hilton (1979) while in the coronary care unit.[47]

The death rate from cardiac disease amongst diabetics is nearly twice that of non-diabetics. Approximately 50% of diabetic patients die from coronary heart disease. One of the major factors

Table 9.1 A review of previous recommendations for bedrest in acute myocardial infarction (after M. Duke, 1971, reprinted from *American Heart Journal*,[31] with permission).

Authors	Year	Recommendations
Lewis[91]	1937	8 weeks bedrest
Levine[88]	1940	4–8 weeks in bed
Levine[89]	1951	4–8 weeks at rest
Levine and Lown[90]	1952	63 of 73 patients in chair by third day
White[156]	1945	1 month bedrest
Irvin and Burgess[68]	1950	2 weeks in bed
Brummer et al.[18]	1956	16 days bedrest
Brummer et al.[17]	1961	12 days bedrest
Wood[162]	1960	3–6 weeks in bed
Wood[163]	1968	2 weeks in bed
Friedberg[49]	1966	2–3 weeks minimum bedrest
Lauper et al.[86]	1966	Armchair treatment beginning second week
Lal and Caroli[81]	1968	Ninth day in chair
Naughton et al.[108]	1969	Up for meals third day; up every 2 hours on fifth day

concerning heart disease in diabetic patients is that not only is the death rate higher but, when the disease occurs, its severity and its rate of progression are so much greater than that in non-diabetic patients.[12] The prognosis following myocardial infarction is also poor,[59,135] and approximately only 50% of those diabetic patients admitted to hospital having survived the initial attack are alive after 4 months.[134]

The development of atheroma and coronary heart disease in diabetics is less clearly understood than that of atheroma in non-diabetics, but such factors as obesity, hyperlipidaemia, hypertension, hypercoagulability of the blood and diseases of the small vessels which are apparent in the retina and elsewhere are probably contributing factors.[58,72,111]

One of the disturbing factors with regard to myocardial infarction in diabetic patients is that it is atypical. Quite commonly, approximately 30% of patients have no chest pain and, when pain is present, it is of a relatively minor character.[13,134] The slow, insidious progression of cardiac failure following the 'silent' myocardial degeneration is seen quite commonly.[26] Some authorities have regarded the painlessness of the ischaemic myocardial disease to be due to an autonomic neuropathy. Faerman et al. (1977)[43] have demonstrated, by detailed histological investigation of the heart of diabetics who died from painless myocardial infarction, that there was degeneration of the sympathetic and parasympathetic nerve fibres in all patients. Similar findings were not present in non-diabetic patients or in diabetics who died after painful myocardial infarction. That this auto-

nomic neuropathy was generalized throughout the body was evident from the findings that there were morphological similarities between the nerve endings in the heart and the abnormalities which had been found previously in the urinary bladder and corpora cavernosa of impotent diabetics (Faerman et al., 1977).[43]

Although cardiac enlargement and cardiac failure are developing in diabetics in the absence of any overt evidence of myocardial infarction, this is frequently due to numerous small infarcts caused by occlusion of the subdivisions of the main coronary vessels. There is evidence that small vessel disease within the myocardial wall is an important factor.[26]

The Differential Diagnosis of Chest Pain

Chest pain is a common presenting symptom and the decision as to whether the condition is of primary importance, even in the young, requires a careful history, a complete physical examination, a series of investigations (physiological and biochemical), and a conscious awareness of the risks associated with a misdiagnosis. Even in the absence of a family history of cardiac disease, severe myocardial ischaemia can be present in the early part of the third decade of life, and sometimes even earlier.

Chest pain can be divided usefully into two

separate entities:

1. pain of cardiac origin,
2. pain of non-cardiac origin.

Cardiac pain

This can occur because of occlusions of the coronary vessels, valve disease or pericarditis.

Angina pectoris

This pain arises because of a decreased blood supply to the myocardium resulting either from partial occlusion of the coronary vessels or from a reduced myocardial blood flow caused by stenosis of the aortic valve.

In its typical form angina pectoris is described as a heavy, crushing, constricting pain located under the sternum, radiating down the **left** arm, sometimes into the fingers. It can also, as in the pain of myocardial infarction, radiate into the neck, the jaw and teeth and the shoulders, sometimes radiating down both arms. It can also radiate into the abdomen, the pain coming on with exercise or excitement. In some instances, the retrosternal pain is absent and the pain is felt only in those sites to which it radiates. The pain may therefore have a shifting nature which can mislead the unwary physician and assuage the anxieties of the patient until it has progressed to a serious degree.

In its typical form, the chest pain is precipitated by exertion; the patient has to stop and rest until the pain disappears. The pain threshold is lowered by such things as eating, emotion, a low ambient temperature, smoking, and an associated disease, especially a condition that is related to a rise in body temperature. A low atmospheric oxygen tension, such as occurs at high altitude, or pneumonia can also initiate angina pectoris.

Relief of pain occurs with rest, the relief of anxiety, an equitable ambient temperature, increase in arterial oxygen tension and the use of sublingual glyceryl trinitrate. The last mentioned may be used as a diagnostic procedure as it may produce immediate relief.

Physical examination of the patient may reveal no abnormality whatsoever, especially when the patient is at rest. During an attack of pain the heart rate may be increased, the blood pressure raised and a 3rd or 4th heart sound may become audible. Most commonly, the 4th heart sound is audible and, if severe myocardial ischaemia is present, it may be palpable.

If the patient is exercised under controlled conditions with continuous monitoring of the ECG, changes in the ST segment and invertion of the T wave may be observed.

The natural progression of a patient with this form of so-called stable angina is for the exercise tolerance to be gradually decreased until cardiac pain occurs at rest. This is called crescendo angina. It is unfortunate that, because of the nature of the disease, angina may present for the first time following an unrelated surgical procedure or an acute infection and present the clinician with a problem with regard to both management and diagnosis.

Management

When the patient presents in the ordinary way, the conventional management is usually relatively simple and consists of reducing the significance of the related factors such as cessation of smoking, loss of weight, reduction of blood pressure, treatment of the hyperlipidaema, and treatment of the diabetes that may be associated. Acute attacks can be treated with glyceryl trinitrate and isosorbide dinitrate (Sorbitrate), which are long-acting nitrate preparations producing coronary vasodilatation. These preparations can be combined with beta-blocking drugs (see p. 375) which reduce myocardial oxygen consumption, effectively reduce the incidence of cardiac pain and also lower the blood pressure (Russek, 1968).[124] Verapamil and nifedipine reduce coronary artery spasm. The addition of one tablet, 120 mg/day, of verapamil, has been shown to increase exercise tolerance in patients receiving high doses of propranolol (Bassan et al., 1982).[6]

Unstable angina pectoris

In this condition the pain tends to be severe, making the patient unhesitatingly report his condition. It is sometimes sharp in character and may be mistaken for a muscular pain. It lasts for much longer and occurs more frequently than stable angina pectoris. It may be so severe that it causes the patient to wake up from sleep, even after sedation. When it occurs postoperatively, changes in the enzyme concentrations in the blood can be either misleading or of little value. In angina, the ECG is usually normal.

Prinzmetal angina

This is an attack of angina pectoris which is associated with severe and prolonged cardiac pain and is associated with a change in the ST segment of the ECG. Elevation or depression of the ST segment can and will vary according to the lead being monitored.[114,115] T wave inversion can also be seen and the ST changes may persist for as long as 48 hours before reverting to normal. The ECG changes are not associated with elevation of enzyme concentrations and, while they occur at rest, Prinzmetal angina can be induced by exercise under controlled conditions during constant monitoring. Under these circumstances the patient is exercised on either a treadmill or a bicycle ergometer. As many as 70% of patients with angina pectoris, who have had no prior myocardial infarction, can have a normal ECG at rest.

Myocardial infarction

In this condition the cardiac pain is usually severe, prolonged and associated with ECG changes and elevation of the cardiac enzymes and it may be associated with cardiac failure.

Small vessel coronary artery disease

The aetiology of small vessel disease is often not known. A number of factors do contribute to this condition, such as drug-induced vasculitis, and it is known to be associated with systemic lupus erythematosus. While small vessel coronary artery disease may be associated with smoking, there is some evidence that in women it can occasionally be related to the taking of oral contraceptives. Certainly, it is recognized that when myocardial infarction occurs in young women, extensive coronary artery disease need not be present.[35,153]

Obstruction to the coronary ostia

In addition to atherosclerosis, confined to the ostia, there are such conditions as syphilitic stenosis, coronary embolism and various forms of arteritis. All these conditions can resemble either angina or, with *transient* but acute occlusion of the vessel, myocardial infarction.

Pericarditis

The pain of pericarditis is different from that of myocardial infarction in that the presence of the pain, its intensity and the frequency with which it occurs are changed by the position of the body and by respiration. It is frequently exacerbated by deep respiration and may be felt in the chest, abdomen, or neck, and may be associated with a pericardial rub. The pericardial rub may, however, be transient and audible for only a very short time. The rub may be of pleuropericardial origin and sometimes can be heard only on deep inspiration. It is often audible in the axilla.

Pericarditis can occur after non-specific viral infections such as those affecting the lungs, after viral infection of the myocardium and pericardium, following trauma, as a result of biochemical changes such as uraemia, and as a result of various bacterial infections.

The Ebstein–Barr infection and Coxsackie viruses are examples of virus infections. Both the clinical signs and X-ray changes of a pericardial effusion may be present, and are more commonly seen following acute myocarditis caused by a viral, staphylococcal or tuberculous infection. Pericardial pain may also be seen in conditions such as leukaemia and collagen diseases.

The ECG shows elevation of the ST segment over a wide area. The changes are usually different from those that occur in myocardial infarction because the alterations in the ST segment are such that they tend to be concave upwards and there is little or no reciprocal depression in those leads which are directionally at right angles to those in which the major changes occur.

The cardiac enzymes are usually not raised to any marked degree, although slight elevations in some components are sometimes seen. Diagnosis is made by chest X-ray, physical signs and, more recently, by echocardiography.

Prolapse of the mitral valve

This is considered to be a condition associated with a defect of the chordae tendineae which allows one or both leaflets of the mitral valve to bulge into the left atrium during contraction of the left ventricle. The condition is more common in females and in those suffering from collagen diseases such as Marfan's syndrome. It produces the typical pain of angina pectoris during exercise which disappears with rest and is largely transient. It may be associated with varying supraventricular arrhythmias.

On auscultation, a midsystolic click may be heard; this is frequently associated with a pansystolic regurgitant mitral murmur. The midsystolic click may be single or multiple. Severe stenosis of the mitral valve rarely causes angina, although Adams-Stokes attacks can occur following vigorous exercise.

Non-cardiac chest pains

These include dissecting aneurysm, hiatus hernia, pleural pain, myositis and bone pain.

Dissecting aneurysm

A serious dissection of the thoracic aorta may occur insidiously with no associated chest pain and no significant symptoms. Conversely, it may present with severe chest pain radiating into both shoulders, the back, lower limbs and upwards towards the neck. It can occur spontaneously as a result of trauma and during cardiac catheterization. The pain is intense and the patient requires immediate sedation. The dissection can progress so that it involves the coronary arteries, producing acute occlusion, or it may rupture into the mediastinum and retroperitoneal tissues. Cardiac tamponade is associated with an abrupt fall in blood pressure. The dissection alone in the presence or absence of tamponade may be associated with a pleural effusion.

Chest X-ray may show widening of the mediastinum and aneurysmal dilatation of the ascending or descending aorta.

Oesophagitis and hiatus hernia
Because of its anatomical location, inflammatory processes in the oesophagus give rise to chest pain; this is deep in character, persistent and can be severe. It can be brought on or exacerbated by lying down, when the acid contents of the stomach regurgitate into the lumen of the oesophagus. This is sometimes the typical, physical sign of hiatus hernia.

There are usually no ECG or enzyme changes and relief is obtained by sitting up and by taking antacids. Diffuse oesophageal spasm of unknown aetiology may occur and may cause, in addition to severe chest pain, obstruction of the oesophagus resulting from a moderately large piece of food such as meat that has been swallowed. This spasm can be relieved by sublingual glyceryl trinitrate, resulting in misdiagnosis of the true cause.

Pleural pain
Inflammatory changes in the diaphragmatic pleura may present as pain in the shoulder, although most commonly pleural pain presents as pain in the chest wall. The pain is usually made worse by inspiration and can be felt when the position of the body is changed. Pleural pain may be felt in association with a partial pneumothorax and, even when this is not present, there may be an associated feeling of restlessness. Pulmonary embolus also produces pleural pain associated with haemoptysis cough, the symptoms and signs of pneumonic consolidation, and a feeling of tightness in the chest. A pleural rub is commonly present in association with pleural pain.

Diagnosis requires X-ray of the chest, investigations to determine the underlying cause which include haematology, serology, lung scan and, in the case of pulmonary embolism, pulmonary angiography.

Myositis
Various viral infections produce myositis of the intercostal muscles. This may be part of a generalized condition in which muscle pain and muscle tenderness are present, or it may be localized as in the case of the Coxsackie virus (Bornholm disease). These virus infections may or may not be associated with a myocarditis or a pericarditis.

Bone pain
Pain in the chest arising from the cervical and thoracic spines is common. It may occur following trauma or degenerative diseases involving the cervical spines or joints in the thoracic wall. The pain is often associated with a change in body position and is sometimes caused by exertion, but it is more closely related to movement. Commonly, degenerative changes may be found on X-ray, and localized tenderness may be elicited on percussion. Lipping of the cervical and thoracic spines, resulting from osteoarthritis, may be seen on X-ray.

Aortic valve disease
Severe aortic stenosis frequently gives rise to angina pectoris. It is commonly seen as a result of calcification having progressed on a congenitally bicuspid aortic valve, so that a marked pressure gradient exists (especially during systoles) between the left ventricle and the aortic arch, distal to the valve. It also follows calcific stenosis resulting from acute chronic rheumatic carditis.

Cardiac Arrhythmias

Sinus rhythm
The normal heart beat, referred to as sinus rhythm, is initiated by impulses which arise from the sino-atrial node (SA node) which is a group of specialized cells situated in the wall of the right atrium close to the junction of the superior vena cava (SVC) with this chamber. This node gives rise to impulses at an average rate of 70/minute and these spread through the muscle of both atria to the atrioventricular node (AV node) which is situated in the wall of the right atrium just above the opening of the coronary sinus.

Recently, the presence of specialized conducting fibres within the atria has been recognized.[71] These fibres are referred to as the middle, anterior and posterior internodal tracts (Fig. 9.4). The anterior tract has fibres that run towards and over

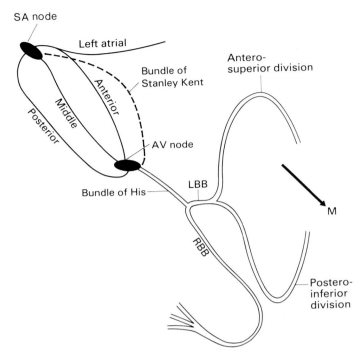

Fig. 9.4 This figure shows the SA node, the conducting bundles from the SA node to the left and right atria which converge upon the AV node, and the bundle of His which divides into a right bundle branch (RBB) and a main left bundle branch (LBB). The left bundle branch subdivides into an antero-superior division (which in life is much smaller than that shown in this diagram) and a left postero-inferior division. The mean spatial left ventricular vector (M) is in health a result of conduction through both divisions of the left bundle and passes to the left, usually slightly downwards and slightly backwards. Damage or ischaemia of either of these divisions results in the hemiblock. The dotted pathway represents an 'accessory pathway' such as the bundle of Stanley–Kent which can bypass the delay that occurs at the AV node resulting in Wolff–Parkinson–White syndrome and other pre-excitation phenomena.

the left atrium as well as towards the AV node. The names given to these tracts or bundles are Wenckebach's, Thorel's and Bachman's, respectively.

The impulse causing contraction of the atria produces the P wave. When the impulse arrives at the AV node (the composition of which was described by Tawara in 1906),[140] the conduction velocity is decreased. The slowing of the impulse and resulting delay in its propagation produce the PR interval.

The AV node consists of fibres, of very small diameter, which form a very complex network with many anastomoses. It is here that co-ordination of the impulse takes place and if, during mitral valve replacement, a tie is accidentally placed around the artery to the AV node, numerous supraventricular and ventricular arrhythmias develop until that tie is removed. The conduction

velocity within the AV node is slow and can be measured in *centimetres* per second, but part of the PR (or, more precisely, PQ) interval is caused by the time taken for conduction through the His bundle, bundle branches and probably the Purkinje network. However, once the impulse has traversed the AV node, conduction velocity is again increased.

It is now known that the AV node, except perhaps for its most distal part, produces no spontaneous electrical activity.* The action potentials that can produce a ventricular contraction at

---

* A number of workers, for example Cranefield and Hoffman (1958)[23] have been unable to find pacemaking cells in the AV node. Some of these cells have been found at the junction between the atria and the AV node and at the junction of the more distal part of the AV node and the bundle of His. Thus junctional rhythms have, as we know, been identified.

approximately 60/minute and are normally suppressed by the impulses originating in the SA node are generated in tissue close to the AV node, called *junctional tissue*. Therefore, rhythms which used to be referred to as *nodal* rhythms are now referred to as *junctional* rhythms, or AV-junctional rhythms.

Many fibres of the His–Purkinje system possess the ability to initiate an electrical impulse and this, as in the SA node and junctional tissue, is termed automaticity. The rate at which a depolarizing impulse can be generated diminishes from the more proximal regions of the system (e.g. 50/minute or more in the His bundle itself) to the more distal regions (e.g. 20/minute in the Purkinje fibres). In the absence of a propagated impulse, these fibres give rise to an idioventricular or ventricular ectopic beat (Lev, 1964).[87]

The diminishing rate of the spontaneously generated impulse is of importance following the insertion of a pacemaker for complete heart block. When the batteries begin to fail, usually after 5 years, the disease may have progressed along the conducting system. While at the time of insertion of the pacemaker the patient had a spontaneous rhythm of, for example, 45 beats/minute, the spontaneous rhythm when seen 5 years later may be only 20 beats/minute or less. If the pacemaker is then disconnected, syncope or death occurs.

After (distal to) the AV node, the bundle of His can be divided into two *penetrating* and *branching* sections. The penetrating portion extends from the distal end of the AV node to the origin of the posterior (postero-inferior) division of the left bundle. It lies in close proximity to the mitral ring, and damage to this ring by infection, fibrosis and calcification may also damage the bundle of His.

The ability of the AV node to slow the velocity of conduction is only partly explained by the phenomena of *decremental* and *inhomogeneous* conduction described below. The normal conduction velocity of the remainder of the His–Purkinje system is very high (3–5 m/second), but the speed of conduction varies in different fibres of the conducting pathway. Having reached the bundle of His, the propagated impulse is conducted more rapidly along the *left* bundle branch (LBB), and the first part of the myocardium to be innervated is the more leftward portion of the thick muscular intraventricular septum.

Functionally, the main branch of the left bundle divides after a very short distance into two branches, an *antero-superior* branch which is thin and broken up into many divisions, and a more robust *postero-inferior* branch.* Following innervation of the left portion of the septum, the impulse which cannot be transmitted without delay to the right portion of the septum, in the normal heart, travels virtually simultaneously through both branches of the left bundle and the right bundle. In this way, a co-ordinated contraction of the ventricles occurs.

The process described above is based on the assumption that the only functioning system for the conduction of the impulse originating in the SA node is that consisting of the AV node and the His–Purkinje system with all its sub-branches. Accessory conducting pathways are, however, sometimes present, including the bundles of Kent, Mahaim and James. The bundle of Kent, for example, largely bypasses the AV node so that there is a short PR interval and rapid excitation of the ventricles forming a QRS with a 'delta'-shaped wave.[76] This combination was described by Wolff, Parkinson and White in 1930.[161] It is well established that the presence of these accessory pathways can be an important factor in the genesis of cardiac arrhythmias. They are referred to as the *pre-excitation syndrome* (Ferrer, 1976).[46]

An electrode placed within the cell allows the action potential to be recorded. If the voltage changes are recorded via the nutritive medium (e.g. the body's extracellular fluid and skin), then we can arrange the electrodes so that an electrical impulse moving towards the electrode produces a positive deflection, and one moving away from an electrode produces a negative deflection. An electrode placed midway so that the impulse moves towards the electrode and then away from it produces first a positive and then a negative deflection recorded on the ECG. This concept is of some importance in understanding not only the ECG but also the subdivisions and various forms of heart block.

Generation of the electrical impulse

The concept of an electrical impulse being generated in the SA node and conducted along specialized tissue to the ventricles, which then contract, is relatively simple, even if delay at the AV node, accessory 'pre-excitation' pathways and distribution along subdivisions of the His–Purkinje

---

* In practice, the *postero-inferior* division is the first branch to arise from the branching section of the His bundle. The terminal portion of the bundle of His bifurcates into the *right* bundle branch (RBB) and the *anterior* division of the *left* bundle. The two branches have in part a common blood supply.

network are more complicated than originally conceived.

The generation of the electrical impulse and the factors that produce the *automaticity* and *rhythmicity* of cardiac muscle contraction are more complicated, but not beyond a working comprehension for clinicians. Without a basic knowledge, the understanding of arrhythmias and their treatment can be limited. Some of the most important aspects of the cardiac cycle are variations in the conduction velocity, the size and length of the action potential, and the variations both natural and abnormal that occur in the refractory period. Let us, therefore, look at the action potential generated within the ventricles. As seen on the end-papers, the spontaneously produced action potential at the SA node is shaped differently from other action potentials and depicts the changes in resting potential that occur during diastole.

These changes, which gradually reach threshold potential, allow spontaneous production of an electrical impulse. This is quite different from ventricular muscle, which is quiescent between beats and, unless damaged, does not normally have the power to produce a spontaneous impulse. The His-Purkinje network, however, does have centres of pacemaker cells which, like the SA node and other tissues, do have the power to generate an impulse.

During the past decade there has been an accumulation of impressive experimental evidence indicating that two distinct inwardly directed currents through the cardiac cell membrane are responsible for the excitation of the heart and the contraction of myocardial muscle.

The first inward current (I_{Na^+}) can be abolished by the removal of external Na ions from the solution veiling the muscle cell. If, for example, choline is made to replace the Na ion, then no action potential can develop. To explain the rapid influx of sodium during depolarization, it is postulated that there are 'gates' in the sarcolemma which open to allow the rapid influx of ions in a selective manner, and these remain closed during the resting state. The mechanism by which this occurs is as yet unknown. However, in addition to physically removing the Na ions, it is possible to block the Na+ gates by means of the toxin, known as tetrodotoxin, obtained from the Puffer fish. It has thus been established that the inward Na+ current of myocardial muscle is at least quantitatively similar to the Na+ currents of nerve and skeletal muscle (Ulbricht, 1977).[143]

The inward sodium current is responsible for the vast upstroke velocity (V_{max}) of the cardiac

action potential (Fig. 9.5). The conduction velocity of the propagated impulse through myocardial tissue is also largely determined by the upstroke velocity V_{max} (Jack *et al.*, 1975).[70]

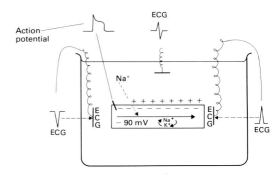

Fig. 9.5   A strip of cardiac muscle lying in Ringer's solution would be in the resting phase, polarized (positively charged on the outside and negatively charged on the inside) so that there is a resting potential of approximately −90 mV. When stimulated, the muscle depolarizes when Na+ passes through the membrane. If electrocardiogram (ECG) plates are placed within the Ringer's solution, the apparatus (electrocardiogram) is arranged so that as the impulse moves away from the electrode it produces a downward-going (negative) deflection and as it moves towards an electrode it produces an upward-going (positive) deflection. If the impulse moves first towards an electrode and then away from it, an initial positive deflection followed by a negative deflection is recorded. If a different type of electrode is placed within the muscle cellular tissue, an action potential is recorded (see p. 301). Repolarization occurs by means of the loss of K+ from the cell and the relatively slow repair of the Na+ : K+ ratio occurs by means of the ordinary sodium pump mechanism.

The second inward current, which is much less rapid and smaller in intensity than the first inward current (I_{Na^+}), is produced by the inward flow of the heavy divalent calcium ion through different 'gates' in the cell membrane (sarcolemma). This current is much more sensitive to variations in the extracellular [Ca++]. The inward flow of calcium ions can initiate a contraction of the myocardium, producing a much slower response during phase 0 of the action potential, and would appear to be the major factor in producing the plateau phase of the cardiac action potential (phase 2) and for initiating the excitation of the myocardium which produces coupling. These aspects have been well reviewed by Fozzard (1977), Langer (1973), Van Winkle and Schwartz (1976), Beeler and Reuter (1977), McAllister *et al.* (1975) and Schwartz *et al.* (1985).[7,48,85,101,128,148]

It can be stated, however, that the existence of two separate inward currents through the cardiac cell membrane is now well established. The inward flow of Na^+, and therefore of V_{max}, is affected by drugs such as quinidine and lignocaine. The number of functional Ca^{++} channels is regulated by the cyclic nucleotides (e.g. cyclic AMP) and therefore by adrenergic–cholinergic transmitters.

Membrane potential

The transmembrane potential (the voltage within the cardiac cell) is approximately −90 mV within the myocardium of most mammals. This is the so-called resting potential. Following stimulation, depolarization of the cell membrane occurs so that a rapid reversal of the transmembrane potential develops and the charge within the cell reaches between +20 and +40 mV.

This phase of rapid depolarization is internationally characterized as 'phase 0' and in mammalian atria, ventricles and the His–Purkinje system this phase occurs over a period of less than 1 millisecond (Fig 9.6). Depolarization, which coincides with systole, is immediately followed by repolarization which begins before systole ends. Repolarization is normally divided into the period of very rapid repolarization (phase 1), the intermediate phase of slow repolarization (phase 2) which forms a plateau in the action potential, and a second phase of rapid repolarization (phase 3). Between periods of depolarization there are phases of membrane stability (phase 4), during which no change occurs in the ventricles in the absence of an electrical stimulus. Before the process of depolarization can occur and a contraction of the myocardium is produced, the potential must fall from +90 mV to −80 or −70 mV, which is the threshold potential. Failure to reach the threshold potential causes a failure in depolarization, or a missed beat, but when threshold potential is reached, depolarization occurs in an 'all or none' manner.

The action potential can be divided into three sections which are loosely complementary to the phases described above. These are: the absolute or effective refractory period (during this the tissue will not respond to a second electrical impulse); the relative refractory period (during this the tissue will respond, but only to an electrical impulse that is greater in magnitude than that which initiated depolarization); and a supersensitive

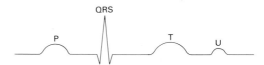

Fig. 9.6   The action potential that is recorded during the depolarization within ventricular muscle that takes place during one cardiac cycle (contraction of the ventricle). The resting potential is approximately −90 mV and this phase is characterized as being phase 4. The period of rapid depolarization is phase 0. When the action potential rises to above +20 mV during phase 1, this is represented by the QRS complex of the scalar electrocardiogram (ECG) shown below the action potential. Phase 2 largely represents the ST segment of the ECG and phase 3 is the T and U wave of the ECG.

(supernormal) period (during this the action potential is approaching threshold and a very small electrical stimulus will stimulate depolarization).

Phase 0 and 1 relate to the QRS complex of the scalar ECG. Phase 2 relates, very largely, to the ST segment. Phase 3 relates to the T wave. This is of some importance in the initiation of ventricular fibrillation (see p. 313). Phase 4 relates to the resting potential and isoelectric portion of the ECG between beats.

The duration of the action potential varies from one fibre to another and from one tissue to another. It tends to be increasingly prolonged from the atria to more distal fibres of the His–Purkinje system. The length of the action potential can also be altered by changes occurring within or around the same tissue or fibre. Hypercalcaemia, for example, both shortens and changes the shape of the action potential; hypocalcaemia lengthens the action potential. Hyperkalaemia causes slowing of the upstroke (phase 0), a reduction in amplitude and shortening of the action potential. Hypokalaemia causes lengthening of the phase 2 plateau and of the action potential.

Depolarization of myocardial muscle is produced by the rapid flow of Na^+ through the cell membrane into the myocardial cell. During the resting phase there appears to be only a very slow inward passage of Na^+ and a very rapid outward flow of K^+.

Phase 1

During the early rapid phase of repolarization (phase 1), the rapid flow of K^+ ceases and the return to zero potential is achieved by outward flow of Cl^-. Regeneration of the ionic equilibrium is restored using a Na^+-K^+ pump mechanism. The ability of the ions to pass through the cell wall, through what are considered to be special channels, changes with the potential difference that is present between the inside and outside of the cell and is therefore considered to be *voltage dependent*.

Phase 2

The most distinctive characteristic of the action potential of cardiac muscle is the phase 2 plateau (the ST segment on the ECG). The maintenance of the plateau is still not fully explained with certainty. This is because it could be achieved either by voltage dependency causing a cessation of the flow of ions across the cell membrane or by an equality of flow of ions so that no potential is produced. There is, in fact, growing evidence that during this period there is a slow inward current produced by the passage of Ca^{++} through the membrane. This can be modified by changes in $[H^+]$, other ions such as Mg^{++} and drugs such as verapamil (Cordilox), nifedipine (Adalat), and diltiazem (Tildiem), that reduce the movement of Ca^{++} through the 'slow channels'.

Phase 3

It is apparent that the outward flow of K^+, which fell to insignificant quantities during phase 1 and was maintained at the same flow during phase 2, returns to the high levels characteristic of the resting cell at the end of the plateau. The cessation of Ca^{++} flow and the rapid loss of K^+ from the cell produce the rapid return of the negative resting potential during phase 3. A second outward flow of ionic exchange is considered to contribute to phase 3 and this is the normal sodium pump which exchanges two sodium ions for three potassium ions.

Concealed conduction

The term *effective* refractory period is now used instead of absolute refractory period because, although no stimulus, whatever its magnitude, can produce a propagated impulse, in the case of myocardial muscle an electrical stimulus, if large enough, can elicit a *local* response. This transient local depolarization is not conducted and, although it does not influence the heart beat that is in the process of being evolved at the time of the stimulus, it can influence the characteristics of subsequent beats. The leads to phenomena such as *concealed conduction* (Langendorf, 1948).[83]

Concealed conduction is now considered to be the cause of the varying intervals between QRS complexes seen in atrial fibrillation (Katz and Pick, 1956; Katz, 1977).[73,75] It can be seen from the above that the two factors inhomogeneity (described below) and concealed conduction can give rise to re-entry phenomena (see p. 304).[105]

Inhomogeneity of depolarization

An electrical impulse which causes localized depolarization of tissue during the refractory period allows the repolarization of the major part of the myocardial tissue to take place in the presence of a small area of tissue that is still refractory. In other words, an area of myocardium repolarizes earlier than the tissue that is adjacent to it and this repolarized myocardium regains its excitability while the tissue around it remains refractory. This phenomenon is known as inhomogeneity of depolarization. It allows re-entry arrhythmias to develop and the stimulation of one part of the myocardial tissue by another to induce a premature systole.

Decremental conduction

A basic electrophysiological mechanism defined as decremental conduction in the AV junctional tissue was first suggested by Hoffman and Cranefield (1960)[63] and supported by Paes de Carvalhò (1961)[110] and Watanabe and Dreifus (1965 and 1967).[151,152] It can be described as the ability of changes in one part of the heart to influence the conduction velocity in another part. Decremental conduction occurs when a normal action potential enters a region of the myocardium in which the conduction velocity is slowed. The rate of rise of the action potential and its amplitude are decreased. In other words, change in electrophysiological characteristics cause the impulse to be propagated at a slower rate.

Decremental conduction occurs in abnormal areas of the heart, for example in the presence of ischaemia when the sodium pump is impaired by lack of oxygen and chemical agents and when partial depolarization has already occurred because some of the intercellular potassium has been replaced. Decremental conduction can be caused by hyperkalaemia, hypokalaemia, hypocalcaemia and by numerous membrane-stabilizing agents such as lignocaine (lidocaine, Xylocaine), beta-blockers and Ca^{++} flux antagonists, for example, nifedipine (Adalat) and verapamil (Cordilox).

Decremental conduction can also occur in certain regions of normal myocardium. For example, the AV node is considered to slow the impulse by this means. This would account for the small, slowly rising action potentials that are seen in this area. Quite typically, after an impulse has passed through a region in which there is decremental conduction, a normal rate of progress of the action potential is resumed. This return of a slowed impulse to one that is propagated at a rapid rate through the rest of the myocardium is characteristic not only of the AV node but also of an ischaemic heart when the impulse, having emerged from the ischaemic area of decremental conduction, penetrates a normally perfused area and is then conducted at a normal rate.

In some circumstances, however, decremental conduction may be of such a degree that the amplitude of the action potential is too small for a sufficiently effective stimulus to excite the normal tissue that lies ahead. Under these circumstances, the impulse is not transmitted and becomes completely blocked. These blocks can occur at the SA node, at the AV node or in one or more of the branches of the His–Purkinje system producing a bundle branch block or hemiblock.

When an area of decremental conduction causes a failure of transmission of an impulse within a small localized area of myocardial tissue, retrograde transmission of the impulses can occur in this tissue, leading to re-entrant arrhythmias.

Re-entry arrhythmias

Between beats, during phase 4 of the cardiac cycle, myocardial excitability remains essentially unchanged. It is referred to as the period of electrical diastole. During systole, however, after onset of the action potential, marked changes occur so that, as we have seen, an effective refractory period is induced. During this period a second impulse cannot be propagated along distal fibres and a conduction block is produced.

During the relative refractory period, however, some stronger stimuli can produce action potentials which have a slower rate of depolarization and reduced conductivity. A significant period of time is required for depolarization, repolarization and the dissipation of the refractory period. However, the permeability of the cell membrane can be altered in a selective manner by external influences, amongst which anoxia is prominent. Quinidine and chlorpromazine can extend the period of relative refractoriness beyond the end of repolarization (Chen and Gettes, 1976).[21] Marked changes in the permeability of the cell membrane can produce a complete or unidirectional block. Conduction delay is also produced in the presence of a tachycardia as successive impulses encroach upon the refractory period of the preceding action potential.

In addition to physiological and pharmacological factors, certain anatomical aspects determine the conduction of an electrical impulse. The larger the diameter of a fibre, the greater its conductivity (Katz, 1948).[74] Branching of a fibre allows an impulse in the normal heart to reach various parts of the myocardium essentially at the same time. If, however, interruption of the system is produced, forward propagation of the impulse becomes impossible, although retrograde conductivity in the opposite direction can be well maintained.

In order to explain the production of coupled premature beats, two main theories are proposed. The first theory postulates the presence of an abnormal ectopic focus which is separate from the SA node. The abnormal focus is stimulated and made to erupt by the action potential of the preceding sinus beat.

The second theory, for which there is accumulating experimental evidence, is that of re-entry. If two channels in close proximity receive an impulse but the first channel has a conduction delay (in that there is decremental conduction), the second channel will transmit the impulse so that it overtakes the impulse in the first channel (which is stopped in the area of the conduction block) and passes onwards to produce contraction of the myocardium. Because there is no electrical impulse within the first channel distal to the block, the impulse in the second channel can spread laterally and then distally along the first channel. This impulse, which has spread indirectly into the first channel, will also contribute to contraction of the myocardium.

There is, however, a delay before the impulse can jump from the second channel to the first channel. In addition, the impulse in the first channel distal to the block (having been derived from the lateral spread from the second channel) can be conducted *retrogradely* when the block in the first channel is unidirectional (Fig. 9.7). If this retrogradely conducted impulse emerges from the area of unidirectional block when the fibre forming channel 2 is no longer refractory, lateral spread back into channel 2 can occur.

Although the correct time intervals are required, if delays in the lateral spread of the impulse and the retrograde conduction through the unidirectional block satisfy the conditions, a continuous flow of current can be generated causing repeated stimulation of the second channel (by lateral spread from the first channel to the second channel) at a time when its refractory period has been dissipated and re-excitation is possible. As this derived impulse passes distally down the second channel, not only will this stimulus spread over and over again into the first channel, but it will also be propagated distally producing repeated contractions of the myocardium. This gives rise to a re-entry arrhythmia and tachycardia. It can also give rise to ectopic beats, for example the regular atrial bigeminy seen on page 308.

A similar re-entry pathway can also be derived when the fibres of the conducting system anastomose (Fig. 9.8) and one portion or one anastomotic fibre develops a unidirectional block, so that the normal distally moving propagated impulse

no longer prevents the retrograde conduction of electrical excitation.

Identification of cardiac arrhythmias

Cardiac arrhythmias can be subdivided into two main categories:

    1. abnormalities in the formation of the impulse,
    2. abnormalities in the conduction of the impulse.

These abnormalities are similar and arise from changes in the myocardial cell membrane and cell membranes of the conducting tissue. The use of His bundle electrocardiography for clinical diagnosis has increased the interest in an electrophysiological approach to cardiology and to the diagnosis and treatment of arrhythmias.

Arrhythmias can be further subdivided into those originating above, in and below the atrioventricular junction. Some of these arrhythmias are dealt with in this chapter.

Sinus rhythm

Sinus rhythm can be identified only by obtaining an ECG. Although its presence may be suggested by clinical examination, one cannot be certain that the regular rhythm felt at a pulse or at the apex of

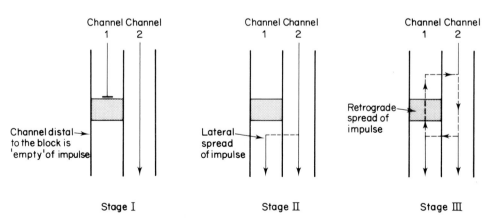

Fig. 9.7 Stage I illustrates a normally conducting fibre or channel which is adjacent to a fibre or channel which is blocked by ischaemia or possibly a molecule of drug situated on its surface. It should be noted that the fibre distal to the block is *not* refractory. Stage II illustrates a lateral transfer of the normal impulse in channel 2 to the non-refractory section of the adjacent fibre channel 1, distal to the block. Stage III illustrates the retrograde spread of the impulse in the adjacent fibre, channel 1, because the block is unidirectional. Lateral spread to channel 2 can occur if the impulse arrives when the channel 2 fibre is no longer refractory. Continuous spread can thus occur and a re-entry arrhythmia is generated.

Note this is only a diagram, and similar re-entry pathways can occur elsewhere on the same principle (e.g. through the slowly conducting AV node and/or accessory pathways).

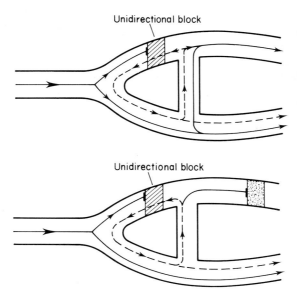

Fig. 9.8 Re-entry pathways can occur within the conducting fibres of the heart very readily when two branches of the His–Purkinje system are joined by an interconnecting branch.

the heart is in fact a normal sinus rhythm. Sinus rhythm is defined as consisting of P waves which arise at fixed intervals and, in the absence of bundle branch block or aberrant conduction, these waves are followed by normal QRS complexes. The PR interval is normally between 0.12 and 0.20 seconds in duration. Upright P waves are always seen in leads I and II and inverted P waves are seen in aVR.

A sinus tachycardia is said to be present when the heart rate is 100 beats/minute or more,* although the pacemaker impulse can arise from sources other than the sinus node. The rhythms

* Note: it is unusual for a patient at rest to have a simple sinus tachycardia at a rate above 140 beats/minute.

are then defined by origin of the pacemaker and are called atrial, AV junctional or ventricular tachycardias.

A sinus bradycardia (Fig. 9.9) is said to be present when the heart rate is 60 beats/minute or less; the impulse originates from the SA node. Here again, the source of the impulse may be other than the SA node. In the elderly, heart rates as low as 38 beats/minute, exhibiting a normal sinus beat, may be observed without any apparent ill-effects and are not the result of any form of therapy. A sinus bradycardia is also present for a relatively short period of our lives during the peak of our athletic prowess, when the weight of the heart increases and its stroke volume can almost double (Fig. 9.10).

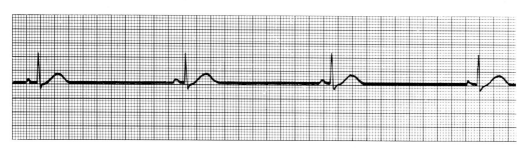

Fig. 9.9 This electrocardiogram (ECG) was taken from a 78-year-old woman who was in no way decompensated and was not dyspnoeic or orthopnoeic.

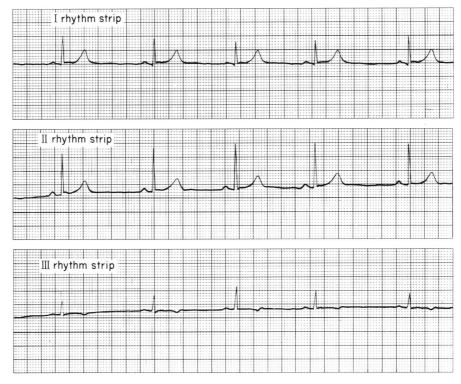

Fig. 9.10   Resting electrocardiogram (ECG) leads I, II and III in a 23-year-old marathon runner. Note the sinus bradycardia and inverted T waves in lead III.

Abnormalities other than those of rate can occur in the production and transmission of the sinus impulse, and some of these abnormalities are discussed below. The sinus beat can be suppressed so that extrasystoles can occur. Extrasystoles may arise from atria, AV junction or the ventricles and assume two forms:

1. premature beats which are extrasystoles, that follow the preceding QRS complex by an interval which is shorter than the normal RR interval;

2. escape beats which are beats that follow the preceding QRS complex by an interval that is longer than the preceding sequence of RR intervals.

Two characteristics of extrasystoles can be observed. These are the *coupling interval*, the time interval between the onset of the preceding QRS complex and the onset of the extrasystole, and the *post-extrasystolic* pause, which is the pause that follows a premature extrasystole before the following R wave is produced. The pause is said to be *complete* when the two complexes on either side of the premature beat are twice the dominant RR interval. Commonly, the postsystolic pause is *incomplete* following an atrial premature beat and complete following a ventricular premature beat, but this is by no means absolute.

Sinus tachycardia can arise in perfectly normal healthy individuals and may reach 180 beats and more/minute, for example in racing drivers at a Le Mans start and in astronauts landing on the moon. There is, however, a tendency towards a poorer prognosis in the cyanosed patient who has a tachycardia lying at rest, following a myocardial infarction. The terms sinus tachycardia and bradycardia therefore have to be defined according to their cause.

Dominant pacemaker
This term is used when two pacemakers are present (one or both of which can be ectopic) and both are capable of exciting the entire heart or a

single chamber. The dominant pacemaker is that which causes ventricular depolarization and is usually the more rapid of the two.

Interpolated beat

Interpolation is said to be present when a QRS complex, which is always an extrasystole, is placed between two normal QRS complexes but there is no compensatory period and the extrasystole in its location on the ECG is normal in time. The importance of interpolated beats lies in the fact that they can give rise to various arrhythmias, including parasystole.

Capture

This term is used to denote the transitory control of ventricular depolarization by a pacemaker which is not the *dominant* pacemaker. Capture can be seen, for example, in a run of ventricular tachycardia when there is the occasional normally conducted beat, a normal QRS preceded by a P wave, (see Fig. 9.15).

Parasystole

When an independent ectopic focus, originating either in the atria, AV junctional tissue or ventricles co-exists with a dominant pacemaker, for example sinus rhythm, and produces ectopic beats (extrasystoles) that have a common interectopic interval, parasystole is said to be present. Often, non-fixed coupling of the extrasystoles and the presence of fusion beats characterize this arrhythmia.

Although the majority of ventricular extrasystoles bear constant relationship to the preceding beat (*fixed coupling*),* ectopic foci sometimes develop within the ventricular conducting system and these give rise to impulses that occur at their own independent rate. When these impulses occur outside the refractory period, an ectopic beat results. For this condition, in which an independent ventricular pacemaker competes with the pacemaker controlling the basic rhythm, the term ventricular parasystole is used. As in other parasystolic rhythms, the impulses arising from the independent focus are in some way shielded or protected so that they can interpose themselves between the beats of the basic rhythm.

* As opposed to ectopic beats that have a variable relationship in time to the preceding beat, known as *variable coupling*.

Aberrant ventricular conduction

Ectopic beats originating in the atria are frequently conducted abnormally through the ventricles (Figs. 9.11, 9.12 and 9.13). They can then sometimes masquerade as premature ventricular extrasystoles, and the complex recorded on the ECG is referred to as an 'aberrant' atrial beat (Gouaux and Ashman, 1947; Langendorf, 1951).[52,84]

The aberrantly conducted supraventricular beat (ACSB) appears to originate above the bifurcation of the bundle of His and is premature enough to arrive at the more distal part of the His–Purkinje system while the major part of the pathway is still refractory. Because the impulse cannot be conducted, or is conducted only very slowly through some fibres of the conduction system, the impulse spreads through the remaining ventricular muscle with delay, which results in a widened QRS complex with a bundle branch block configuration. Commonly, the complex is not unlike that produced by an ectopic beat originating in the ventricular portion of the His–Purkinje system, producing a ventricular beat (ventricular extrasystole).

The refractory period is common to all portions of the myocardium but it varies in duration from one part of the myocardium to another and even within the conducting system itself. The right bundle, for example, even in the normal heart, tends to have a longer refractory period than the left bundle. In addition to this basic difference, the period of refractoriness is influenced by numerous factors including the heart rate and the ionic concentration of, for example K^+ and Ca^{++} in the tissue fluid. The increase in the heart rate reduces and shortens the speed at which repolarization takes place and therefore shortens the refractory period. A decreased heart rate thus prolongs the refractory period.

When the heart beat is irregular, such as in atrial fibrillation, the sequence of ventricular activation results in aberrantly conducted beats because the propagated electrical impulse from the atria arrives at a part of the conducting pathway that is still in the refractory phase.

When the impulses are conducted aberrantly at a markedly increased heart rate, they are referred to as 'rate-related aberrant beats'. There is commonly a 'critical rate' at which aberrancy occurs.

Ischaemia causes a reduction in the rate of repolarization and, therefore, in the critical rate at which aberrancy can be produced. The critical rate is very much slower in the ischaemic heart than that required when the conducting system is well supplied with oxygenated blood and is not affected by drugs.

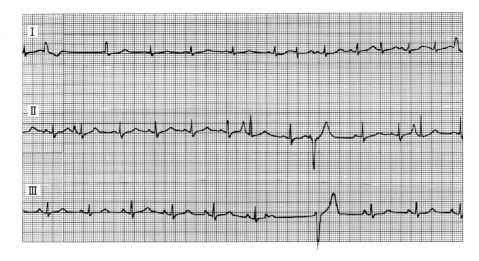

Fig. 9.11 Electrocardiogram (ECG) demonstrating abnormal complexes described in the preceding pages. The first complex is a sinus beat.

Lead I: the second complex is a ventricular extrasystole which has a *complete* extrasystolic pause. The third complex is initiated by an atrial beat which is conducted aberrantly. Aberrant conduction of a premature atrial beat is also seen in lead I in the eighth complex in this rhythm strip. The last complex is a ventricular extrasystole.

Lead II: the third complex is an atrial premature beat demonstrating P-on-T with minimal aberrancy. The eighth complex again demonstrates a premature atrial beat with P-on-T, the prematurity of the beat and the degree of aberrancy being greater. The tenth beat is an ectopic ventricular, possibly fusion, beat being a combination of a premature ventricular extrasystole and a premature atrial beat. Partial conduction down the His–Purkinje system ensures narrowing of the QRS complex. Once again, the compensatory pause is complete. The penultimate (13th) complex is a premature atrial systole with P-on-T and aberrant conduction.

Lead III: after the sixth QRS complex, a P wave can be seen emerging from and superimposed upon the upstroke of the T wave and this is not propagated. There is therefore a pause following a complex which is not an ectopic beat. Only partial penetration has occurred and this can be considered to be concealed conduction. Although the premature atrial impulse manifests itself on the ECG and is not conducted, it has depolarized pacemaker centres lower down in the His–Purkinje system. There is therefore a pause until an escape ventricular, possibly fusion, beat is seen in the seventh complex of lead III.

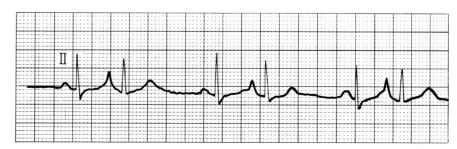

Fig. 9.12 Atrial bigeminy; premature atrial ectopic beats occur after every sinus beat. The ectopic atrial impulse falls on the preceding T wave, P-on-T phenomenon so that it is enlarged and distorted. The ectopic atrial beat is also conducted aberrantly so that the QRS complex in every second (aberrant) beat is abnormal.

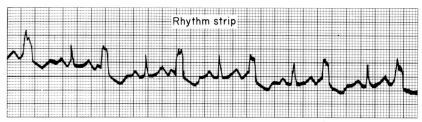

Fig. 9.13   Atrial bigeminy demonstrating P-on-T and aberrant conduction with RBBB formation.

Aberrantly conducted supraventricular impulses through the right bundle usually have an RBB morphology. A ventricular 'fusion beat' is produced when impulses arise, within the same short period, from two pacing sites—one supraventricular and the other ventricular. When the initial supraventricular impulse meets the wave of depolarization that has originated from the ventricular impulse, the QRS morphology lies between that of a normally conducted supraventricular beat and an ectopic ventricular extrasystole. In this way a 'fusion beat' is a reliable indicator that a pure supraventricular ectopic beat is not the sole originator of the impulse, and that a ventricular beat is also present. There are a number of other factors which help diagnosis and assist in the differentiation between an aberrantly conducted supraventricular beat and a ventricular ectopic beat.

1. The degree of aberrancy of a premature atrial beat (PAB) varies, depending upon the degree of prematurity of the atrial impulse. This results in a minor or major difference in QRS morphology. Ventricular ectopic beats originating from the same focus tend to have a uniform morphology.
2. The time interval between the preceding normal beat and the supraventricular beat—the coupling interval—is frequently variable, giving rise to the aberrancy described above. Most commonly, ventricular ectopic beats have a fixed coupling interval.
3. Beats originating in the atria frequently alter the sinus rhythm. Ventricular ectopic beats usually have no effect on the regularity of the sinus beats unless they give rise to a ventricular tachycardia as in Fig. 9.15. Therefore, isolated ventricular ectopic beats with a compensatory pause followed by a sinus beat or beats appearing at the correct time interval suggest ventricular beats.
4. A slow heart rate produces a lengthening of the refractory period. Therefore, when there

are variations in the heart rate so that a pause that is longer than the intervals between preceding beats is produced and this is followed by another beat after a short pause, the variations in rate favour the production of a beat that meets refractory conducting tissue as it passes along the His–Purkinje system. An aberrantly conducted beat is then frequently seen and can lead to a re-entry rhythm. This phenomenon, a 'slow' beat followed by a 'quick' beat resulting in a re-entry rhythm, is referred to as the 'Ashman effect'.

Bigeminal rhythm

This is said to occur when every second beat is an extrasystole originating from an ectopic focus. The ectopic impulse may arise in the atria, AV junctional tissue and the ventricles. The origin of the ectopic beat can only be diagnosed by means of the ECG.

Premature atrial systoles may have a constant coupling interval followed by a compensatory pause which may be complete or incomplete (see p. 306). When the atrial beat arrives early it may impinge on the preceding T wave, increase its size and deform its shape; this condition is known as P-on-T phenomenon. Aberrant conduction deforming the QRS complex then frequently occurs (see Figs. 9.12 and 9.13). As can be seen, aberrant conduction may give rise to a right bundle branch block (RBBB) pattern.

As in the case of ventricular ectopic beats, the main importance of bigeminy lies in the possible development of a more serious arrhythmia. (Fig. 9.14).

Usually, isolated ventricular beats do not require treatment, but following myocardial infarction when the dangers of R-on-T are apparent, immediate treatment is necessary. Ventricular bigeminal rhythm requires urgent active and continous treatment when it is a consequence of myocardial infarction. It may also require early active treatment when it is the result of digitalis intoxication.

The most usual and generally acceptable form

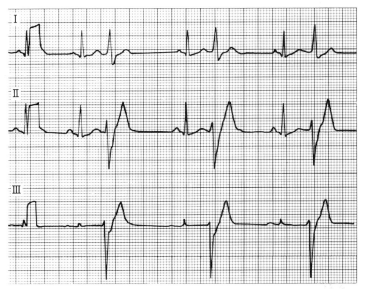

Fig. 9.14 Every second beat is a ventricular ectopic beat. These are called coupled beats, pulsus bigeminus or bigeminal rhythm and may in some circumstances herald ventricular fibrillation.

of medication at this time is the injection of lignocaine (lidocaine, Xylocaine) 100–200 mg i.v. When this is not possible, 200–300 mg of lignocaine should be given intramuscularly. This is said to result in therapeutic concentrations in the blood within 15 minutes which persist for at least 1 hour (Bellet *et al.*, 1971; Fehmers and Dunning, 1972; Bernstein *et al.*, 1972).[8,10,45] Because of the achievement of therapeutic blood levels, lignocaine has been used prophylactically in the pre-hospital phase of acute myocardial infarction (Valentine *et al.*, 1971 and 1974).[145,146]

The half-life of lignocaine when given intravenously is only 8–10 minutes. To maintain a concentration of 2 µg/ml in the blood, an infusion of lignocaine at a rate of 1–2 mg/minute is required (Hollinger, 1960).[64] To infuse the minimal amount of fluid, it is therefore convenient to add sufficient lignocaine to the infusion solution, usually 5% glucose (dextrose), to make a concentration of 4–8 mg/ml. Thus 500 ml of solution would contain 2–4 g of lignocaine, and 1 litre would contain 4–8 g.

Procainamide is also a valuable agent in the treatment of ventricular bigeminy. It is given in doses of 200–300 mg i.v., and it is usually safe if it is administered at a rate that is no greater than 25–50 mg/minute (Koch-Weser, 1974).[80] It is important not to exceed a loading dose of 12 mg/kg body weight, which in a 70-kg man is 840 mg. When given orally there is a delay of 15–30 minutes

before absorption occurs. Ventricular bigeminy can also be treated with quinidine 200–300 mg q.d.s.

Tocainide and flecainide

These oral anti-arrhythmic agents have been demonstrated (see p. 289) to effectively abolish ventricular ectopic beats (see p. 286).

R-on-T phenomenon

The R-on-T phenomenon refers to ventricular depolarization from an ectopic source (producing the R wave of an ectopic beat) being superimposed on the preceding beat. Numerous ECGs have demonstrated that the coupling of extrasystoles has been implicated in the initiation of abnormal ventricular rhythms. Although the importance of the R-on-T phenomenon in the production of tachyarrhythmias was first demonstrated by Smirk (1949) and Smirk and Palmer (1960),[129,130] it was shown by Lown *et al.* (1963 and 1969)[93,94] that the early coupling of the ectopic beat could be a cause of sudden death. This was confirmed by Epstein *et al.* (1973)[39] who referred to the malignant nature of the R-on-T phenomenon.

Because of the dangers associated with the R-on-T phenomenon, numerous authors have justified the prescription of anti-arrhythmic drugs, such as lignocaine, to patients with ischaemic heart disease following myocardial infarction, and these have been demonstrated to be effective.

There is no doubt that because of the nature of the action potential the prevention of the R-on-T phenomenon is of great importance and early treatment can be life saving.

More recently, however, some observations have cast doubt on the uniqueness of the R-on-T phenomenon in predicting, and indeed causing, the onset of a malignant arrhythmia.

Originally, Smirk believed that R-on-T was associated with supernormal excitability during myocardial disease, but the patients he described had not only numerous ectopic foci, but also severe and extensive heart disease. However, animal experimentation, in which acute infarcts were produced, demonstrated a reduced threshold for ventricular fibrillation (Han, 1969).[56] Experience with patients in the coronary care unit lead Lown et al. to predict that when myocardial infarction and an ectopic beat with a coupling interval of 60–85% of the preceding RR interval occurred, ventricular fibrillation would probably follow. Lown and Wolfe (1971)[95] concluded that even when chronic ischaemic heart disease was present, R-on-T was more important in the causation of sudden death than numerous repetitive episodes of ectopic beats.

Epstein et al. demonstrated that in the dog with induced acute myocardial infarction, ventricular fibrillation occurred when ventricular ectopic beats were initiated within 0.43 seconds of the preceding QRS complex.[39,40] When dogs had ventricular ectopic beats that occurred later than 0.43 seconds after the preceding QRS complex, ventricular fibrillation did not result. An important factor to note, however, is that 6 of the 15 dogs who developed ectopic beats within 0.43 seconds of the preceding QRS complex did not fibrillate. This accentuated the question as to why (as observed in patients) R-on-T occurring within the vulnerable period frequently does not give rise to a tachyarrhythmia, and it raises some doubt as to the critical nature of the timing of the ectopic beat in inducing a malignant or non-malignant ventricular arrhythmia.

In quite heroic investigations, Wellens et al. (1974 and 1976)[154,155] investigated seven patients with ventricular tachycardia following acute myocardial infarction. After the patients had been converted to a sinus rhythm, extrasystoles were produced by means of a pacemaker inserted into the right ventricle. The electrical impulse was applied so that it scanned the whole of diastole including the QT interval. The artificially produced ventricular ectopic beats failed to produce ventricular tachycardia, even when they were placed on the T wave. While these experiments have been criticized in that there was probably a failure of the impulse to enter the 're-entry' pathway, it would appear from other evidence (some of which is described below) that this was not a critical factor.

Several centres have reported delayed epicardial activation with increased duration of electrograms when bipolar electrograms were recorded from areas of infarction in the acutely infarcted dog's heart (Williams et al., 1974; El-Sherif et al., 1975; Dhurandhar et al., 1971).[29,30,34,158] The prolonged electrograms were associated with the initiation of cardiac arrhythmias, the sustained myocardial excitation was apparently caused by the re-entrant ectopic contractions.

Williams et al. (1974)[158] observed that spontaneous ventricular tachyarrhythmias were almost always initiated by ectopic beats which had coupling intervals that were longer than that which would produce R-on-T. Ventricular tachycardia followed ectopic beats which produced the greatest delay in ventricular activation time. When the ventricular tachycardia degenerated into fibrillation, it was associated with a ventricular activation time which was progressively prolonged. The recordings of Williams et al. (1974)[158] showed that delayed ventricular activation of a premature beat, emanating from ischaemic myocardial tissue, could result in the beat appearing as a late ectopic beat but still initiating a tachycardia.

Clinical observations

It was found by Dhurandhar et al.[29,30] that in 8 out of 20 patients with primary ventricular fibrillation observed in the coronary care unit, no warning arrhythmias, such as ectopic beats, were present. While 16 of the 20 patients did in fact have R-on-T as the initiating beat of the ventricular fibrillation, 8 patients did not have earlier and warning R-on-T beats to alert the clinician to the need for treatment. De Sanctis et al. (1972)[27] found that ventricular tachycardia could be initiated by ectopic beats which fell outside the so-called vulnerable area of the ECG. De Soyza et al. (1974)[28] found that ventricular tachycardia following acute myocardial infarction in patients could be initiated by ectopic beats, the mean coupling interval of which was 0.59 seconds, or 152% of the preceding QT interval. There was, therefore, no significant difference between the mean coupling interval in these patients in whom ventricular tachycardia developed and the mean coupling interval of isolated ectopic beats which did not produce paroxysms of ventricular tachycardia. The findings were the same whether myocardial infarction was present or not. It was also found that only 12% of the ventricular tachycardias observed were initiated by the R-on-T, while in other patients 16% of ectopic beats exhibited R-on-T, but in no way initiated ventricular tachyarrhythmias.

Later, Rothfield et al. (1977)[122] observed that only 25% of ventricular tachycardias following acute myocardial infarction were initiated by R-on-T. They did note, however, that when the arrhythmia was initiated by R-on-T, it tended to be more prolonged, more often failed to respond to intravenous lignocaine (lidocaine, Xylocaine), and more often degenerated into ventricular fibrillation.

The reports by Lie et al. (1974)[92] are therefore similar to the observations of many clinicians.

1. That ectopic beats are common following myocardial infarction.
2. That primary ventricular fibrillation can occur without any warning arrhythmia.
3. That while R-on-T does appear to initiate ventricular fibrillation, this arrhythmia can be initiated by an ectopic beat which does not fall on the T wave.

Lie et al.[92] monitored 262 patients who had acute myocardial infarction; 20 of these patients developed primary ventricular fibrillation. Nine of the 20 episodes of fibrillation were not initiated by R-on-T ectopic beats. Only 2 of the 20 cases of ventricular fibrillation had warning R-on-T arrhythmias. While arrhythmias of various kinds were present in 60% of those patients who developed ventricular fibrillation, and would therefore act as a warning of the potential danger, arrhythmias were also present in 59% of the 242 patients who did not have ventricular fibrillation.

These findings are of immense clinical importance. They indicate the growing evidence that antiarrhythmic therapy should be administered to all patients with acute myocardial infarction regardless of whether ectopic beats or any other arrhythmia develops. In the reports from Lie and his colleagues, when prophylactic lignocaine (lidocaine, Xylocaine) was given to patients with acute myocardial infarction, ventricular fibrillation was eliminated, but warning arrhythmias persisted in 34% of patients.

Support for the above conclusions is given by the observations of El-Sherif et al. (1976)[33] who later reported their studies on 20 patients who developed primary ventricular fibrillation after

acute myocardial infarction. In only half of these patients was ventricular fibrillation initiated by R-on-T ectopic beats. Only 5 of these patients had 'warning' R-on-T beats prior to the onset of ventricular fibrillation.

It would therefore appear from observations in cardiac care units that while R-on-T is of great importance in initiating a fatal arrhythmia, any late ectopic beat is capable of initiating ventricular fibrillation, whether there are the premonitory signs of arrhythmias or not. The clinical significance of these observations is that death following myocardial infarction is due to the apparent sensitivity of the myocardial muscle and its inability following an abnormal electrical phenomenon to sustain an organized repetitive contraction. There is, therefore, an apparent need for prophylactic antiarrhythmic therapy in all patients following myocardial infarction. This can be extended to include patients suffering from myocardial ischaemia.

While it is well recognized that R-on-T can produce clinically significant (Fig. 9.15) and sometimes fatal arrhythmias in the diseased heart, the question has to be asked whether a similar ectopic beat can produce an arrhythmia in patients who have a normal myocardium, and whether this is more probable in patients who, although they have a normal myocardium, are undergoing some form of drug therapy, the nature of which is not associated with treatment for a cardiac condition.

The ECG can be monitored in the ambulatory patient by means of tape recording. A prospective study was performed in patients suffering from paroxysmal ventricular tachycardia by Winkle et al. in 1977.[159] They observed 94 episodes of ventricular tachycardia in 23 patients. In only 15% of these episodes was ventricular tachycardia initiated by R-on-T. Kleiger et al. (1974),[79] having observed 19 cases of paroxysmal ventricular tachycardia, found only one episode in which it was initiated by R-on-T. Bliefer et al. (1973)[11] used ambulatory tape-recorded monitoring and observed 58 sequences of paroxysmal ventricular tachycardia. They found that in no instance did R-on-T alone produce the arrhythmia and, when it did occur, the R-on-T was associated with a pair of ectopic beats. The work of Van Durme and Pannier (1976)[147] also gives some indication as to the importance of R-on-T. They carefully monitored patients at monthly intervals after myocardial infarction. Of the 138 patients who survived for 1 year, only 4% exhibited R-on-T phenomena. During the study 12 patients died suddenly, 9 of whom had had previous paroxysms of ventricular

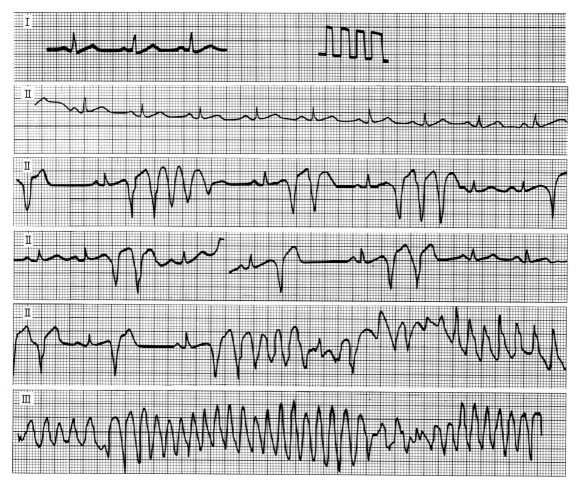

Fig. 9.15 This electrocardiogram (ECG), which is a continuous trace, reveals a sinus rhythm with a prolonged PR interval (first degree AV block) of 0.21 seconds in the first short strip and second strip. The complex of the third strip begins with a ventricular extrasystole, a compensatory pause and a normal sinus beat. This is followed by a ventricular extrasystole with R-on-T. The latter causes a run of ventricular tachycardia followed by a sinus beat. This is a *capture* beat. A ventricular extrasystole with R-on-T occurs again but ventricular tachycardia is not sustained and a second capture beat is visible, but R-on-T follows immediately. Ventricular tachycardia is not sustained. R-on-T with subsequent capture beats is seen three times in the fourth strip. By definition, ventricular tachycardia has not developed in this strip because it is defined as three or more ventricular ectopic beats in sequence. It is readily apparent, however, that R-on-T is threatening the development of a fatal arrhythmia.

In the fifth strip, R-on-T initiating ventricular tachycardia is apparent after the fifth complex, which is a capture beat. Ventricular tachycardia is followed by ventricular flutter and fibrillation in the sixth strip (lead III).

It should be noted that capture beats indicate that if more refined anti-arrhythmic medication is available and is instituted early, the development of a serious arrhythmia can be avoided.

tachycardia. Not one of these patients had exhibited the R-on-T phenomenon. Engel *et al.*, [36,38] using induced electrical stimulus, found that in very few patients was the coupling interval restricted to the area of the QT interval in order to produce ventricular tachycardia in susceptible patients.

They also concluded that unless there was a pre-existent propensity for the tachyarrhythmia to be induced, it was virtually impossible to initiate an arrhythmia. In 1977, Engel *et al.*[37] together with Spear and Moore in 1976,[137] concluded that the supernormal phase of myocardial excitement did not exist in the way that had been suggested by previous observations. The following conclusions can therefore be drawn.

1. R-on-T phenomenon is unlikely to initiate an arrhythmia in patients unless there is active ischaemic disease, such as immediately following a myocardial infarction.

2. R-on-T is most unlikely to initiate an arrhythmia in a biochemically normal person with a normal heart.

3. Even following myocardial infarction, ectopic beats which do not fall within the QT interval are more likely to initiate an arrhythmia than those falling on the T wave.

4. The coupling interval that will induce a tachyarrhythmia can vary markedly according to the condition of the myocardium, the nature of disease, and the therapy that the patient is receiving.

5. The supression of all ectopic beats by antiarrhythmic agents is important following myocardial infarction and other cardiac conditions no matter where the ectopic beats occur in the cardiac cycle.

References

1. Abitbol, H., Califano, J. E., Abate, C., Beilis, P. and Castellanos, H. (1983). Use of flecainide acetate in the treatment of premature ventricular contractions. *Amer. Heart J.*, **105**, 227.

2. Achuff, S. C., Campbell, R. W. F., Poggate, A., Murrary, A., Prescott, L. and Julian, D. G. (1975). Mexiletine in the prevention of ventricular dysrhythmias in acute myocardial infarction. *Circulation*, **51/52**.II, 147.

3. Altura, B. M. and Altura, B. T. (1974). Peripheral vascular actions of glucocorticoids and their relationship to protection in circulatory shock. *J. Pharmacol & Exper. Therapeutics*, **190**, 300.

4. Barber, J. M., Boyle, D. McC., Hussain, Z., Kelly, J. G. and McDevitt, D. G. (1977). Simple lignocaine regimen for transit to hospital after myocardial infarction. *Brit. Heart J.*, **39**, 1361.

5. Barzilai, D., Plavnick, J., Hazani, A., Einath, R., Kleinhaus, N. and Kantery, A. (1972). Use of hydrocortisone in the treatment of acute myocardial infarction. *Chest*, **61**, 488.

6. Bassan, M., Weiler-Ravell and Shalev, O. (1982). Additive antianginal effect of verapamil in patients receiving propranolol. *Brit. med. J.*, **284**, 1067.

7. Beeler, G. W. and Reuter, H. (1977). Reconstruction of the action potential of ventricular myocardial fibres. *J. Physiol. London*, **268**, 177.

8. Bellett, D., Roman, L., Kostis, J. B. and Fleischman, D. (1971). Intramuscular lidocaine in the therapy of ventricular arrhythmias *Amer. J. Cardiol.*, **27**, 291.

9. Berk, J. L. (1975). Use of vasoactive drugs in the treatment of shock. *Surgical Clinic of N. America*, **55**, 721.

10. Bernstein, V., Berstein, B., Griffiths, J. and Peretz, D. I. (1972). Lidocaine intramuscularly in acute myocardial infarction. *J. Amer. med. Ass.* **219**, 1027.

11. Bliefer, S. B., Karpman, H. L., Sheppard, J. J. and Bliefer, D. J. (1973). Relation between premature ventricular complexes and development of ventricular tachycardia. *Amer. J. Cardiol.*, **31**, 400.

12. Bradley, R. F. (1971). In *Joslin's Diabetes Mellitus*, p. 417. Edited by A. Marble, P. White, R. F. Bradley and L. P. Krall. Philadelphia: Lea & Febiger.

13. Bradley, R. F. and Schonfield, A. (1962). Diminished pain in diabetic patients with acute myocardial infarction. *Geriatrics*, **17**, 322.

14. Braunwald, E. (1980). *Heart Disease: A Textbook of Cardiovascular Medicine*. Philadelphia: W. B. Saunders.

15. British Medical Journal (1979). Leading article. *Brit. med. J.*, **1**, 969.

16. Brodsky, S. J., Cutler, S. S., Weiner, D. A. and Klein, M. D. (1981). Hepatotoxicity due to treatment with verapamil. *Ann. Int. Med.*, **94**, 490.

17. Brummer, P., Linko, E. and Kallio, V. (1961). Myocardial infarction treated by early ambulation. *Amer. Heart J.*, **62**, 478.

18. Brummer, P., Linko, E. and Kasanen, A. (1956). Myocardial infarction treated by early ambulation. *Amer. Heart J.*, **52**, 269.

19. Carey, J. S., Brown, R. S., Mohr, P. A., Monson, D. O., Yao, S. T. and Shoemaker, W. C. (1967). Cardiovascular function in shock: responses to volume loading and isoproterenol infusion. *Circulation*, **35**, 327.

20. Charles, S., Ketelslegers, J-M., Buysschaert M. and Lambert, A. (1981). Hyperglycaemic effect of nifedipine. *Brit. med. J.*, **283**, 19.

21. Chen, C. M. and Gettes, L. S. (1976). Combined effects of rate membrane potential and drugs on maximum rate of rise (Vmax) of action potential upstroke of guinea pig papillary muscle. *Circ. Res.*, **38**, 464.

22. Coltart, D. J., Bremdt, T. B., Kernoff, R. and Harrison,

D. C. (1974). Antiarrhythmic and circulatory effects of Astra W36095 (a new Lidocaine-like agent). *Amer. J. Cardiol.*, **34**, 35.

23. Cranefield, P. F. and Hoffman, B. F. (1958). Propagated repolarization in heart muscle. *J. Gen. Physiol.*, **41**, 633.

24. Cronin, R. F. P., Moore, S. and Marpole, D. C. (1965). Shock following myocardial infarction. A clinical survey of 140 cases. *Canad. Med. Assoc. J.*, **93**, 57.

25. Cronin, R. F. P. and Zsotér, T. (1965). Hemodynamic effects of rapid digitalization in experimental cardiogenic shock. *Amer. Heart J.*, **69**, 233.

26. Dash, H., Johnson, R. A., Dinsmore, R. E., Francis, C. K. and Harthorne, J. W. (1977). Cardiomyopathic syndrome due to coronary artery disease II. Increased prevalence in patients with diabetes mellitus: a matched pair analysis. *Brit. Heart J.*, **39**, 740.

27. De Sanctis, R. W., Block, R. and Hutter, A. M. (1972). Tachyarrhythmias in myocardial infarction. *Circulation*, **45**, 682.

28. De Soyza, N., Bissett, J. K., Kane, J. J., Murphy, M. L. and Doherty, J. E. (1974). Ectopic ventricular prematurity and its relationship to ventricular tachycardia in acute myocardial infarction in man. *Circulation*, **50**, 529.

29. Dhurandhar, R. W., MacMillan, R. L. and Brown, K. W. G. (1971). Primary ventricular fibrillation complicating acute myocardial infarction. *Amer. J. Cardiol.*, **27**, 347.

30. Dhurandhar, R. W., Teasdale, S. J. and Mahon, W. A. (1971). Bretylium tosylate in the management of refractory ventricular fibrillation. *Can. Med. Assoc. J.*, **105**, 161.

31. Duke, M. (1971). Bed rest in acute myocardial infarction. *Amer. Heart J.*, **82**, 486.

32. Eichna, L. W. (1967). Treatment of cardiogenic shock: III. Use of isoproterenol in cardiogenic shock. *Amer. Heart J.*, **74**, 848.

33. El-Sherif, N., Myerbury, R. J., Scherlag, B. J., Befeler, B., Aranda, J. M., Castellanos, A. and Lazzara, R. (1976). Electrocardiograph antecedents of primary ventricular fibrillation. Value of the R-on-T phenomenon in myocardial infarction. *Brit. Heart J.*, **38**, 415.

34. El-Sherif, N., Scherlag, B. J. and Lazzara, R. (1975). Electrode catheter recordings during malignant ventricular arrhythmia following experimental acute myocardial ischaemia. Evidence for re-entry due to conduction delay and block in ischaemic myocardium. *Circulation*, **51**, 1003.

35. Engel, H. J., Hundeshagen, H. and Lichtlen, P. (1977). Transmural myocardial infarction in young women taking oral contraceptives. Evidence of reduced regional coronary flow in spite of normal coronary arteries. *Brit. Heart J.*, **39**, 477.

36. Engel, T. R., Frankl, W. S. and Meister, S. (1976). Premature ventricular stimulation during sinus rhythm (abstract). In *Proceedings of the VIth Asian Pacific Congress of Cardiology*, p. 96.

37. Engel, T. R., Meister, S. G. and Frankl, W. S. (1977). The extent of supernormal ventricular excitability in man. *J. Electrocardiol.*, **10**, 13.

38. Engel, T. R., Mendizabal, R., Meister, S. G., Bentivoglio, L. G. and Frankl, W. S. (1975). Testing for ventricular tachycardia with programmed extrasystoles in sinus rhythm (abstract). *Circulation*, **52** (Suppl. II), 11.

39. Epstein, S. E., Beiser, G. D., Rosing, D. R., Talano, J. V. and Karsh, R. B. (1973). Experimental acute myocardial infarction. Characterization and treatment of the malignant premature ventricular contraction. *Circulation*, **47**, 446.

40. Epstein, S. E., Goldstein, R. E., Redwood, D. R., Kent, K. M. and Smith, E. R. (1973). The early phase of acute myocardial infarction: pharmacologic aspects of therapy. *Ann. Int. Med.*, **78**, 918.

41. Erhardt, L. R. (1974). Clinical and pathological observations in different types of acute myocardial infarction. *Acta. Med. Scand.*, **Suppl. 560**.

42. Erhardt, L. R., Sjogren, A. and Wahlberg, I. (1976). Single right-sided precordial lead in the diagnosis of right ventricular involvement in inferior myocardial infarction. *Amer. Heart J.*, **91**, 571.

43. Faerman, I., Faccio, E., Milei, J., Nunez, R., Jadinsky, M., Fox, D. and Rapaport, M. (1977). Autonomic neuropathy and painless myocardial infarction in diabetic patients, Histologic evidence of their relationship. *Diabetes*, **26**, 1147.

44. Farrer-Brown, G. (1968). Vascular pattern of myocardium of right ventricle of human heart. *Brit. Heart J.*, **30**, 679.

45. Fehmers, M. C. O. and Dunning, A. J. (1972). Intramuscularly and orally administered lidocaine in the treatment of ventricular arrhythmias in acute myocardial infarction. *Amer. J. Cardiol.*, **29**, 514.

46. Ferrer, M. I. (1976). *Pre-excitation*. New York: Futura Publishing Co.

47. Flear, C. T. G. and Hilton, P. (1979). Hyponatraemia and severity and outcome of myocardial infarction. *Brit. med. J.*, **1**, 1242.

48. Fozzard, H. A. (1977). Heart: excitation-contraction coupling. *Ann. Rev. Physiol.*, **39**, 201.

49. Friedberg, C. K. (1966). *Diseases of the Heart.*, 3rd edn. Philadelphia: W. B. Saunders.

50. Gillespie, T. A., Ambos, H. D., Sobel, B. E. and Roberts, R. R. (1977). Effects of dobutamine in patients with acute myocardial infarction. *Amer. J. Cardiol.*, **39**, 588.

51. Giugliano, D., Torella, R., Cacciapuoti, F., Gentile, S., Verza, M. and Varriescho, M. (1980). Impairment of insulin secretion in man by nifedipine. *Eur. J. Clin. Pharmacol.*, **18**, 395.

52. Gouaux, J. L. and Ashman, R. (1947). Auricular fibrillation with aberration simulating ventricular paroxysmal tachycardia. *Amer. Heart J.*, **34**, 366.

53. Gunnar, R. M. and Loeb, H. S. (1972). The use of

drugs in cardiogenic shock due to acute myocardial infarction. *Circulation*, **45**, 1111.

54. Gunnar, R. M., Loeb, H. S., Pietras, R. J. and Tobin, J. R. (1967). Ineffectiveness of isoproterenol in shock due to acute myocardial infarction. *J. Amer. med. Ass.*, **202**, 1124.

55. Haglund, U. (1974). Effect of large doses of methyl-prednisolone on the cardiovascular derangement induced by simulated intestinal shock. *Europ. Surg. Res.*, **6**, 277.

56. Han, J. (1969). Mechanisms of ventricular arrhythmias associated with myocardial infarction. *Amer. J. Cardiol.*, **24**, 800.

57. Harlan, W. R., Oberman, A., Grimm, R. and Rosati, R. A. (1977). Chronic congestive heart failure in coronary artery disease: clinical criteria. *Ann. Int. Med.*, **86**, 133.

58. Harrower, A. D. B. (1977). Cardiovascular disease in diabetes mellitus. *Br. J. Clin. Pract.*, **31**, 47.

59. Harrower, A. D. B. and Clarke, B. F. (1976). Experience of coronary care in diabetes. *Brit. med. J.*, **i**, 126.

60. Heaseman, M. A. and Carstairs, V. (1971). Inpatient management variations in some aspects of practice in Scotland. *Brit. med. J.*, **i**, 495.

61. Hellestrand, K. (1981). The electrophysiological effects of flecainide acetate on the cardiac conduction system. *Proceedings of the British Pharmaceutical Society,* 16–18 September.

62. Hirschfeld, J. W., Borer, J. S. and Goldstein, R. E. (1973). Reduction in extent of myocardial infarction when nitroglycerin and methoxamine are administered during coronary occlusion. *Clin. Res.*, **21 (Abst.)** 426.

63. Hoffman, B. F. and Cranefield, P. F. (1960). *Electrophysiology of the Heart.* New York: McGraw-Hill.

64. Hollinger, G. (1960). On the metabolism of lidocaine. II. The biotransformation of lidocaine. *Acta. Pharmacol. et Toxicol.*, **17**, 365.

65. Holzer, J., Karliner, J. S., O'Rourke, R. A., Pitt, W. and Ross, J. (1973). Effectiveness of dopamine in patients with cardiogenic shock. *Am. J. Cardiol.*, **32**, 79.

66. Hood, W. B., Yenikomshian, S., Norman, J. C. and Levine, H. D. (1968). Treatment of refractory ventricular tachysystole with hyperbaric oxygenation. *Am. J. Cardiol.*, **22**, 738.

67. Horwitz, D., Fox, S. M. and Goldberg, L. I. (1962). Effects of dopamine in man. *Circulation Research*, **10**, 237.

68. Irvin, C. W. and Burgess, A. M. (1950). The abuse of bed rest in the treatment of myocardial infarction. *N. Engl. J. of Med.*, **243**, 486.

69. Isner, J. M. and Roberts, W. C. (1978). Right ventricular infarction complicating left ventricular infarction secondary to coronary heart disease: frequency, location, associated findings and significance from analysis of 236 necropsy patients with acute or healed myocardial infarction. *Am. J. Cardiol.*, **42**, 885.

70. Jack, J. J. B., Noble, D. and Tsien, R. W. (1975). *Electric current flow in excitable cells*, p. 502. Oxford: Clarendon Press.

71. James, T. N. (1963). The connecting pathways between the sinus node and the AV node and between the right and left atrium in the human heart. *Amer. Heart J.*, **66**, 498.

72. Jarrett, J. (1977). Diabetes and the heart: coronary heart disease. *Clin. Endocr. Metab.*, **6**, 389.

73. Katz, A. M. (1977). *Physiology of the heart*, p. 239. New York: Raven Press.

74. Katz, B. (1948). Electrical properties of the muscle fiber membrane. *Proc. R. Soc.*, **135**, 506.

75. Katz, L. N. and Pick, A. (1956). *Clinical Electrocardiography: The Arrhythmias.* Philadelphia: Lea & Febiger.

76. Kent, A. F. S. (1893). Researches on structure and function of mammalian heart. *J. Physiol.*, **14**, 233.

77. Kent, K. M., Smith, E. R., and Redwood, D. R. (1973). Electrical stability of acutely ischaemic myocardium. *Circulation*, **47**, 291.

78. Kinlen, L. J. (1973). Incidence and presentation of myocardial infarction in an English community. *Brit. Heart J.*, **35**, 616.

79. Kleiger, R. E., Martin, T. F., Miller, J. P. and Iliver, G. G. (1974). Ventricular tachycardia and ventricular extrasystoles during the later recovery phase of myocardial infarction (abstract). *Amer. J. Cardiol.*, **33**, 149.

80. Koch-Weser, J. (1974). Clinical application of the pharmocokinetics of procainamide. *Cardiovasc. Clin.*, **6**, 63.

81. Lal, H. B. and Caroli, R. K. (1968). A study of myocardial infarction. *Indian J. Med. Res.*, **56 (Suppl.)**, 1107.

82. Lalka, D., Meyer, M. D., Duce, B. R. and Elvin, A. T. (1976). Kinetics of the oral antiarrhythmic lidocaine congener, tocainide. *Clin. Pharmacol. Ther.*, **19**, 757.

83. Langendorf, R. (1948). Concealed A-V conduction. The effect of blocked impulses on the formation and conduction of subsequent impulses. *Amer. Heart J.*, **35**, 542.

84. Langendorf, R. (1951). Aberrant ventricular conduction. *Amer. Heart J.*, **41**, 70.

85. Langer, G. A. (1973). Heart: excitation-contraction coupling. *Ann. Rev. Physiol.*, **35**, 55.

86. Lauper, N. T., Lichtlen, P. and Rossier, P. H. (1966). Modified armchair treatment as a safe routine procedure in the therapy of acute myocardial infarction. *Helv. Med. Acta*, **4**, 279.

87. Lev, M. (1964). The normal anatomy of the conduction system in man and its pathology in atrioventricular block. *Ann. N. Y. Acad. Sci.*, **111**, 817.

88. Levine, S. A. (1940). *Clinical Heart Disease*, 2nd edn. Philadelphia and London: W. B. Saunders.

89. Levine, S. A. (1951). *Clinical Heart Disease*, 4th edn. Philadelphia: W. B. Saunders

90. Levine, S. A. and Lown, B. (1952). 'Armchair' treatment of acute coronary thrombosis. *J. Amer. med. Ass.*, **148**, 1365.

91. Lewis, T. (1937). *Diseases of the Heart.* New York: The Macmillan Co.

92. Lie, K. I., Wellens, H. J., Van Capelle, F. J. and Durrer, D. (1974). Lidocaine in the prevention of primary ventricular fibrillation. A double-blind randomized study of 212 consecutive patients. *N. Engl. J. of Med.*, **291**, 1324.

93. Lown, B., Clien, M. D. and Hershberg, P. I. (1969). Coronary and precoronary care. *Amer. J. Med.*, **46**, 705.

94. Lown, B., Kaid Bey, S., Periroth, M. G. and Abe, T. (1963). Comparative studies of ventricular vulnerability to fibrillation. *J. Clin. Invest.*, **42**, 953.

95. Lown, B. and Wolfe, M. (1971). Approaches to sudden death from coronary heart disease. *Circulation*, **44**, 130.

96. MacLean, L. D., Duff, J. H., Scott, H. M. and Peretz, D. I. (1965). Treatment of shock in man based on haemodynamic diagnosis. *Surg. Gynecol. & Obstet.* **120**, 1.

97. Maley, T., Gulotta, S. and Morrison, J. (1966). Effect of methylprednisone on predicted infarct size in man. *Clin. Res.*, **14**, 193.

98. Maroko, P. R., Kjekshus, J. K., Sobel, B. E., Watanabe, T., Covell, J. W., Ross, J. and Braunwald, E. (1971). Factors influencing infarct size following experimental coronary artery occlusions. *Circulation*, **43**, 67.

99. Mather, H. G., Pearson, N. G., Read, K. L. O., Shaw, D. B., Steed, G. R., Thorne, M. G., Jones, S., Guerrier, C. J., Eraut, C. D., McHugh, P. M., Chowdhury, N. R., Jafary, M. H., Wallace, T. J., (1971). Acute myocardial infarction, Home and hospital treatment. *Brit. med. J.*, **3**, 334.

100. Matsumoto, S., Takashi, I., Sada, T., Takahashi, M., Su, K-M., Ueda, A., Okabe, F., Sato, M., Sekine, I. and Ito, Y. (1980). Hemodynamic effects of nifedipine in congestive heart failure. *Am. J. Cardiol.*, **46**, 476.

101. McAllister, R. E., Noble, D., Tsien, R. W. (1975). Reconstruction of the electrical activity of cardiac Purkinje fibres. *J. Physiol. London.*, **251**, 1.

102. McGee, D. and Gordon, T. (1976). *The Framingham Study, Section 31,* (DHEW). Publ. No. NIH 76–1083. Washington: Government Printing Office.

103. Miller, G. J. and Miller, N. E. (1975). Plasma-high-density-lipoprotein concentration and development of ischaemic heart disease. *Lancet*, **i**, 16.

104. Miller, N. E., Førde, A. H., Thelle, D. S. and Mjøs, O. D. (1977). The Tromsø heart study. High density lipoprotein and coronary heart disease: a prospective case-control study. *Lancet*, **i**, 965.

105. Moe, G. K., Abildskov, J. A. and Mendez, C. (1964). An experimental study of concealed conduction. *Amer. Heart J.*, **67**, 338.

106. Moon, A. J., Williams, K. G. and Hopkinson, W. I. (1964). A patient with coronary thrombosis treated with hyperbaric oxygen. *Lancet*, **i**, 18.

107. Moore, E. N., Spear, J. F., Horowitz, L. N., Feldman, H. S. and Moller, R. A. (1978). Electrophysiologic properties of a new antiarrhythmic drug—tocainide. *Amer. J. Cardiol.*, **41**, 703.

108. Naughton, J., Bruhn, J., Lategola, M. T., and Whitsett, T. (1969) Rehabilitation following myocardial infarction, *Amer. J. Med.*, **46**, 725.

109. Opie, L. H. (1980). Drugs and the heart. Calcium antagonists. *Lancet*, **i**, 806.

110. Paes de Carvalho, A. (1961). Cellular electrophysiology of the atrial specialized tissues. In *The specialised tissues of the heart.* Edited by A. Paes de Carvalho, W. C. De Mello and B. F. Hoffman. Amsterdam: Elsevier.

111. Page, M. M. and Watkins, P. J. (1977). The heart in diabetes: autonomic neuropathy and cardiomyopathy. *Clin. Endocr. Metab.*, **6**, 377.

112. Pantridge, J. F. and Geddes, J. S. (1967). A mobile intensive-care unit in the management of myocardial infarction. *Lancet*, **ii**, 271.

113. Perlow, G. M., Jain, B. P., Pauker, J. G., Zarren, H. S., Wistran, D. C. & Epstein, R. L. (1981). Tocainide—associated interstitial pneumonitis., *Ann. Int. Med.*, **94**, 488.

114. Prinzmetal, M., Ekmekci, A., Kennamer, R., Kwoczynski, J. K., Shubin, H. and Toyoshima, H. (1960). Variant form of angina pectoris previously undelineated syndrome. *J. Amer. med. Ass.*, **174**, 1094.

115. Prinzmetal, M., Kennamer, R., Merliess, R., Wada, T. and Bor, N. (1959). Angina pectoris. I. A variant form of angina pectoris preliminary report. *Amer. J. Med.*, **27**, 375.

116. Puri, P. S. (1974). Modification of experimental myocardial infarct size by cardiac drugs. *Amer. J. Cardiol.*, **33**, 521.

117. Rhoads, G. G., Gulbrandsen, C. L. and Kagan, A. (1976). Serum liproproteins and coronary heart disease in a population study of Hawaii Japanese men. *N. Engl. J. of Med.*, **294**, 293.

118. Richmond, D. R. (1980). Coronary artery spasm: a review. *J. Roy. Soc. Med.*, **73**, 570.

119. Rosenbaum, R. and Frieden, J. (1972). Intravenous dopamine in the treatment of myocardial infarction after open-heart surgery. *Amer. Heart J.*, **83**, 743.

120. Rosenblum, R., Berkowitz, W. D. and Lawson, D. (1968). Effect of acute intravenous administration of isoproterenol on cardiorenal hemodynamics in man. *Circulation*, **38**, 158.

121. Rosenblum, R., Tai, A. R. and Lawson, D. (1972). Dopamine in man: cardiorenal hemodynamics in normotensive patients with heart disease. *J. Pharmacol. Exp. Ther.*, **183**, 256.

122. Rothfeld, E. L., Parsonnet, J., McGorman, W. and

Linden, S. (1977). Harbingers of paroxysmal ventricular tachycardia in acute myocardial infarction. *Chest*, **71**, 142.

123. Rotman, M., Ratliff, N. B. and Hawley, J. (1974). Right ventricular infarction: a haemodynamic diagnosis. *Brit. Heart J.*, **36**, 941.

124. Russek, H. I. (1968). Propranolol and isosorbide dinitrate synergism in angina pectoris. *Am. J. Cardiol.*, **21**, 44.

125. Sakamoto, T. and Yamada, T. (1977). Hemodynamic effects of dobutamine in patients following open heart surgery. *Circulation,* **55**, 525.

126. Sayen, J. J., Katcher, A. H., Sheldon, W. F. and Gilbert, C. M. (1960). The effect of levarterenol on polarographic myocardial oxygen, the epicardial electrogram and contraction in non-ischemic dog hearts and experimental acute regional ischemic dog hearts and experimental acute regional ischemia. *Circ. Res.,* **8**, 109.

127. Schuelke, D. M. and Mark, A. L. (1971). Coronary vasodilation produced by dopamine after adrenergic blockade. *J. Pharmacol. Exp. Ther.*, **176**, 320.

128. Schwartz A., Matlib, A., Balwierczak, J. and Lathrop, D. A. (1985). Pharmacology of calcium antagonists. *Am. J. Cardiol.*, **55**, 30.

129. Smirk, F. H. (1949). R waves interrupting T waves. *Brit. Heart J.*, **11**, 2.

130. Smirk, F. H. and Palmer, D. G. (1960). A myocardial syndrome: with particular references to the occurrence of sudden death and of premature systoles interrupting antecedent T waves. *Amer. J. Cardiol.*, **6**, 620.

131. Smith, E. R., Redwood, D. R., McCarron, W. E. and Epstein, S. E. (1973). Coronary occlusion in the conscious dog. *Circulation*, **47**, 51.

132. Smith, G. (1964). Therapeutic applications of oxygen at two atmospheres pressure. *Dis. Chest.*, **45**, 15.

133. Smith, H. C., Oriol, A., March, J. and McGregor, M. (1967). Hemodynamic studies in cardiogenic shock. Treatment with isoproterenol and metaraminol. *Circulation*, **35**, 1084.

134. Soler, N. G., Bennett, M. A., Pentecost, B. L., Fitzgerald, M. G. and Malins, J. M. (1975). Myocardial infarction in diabetics. *Quart. J. Med.*, **44**, 125.

135. Soler, N. G., Pentecost, B. L., Bennett, M. A., Fitzgerald, M. G., Lamb, P. and Malins, J. M. (1974). Coronary care for myocardial infarction in diabetics. *Lancet*, **i**, 475.

136. Spath, J. A., Lane, D. L. and Lefer, A. M. (1974). Protective action of methylprednisolone on the myocardium during experimental myocardial ischemia in the cat. *Circulation Research*, **35**, 44.

137. Spear, J. F. and Moore, E. N. (1976). Supernormal excitability and conduction. In *The Conduction System of the Heart*, p. 111. Edited by H. J. J. Wellens, K. I. Lie and M. J. Janse. Philadelphia: Lea and Febiger.

138. Stanhope, J. M., Sampson, V. M. and Clarkson, P. M. (1977). High-density-lipoprotein cholesterol and other serum lipids in a New Zealand biracial adolescent sample. *Lancet*, **i**, 968.

139. Talley, R. C., Goldberg, L. I., Johnson, C. E. and McNay, J. L. (1969). A hemodynamic comparison of dopamine and isoproterenol in patients in shock. *Circulation*, **39**, 361.

140. Tawara, S. (1906). *Das Reizleitunzssytem des Saugetierherzens*. Jena: Gustav Fischer.

141. Thibault, G. E., Farham, G. S. and Myers, R. W. (1973). Increased myocardial ischaemia caused by reflexly induced hypotension during coronary occlusion in the conscious dog. *Clin. Res.*, **21 (Abst.)**, 54.

142. Thurston, J. G., Greenwood, T. W. and Bending, M. R. (1973). A controlled investigation into the effects of hyperbaric oxygen on mortality following acute myocardial infarction. *Quart. J. Med.*, **42**, 751.

143. Ulbricht, W. (1977). Ionic channels and gating currents in excitable membranes. *Ann. Rev. Biophys. Bioeng.*, **6**, 7.

144. Underwood, D. A., Proudfit, W. L., Lim, J. and MacMillian, J. P. (1985). Symptomatic coronary artery disease in patients aged 21 to 30 years. *Am. J. Cardiol.*, **55**, 631.

145. Valentine, P. A., Frew, J. L., Mashford, M. L. and Sloman, J. G. (1974). Lidocaine in the prevention of sudden death in the pre-hospital phase of acute infarction: a double-blind study. *N. Engl. J of Med.*, **291**, 1327.

146. Valentine, P. A., Sloman, J. F. and McIntyre, M. (1971). A double blind trial of lidocaine in acute cardiac infarction. In *Lidocaine in the treatment of ventricular arrhythmias*. Edited by D. B. Scott and D. G. Julian. Edinburgh: E. & S. Livingstone.

147. Van Durme, J. P. and Pannier, R. H. (1976). Prognostic significance of ventricular dysrhythmias 1 year after myocardial infarction. *Amer. J. Cardiol.*, **37 (Abst.)**, 178.

148. Van Winkle, W. B. and Schwartz, A. (1976). Ions and inotropy, *Ann. Rev. Physiol.*, **38**, 247.

149. Wackers, F. J. T., Lie, K. I., Sokole, E. B., Res, J., Van der Schoot, J. B. and Durrer, D. (1978). Prevalence of right ventricular involvement in inferior wall infarction assessed with myocardial imaging with thallium-201 and technetium-99m pyrophosphate. *Amer. J. Cardiol.*, **42**, 358.

150. Wartman, W. B. and Hellerstein, H. K. (1948). The incidence of heart disease in 2,000 consecutive autopsies. *Ann. Int. Med.,* **28**, 41.

151. Watanabe, Y. and Dreifus, L. S. (1965). Inhomogeneous conduction in the A-V node: a model for reentry. *Amer. Heart J.*, **70**, 505.

152. Watanabe, Y. and Dreifus, L. S. (1967). Second degree atrioventricular block. *Cardiovasc. Res.*, **1**, 150.

153. Waxler, E. B. (1971). Myocardial infarction and oral contraceptive agents. *Amer. J. Cardiol.*, **28**, 96.

154. Wellens, H. J., Duren, D. R. and Lie, K. I. (1976). Observations on mechanisms of ventricular tachycardia in man. *Circulation*, **54**, 237.

155. Wellens, H. J. J., Lie, K. I., Durrer, D. (1974). Further observations on ventricular tachycardia as studied by electrical stimulation of the heart. Chronic recurrent ventricular tachycardia and ventricular tachycardia during acute myocardial infarction. *Circulation*, **49**, 647.

156. White, P. D. (1945) *Heart disease*, 3rd edn. New York: The Macmillan Co.

157. Wilkinson, J. H. (1962). *An introduction to diagnostic enzymology*, p. 246. London: Edward Arnold.

158. Williams, D. O., Scherlag, B. J., Hope, R. R., El-Sherif, N. and Lazzara, R. (1974). The pathophysiology of malignant ventricular arrhythmias during acute myocardial ischaemia. *Circulation*, **50**, 1163.

159. Winkle, R. A., Derrington, D. C. and Schroeder, J. S. (1977). Characteristics of ventricular tachycardia in ambulatory patients. *Amer. J. Cardiol.*, **39**, 487.

160. Winkle, R. A., Meffin, P. J., Fitzgerald, J. W. and Harrison, D. C. (1976). Clinical efficacy and pharmokinetics of a new orally effective antiarrhythmic, tocainide. *Circulation*, **54**, 884.

161. Wolff, L., Parkinson, J., White, P. D. (1930). Bundle-branch block with short P-R Interval in healthy young people prone to paroxysmal tachycardia. *Amer. Heart J.*, **5**, 685.

162. Wood, P. (1960). *Diseases of the heart and circulation*, 2nd edn. London: Eyre and Spottiswoode.

163. Wood, P. (1968). *Diseases of the heart and circulation*, 2nd edn. London: Eyre and Spottiswoode.

164. Yater, W. M., Aaron, H. T., Brown, W. G., Fitzgerald, R. P., Geisler, M. A. and Wilcox, B. B. (1948). Coronary artery disease in men 18 to 39 years of age: Part 3. *Amer. Heart J.*, **36**, 683.

165. Zeluff, G. W., Caskey, C. T. and Jackson, D. (1978). Heart attack or stroke in a young man? Think Fabry's disease. *Heart & Lung*, **7**, 1056.

Further Reading

De Feyter, P. J., Serruys, P. W., van den Brand, M., Balakumaran, K., Mochtar, B., Soward, A. L., Arnold, A. E. R. and Hugenholtz, P. G. (1985). Emergency coronary angioplasty in refractory unstable angina. *N. Engl. J. of Med.*, **313**, 342.

Goenen, M., Pedemonte, O., Baele, P. and Col, J. (1985). Amrinone in the management of low cardiac output after open heart surgery. *Amer. J. Cardiol.*, **56**, 33B.

Greenberg, H. M., Kulbertus, H. E., Moss, A. J. and Schwartz, P. J. (1984). Clinical aspects of life-threatening arrhythmias. *Ann. N.Y. Acad. Sci.*, **427**.

Remme, W. J., Diederick, C. A., Van Hoogenhuyze, X., Krauss, H., Hofman, A., Kruyssen, A. C. M. and Storm, C. J. (1985). Acute hemodynamic and antiischemic effects of intravenous amiodarone. *Amer. J. Cardiol.*, **55**, 639.

Taylor, S. H., Verma, S. P., Hussain, M., Reynolds, G., Jackson, C., Hafizullah, M., Richmond, A. and Silke, B. (1985). Intravenous amrinone in left ventricular failure complicated by acute myocardial infarction. *Amer. J. Cardiol.*, **56**, 29B.

Chapter 10
Cardiac Disease II: acute problems and their treatment

THE TACHYARRHYTHMIAS

The causes of tachyarrhythmias have been divided by De Sanctis *et al.*[36] into five categories which overlap to some degree. These are metabolic, anatomic, autonomic, haemodynamic and iatrogenic. The author would prefer to add endocrine to the De Sanctis classification as a separate category.

The tachyarrhythmias commonly found in critical care areas of the hospital are listed in Table 10.1.

Paroxysmal Tachycardia

These tachycardias are characteristically of sudden onset and sudden cessation, beginning and ending without warning. Although they may occur in some people with no organic myocardial disease, they constitute a danger to those who have acquired or congenital cardiac abnormalities. The attacks may last for only a few seconds or may continue for some hours and have been known to extend over a period of weeks; however, with the introduction of anti-arrhythmic agents and DC countershock, this is now rarely allowed to occur.

Disturbances of rhythm are commonly divided into supraventricular and ventricular forms. Supraventricular arrhythmias that can be seen on ECG to be originating in the auricle or atrioventricular (AV) node and, therefore, unless conducted aberrantly (see p. 307), they have a normal QRS complex. Ventricular arrhythmias originate in the ventricles and, as seen on ECG, have a deformed QRS-T complex with a prolonged QRS interval.

Differentiation rests on the identification of the P wave. Although in most cases the P wave can be identified (albeit occasionally with difficulty), serious tachyarrhythmias develop, causing profound hypotension in which identification of the

Table 10.1 The major causes of the tachyarrhythmias

A Metabolic	Electrolyte imbalance Acid–base imbalance Hypoxia Hypocarbia Anaemia
B Endocrine	Phaeochromocytoma Thyroid disease Diabetes Addison's disease
C Autonomic	Emotional stress Pain Pyrexia Sympathomimetic drugs Toxins Central nervous system abnormalities Hypoxia Hypovolaemia
D Anatomic	SA node abnormalities and ischaemia AV node abnormalities and ischaemia Pericardial disease Myocardial ischaemia Re-entrant, pre-excitation pathway activity Trauma to the heart
E Haemodynamic	Hypotension and hypertension Pulmonary embolus Left ventricular failure Mitral and tricuspid valve disease Pericardial effusion Constrictive pericarditis Cardiac tamponade
F Iatrogenic	Digitalis (excess) Diuretics Anorexants Decongestants Antidepressants Thyroid preparations Bronchodilators Excess fluid administered intravenously

P wave is impossible. Synchronized DC shock is then commonly the treatment of choice.

Clinical characteristics of paroxysmal atrial tachycardia

In the short, acute attack the symptoms may be mild or severe. The patient complains of palpitations appearing suddenly, a feeling of fullness in the neck and mouth, weakness, dizziness, faintness and marked depression. If the attack is prolonged, the patient may become severely breathless because of cardiac failure, and substernal pain of an ischaemic nature may develop in patients who have no ischaemic heart disease. Severe pain may be felt in the back between the shoulder blades. Profuse sweating sometimes occurs and the patient may vomit. Syncope can occur. The attack can produce and, conversely, is sometimes caused by, an epileptiform attack.

When the symptoms are mild some patients become accustomed to the condition and may be unaware of its presence. In the severe attack the patient has a greyish pallor, is mildly dyspnoeic and, if the blood pressure has fallen to low levels, may be disorientated or comatose because of cerebral ischaemia.

The pulse rate is found to be between 150 and 250/minute, is perfectly regular and, on the electrocardiogram (ECG), each QRS complex is normal and preceded by a P wave.

Atrial tachycardia can be seen in conjunction with bundle branch block (which is present only during the tachycardia) when the P wave is difficult or impossible to identify. It can be seen also with each impulse conducted aberrantly, when not only is the P wave unidentifiable but the ECG has the appearance of *ventricular tachycardia*.

Some workers, such as Schamroth (1980),[132] are of the opinion that, because of these difficulties, the diagnosis of ventricular tachycardia can never be made with certainty. Help in making the differentiation frequently lies in the field of clinical examination, and a knowledge of the previous history of the patient, for example, the presence of Wolff–Parkinson–White syndrome or the existence of an earlier ECG demonstrating R on T phenomena (see p. 310).

In the young adult paroxysmal atrial tachycardia (PAT) may be asymptomatic or the symptoms may be limited to palpitations and a vague feeling of tiredness. It is subject to abrupt onset and abrupt termination, which can be achieved by no action at all or by simple manoeuvres such as taking a deep breath and holding it against a closed glottis (the Valsalva manoeuvre) aided by increasing the intra-abdominal pressure or by carotid sinus massage or pressure on the eyeball.

In adults where the origin of the PAT is more commonly due to intrinsic heart disease, the patient frequently presents with hypotension, ischaemic chest pain and congestive cardiac failure. When these factors are present, electrical cardioversion is almost always indicated.

Pressure on a carotid sinus may terminate the event. Pressure on both carotid sinuses may cause the patient to faint, but when performed intermittently so fainting is avoided, this is much more effective than pressure on a single carotid sinus alone. Eyeball pressure is similarly sometimes effective in terminating the arrhythmia.

Treatment of supraventricular tachycardias

Paroxysmal atrial tachycardia (PAT)*

Raising the blood pressure is often effective, with an agent such as phenylephrine (Neosynephrine, Neophryn) 1 mg diluted in 10–20 ml of saline given slowly intravenously, or metaraminol (Aramine) 100 mg diluted in 200 or 250 ml of 5% glucose or glucose/saline infused at a rate which is sufficient to raise the blood pressure by 30–40 mmHg. The ECG should be monitored so that the infusion can be stopped if severe ischaemic changes appear.

Edrophonium (Tensilon), by allowing the accumulation of acetylcholine at the nerve endings as a result of its anticholinesterase effect, and by causing an increase in vagal tone, can induce cessation of the arrhythmia. A test dose of 1 mg should be given, followed by the slow injection of 5–10 mg i.v. If unpleasant cholinergic effects develop, 0.6 or 1 mg of atropine can be administered intravenously.

Summary of treatment of PAT
1. Carotid sinus massage.
2. Eyeball pressure.
3. Valsalva manoeuvre.
4. Sedation—diazepam, 5–10 mg p.o. or i.v.
5. Increase of systemic blood pressure.
6. Propranolol.
7. Digoxin.
8. Electrical cardioversion.
9. Edrophonium (Tensilon).
10. Verapamil.
11. Amiodarone.

* *Note:* the treatment of multifocal atrial tachycardia is the same as that for PAT.

Supraventricular tachycardias are usually due to re-entry mechanisms at the AV junction level. Increased automaticity is, however, another common cause. They are commonly associated with a functioning pre-excitation pathway.

It is therefore apparent that treatment should be directed at interrupting the re-entry mechanism with either vagal stimulation or drugs that slow AV conduction.

These drugs include digitalis, verapamil (Cordilox) and beta-blockers. The anti-arrhythmic agents that decrease myocardial excitability and automaticity are also effective. These include disopyramide (Norpace, Rythmodan), phenytoin (diphenylhydantoin, Epanutin) and quinidine. When these measures fail cardioversion or artificial cardiac pacing should be instituted.

In a small number of cases the tachycardia is due to an ectopic focus which has an enhanced automaticity caused by drugs or generalized disease. In these circumstances attempts to terminate the arrhythmia by vagal stimulation is ineffective and the extracardiac cause of the arrhythmia should be identified and treated. Digitalis intoxication can, however, be treated with beta-blockers and, if the generalized disease cannot be correctly treated, surgical intervention, breaking the accessory pathway, is sometimes necessary.

Verapamil is the treatment of choice and is given intravenously in doses of 5–10 mg. It is effective in 90% of patients. The beta-blocker propranolol (Inderal), which is not cardioselective, is given in doses of 1 mg i.v., and practolol (Eraldin) is given in doses of 5 mg i.v. Practolol is cardioselective but should be used with the precautions mentioned on page 331 with regard to having an isoprenaline (isoproterenol) infusion readily available. Amiodarone (see p. 332) is also a valuable and effective agent.

Paroxysmal (AV) junctional tachycardia

This arrhythmia is defined as three or more consecutive premature beats that are AV junctional in origin. Paroxysmal junctional tachycardia (PJT) closely resembles paroxysmal atrial tachycardia (PAT) when seen on the ECG for the first time. The ventricular rate is approximately 160–200 beats/minute, with a precisely regular response.[123] The P waves, which are sometimes inverted, have no constant relationship to the QRS complex and occur before, after or in the R waves. Commonly, no P waves are visible as they are buried in the QRS complex. PJT can occur in the absence of any form of heart disease, and the treatment is identical to that of PAT.

Non-paroxysmal junctional tachycardia

Non-paroxysmal junctional tachycardia has a gradual onset and gradual termination.[123,126] It has a slower rate than PJT, the ventricular rate is 70–130 beats/minute. It does not usually respond to carotid sinus massage. AV dissociation is commonly present, with the junctional rate faster than the atrial rate, and the relationship of atrial activity to the R wave is not constant.

The arrhythmia may result from disease depressing the function of the sinoatrial (SA) node, though it can be induced by the enhancement of automaticity in the junctional tissue as a result of infection (e.g. rheumatic carditis), digitalis toxicity, ischaemia, myocardial infarction, and metabolic and biochemical disorders. It commonly occurs as an *escape rhythm* secondary to a sinus bradycardia or SA or AV block. It is often seen following cardiac surgery. If it produces no significant haemodynamic effect which, because of the slower rate, is usually so, no specific treatment is necessary. If, however, it is seen following myocardial infarction, anti-arrhythmic treatment should be instituted. Digitalis intoxication may also require more active intervention than simple withdrawal of the drug. The treatment for non-paroxysmal junctional tachycardia is the same as that which is used for PAT.

Pre-excitation syndrome with re-entry arrhythmias

In this condition stimulation of the vagus nerve is frequently effective, as are drugs that lengthen the conduction time to the AV node (e.g. digitalis, verapamil, the beta-blockers and amiodarone). By prolonging the refractory period of the AV node, digitalis can frequently be used to terminate a re-entry arrhythmia. Digitalis may, however, facilitate conduction through the accessory pathway, and it is therefore sometimes contraindicated. Drugs that slow conduction along the accessory pathway are procainamide, disopyramide, quinidine, amiodarone, aprindine and ajmaline.

Treatment of atrial flutter

Attacks of atrial flutter, or flutter fibrillations with a rapid ventricular response resulting from anterograde transmission through accessory pathways, are usually the most serious complication of pre-excitation syndrome. These attacks can often result in ventricular tachycardia and ventricular fibrillation.[42,168] Frequent attacks should be treated by surgical intervention.[32] Prior to surgical intervention a combination of the drugs mentioned above may be used, and cardiac pacing may be necessary while surgery is being arranged.

Digitalis and beta-blockers, used in combination, can be employed to increase the degree of AV block and therefore reduce the ventricular rate. They may also terminate the arrhythmia. Verapamil, nifedipine, diltiazine and disopyramide can be used to terminate the arrhythmia. Both quinidine and procainamide are of value, and quinidine particularly can be used, once digitalization has been achieved. Cardioversion with synchronized DC shock should be performed when the arrhythmia is causing a profound haemodynamic change which is persistent and when drug therapy is ineffective.

Atrial Fibrillation

This is a condition in which impulses from ectopic foci exceed 350/minute and only unorganized contraction of the atria can occur. Except in those cases resulting from extremely severe rheumatic carditis or congenital heart disease, it rarely occurs in patients of the younger age-groups. Almost always, established organic myocardial disease is present and this results in a sudden worsening of the patient's condition. Onset of atrial fibrillation may be caused by a sudden acute infection or increased physical stress, such as pregnancy, surgery or unaccustomed physical activity. Once it has appeared it is likely to re-appear after reversion to a normal rhythm has been obtained. Most commonly, atrial fibrillation is associated with mitral disease, either stenosis or incompetence, or mitral insufficiency combining both factors. It occurs also in ischaemic myocardial disease in the older age-groups, in hypertensive heart disease, atrial septal defects, constrictive pericarditis, thyrotoxicosis, cardiac tamponade resulting from periarteritis nodosa, diagnostic puncture of the left ventricle in the presence of a phaeochromocytoma and following open heart surgery. Very rarely it may occur in the absence of any disease process, either in the myocardium or elsewhere.

Clinical manifestations

Atrial fibrillation (Fig. 10.1) may be present in a symptomless form. Patients may have heart (ventricular) rates of 120 beats/minute or more which can be present without significant cardiac decompensation, limitation of exercise, orthopnoea or dyspnoea. The atrial rate may be 400/minute or more.

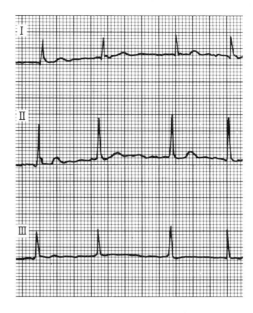

Fig. 10.1   Atrial fibrillation. The normal P waves are replaced with 'f' waves and the QRS complexes occur at irregular intervals.

The onset of atrial fibrillation is often characterized by a sudden feeling of irregular palpitation (conscious awareness of the beating of the heart) and a feeling of being unwell. It always precipitates some degree of heart failure, even though the degree of failure may be such that it is not of immediate danger to the patient. In other cases the degree of failure is so great that it requires immediate treatment. When it occurs in the undigitalized or underdigitalized patient (i.e. in someone suffering from valvular disease originating from rheumatic carditis and maintained on only 0.125 mg/day of digoxin), the fibrillation may occur in paroxysms and the treatment required and the diagnosis may be missed by the clinician. In response to the rapid atrial contractions the ventricles also contract in a chaotic manner at 120–180/minute, many of the contractions are of insufficient strength for the projected impulse to reach the wrist. There is, therefore, an apex–pulse deficit and the pulse felt at the wrist is slower than that at the apex. On inspection, the patient may be in the partially controlled condition, merely pale and anxious with a slightly raised respiratory rate, or in the completely uncontrolled state, disorientated, restless, unable to take food or drink, incapable of holding a glass that is handed to him, and the rapid pulsation of the ventricle may be seen at the neck or at the apex and appear to make the whole of the thorax vibrate. In very severe cases, even the pillows on the bed appear to shake.

The jugular venous pulse (JVP) shows flutter waves and the normal 'a' wave is absent. On auscultation the heart sounds are rapid and completely irregular (sometimes called 'irregularly irregular'), the sounds vary in intensity, some are louder than others when a number of atrial contractions happen to synchronize with a ventricular contraction. A third sound is commonly present, but it is sometimes clinically undetectable in the chaotic beating of the heart.

Differential diagnosis

The condition must be differentiated from numerous extrasystoles which also produce a dropped beat at the wrist and auricular flutter with varying degree of AV block. When dropped beats are a result of numerous extrasystoles, the basic rhythm of the heart is regular, but if these appear too frequently, the diagnosis may have to be made by electrocardiogram. In atrial flutter the jugular pulse usually shows flutter waves and in the electrocardiogram, abnormal P waves or flutter waves are present with some degree of block so that the atria beat in the region of 250–350/minute and the ventricles beat at 80–200/minute.

Electrocardiogram taken during atrial fibrillation shows that the P waves are replaced by small and irregular flutter of 'f' waves. They are irregular in shape, size and distribution and can, therefore, be easily distinguished from normal P waves. The QRS complexes appear at completely irregular intervals.

Treatment

In the severe case, intravenous digoxin should be given, but if the patient is known to have previously been given only small doses of digitalis, digoxin should be given intramuscularly 0.5 mg every 4 hours until the apex beat falls to 80/minute. The situation may then be re-assessed and oral administration of digitalis and its derivatives can be instituted. Occasionally, a patient is left untreated for 2 or 3 days, because the acute onset of atrial fibrillation has not been considered to be the cause of the patient's sudden deterioration. When first seen, therefore, marked biochemical changes may be observed in the blood. The plasma $[Na^+]$ has frequently fallen and K^+ depletion produced by vomiting is often present. The plasma $[PO_4^{---}]$ is raised and a metabolic alkalosis is reflected in high plasma $[HCO_3^-]$ and low $[Cl^-]$. Potassium depletion should, therefore, be treated by means of KCl in doses of 2–8 mg/day in divided doses. In this way the sudden onset of digitalis intoxication may be avoided. Although carotid sinus massage may be effective in terminating an attack of atrial flutter, it has no action on atrial fibrillation.

The underlying disease should be treated. If mitral stenosis is present, mitral valvotomy may be necessary, and thyrotoxicosis requires either medical or surgical treatment, as does a phaeochromocytoma.

Reversion to a normal rhythm should be attempted by means of quinidine, but digitalization must be performed in all cases prior to this treatment. When reversion has occurred an unfortunate consequence may be the dislodgement of a clot from the left atrium giving rise to cerebral emboli; under these circumstances reversion may best be performed when the fibrillation has been long standing and attachment has occurred to the atrial wall. When atrial fibrillation is of acute onset and results in severe cardiac decompensation, electric cardioversion should be employed. Although this can be achieved with 50–100 Joules (watt seconds), when it has to be performed because the patient is deteriorating rapidly, a charge of 300–400 Joules (watt seconds) should be used at the first attempt.

The major contraindications to electric cardioversion are as follows.

1. Long-standing atrial fibrillation. However, when a patient is going downhill rapidly and is in intractable cardiac failure, cardioversion may be necessary. For example, dramatic improvement occurred in a 48-year-old woman following cardioversion. She had been in atrial fibrillation for more than 5 years, digitalized and receiving quinidine in the intensive care ward for 4 weeks. Cardioversion was achieved with a single shock of 300 Joules (watt seconds) under sedation with diazepam (Valium) 10 mg i.v. There were no complications.
2. A heart rate of 60/minute or less while receiving digitalis.
3. Slow ventricular response in the absence of medication.
4. Reversion to atrial fibrillation which continues to occur even after lengthy medication with quinidine. The patient may need to receive quinidine in maintenance doses for 6 weeks before stable cardioversion can be achieved.
5. If no significant improvement occurs in cardiac output following cardioversion.

6. When there is a primary cause for atrial fibrillation which can be diagnosed such as thyrotoxicosis or phaeochromocytoma.

Whatever the means of causing reversion to a sinus rhythm, small doses of quinidine may be required for an indefinite period (Hurst *et al.*, 1964).[73] When the arrhythmia is associated with a phaeochromocytoma it may be reverted with propranolol (Inderal) (Rowlands *et al.*, 1965).[127]

Elective Cardioversion

The use of a synchronized DC shock across the heart avoiding the vulnerable segment of the cardiac cycle (see p. 310) has been a major advance in the treatment of arrhythmias resistant to medical treatment and when the haemodynamic effect of the arrhythmia causes the patient's condition to worsen. The negative electrode should be placed on the apex of the heart. The positive electrode can be placed in the right pectoral region or posteriorly when a flat or posterior electrode is available.

Although a general anaesthetic is ideal, the procedure can be performed within 15 minutes of giving diazepam (Valium) 10–20 mg i.v. Although patients may give a little cry when receiving the shock, they have complete amnesia for the event.

The following rules must be followed.

1. Withhold digoxin for 24–36 hours and digitoxin for 4–5 days prior to cardioversion. This is often not possible following open-heart surgery. It only very rarely causes a problem. The slow intravenous infusion of isoprenaline will correct the bradycardia if it occurs.
2. Have the means to perform the usual resuscitation procedures (e.g. intubation, ventilation of the lungs, appropriate drugs) available.
3. An intravenous infusion using a plastic cannula should be *in situ* and firmly anchored to the skin before cardioversion is performed.
4. Ensure the discharge from the defibrillator synchronizes with the R wave of the patient's electrocardiogram. An experimental discharge before placing the electrodes on the patient's chest usually allows a 'blip' to be seen on the cardiac monitor (cathode ray oscilloscope).
5. If the antero-posterior location is chosen, a starting energy value of 100 Joules (watt seconds) can be used. If the shock is placed transversely across the chest, the energy level should be at least 200 Joules (watt seconds). Some clinicians would consider these values to be high for starting energy values, but the author's opinion is that more damage occurs when repeated shocks are given than when a single shock of adequate power is administered. It should be noted, however, that atrial flutter can be converted with 25 Joules (watt seconds) and atrial fibrillation with 50 Joules (watt seconds).
6. The patient should be monitored for at least 24 hours following cardioversion and for longer if the elective cardioversion has been performed more than once. Patients with recurrent atrial fibrillation sometimes benefit from having quinidine for a long period (e.g. 6 weeks) prior to cardioversion. It appears that little benefit is derived from quinidine given 24 or 48 hours prior to cardioversion. Amiodarone is also of value in recurrent atrial fibrillation and flutter.[171]

Paroxysmal Ventricular Tachycardia

Ventricular tachycardia is defined as consisting of three or more successive beats originating in the ventricle at a rate that is greater than 100 beats/minute. The ventricular rate is usually between 150 and 200 beats/minute.

Although this arrhythmia may occur following overdosage with digitalis or quinidine and excessive administration of adrenaline and may appear in the terminal stages of acute renal failure when the potassium concentration has risen to cardiotoxic levels, it is almost always a result of organic myocardial disease. It is, however, being seen with increasing frequency following treatment with tricyclic antidepressant drugs (see p. 327).

It can suddenly appear in patients, who have a normal myocardium, following an emotional experience of great intensity or an episode of intense fear when it may cause sudden death. It most commonly appears following coronary occlusion and open-heart surgery.

When it occurs it may last for only a few seconds or for many hours. It may recur at varying time intervals. It is a much more severe condition than a supraventricular tachycardia; the patient feels subjectively very much worse and the degree of hypotension is very much greater.

The patient has a shocked, anxious appearance, is dyspnoeic and complains of pain and discomfort, typical of those described occurring as a result of myocardial ischaemia (see p. 282). When the atrium beats with the tricuspid valve closed, cannon waves may be seen in the jugular pulse. The heart rate is usually betweeen 150 and 250 beats/minute and the apical first sound is of variable intensity, being loudest when ventricular contraction is just preceded by atrial contraction. The apical first sound and the pulmonary second sound are widely split.

Electrocardiogram

The QRS complex is widened (greater than 0.12 s) as in a bundle branch block. Superimposed upon the abnormal ventricular complexes may be P waves at a slower rate (e.g. 80/minute), but quite commonly they are not identifiable. Probably, the most difficult electrocardiographic diagnosis to be made is the differentiation between ventricular tachycardia and supraventricular tachycardia with aberrant ventricular conduction. Although fusion beats are sometimes seen, they are usually not identifiable unless the ventricular rate is below 150 beats/minute. When fusion beats are seen, however, they do identify the ventricular nature of the arrhythmia so that differentiation can be made. R-on-T frequently initiates the arrhythmia (see p. 313).

The diagnosis of ventricular tachycardia is difficult and sometimes cannot be made with certainty. The differentiation from supraventricular tachycardia with aberrant conduction has to be made by other means.

If there is marked haemodynamic impairment with a low blood pressure, cardioversion by synchronized DC shock should be instituted as soon as possible. An injection of lignocaine (lidocaine, Xylocaine), 100–250 mg i.v., can be attempted if this causes no delay in making preparation for cardioversion. Alternative treatment is procainamide (Pronestyl) given slowly in doses of 100–200 mg i.v. and repeated at 5-minute intervals to a total of 1 g. Procainamide may be given orally in doses of 200–600 mg 4-hourly. Quinidine dihydrochloride or quinidine gluconate injection has been recommended and can be given intravenously in doses of 200–500 mg diluted in 20–40 ml of glucose or saline and injected over a period of 10–15 minutes. The dangers of quinidine therapy cannot be overstressed and procainamide must be preferred. A much safer method of administration of quinidine sulphate is by mouth, beginning with 0.2–0.4 g every 2 hours for five doses, then 6-hourly. A test dose of 0.2 g should be given first to detect serious sensitivity reactions.

Ventricular tachycardia developing from an overdose of tricyclic antidepressant (TCA) does not require R-on-T to initiate the arrhythmia. Indeed, when *torsade de pointes* develops, it does so as a result of a 'late' (escape) ventricular extrasystole (see p. 306). Furthermore, it has been observed by Krikler and Curry,[83] and by the author, that anti-arrhythmic drugs which further prolong the Q–T interval are probably contraindicated in the treatment of TCA–induced arrhythmias. Isoprenaline (isoproterenol, Isuprel) is probably the treatment of choice in the tachyarrhythmias produced by tricyclic antidepressants, both as an anti-arrhythmic agent, surprisingly slowing the heart rate and by inducing conversion to a supraventricular rhythm, either spontaneously or by assisting the action of other anti-arrhythmic agents when they are used concomitantly, and by raising the blood pressure.

Case history. The patient, a 20-year-old female, was seen in the emergency department at 7.00 a.m. She had taken a full bottle of amitriptyline 25-mg tablets, at approximately 6.30 a.m. with vodka. Gastric lavage was performed. At 8.00 a.m. she was unconscious, had no reaction to pain and her pupils were dilated with no reaction to light. Muscle tone was flaccid. Her optic fundi were normal. No reflexes could be elicited except the plantar reflexes which were down going. Her pulse rate was 130/minute and her blood pressure was 90/70 mmHg. At 8.25 a.m. she convulsed for approximately 15 seconds, and this was repeated at 8.40 a.m. and 8.45 a.m. An intravenous infusion of dextrosaline was begun but her blood pressure fell to 60 mmHg. The cardiac monitor showed that a ventricular tachycardia was present (Fig. 10.2). She was ventilated artificially with oxygen via an endotracheal tube. Blood gas analysis revealed the following: pH = 7.52, PCO_2 = 25 mmHg, PO_2 = 280 mmHg, $[HCO_3^-]$ = 20 mmol/l. $[Na^+]$ = 136 mmol/l (mEq/l), $[K^+]$ = 3.3 mmol/l (mEq/l), urea = 25 mmol/l, blood sugar = 7.5 mmol/l (149 mg%). While the patient was hypotensive she was infused with isoprenaline 4 mg in 700 ml. The heart *slowed* and there was a rise in blood pressure to 90 mmHg systolic. Paraldehyde, 10 ml i.m., was injected in divided doses to control the convulsions. Lignocaine 50 mg i.v. was given three times. The tachycardia reverted to sinus rhythm following the third intravenous injection. Diazepam 10 mg i.v. was also given in two divided doses. The blood pressure rose to 120/70 mmHg following the appearance of the sinus rhythm, and the isoprenaline (isoproterenol) was discontinued.

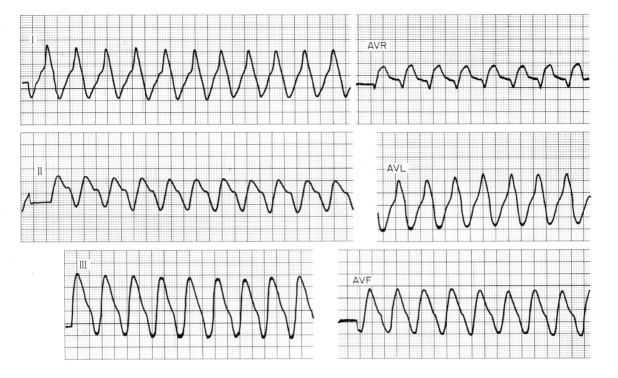

Fig. 10.2 Ventricular tachycardia. The electrocardiogram (ECG) taken from a 20-year-old female seen in the emergency department. She had taken a large number of 25 mg amitriptyline tablets approximately 3 hours earlier. She convulsed and was treated with 10 ml of paraldehyde injected intramuscularly, 5 ml into each thigh. She was treated for the ventricular tachycardia that was present, with an intravenous infusion of isoprenaline (5 mg in 1 litre of 0.9% saline) and a bolus of 50 mg of lignocaine (lidocaine) repeated twice. Following this treatment she reverted to sinus rhythm. Artificial ventilation of the lungs was necessary during this period.

Ventricular tachycardia caused by tricyclic antidepressants

The sudden death of patients receiving amitriptyline was reported by Coull *et al.* in 1970.[33] A further report from the same centre[107] substantiated the findings of Thorstrand,[156] Burrows *et al.*,[23] and Boulos and Brooks.[15] It is now well established that numerous psychotropic agents give rise to abnormalities of conduction of cardiac impulses and the control of rhythmicity. In the presence of psychotropic agents, abnormal action potentials can be initiated.

Among the characteristic effects that influence the myocardium are a more rapid repolarization of the S–A node, impaired conduction through the His–Purkinje system, prolongation of the Q–T interval and *torsade de pointes*.[82] The last-mentioned is characterized by an undulating QRS axis occurring in successive episodes (5–20 beats). It is associated with a prolongation of the Q–T interval.[83]

Electrocardiograph disturbances that have been observed following overdosage with tricyclic antidepressants and other psychotropic agents include:

P–R interval prolongation
Q–T interval prolongation
tachycardia—supraventricular and ventricular
bradycardia
premature atrial contractions
ST and T abnormalities
torsade de pointes
progressive intraventricular conduction abnormality with left anterior hemiblock.

There are a number of unwanted reactions associated with overdoses of psychotropic agents. Convulsions occur during which ventricular fibrillation may develop, possibly as a result of anoxia. Respiratory depression often occurs and hypotension and hyperpyrexia can be observed.

Very soon after taking an excess of tricyclic antidepressant, a metabolic acidosis can be detected before convulsions or cardiac arrhythmias have developed. Correcting the metabolic acidosis can alone terminate the arrhythmia without any specific anti-arrhythmic treatment being given.

Because of the prolongation of the action potential, and therefore of the Q–T interval, by the psychotropic agents, a problem with regard to treatment arises. The commonly used anti-arrhythmic agents themselves prolong the action potential. These include lignocaine, procaine and its amide, disopyramide, mexiletine and verapamil. Therefore, the administration of these agents tends to worsen the condition. An agent that shortens the Q–T interval should thus be used prior to the administration of the anti-arrhythmic agent, and in some cases anti–arrhythmic agents should be avoided completely.[15]

Case history. A 20-year-old female came to the hospital having been found semiconscious and collapsed 1 hour earlier. She had numerous grand mal seizures in the ambulance and on arrival had no recordable blood pressure. Her blood pressure did, however, return periodically so that a value of 80/40 mmHg was obtained on one occasion. The heart rate at the apex by palpatation was 150/minute and at the radial pulse 100/minute. Irregularities of rate and rhythm were observed at both sites. An endotracheal tube was passed and gastric lavage performed. It transpired that she had taken 50 tablets of 2.5 mg orphenadrine (Disipal, Norflex, Norgesic).

An infusion of 150 ml of 8.4% (150 mmol) NaHCO$_3$ was begun, although no acid–base data were obtained. When an electrocardiogram (ECG) was recorded it was considered to be ventricular tachycardia with *torsade de pointes* (Fig. 10.3). Because the patient had virtually no cardiac output, an intravenous injection of 1 mg of isoprenaline (Isuprel, isoproterenol, Saventrine) was given while observing the ECG. The rhythm suddenly changed at the end of the injection to atrial fibrillation and the volume of the pulse improved, even though the heart rate was still rapid. An intravenous injection of neostigmine was given slowly and the heart reverted to a sinus rhythm after the

patient had received 1.5 mg. Neostigmine was preferred because of the atropine-like nature of orphenadrine.

The patient recovered well and left hospital 1 week later.

As noted above, ventricular tachycardia was not present, and in addition to defects in automaticity and rhythmicity there were defects in conduction so that the transitory left anterior hemiblock was present.

In summary, therefore, the ECG demonstrates that:

(a) the aberrant beats resemble a left bundle branch block (LBBB) pattern;

(b) the degree of aberration in consecutive beats becomes progressively greater so that the widening of the QRS complex increases and the degree of LBBB becomes progressively more pronounced;

(c) the axis of the aberrant complexes represents a change from that of the basic normal axis to that of approximately −60°, indicating the presence of left anterior hemiblock, and that the major defect of conduction was in the anterosuperior division of the left bundle.

Anti-Arrhythmic Drugs

It would be so simple if the agents used for either treating or preventing cardiac arrhythmias could be classified so that any one drug would correct a disturbance of rhythm with predictable certainty every time it is used under all circumstances. Unfortunately, the classification of drugs is almost entirely empirical, although the electrophysical and electrophysiological characteristics of many properties of these drugs have been investigated and are known. It has, however, been clearly demonstrated by every clinician in the field that no one drug will always revert a cardiac arrhythmia, and indeed many of the agents used give rise to serious and life-threatening arrhythmias in their own right. Included in the latter group is, of course, digitalis. In spite of the advances that have been made using His bundle potential measuring techniques in man and ultramicroelectrode techniques, there is still incomplete understanding of the genesis of various arrhythmias, the pathway taken by the abnormal impulses or the action to be taken. The clinician has no certain method of knowing whether a drug will be beneficial or will precipitate a more undesirable and dangerous problem.

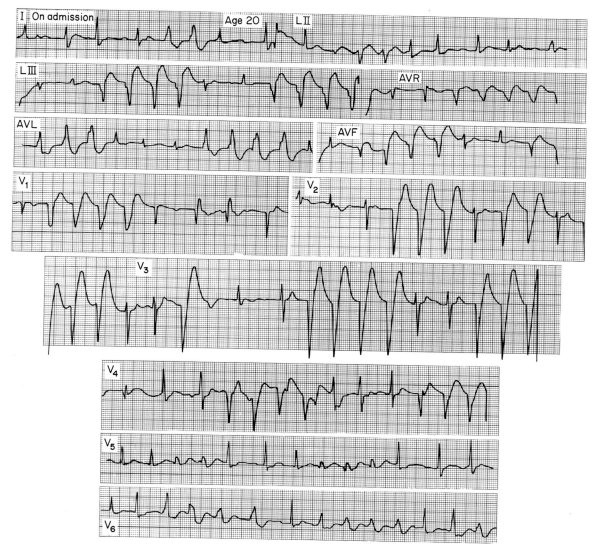

Fig. 10.3 The basic rhythm is probably sinus with a prolonged P-R interval of 0.32 seconds. These sinus beats are seen in the 4th beat in lead 1, the 7th beat in AVF, the 7th and 14th beats in V3, the 10th beat in V4, and the 7th and 12th beats in V6. Other beats demonstrating a junctional AV nodal origin are seen in the 1st and in numerous other leads. AV junctional beats with markedly aberrant conduction are observed in a varying repetitive manner masquerading as ventricular tachycardia in the 5th and 6th beats of lead 1, the 2nd, 3rd, and 4th beats of lead II, the 3rd, 4th, 5th and 6th beats of lead III and followed by the same aberrant conduction in the 9th, 10th, 11th, 12th, 15th, 16th, 17th and 18th beats of the same lead. Similar aberrant conduction of junctional beats is seen in all the subsequent leads. The following factors can be noted.

(a) The aberrant beats resemble a LBBB pattern.

(b) The degree of aberration in consecutive beats becomes progressively greater so that the widening of the QRS complex increases and the degree of LBBB becomes progressively more pronounced.

(c) The axis of the aberrant complexes represents a change from that of the basic normal axis to that of approximately −60°, indicating the presence of LAH, and the major defect of conduction was in the antero-superior division of the left bundle.

Cardiac function and the blood pressure improved when the rhythm converted to atrial fibrillation and improved markedly following the injection of neostigmine. Blood pressure recorded at that time was 105/60 mmHg, rising to 130/70 mmHg a short while later. The patient's level of consciousness began to improve approximately 6 hours later and during continuous monitoring she remained in sinus rhythm with a steady blood pressure. She was discharged from hospital totally physically fit 1 week later.

Almost 40 drugs are now available for treatment of disturbances of cardiac rhythm. The number is growing very rapidly and some drugs that have been previously discarded (e.g. hypotensive agents in the case of bretylium tosylate) are being used some 20 years after being introduced as effective anti-arrhythmic drugs.

The first attempt to classify anti-arrhythmic drugs was made by Vaughan Williams[159] and is still widely used, although there are several other classifications that have been, or are in the process of being, presented. The Vaughan Williams' classification (revised in 1980)[160] is based on the electrophysiological effects on the action potentials of various tissues under different conditions. For an understanding of this classification one has to refer to the action potential on page 301. It is unfortunate that there is no reliable animal model available, and the methods used for producing an arrhythmia are varied and include coronary blood vessel ligation, ischaemia, chloroform, adrenaline (epinephrine), aconitine, digitalis intoxication and electrical stimulus.

The Vaughan Williams' classification Class 1 contains the local anaesthetic agents which depress both the membrane responsiveness and conduction velocity. These drugs also depress the speed with which diastolic depolarization (Phase 4) takes place, therefore reducing the possibility of spontaneous automaticity. Class 1 can be subdivided into three groups based upon the electrophysiological response.

Subgroup A includes those drugs which lengthen the duration of the action potential.

Subgroup B includes those drugs which shorten the duration of the action potential.

Subgroup C includes those drugs which do not affect the duration of the action potential.

Class 2 contains drugs which effectively block the actions of catecholamines on the action potential. Most of these are beta-adrenergic receptor blockers which, except for very high concentrations of some preparations such as propranolol (Inderal), have no central effect upon the action potential.

Class 3 comprises a small group of drugs which prolong the duration of the action potential but do not depress membrane responsiveness. In other words, they have largely no effect upon the rate of rise of phase 0.

Class 4 drugs impair the transport of calcium into the cell; this results in depression of the plateau phase of the action potential which includes the phases 2 and 3.

Class 5 includes anti-arrhythmic agents which appear to impede the movement of the chloride ion through the membrane. There is only one member of this class to date and this is alnidine, which is not generally available for clinical use as it may be metabolized to chlorine.[103]

While in some ways this classification is of enormous value, it has several important drawbacks. For example, it cannot be applied in a direct clinical setting, and the digitalis glycosides cannot be included.

Table 10.2 is based on the classification of Vaughan Williams.[159]

It can be readily appreciated that no single classification is ideal, but together with a basic knowledge of the generation of the heart beat, an understanding of the action of an anti-arrhythmic agent can help the clinician when an arrhythmia is life-threatening.

Table 10.2 A classification of anti-arrhythmic agents

I	II	III	IV
Quinidine	Beta blockers	Bretylium	Verapamil
Procainamide		Amiodarone	Diltiazem
Propranolol		Sotalol	Bepridil
Aprindine		Nifenalol	
Disopyramide		Bethanidine	
Mexiletine		Clofilium	
Lidocaine			
Tocainide			
Encainide			
Phenytoin			

The drug treatment of cardiac arrhythmias

A sustained tachycardia, whether of supraventricular or ventricular origin, may require urgent treatment. Even when the haemodynamic effect is minimal when the patient is seen for the first time, it is well recognized that persistent rapid beating of the heart over a period of days, and in some cases hours, will often lead to cardiac failure and ventricular fibrillation. The latter especially can readily develop from a pre-existing supraventricular tachycardia of either brief or prolonged existence.

Supraventricular tachycardias

The electrophysiological mechanisms that give rise to supraventricular tachyarrhythmias are enhanced atrial or atrioventricular (AV) nodal automaticity and re-entry mechanisms.

By slowing the conduction through the AV node and producing a first-degree AV block (see p. 335) using manoeuvres such as carotid sinus massage, not only can the supraventricular origin of the arrhythmia be established, but the re-entry circuit can be broken and a sinus-nodal* or AV junctional re-entry rhythm can be terminated.

Digitalis

It has been demonstrated that digitalis has a marked effect on conduction through the AV node and this appears to be dependent upon innervation by fibres of the autonomic nervous system.[58] Both the delay at the AV node and the effective refractory periods are prolonged by digitalis in a manner unrelated to the length of the cardiac cycle. Prolongation of the effective refractory period appears to be mediated by vagal activity and therefore no significant changes occurred in patients who have denervated hearts. Digitalis decreases the rate of rise of phase 0 in the action potential of the AV node, magnifying its intrinsic quality of decremental conduction.

Beta-adrenergic blocking agents

These agents are well covered elsewhere in this book, but it can be stated here that their anti-arrhythmic action is a result of their ability to reduce automaticity and to delay conduction, most markedly at the AV node. They are effective, therefore, in decreasing response of the ventricle to atrial tachyarrhythmias and will control arrhythmias caused by digitalis toxicity, myocardial ischaemia and high concentrations of catecholamines as in phaeochromocytoma (Benfey and Varma, 1966).[8]

Propranolol (Inderal) and to a lesser extent practolol (Eraldin) have marked negative inotropic effects (Bett, 1968).[9] So that, for example, 1 mg of propranolol given intravenously may cause the sudden collapse of the patient with hypotension and respiratory embarrassment; respiratory embarrassment is not caused by the effect of the agent on the bronchi. It is the practice of the author never to give either of these agents intra-

* The term sinus-nodal is given to those rhythms that arise from the more distal portion of the SA node in the vicinity of the coronary sinus. In these rhythms the P waves are upright in leads I and aVF, but the PR interval is 0.11 seconds or less. In the absence of bundle branch block or aberrant ventricular conduction the QRS configuration is normal. Although the term is applied to this portion of the SA node, there is no evidence that rhythms of this kind do in fact originate at this site.

venously without preparing an infusion of iso-prenaline (isoproterenol, Suscardia, Saventrine) 5 mg in 1 litre of solution which can be infused to exert its beta-stimulating effects so that the cardiac output is restored.

Esmolol, a new short-acting beta-adrenergic blocking agent for controlling postoperative supraventricular tachyarrhythmias has been demonstrated to be effective by Gray et al. (1985). They infused this substance at a rate of 500 µg/kg/min, but the rate of infusion was limited by the hypotension that esmolol produced.

Digitalis and propranolol combined therapy

Experimental evidence that there is a complimentary and synergistic action when digitalis glycosides and propranolol are used together has grown, and there is some evidence that this synergism is seen in man. Some investigators consider that the combination therapy is a major advance in the control of supraventricular arrhythmias.[45,115] The rate of both atrial flutter and atrial fibrillation is markedly slowed.

Disopyramide phosphate (Norpace, Rythmodan)

This anti-arrhythmic agent has been used successfully in the treatment of both supraventricular and ventricular arrhythmias. However, its value has been most marked in the control of ventricular arrhythmias and it is apparent that this can be achieved in the presence of paroxysmal atrial and AV junctional tachycardias.[43,44,128,162] The drug has a quinidine-like action on the His–Purkinje system and upon the action potential.[85,177] The membrane effects of disopyramide include an increase in the duration of the action potential and of the refractory period. The duration and rate of rise of phase 0 in the depolarization cycle are decreased. This effect is similar to that produced by both quinidine and other quinidine-like anti-arrhythmic agents. Decrease in the plasma $[K^+]$ tends to reverse these membrane effects.

While disopyramide increases the delay in conduction through the AV node, it is also known to slow the conduction velocity through the His–Purkinje system. Clinically, therefore, disopyramide in pharmacological doses increases the duration of the P–R, QRS and Q–T intervals. The refractory period of the atria is also increased, although it has an apparent variable effect on the A–H and H–V intervals.[7,74,99]

Karim (1975)[76] and Ward (1976)[165] found that the half-life of disopyramide was 5–7 hours. However, this half-life is extended by approximately

10–20 hours in some patients.[71,72,76,118,119,165] The excretion of disopyramide is largely via the kidneys so that there are significant increases in the half-life of the drug in the plasma in those patients who have a reduced creatinine clearance.

The resting cardiac output is decreased by 10–28% after intravenous disopyramide. The largest decrease is found in those patients with severe myocardial insufficiency.[6,7,161]

Disopyramide has been found to be effective in patients who have ventricular arrhythmias that are refractory to other anti-arrhythmic agents.[53,131,163] Therapeutically effective levels have been found by a number of authors to be similar to those of lignocaine (lidocaine) and are in the region of 2–4 µg/ml.

Disopyramide has side-effects which are unwanted with an anti-arrhythmic drug. These include severe hypotension, especially in patients with a pre-existing low cardiac output, the development of AV block and hemiblock, and the anticholinergic effects. The anticholinergic effects include blurred vision, urinary retention and constipation. The drug is prepared in doses of 150 mg to be administered orally every 6 hours. The maximum dose usually given is 800 mg/day. When intravenous medication is necessary during an acute ventricular arrhythmia, disopyramide phosphate is administered slowly to a maximum dose of 150 mg or approximately 2 mg/kg body weight. Care should be taken in the presence of myocardial insufficiency and a loading dose of less than 200 mg should always be given.

Disopyramide may give rise to collapse and to asystole after a loading dose of 400 mg p.o.[96]

Nifedipine

An account of this calcium channel blocker is given on page 285.

Verapamil

It has been demonstrated that verapamil blocked the slow inward current of Ca^{++} and possibly the slow flux of Na^+ during the diastolic phase, but not the rapid Na^+ current which produces phase 0 of the action potential.[78] Verapamil prolongs the action potential.

The effective refractory period of the fibres of the AV node was lengthened when the slow inward current in phase 2 of the cardiac cycle (see p. 301) was investigated by Wit and Cranefield.[175] The amplitude of the action potential in the AV node was reduced. No effect was found with regard to the atrial or His bundle action potentials.

Verapamil would appear, on theoretical as well as empirical grounds, to be effective in re-entry arrhythmias. The observation by Schamroth et al.[133] that the agent is particularly effective in slowing the rate in atrial fibrillation and atrial flutter and suppressing supraventricular arrhythmias, appears to be confirmed by electrophysiological studies.

Diltiazem

This substance is a calcium channel antagonist with an action very similar to that of verapamil. The SA and AV nodes which are predominantly dependent on the slow Ca^{++} current responses are largely affected. Peripheral vasodilatation also occurs. Diltiazem is given in doses of 15–25 mg i.v. and orally in doses of 60–90 mg, preferably at 6-hourly intervals. In addition to its anti-arrhythmic action, it is used for the treatment of angina pectoris and hypertension. It is also used in malignant hyperthermia.

Amiodarone (Cordarone X)

In the Vaughan Williams' classification, amiodarone, which is a benzfuran derivative with anti-anginal and anti-arrhythmic qualities, is placed in Group III. This is because its anti-arrhythmic actions appear to be produced by its prolongation of the action potential without suppressing automaticity (phase 4 of the action potential) (Singh and Vaughan Williams, 1970),[141] a characteristic also of Group I agents.

Later studies (Wellens et al., 1976)[171] in man demonstrated that amiodarone increased the refractoriness of the atrial muscle, the AV node, the ventricular muscle and the anomalous conducting pathways that can give rise to Wolff–Parkinson–White and other pre-excitation phenomena.

Its use in paroxysmal tachycardia was studied by Ward et al. (1980).[164] They concluded that it was of great value as an anti-arrhythmic agent and was effective in the treatment of recurrent paroxysmal arrhythmias that were resistant to other anti-arrhythmic drugs.

The efficacy of amiodarone when given intravenously has been confirmed by Strasberg et al. (1985).[151] These workers treated patients with paroxysmal and recent onset atrial fibrillation producing a rapid ventricular rate. They gave 5 mg per kilogram body weight (mean dose 348 mg) over a period of 3–5 minutes to 26 patients suffering from various myocardial conditions. No serious side-effects were noted, although frequent blood pressure measurements were made.

Amiodarone-induced refractoriness to electrical cardioversion has been suggested (Fogoros,

1984)[50] as in other anti-arrhythmic agents such as encainide (Winkle *et al.*, 1981),[174] but this has not been firmly documented.

The effects of amiodarone including its pharmacology have been reviewed by Bexton and Camm (1982)[10] together with other class III anti-arrhythmic drugs such as bretylium tosylate, sotalol, meobentine and clofilium.

Amiodarone used alone in therapeutic doses has few adverse cardiovascular manifestations,[98] but in association with other drugs serious unexpected reactions have occurred. Amiodarone has interacted with digoxin causing increased serum digoxin concentrations[110] and has led to ventricular fibrillation.[101] When given with quinidine,[153] amiodarone has given rise to increased serum quinidine concentrations causing ventricular tachycardia, prolongation of the Q–T interval and *torsade de pointes*. In one patient an intravenous dose of 150 mg precipitated the arrhythmia, and in another receiving amiodarone 200 mg/day, an exercise test initiated the arrhythmia that developed into ventricular fibrillation which required cardiopulmonary resuscitation.

Amiodarone is normally given in doses of 200 mg p.o. three times a day until the rhythm is controlled, which may take up to 4 weeks, but often only 2 weeks. Many patients can then be controlled by 200 mg/day taken 5 out of 7 days of each week.

In addition to slate-grey skin discolouration, photosensitivity, thyroid dysfunction (both hypo- and hyperthyroidism), corneal microdeposits (cataracts), neurotoxicity which includes muscle weakness, peripheral neuropathy and extrapyramidal symptoms, diffuse reticular pulmonary infiltrates occur that can be identified radiologically. Basilar râles, pleural rubs and decreased arterial PO_2 are associated with a fall in PCO_2. Pulmonary function tests demonstrate impairment of lung function.[97]

Aprindine

The properties of this anti-arrhythmic agent are very similar to those of lignocaine (lidocaine) (Van Durme *et al.*, 1974).[158] It binds preferentially to the myocardium very soon after intravenous injection. The serum aprindine level is therefore not critical with regard to its anti-arrhythmic action and represents only 1% or 2% of the total dose given.[178] Aprindine was found to depress the rate of rise of phase 0 of the action potential,[65] and therefore its amplitude and duration. The resulting depression of automaticity and slowing of conduction could therefore slow a tachycardia. It is given intravenously in doses of 200 mg at a rate not

exceeding 20 mg/minute. Aprindine is given orally in a loading dose of 200–400 mg, followed by 100 mg twice daily.

Bretylium tosylate

Bretylium tosylate is an anti-arrhythmic drug with an action that differs signficantly from those of other drugs used for this purpose. It was introduced into clinical medicine in the 1950s as a hypotensive agent. However, because of the development of tolerance and undesirable side-effects when given orally, its use was limited.[40,41] In 1965 Leveque[89] reported that bretylium tosylate had anti-arrhythmic activity. He found that it protected dogs, who had been made hypokalaemic, against acetylcholine-induced atrial fibrillation. The effect was maximum at approximately 4 hours and lasted for approximately 8 hours.

Since that time numerous clinical reports have noted that bretylium tosylate has been particularly effective against ventricular arrhythmias such as paroxysmal ventricular tachycardia or ventricular fibrillation.

Pharmacology
When bretylium tosylate is injected it appears to be taken up by the peripheral adrenergic nerve endings where it exerts two effects. Initially, there is a release of noradrenaline (norepinephrine) producing a sympathomimetic effect.[16,57,80] After about 30 minutes, a second effect appears which is the inhibition of noradrenaline (norepinephrine) release, producing adrenergic neuronal blockade.[16,17,57,80] In the anaesthetized cat sympathomimetic effects can be observed, for example hypertension, tachycardia and increased vascular resistance; and in the anaesthetized dog, hypertension, tachycardia, increased myocardial contractility and increased venous catecholamine concentrations can be seen.[55] These sympathomimetic effects can be blocked by the appropriate alpha- or beta-adrenergic blocking drug.[80]

Adrenergic neuronal blockade is manifested by a fall in systemic arterial blood pressure, leading to orthostatic hypotension and increased response to circulating catecholamines.[56]

Cardiac effects
Because bretylium tosylate is effective against ventricular arrhythmias, studies have been performed on its affect upon ventricular muscle and Purkinje fibres.[13,176] It would appear that in therapeutic concentrations (0.6–20 μg/ml) bretylium tosylate produces an increase in the duration of the action potential (see p. 301) and the refractory period of both the ventricular muscle and the

Purkinje fibres. Prolongation of the action potential occurs largely by the lengthening of phase 2 (see p. 301). The drug does not appear to alter the relative lengths of the duration of the action potential and the refractory period because both components are prolonged and to the same degree. The change in potential during depolarization is not altered, nor is the rate of depolarization phase 0, the conduction velocity or the intrinsic automaticity of the Purkinje fibre. However, some changes do occur when the concentration of the drug is high (e.g. 40 μg/ml or more) when there is a significant decrease in the membrane resting potential, conduction velocity and rate of depolarization of the Purkinje fibres. Changes in membrane responsiveness (the relationship between transmembrane potential and rate of phase 0 depolarization) also occur at high concentrations.[13]

This drug is quite different from the other preparations used for the treatment of ventricular arrhythmias. Quinidine,[13,69] procainamide,[69] propranolol,[34] lignocaine (lidocaine)[14] and phenytoin[12] have all been studied and found to depress the automaticity of cardiac tissue, prolonging the refractory period relative to the duration of the action potential. Bretylium tosylate lengthens the refractory period and prolongs the action potential *without slowing conduction*. By this means the drug can alter the electrophysiology of a re-entrant pathway and thus prevent re-entry arrhythmias.

When the effects of bretylium were investigated following myocardial infarction produced in the dog,[25] it was found that there was an increase in the duration of the action potential and the duration of the refractory period and this was greater in the Purkinje fibres of normal tissue than in those of the infarcted area. Those fibres in the infarcted area had multiple prolonged action potentials as a result of the infarction. Bretylium tosylate produced improved automaticity, improvement in phase 0 depolarization and increased conduction velocity in the depressed Purkinje fibres in the infarcted areas. These factors would also have an anti-arrhythmic effect.

In 1972 Waxman and Wallace gave bretylium tosylate in doses of 10 mg/kg body weight intravenously to non-anaesthetized dogs.[170] Electrodes had been implanted earlier over the sinoatrial (SA) node, bundle of His and right bundle branch. Within the first 15 minutes following the injection of bretylium tosylate, a decrease in the rate of sinus discharge appeared which amounted to a 24% reduction in the heart rate. The AV conduction time increased by 30% and second degree atrioventricular block was observed frequently.

The refractory period in the atria and ventricles increased and the Q–T interval was prolonged. Surgical denervation of the heart in these experiments did not alter the electrophysiological changes. It was therefore concluded that these changes were due to the direct action of bretylium tosylate upon the heart rather than a response mediated by adrenergic blockade.

Clinical use

Bretylium tosylate has been used for treating ventricular arrhythmias that have followed myocardial infarction.[38,154] It has also been used for prophylaxis against arrhythmias after myocardial infarction, sometimes causing hypertension (Luomanmake et al., 1975),[95] and during cardiopulmonary resuscitation when it has been particularly effective. It has been found to be effective in doses of 5 mg/kg body weight.

Serum digitalis levels in clinical practice

Serum digitalis concentration is measured almost exclusively by radioimmunoassay. The technique of measurement was introduced by Smith et al. in 1969,[142] and the most commonly used preparations that are estimated are digoxin, digitoxin, acetylstrophanthidin and ouabain. In its natural state, none of these preparations is antigenic, and therefore no immunological action develops. However, in 1967, a technique by which digoxin could be coupled to a protein carrier was devised in which the complex was rendered antigenic.[24]

By this means it was possible to produce an antibody which had an extremely high affinity for digoxin. It has been demonstrated that not only is the steroid portion of the molecule the main site of antigenicity, but there is no significant antigenicity to other steroidal structures.

The radioimmunoassay is based upon competition between the known quantity of tritiated digoxin and the digoxin found in the serum (for a constant number of digoxin antibody-binding sites).

With the increasing concentration of digoxin in the serum, the number of reactions that can occur between a known quantity of added tritiated digoxin and the antibody decreases. When a standard curve for serum digoxin concentration is produced, with which serum samples from the patient can be compared, the amount of digoxin present in the patient's serum can be calculated.[142] The test is very accurate and concentrations of digoxin which are as low as 0.2 ng/ml can be determined.[144]

The test is fairly easy to perform and the results can commonly be made available within 1 hour.

Antibodies to all four of the most commonly used digitalis glycosides are now available.

Errors in assay procedure

Because the test depends upon the affinity of the antibody, any variability in the binding characteristics of the antibody being used will result in an abnormal value being obtained. Unfortunately, some variability does exist in the commercially available kits used for radioimmunoassays.[84] A further factor is important in the estimation of the serum digoxin level. It is assumed that no marked change in the concentrations is occurring over the period of time that the test is being performed, and that a steady state exists with regard to the equilibrium between the serum and the tissues. In a patient who is receiving increasing or decreasing doses of digitalis glycosides, this presumption may not be true. Once a steady state is established, the ratio that exists between the serum concentrations and myocardial concentration of the drug is relatively stable and predictable for the individual patient. It has been established that there is a reasonably good, but by no means absolute, correlation between the serum digitalis concentration and the positive inotropic and toxic effects of the drug.[143]

In order to avoid some of the problems, blood should be obtained prior to the normal regular daily dose of the preparation. If an intravenous injection of a digitalis is given, a minimum of 2 hours should elapse before a blood sample is taken. Another factor that can contribute to a misleading value is the presence of other radioisotopes used for other diagnostic purposes. The digitalis antibody has been used inappropriately in the past when it was not appreciated that a digitalis preparation other than that thought to have been prescribed had been used or when two different digitalis glycosides had been prescribed.

It should therefore be apparent, that great care must be taken in interpreting the digitalis levels, especially when the clinical responses do not correlate well with the measured digitalis level.

It should be remembered that Doherty and his co-workers have demonstrated that equilibrium of serum and tissue digoxin occurs 2 hours after an i.v. dose and 6 hours after an oral dose of digitalis.[39]

Heart Block

When conduction within the AV node is impaired, the conduction of impulses from the atria to the ventricles is reduced in rate or stopped completely. We refer to this condition as AV block (atrioventricular block). It is sometimes diagnosed in the fetus *in utero*, when it occurs congenitally, but is most commonly seen in association with ischaemic heart disease, rheumatic carditis, hypertension, degenerative changes occurring as the result of syphilis, inflammatory processes produced by acute virus infections, or diphtheria. It appears during digitalis overdosage or potassium depletion or as a result of overdosage with quinidine. It occasionally arises from localized disease processes, such as secondary neoplasia of the septum, gumma and hydatid disease and isolated fibrosis of the bundle. When it arises congenitally it may be associated with a ventricular septal defect (VSD), idiopathic endomyocardial fibrosis and fibroelastosis.

In 1827, Adams produced his original description of attacks of syncope associated with a slow heart rate.[1] Subsequent observations by Stokes in 1846 and 1854 confirmed the clinical entity.[149,150] Wenckebach in 1899 described a progressive prolongation of 'a–c' interval (the interval between atrial and ventricular contractions) until one ventricular contraction failed to occur.[172] Following a pause, the a–c interval was short and indeed shortest in the series of beats. When the degree of impairment of conductivity was judged by the increase in the a–c interval, it appeared to be most marked in the second conducted beat, and much smaller increases were observed in subsequent beats. When, in 1924, Mobitz originated the very first classification of incomplete AV conduction disturbances, he called what we now know as Wenckebach conduction abnormality, Type I.[106] Another type of conduction block in which an atrial beat was not conducted and the preceding P–R intervals, even when prolonged, were of the same length, he called Type II. This 'fixed type' of AV block, as in the case of the Wenckebach block, was based entirely on the variations or regularity of the AV conduction time.

Heart block can be divided into three grades as follows.

Grade I. Where the P–R interval is prolonged to more than 0.2 of a second (Fig. 10.4). This is sometimes the only indication of a frequently recurring total block resulting in Adams–Stokes attacks. It may also be associated with paroxysmal atrial tachycardia.

Grade II heart block. Not uncommonly, Adams–Stokes attacks are associated with the Wenckebach phenomenon in which the P–R interval progressively lengthens beat by beat until

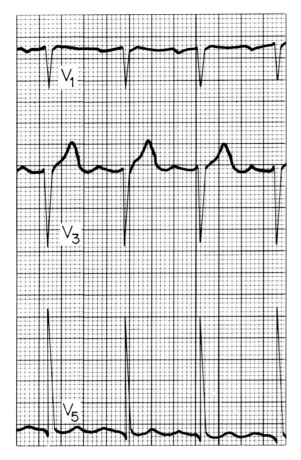

Fig. 10.4 Prolonged P-R interval. The distance between two thick lines equals 0.2 seconds and the distance between the thin lines equals 0.04 seconds. The P-R interval in this case is 0.24 seconds.

finally the P wave arrives during the refractory period of the previous ventricular beat and is, therefore, blocked and a 'missed beat' occurs. This cycle is repeated over and over again, the 'missed beat' appearing either at regular intervals or irregularly. This is also called the Mobitz type I block. Another form of Grade II block occurs when a ventricular beat is missed every second, third or fourth time with a prolonged P–R interval of fixed length. This is the Mobitz type II block. This and other forms of heart block are of interest, like the Grade I form, only because of their association with underlying myocardial disease which may require emergency treatment.

Grade III complete heart block. This occurs when there is complete dissociation between the atrial contractions and the ventricles which adopt their own intrinsic rate of contraction of 30–40/minute in the adult. In the very young, when the heart rate is normally much faster (130/minute in the infant), the ventricular rate may be much faster (e.g. 60–80/minute), but still inadequate for the needs of the body. The atria in both cases continue to contract at their normal rate of 70–80/minute in the adult and at faster rates in the young.

The condition can rapidly give rise to congestive cardiac failure, and digitalis therapy is then required, even when artificial electrical stimulation is maintained by means of an artificial pacemaker. This is because even when an electrical impulse is provided in order to initiate a heart beat, the ventricles still have to contract forcibly to expel blood and the improvement in myocardial function obtained in the failing heart by digitalis therapy is still necessary. The patient with complete heart block may complain of faintness and dizziness and may be observed to behave in an irrational and bizarre manner which can be confused with petit mal. Attacks of syncope are a common occurrence.

On examination, the pulse rate is slow, irregular and of 'increased' volume, because of the large pulse pressure. Irregular 'cannon' waves may be seen in the jugular pulse as the rapidly beating atria contract against a closed tricuspid valve. The first heart sound varies greatly in loudness, being maximum when the situation approximates to normality and the atria contract completely just before the AV valves close and a ventricular beat is initiated.

Electrocardiogram
The ECG shows a complete dissociation of the P waves and QRS complexes, the P waves appear at 70–80/minute and the ventricular rate is in the region of 40/minute.

Although complete heart block can develop suddenly without warning with no or minimal ECG changes, in most patients various blocks occur in the separate branches that arise from the bundle of His.

Bundle Branch Block (intraventricular conduction delay)

As we have seen when discussing the conduction of the propagated electrical impulse through the His–Purkinje system, bundle branch block was previously divided simply into 'complete right bundle branch block' and 'left bundle branch block'. However, we now subdivide the blocks so that we talk of monofascicular, bifascicular and trifascicular blocks of the bundle branches.

Right bundle branch block (RBBB)
When a block develops in the right bundle branch the following observations can be made.

1. Depolarization of the left ventricular septum occurs in a normal manner.
2. This is followed by depolarization of the left ventricular wall.
3. Depolarization of the right ventricular portion of the septum occurs after delay so that a second 'R' wave is produced on the ECG.
4. Delayed depolarization of the right ventricular wall occurs and an 'M'-shaped wave is therefore produced in the right ventricular leads V_1, V_2 and V_3.

The QRS is widened to 0.12 seconds or more and this is most probably due to the delay in the electrical impulse which occurs in the presence of a bundle branch block across the wall of septum. This explanation is favoured as a result of the work performed by Sodi-Pallares and his colleagues (1970).[146] There is increased amplitude of the intrinsicoid deflection (R1) in the right precordial leads. Because depolarization of the septum in RBBB occurs from left to right, there is initial positivity of the QRS complex to a greater degree than that observed in the normal subject.

The left precordial leads show the normal small Q waves, a slurred broad S wave caused by the late depolarization of the right portion of the septum and right ventricle, and a normal QRS activation time. The T wave in the absence of any other abnormalities is upright in V_5 and V_6.

Incomplete right bundle branch block
Incomplete right bundle branch block demonstrates that there is a change in the right bundle which slows but does not interrupt the transmission of the propagated impulses from the atria to the ventricles. This change may be either functional or organic and can occur in the completely normal heart as a congenital deviation from the general pattern. The QRS complex, although prolonged, is less than 0.12 seconds. Incomplete RBBB can be seen and diagnosed in the standard chest leads by a broad S wave in lead I (Fig. 10.5) and in the precordial lead V_6. Early R

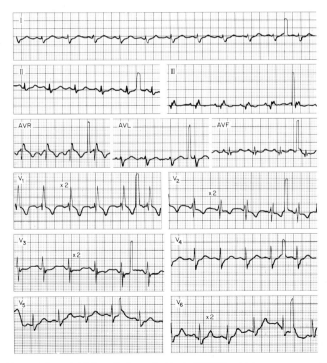

Fig. 10.5 An example of incomplete right bundle branch block (RBBB) which was present in a patient suffering from myxoedema. Some of the leads, therefore, are calibrated at twice the normal standard (1 mV = 2 cm). Note also the deep S waves in lead 1 and the M-shaped waves in the right chest leads.

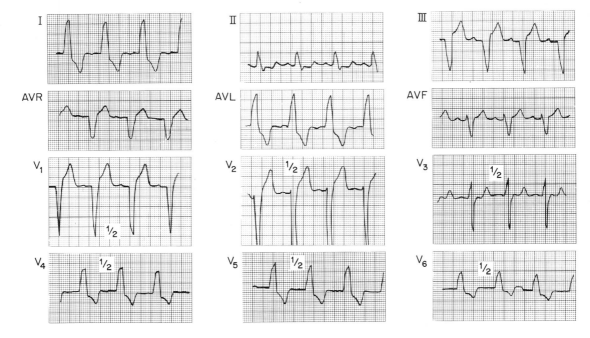

Fig. 10.6   Electrocardiogram (ECG) showing left bundle branch block (LBBB). Note the wide QRS complexes, the almost M-shaped waves in the left chest leads, and the absence of a Q wave in these leads. There is, however, S-T depression in these leads with reciprocal elevation of the S-T segment in the right chest leads. Diagnosis of myocardial infarction is electrocardiographically made more difficult.

and late RI waves are observed in the right precordial leads. One would expect a QRS complex of at least 0.10 seconds. However, incomplete RBBB can occur when the QRS is 0.08 seconds or less.

Complete left bundle branch block (LBBB)

When the main left bundle is blocked, the sequence of depolarization is such that the initial portion of the myocardium to be activated is the *right* side of the intraventricular septum. This begins low down, close to the base of the right ventricular anterior papillary muscle. Activation then proceeds to the left septal mass and the left ventricle. Because of the delay, slurring and the formation of a biventricular 'M'-shaped wave is formed.

Characteristics of left bundle branch block (Fig. 10.6)

1. The QRS is widened to 0.12 seconds or more.
2. There is late onset of intrinsicoid deflection in those leads over the left ventricle. This is because the ventricular activation time (onset of the intrinsicoid deflection) in the left precordial leads may be as late as 0.1 seconds or more.

3. The S–T segment in the left precordial leads is depressed and the T wave is inverted. Reciprocal changes, elevated S–T segments, are seen in the *right* precordial leads.
4. A small R wave is seen in the right chest leads due to septal depolarization from right to left. This prevents the formation of a Q wave except in those cases in which there is a minimal degree of LBBB or in the presence of an associated septal myocardial infarction.
5. The right precordial leads also show a broad slurred S wave due to the delay in left ventricular activation.

Clinical significance of left bundle branch block

Numerous studies have tried to indicate the clinical significance of newly acquired LBBB and its importance with regard to the patient's prognosis. However, these studies have produced conflicting results and have been well reviewed by Schneider *et al.*[134] The long-term prospective study at Framingham indicated that the mean age of onset of LBBB was 62 years; it occurred largely in people who had suffered from hypertension, cardiac enlargement and coronary artery disease or a combination of these. Of the patients studied, 48% developed clinical coronary artery disease or congestive cardiac failure either at the time of onset of LBBB or subsequent to it. During the 18-year period of observation, only 11% of patients remained free of clinically obvious cardiac disease, and within 10 years of the onset 50% of patients who developed LBBB died from a cardiovascular cause. Schneider *et al.*, concluded that newly acquired LBBB commonly indicates advanced hypertensive and/or ischaemic heart disease.

Intermittent left bundle branch block

As can be seen in Fig. 10.7, intermittent LBBB can occur as a result of myocardial ischaemia and is sometimes caused by drugs such as digitalis or psychotropic agents.

The electrical axis

The electrical axis refers to the position of the sum of the cardiac vectors in the frontal plane, although it is known that the vectors that form this axis are

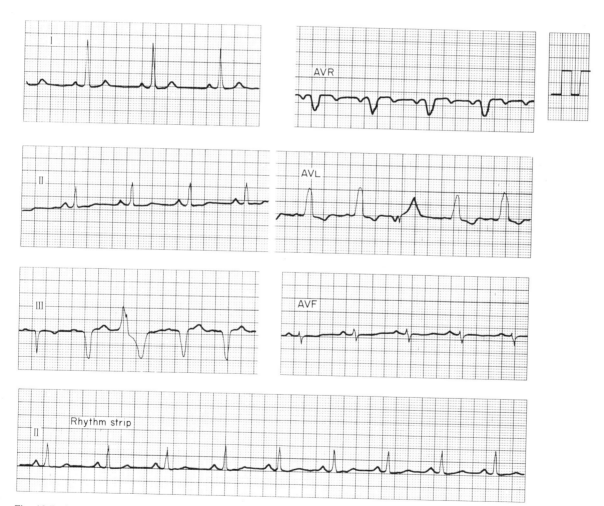

Fig. 10.7 Intermittent left bundle branch block (LBBB). In leads I, II and the first complex in III a normal QRS configuration is evident. The second, fourth and fifth complexes in III demonstrate LBBB pattern. The third complex in III is a ventricular extrasystole with an incomplete compensatory pause. LBBB is evident in AVR and AVL with a return to normality in AVF. (Fig. 10.7 is continued on p. 340).

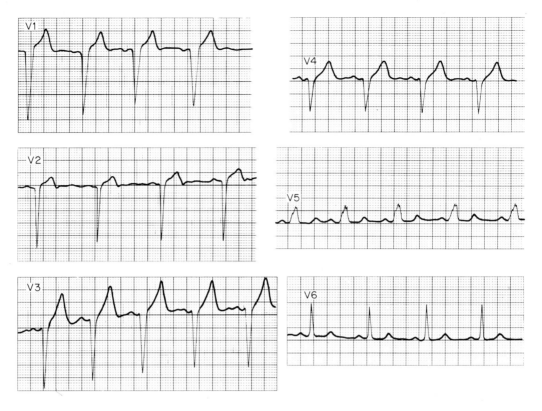

Fig. 10.7 (continued) Normality continues through V_1, V_2, V_3 and V_4 but only minute R waves are present in V_1 and V_2 and very small R waves are present in V_3 and V_4. There is therefore poor progression of the R wave which should be largely upright in V_4, and this indicates anterior myocardial infarction. LBBB returns in V_5. The QRS complexes are normal in V_6. This electrocardiogram (ECG) was recorded in the normal way with the normal brief time intervals required for switching from one lead to another.

three dimensional. It is derived from the magnitude of the QRS complexes in the first six leads of the 12-lead electrocardiogram (I, II, III, aVR, aVL and aVF). Einthoven put forward the concept that the heart lay within an equilateral triangle. The electrical impulses were assumed to emanate from a central point within the equilateral triangle, the extremities of which were considered to be formed by the left arm, the right arm, and the left leg. The sides of the triangle were analogous to the standard leads, I, II and III (Fig. 10.8). The heart was also considered to consist of several single dipoles or batteries and the directions in which these were pointed were called the 'cardiac vectors'. Because these vectors have both magnitude and direction, the average of all the vectors was called the mean electrical axis, thus any portion of the ECG (e.g. the P wave, QRS complex and the

T wave) must have its own mean electrical axis.

The Einthoven triangle is an inconvenient way of measuring the mean electrical axis so that the lines formed by the sides of the equilateral triangle (Fig. 10.8a) are moved in order to form a tri-axial system (Fig. 10.8b). The vectors formed by the vector leads aVR, aVL, aVF (Fig. 10.8c) can be superimposed upon the tri-axial system. This system can now be subdivided into quadrants, as shown in Fig. 10.9. It is divided into the normal axis extending from $-30°$ to $+90°$, the left access extending from $-30°$ to $-90°$, the right axis extending from $+90°$ to $+180°$, and an intermediate axis extending from $-90°$ to $-180°$. Some authors prefer the normal axis to lie between 0 and $+90°$, and for an axis lying in the upper right-hand quadrant between 0 and $-90°$ to be called left axis deviation. However, it is now almost universally accepted that the

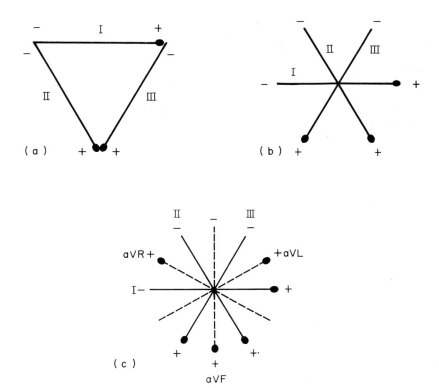

Fig. 10.8 (a) The three leads forming the equilateral triangle can be formed from three matchsticks and the heads are denoted as having a positive electrical charge. (b) The three are moved to form a tri-axial system. The axis can be calculated from this form. (c) The augmented (a) vector (V) leads are superimposed upon the tri-axial system forming a hexaxial system. .

axis that lies between −30° and −90° (see Fig. 10.9) should be called 'abnormal left axis deviation' and that an axis between 0 and −30° should be called 'normal left axis deviation'. Different opinions, however, will still be found. Understanding of the axis in the frontal plane is essential for the diagnosis of the various forms of conduction block within the myocardium.

In practice, only two leads are required to derive the mean cardiac axis in the frontal plane (Fig. 10.10). These are leads I and aVF. Although the *area* encompassed by the QRS complex is required, it is usual to measure the lengths of the positive and negative waves (in millimetres) and, by subtracting the one from the other, arrive at an algebraic sum. When this is plotted in the quadrants formed by I and aVF and perpendicular lines are drawn so that they meet within the appropriate quadrant, the axis in the frontal plane can be measured. In clinical practice it is possible merely

to look at the ECG and perform a mental calculation. Further assistance can be obtained in deciding whether the axis is normal or abnormal by inspection of other standard leads (e.g. lead II) (Fig. 10.11), and the knowledge that the axis is approximately at right angles to that lead which is of smallest magnitude.

The clinical significance of left axis deviation (LAD) has been a subject of discussion and controversy for many years. Even the degree of LAD which is considered to be abnormal has been a subject of great debate. In 1937, Ashman and Hull[4] indicated with some emphasis that LAD could be caused by disease of the coronary arteries. Up to that time, LAD had been considered to be a manifestation of left ventricular hypertrophy. In 1951 Moll and Lotterotti[108] reported that marked LAD could be caused by an anterior myocardial infarction. Grant and his co-workers (1956, 1958, 1959)[62–64] observed that LAD was associated with

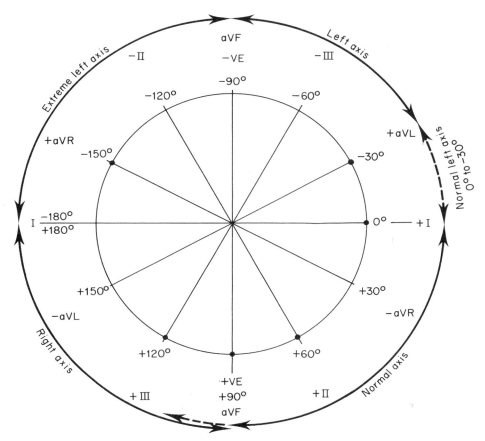

Fig. 10.9   The cardiac axis in the frontal plain. Note the normal adult axis is between 0° and +90°, although we are born with an axis that is in the lower right quadrant between +90° and +180°. As the left ventricle becomes of greater significance the axis moves anticlockwise into the normal axis. This has usually occurred by the age of 8–10 years. The upper left quadrant 0° to −90° is the left axis. Between 0° and −30° it is normal left axis. The upper right quadrant −90° to −180° represents extreme left axis.

myocardial damage, Bayley *et al.* (1944)[5] having introduced the term *peri-infarction block* in which they described a form of intraventricular conduction defect associated with myocardial infarction. Not only was the duration of the QRS complex prolonged, but there was also a shift of axis. The forms of peri-infarction block that were described by First *et al.* (1950)[48] now largely conform with left antero-superior and left postero-inferior hemiblock.

Many workers in the field of electrophysiology and electrocardiology had observed the two major divisions of the left bundle branch. Pryor and Blount in 1966[117] stated and emphasized the fact that it was important 'to at least conceptualize the fiber of the left bundle as being arranged into superior and inferior divisions in order to rationally approach the diseases that alter the sequence of depolarization of the myocardium supplied by these radiations'. These two divisions of the left bundle freely anastomose peripherally in the sub-endocardial layers of the ventricle via a network of Purkinje fibers. These workers coined such terms as '*left superior peri-infarction block*' (LSPIB).

The term peri-infarction block was not accepted by workers such as Sodi-Pallares (1952, 1960)[145,147] in view of the fact that the slurring of the QRS complex is caused by the block occurring *in*, not around, the infarcted area. He therefore preferred the term '*intra-infarction block*'. Other workers,

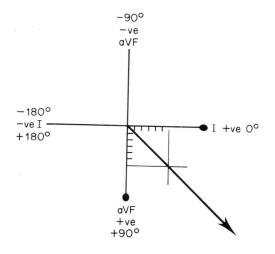

Fig. 10.10 Two leads are depicted in this diagram, 'I and aVF'. By adding up the height of the R wave from the upper edge of the isoelectric line and subtracting the sum of the negative waves Q and S, measured from the bottom edge of the isoelectric line, a figure of 6 mm has been derived, which is positive. A similar value has been obtained for aVF and perpendiculars drawn from the two leads. The mean spacial vector or axis in the frontal plain can be obtained by drawing a line from the zero point, where the two *leads* intersect, through the point at which the lines drawn perpendicular to the two leads intersect. The line with the arrow therefore depicts the axis in the frontal plain. The positivity and size (area) encompassed by these two leads determine the position or quadrant in which the axis falls.

	Lead I	Lead II	Lead aVF
Normal axis			
'Normal' left axis			
'Abnormal' left axis and LAH			
Diaphragmatic (inferior) MI			
Pacemaker placed in apex of right ventrical			

Fig. 10.11 As described in the text, an approximate guide to the cardiac axis in the frontal plane can be obtained by merely looking at two or three leads. This is particularly important when deciding whether left anterior hemiblock (abnormal left axis deviation) is present. Although (as shown) abnormal left axis deviation can occur in the presence of an acute inferior (diaphragmatic) myocardial infarction. The insertion of a pacemaker so that it impinges low down at the apex of the right ventricle will by the very origin of the electrical impulse induce grossly abnormal left axis deviation preceded by a 'blip' seen on the electrocardiogram (ECG) preceding the ventricular complex.

as in the case of Pryor and Blount, prefer the term *post-infarction block*'.

The characteristic changes in the electrocardiograms recognized in peri-infarction block are as follows.

1. There is evidence of myocardial infarction in terms of abnormal Q waves and, if the lesion is anterior, the ECG suggests LBBB.
2. The duration of the QRS is prolonged to at least 0.11 seconds.
3. Those leads that have evidence of myocardial infarction, in that abnormal Q waves are present, typically have wide R waves of late onset.
4. The onset of the intrinsicoid deflection in the precordial leads which overlie the undamaged portions of the left ventricle occurs normally, but there is delay in those leads which overlie the zone of infarction.
5. There must be abnormal right or left axis deviation in addition to the conduction defect.

Although the term peri-infarction block is still used it has largely been replaced by 'hemiblock'.

The Hemiblocks

The basic differences between a right bundle branch block (RBBB) and a left bundle branch block (LBBB) have been noted. The calculation involving two commonly used leads, I and aVF, and some relevant aspects of electrical axis of the heart in the frontal plane have also been discussed. We can therefore investigate the changes in the common forms of hemiblock.

It was recognized that when RBBB developed it was frequently associated with right axis deviation (RAD); LBBB was associated with left axis deviation (LAD). The situation was therefore relatively simple, except for the fact that in some patients when RBBB developed it could be associated with *left* axis deviation. It was also recognized, a considerable time ago, that patients who developed RBBB with *left* axis deviation frequently suffered from acute syncopal attacks. The aetiology of these syncopal attacks was then unclear, but it is now realized that they are due to the development of complete heart block.

The term 'hemiblock' was originated by Rosenbaum in 1968.[124] The term related to blocks occurring in the two branches or fascicles of the left bundle. If a block occurs in either division of the left bundle, that part of the left ventricle which is no longer supplied with conducting tissue is activated through the remaining division, but after a delay. Trifascicular blocks can also occur (Rosenbaum, 1969).[125]

As we have already seen, the left bundle has two divisions (or fascicles). The origin of the anterior division of the left bundle has a common origin with the *right* bundle branch. It is, therefore, possible for a relatively small lesion to impair the function of both fascicles. The anterior division can, therefore, be said to have the following characteristics.

1. It has virtually a single blood supply, almost entirely derived from the left coronary artery.
2. Damage occurs as a result of anterior myocardial infarction, especially anteroseptal and anterolateral myocardial infarction.
3. Because it is a relatively thin structure having only a single blood supply, it is the most vulnerable of the three fascicles to ischaemic damage.
4. Left anterior hemiblock (LAH) and RBBB frequently occur together.

Anatomically, the first branch to arise from the bundle of His is the posterior division of the left bundle.* It can be said to have the following characteristics.

1. It has a dual blood supply, the proximal part from the right and the distal part from the left coronary artery.
2. It is thicker and anatomically more prominent than the anterior division of the left bundle.
3. Because of its structure and anatomical location it is the least vulnerable of the three fascicles that contribute to the His–Purkinje system.

---

*This may contribute to the early activation of the *left* portion of the septum.

Left anterior hemiblock (LAH)

This condition may be found as an isolated occurrence in the electrocardiograms of the more elderly patient or in association with other blocks in the trifascicular conduction system that we have already examined. A most common cause of LAH is coronary heart disease; other causes are hypertension, aortic valve disease, and cardiomyopathies. Generally, the most common cause of left axis deviation (LAD) is myocardial ischaemia.

Although when Rosenbaum first elucidated the hemiblock he considered that in order to establish the diagnosis an axis of greater than −60° was required, other authors now consider that LAH is present when the rotation of the axis to the left is greater than −30°.

When a block occurs in the anterior division of the left bundle, the axis of the heart shifts *superiorly* and to the left. This results in the production of large S waves in leads II, III, and aVF (see Fig. 10.11). Prolongation or widening of the QRS does not need to be outside normal limits for the diagnosis of LAH to be made.[26]

To summarize LAH, therefore, we can say:

(1) it is associated with myocardial ischaemia (Fig. 10.12), especially that which results from occlusion of the left coronary artery;
(2) it is diagnosed by the presence of abnormal left axis deviation of greater than −30°;
(3) electrocardiographic diagnosis is made by the presence in lead I of positivity and of negativity in leads II and aVF;
(4) in the absence of other ECG abnormalities, the QRS complex and the P–R interval are normal.

We have seen that there are a number of causes for abnormal left axis deviation other than left anterior hemiblock.

Left posterior hemiblock (LPH)

For reasons that have already been examined, that is to say the dual blood supply of the posteroinferior branch of the left bundle, the development of isolated LPH is uncommon. Nevertheless, the diagnosis of LPH from the ECG is by no means satisfactory, and it may well be that it occurs in isolation more commonly than is at present thought.

The electrocardiographic criteria used for the diagnosis of LPH are also used in the diagnosis of right ventricular hypertrophy, cor pulmonale, vertically positioned heart and marked right axis deviation. The last two conditions can, of course, occur in the normal heart.

Left posterior hemiblock is, however, usually

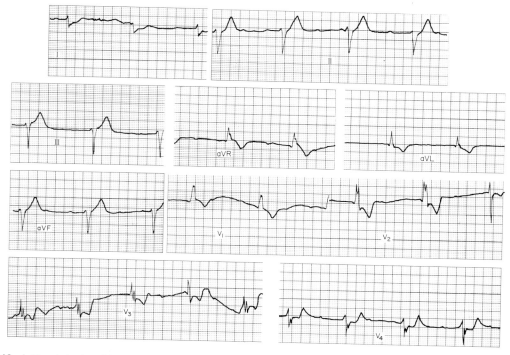

Fig. 10.12   Left anterior hemiblock. The electrocardiogram (ECG) of a 64-year-old male who presented with intermittent collapse and intermittent ventricular fibrillation.

The patient from whom this recording was taken has a complete conduction block, P waves being seen most readily in aVF. The heart rate is 43 beats/minute. Deep S waves are seen in leads I and II and the axis in the frontal plane is extreme 'left axis'. The left precordial leads demonstrate the M-shaped waves of RBBB and the abnormal left axis deviation (ALAD) indicates left anterior hemiblock.

It was apparent that the patient had been suffering from a bifascicular block, that of the right bundle and the antero-superior division of the left bundle, the latter giving rise to abnormal LAD. Intermittently, a block had developed also in the postero-inferior division of the left bundle, so that the patient passed into complete block and his syncopal attacks were Adams–Stokes. Just before the patient was admitted, the Adams–Stokes attacks increased in length and he passed into ventricular fibrillation. Initially, he reverted spontaneously, but in hospital electrical cardioversion became necessary, prior to inserting a pacemaker.

associated with RBBB and atrioventricular (AV) blocks. LPH is also quite commonly seen in association with right ventricular block and left anterior hemiblock. When LPH occurs, therefore, it indicates extensive myocardial disease and is associated with a very poor prognosis (Fig. 10.13).

The diagnosis of LPH, as in the case of LAH, is made from the standard leads (Fig. 10.14). The cardiac vector is the lower image of LAH, because the lead vector is changed so that it points inferiorly and to the right.

Large S waves are produced in lead I and large R waves are present in leads II and aVF. Because, initially, a normal vectorial pattern occurs, a small 'r' wave occurs in lead I and small 'q' waves are produced in leads II and aVF.

We can therefore summarize the characteristics of LPH as follows.

1. Isolated LPH is an uncommon finding.
2. When LPH occurs it is associated with severe myocardial disease.
3. The ECG alone cannot be used to diagnose LPH, although it can be inferred by the association of other blocks.
4. Because the blood supply to the right posterior division of the left bundle is the same as that supplying the AV node, LPH is commonly associated with first degree AV block.
5. LPH is commonly associated with RBBB.
6. Right axis deviation, that is to say, an axis in the frontal plane of +100° or more, must be present.
7. Lead I is negative (rS) while leads II and aVF are positive (qR).

The following make the diagnosis of LPH more

	Lead I	Lead II	aVF
Right axis deviation			
Left posterior hemiblock			
Right ventricular hypertrophy			
Antero-lateral myocardial infarction			

Fig. 10.13 The salient changes seen in leads I, II and aVF in the presence of right axis deviation, left postero-inferior fascicular block, right ventricular hypertrophy and antero-lateral myocardial infarction.

difficult. These are inferior myocardial infarction, Wolff–Parkinson–White syndrome, complete LBBB, emphysema and congenital deformities,

for example corrected transposition, Ebstein's disease, and S1S2S3 syndrome.

The fascicular blocks

We have now seen how conduction block can occur in one or all three of the conducting fascicles. The term monofascicular block is used when only one fascicle is diseased. The most commonly found monofascicular blocks are RBBB and LAH.

When two fascicles are involved the term used is *bifascicular* block, the most common being that of the combination of RBBB and LAH.

When all three fascicles are diseased this leads usually to complete block; but both temporary and permanent block of the three fascicles can occur, and the term *trifascicular block* is used.

When a trifascicular block is indicated by the presence of RBBB associated with first degree AV block (LPH) and left axis deviation of greater than −30° (LAH), the insertion of an artificial pacemaker is probably indicated. If a syncopal or an Adams–Stokes attack occurs in the presence of a trifascicular or bifascicular block, the insertion of a pacemaker is even more strongly indicated and in some cases is mandatory.

The recommendations of the Criteria Committee of the New York Heart Association (1969)[113] for

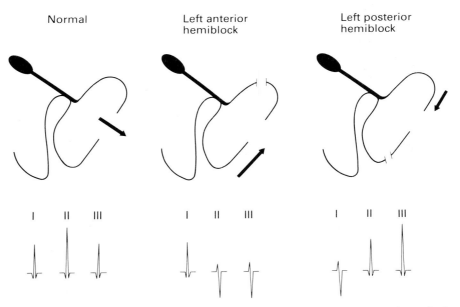

Normal   Left anterior hemiblock   Left posterior hemiblock

I   II   III   I   II   III   I   II   III

Fig. 10.14 This depicts the direction of the mean spatial vector in the normal heart in the presence of a conduction block in the left antero-superior division of the left bundle, and a conduction block in the left postero-inferior division of the left bundle. The changes that arise in the configuration of the three standard leads are also shown. Isolated LPH cannot be differentiated from right ventricular hypertrophy by the ECG alone.

the various types of block were as follows.

Right bundle branch block. The criteria for electrocardiographic diagnosis of right bundle branch block included a QRS duration of 0.12 seconds or greater with an rSR or with qR configuration of the QRS in lead V_1.

Left anterior hemiblock. When the mean frontal QRS axis was more negative than $-30°$, left anterior hemiblock was diagnosed.

Left posterior hemiblock. Criteria for diagnosis of left posterior hemiblock with right bundle branch block included a mean frontal QRS axis more positive than $+110°$ and absence of right ventricular hypertrophy.

Left bundle branch block. Diagnosis of left bundle branch block used the following criteria: (1) QRS duration of 0.12 seconds or greater; (2) the presence of a broad monophasic R wave in lead V_6; and (3) S–T depression and T wave inversion in V_6.

Clinical significance of right axis deviation

Right axis deviation is found in: (1) right ventricular hypertrophy; (2) anterolateral infarction; and (3) left posterior hemiblock. Lead I is negative and leads II and aVF are positive.

In anterolateral infarction, the development of a deep abnormal Q in lead I causes the frontal plane axis to move to the right.

Adams–Stokes Attacks

These are acute syncopal attacks of sudden onset occurring without warning. They are produced when the heart changes from a partial to a complete block resulting in a pronounced bradycardia or when the heart, which may or may not be in complete block, passes momentarily into asystole or ventricular fibrillation.

The block may be initiated by exercise, excitement or anoxia and sometimes by hypokalaemia (Guyer, 1964)[66] and is the result of temporary ventricular standstill producing cerebral ischaemia. On examination during an attack the patient is deathly pale or yellowish in colour, no pulse can be felt and no heart sound heard. Convulsions occur frequently and breath sounds are noisy, infrequent and stertorous, and if the patient is half or completely rotated onto the back, respiratory obstruction may result (see p. 392). The patient is likely to die during such an attack and one of the reasons for this is anoxia superimposed upon intrinsic depression of the ventricular pacemaker.

Usually after a few seconds, flushing of the skin occurs and the patient regains consciousness and is often able to hold a normal conversation almost immediately and to continue with what he was doing before the onset of the attack. In others, a feeling of weakness and anxiety persists and they continue to appear pale and lethargic for some hours afterwards.

Sometimes the ECG shows no evidence of partial block and may even appear to be normal, and in these circumstances the differentiation of the condition from grand mal is difficult. While congenital heart block has a relatively good prognosis, acquired heart block, resulting from either myocardial disease or open-heart surgery, has a poor prognosis, the average time of survival following its presentation being 2 years if a cardiac pacemaker is not inserted.

Treatment of Adams–Stokes attacks

The chest should be thumped immediately and vigorously at the lower part of the sternum. This will often terminate an attack.

External cardiac massage may also sometimes terminate an attack and should be instituted if respiration ceases and there is a danger of developing ventricular fibrillation. Cardiac output is commonly so poor that spontaneous respiration is not maintained. If artificial ventilation is started, preferably using an endotracheal tube (to avoid the inhalation of vomit), this alone will sometimes be sufficient to resuscitate the patient and maintain the blood pressure. Ventilation of the lungs with air can, following three or four breaths, return an apparently dead person to a non-cyanosed, pink patient with amazing rapidity, although the heart rate is slow.

Infusions of isoprenaline (isoproterenol, Suscardia, Saventrine) 4 or 5 mg in 1 litre of 5% dextrose or 0.9% saline increase the heart rate, return the blood pressure to normal and induce the return of spontaneous ventilation.

If complete asystole occurs, the chest should be thumped repeatedly and an injection of 0.5–1 ml of 1 : 10 000 adrenaline (epinephrine) may be given directly into the heart through a long needle passed through the chest wall to the left of the sternum through the fourth or fifth left intercostal space (i.e. into the right ventricle).

In medical practice therefore, the measures described to cope with cardiac arrest should be instituted. It is of great importance that obstruction of the respiratory airway should be relieved and artificial ventilation maintained (Chapter 11).

Treatment of recurrent attacks

Recurrent attacks frequently occur following the onset of myocardial failure because inadequate perfusion of the tissues gives rise to an increased arteriovenous oxygen gradient which tends to initiate suppression of the intrinsic ventricular pacemaker in much the same way as increased physical effort. It is often stated that digitalization, because of its ability to produce heart block on its own account, may convert a partial block into a complete block and this, therefore, should not be used in these circumstances. The relief of myocardial failure is by far the most important factor in the relief of heart block and in one case treatment with digitalis produced relief of attacks that were occurring once every 1 or 2 weeks so that they disappeared completely for a period of 6 months.

The treatment of choice is the insertion of an artificial pacemaker. This can be introduced via an antecubital vein or, preferably, via the subclavian vein, and passed either under fluoroscopic or ECG control into the right ventricle. This allows time for elective surgical intervention and the implantation of a 'permanent' pacemaker.

Adrenaline may be given intramuscularly in the form of an oily solution 1 : 1000, the long-acting adrenaline mucate (hyperduric adrenaline) at 4- to 12-hourly intervals, or it may be given subcutaneously or intramuscularly in the 1 : 1000 solution every 3–4 hours. Subcutaneous isoprenaline sulphate (Isuprel, Isoproterenol) 0.2 mg every 6 hours may assist in warding off recurrent attacks. This substance may also be given sublingually four or five times daily in doses of 10–20 mg. A sustained action tablet (Saventrine) containing 30 mg of isoprenaline hydrochloride is available and is suitable for treatment and maintenance therapy. Initially, 2–4 tablets can be swallowed every 8 hours and when tolerance has been established the same dose may be taken more frequently (e.g. every 3 hours if necessary). If the dose of this preparation is too large, it may give rise to tremor, tachycardia, anginal pain and vomiting.

Ephedrine 30–60 mg t.d.s. is frequently used in this condition. Very rarely, intravenous adrenaline may be needed to overcome recurrent Adams–Stokes attacks. Three millilitres of 1–1000 solution is added to 1 litre of 5% dextrose in water and is administered at a rate of 20–30 drops/minute and the infusion stopped when a regular heart rate of 50–60/minute is achieved.

A period of myocardial inadequacy follows a severe Adams–Stokes attack and hypotension may develop. During the attack a grave biochemical and biophysical upset develops so that a marked metabolic acidosis is present and adrenocortical activity is reduced. The use of pressor agents (see p. 226) should, therefore, be instituted and the metabolic acidosis corrected by the infusion of sodium bicarbonate solution 2.74% (the most useful solution), and hydrocortisone given intravenously in doses of 100–300 mg. A maintenance dose of cortisone or prednisone (Delta–Cortelan, Meticorten) 20–30 mg/day should be given.

When digitalis is the cause of heart block it must be withdrawn immediately for at least 48 hours. This is essential, even when the digitalis intoxication is a result of potassium depletion caused by inadequate replacement following diuretic therapy. Potassium depletion of this nature cannot be adequately corrected by oral administration of KCl in less than 48 hours. This is probably because the K^+ requires 24 hours to equilibrate with some tissue cells. Potassium chloride (6–8 g) should be given daily in divided doses in non-enteric coated capsules or dissolved in water and made palatable with orange juice or other sweetened beverages. The effervescent form (potassium bicarbonate) or the mixture consisting of potassium acetate, potassium bicarbonate and potassium citrate should not be used because its retention by the body is variable. Effervescent preparations containing KCl can, however, be used.

Atropine potentiates the effect of sympathomimetic drugs, such as ephedrine and isoprenaline, and therefore can be administered by subcutaneous injection, 0.5 mg 4-hourly.

Syncope

Syncope is the term applied to a sudden transitory loss of consciousness often associated with hypotension. It usually occurs to people who are standing upright, and hypotension results in an insufficient supply of blood to the brain. Cerebral hypoxia, therefore, is considered to be the cause. Syncope, can, however, occur when a patient is in bed. This applies to all forms of syncope, including the ordinary vasovagal syncope or simple faint. It sometimes occurs as a result of hypoglycaemia arising especially in either uncontrolled diabetics or those who have a varying blood glucose level in response to stress and exercise. Fainting is more common in epileptics and the flaccid state following a grand mal attack is sometimes mistaken for fainting. Syncope, therefore, assumes various forms including the following.

Vasovagal syncope
Orthostatic hypotension
Drug syncope
Syncope arising from
    metabolic disorders
Anaemia
Cough syncope
Cardiogenic syncope
Subclavian steal
    syndrome

Quinidine syncope
Micturition syncope
Swallow syncope
Weightlifter's syncope
Pulmonary embolus
Coronary occlusion
Syncope arising from
    pregnancy

Vasovagal syncope

This is probably the most common form of syncope and may occur in anyone at any time, but it usually occurs when a person is standing upright in a hot stuffy atmosphere, such as a theatre, or when there has been a sudden emotionally unpleasant episode, such as the viewing of a severe accident or the hearing of unpleasant news. Extreme pain, or the psychological overlay associated with minor discomfort or potential danger, such as a small electric shock or a cut finger, may also cause syncope. Syncope is most likely to occur after an acute illness, even of moderate severity, such as influenza, and in those who are anaemic either from malnutrition and pregnancy or from a chronic bleeding lesion.

The mode of onset almost always gives warning to the patient that it is about to happen and if it is occurring repeatedly, they are sometimes able to avoid it by breathing deeply while lying down. This differs markedly from syncope of the cardiogenic type and also from the metabolic or drug-induced type of syncope.

The patient suffering from vasovagal syncope feels completely exhausted and often tries to sit down. Sometimes hyperventilation occurs and almost invariably profuse sweating develops. There is a feeling of nausea and the patient may vomit. When it occurs during screening the stomach, and barium is swallowed, the stomach can be seen to dilate suddenly. When observed the patient is extremely pale—'as white as a sheet',—and often is green in colour at the onset of the condition. This is especially true when syncope is the result of pain, as on the battle field. The blood pressure is very low and may be unrecordable; the pulse is often not palpable at the wrist, but is always palpable over the carotid arteries and usually over the brachial artery. The pulse rate is usually slow at first, gradually increasing until a tachycardia can be detected. This is quite different from an Adams–Stokes attack or epilepsy. In the former the pulse rate is slow, in the latter the pulse rate is rapid throughout the whole episode. On recovery

vomiting is not uncommon, the patient feels weak and lethargic, but the more determined subjects can overcome this if they deliberately set out to do so. They continue, however, to look extremely pale and ill for a further 10 minutes or more.

Treatment
Great care must be taken to differentiate vasovagal syncope from that of cardiac origin as the treatment is often different. Fainting due to psychological shock usually corrects itself very shortly after the patient reaches a horizontal position. If there is sufficient time, the patient should be made to lie down before fainting has fully developed. When the cause of fainting is complete exhaustion and is of a metabolic nature, the episode may last a frighteningly long time (e.g. 5 or 10 minutes). It is syncope of this type, together with that caused by haemorrhage, that is most likely to occur in bed. For this reason it is important that the airway should be kept patent and steps should be taken to avoid the inhalation of vomit. The patient should be placed on the side with the lower end of the body raised. This can be achieved on the ground by placing a cushion or pillow under the pelvis and placing the legs on a chair. Alternatively the patient can be placed head down in the prone position, leaning over a chair or suitcase etc. Ideally, the patient should be placed in bed, the foot of which is raised. In the majority of cases recovery is inevitable and no special treatment is required, but every now and then fainting is the first sign of important, usually slowly progressing, pathological change. When the heart rate remains slow, atropine 0.6–1 mg i.v. can be given with safety unless the bradycardia is due to anoxia (see p. 383).

Orthostatic hypotension (postural hypotension)

This is becoming a more common condition in this era of addiction to television viewing. It is produced by a marked fall of blood pressure on assuming the upright position and is more likely to appear when this is performed abruptly. This type of syncope is also more likely to occur in hot stuffy surroundings and is largely due to the inability of the autonomic nervous system to compensate for the abrupt changes in hydrostatic pressure occurring within the vascular system. When the viewer rushes from a warm room having changed from the semi-supine to the upright position and has walked a few steps, syncope occurs. It is sometimes repeated on numerous occasions. Collapse in the lavatory is not an uncommon history.

When the history is carefully taken it is almost

invariably found that attacks of dizziness and faintness have been experienced previously and sometimes weakness in one arm or one leg and a feeling of numbness in these limbs and on one side of the chest of a transitory nature are described. These latter phenomena are more common in men and are frequently relieved completely when a tight collar is loosened (carotid sinus syncope).

Sometimes postural hypotension is a manifestation of diseases of the autonomic nervous system. It has been observed to occur in a patient who was an untreated diabetic who had developed a peripheral neuritis and a spontaneous degeneration of the thoracolumbar sympathetic system which produced pooling of blood in the lower limbs. It may also be associated with underlying disease processes such as Addison's disease, diabetes mellitus (even in the absence of neurological manifestations), Parkinson's disease, tabes dorsalis, peripheral neuritis, syringomelia and cerebral tumours. In both Addison's disease and diabetes the total body water is reduced, and so therefore is the blood volume. A fall in blood pressure can be observed using a sphygmomanometer, when the measurement is made first in the supine and then in the erect position.

Shy–Drager syndrome

This form of hypotension is a disorder of unknown aetiology. It is characterized by autonomic nervous system insufficiency, which causes a reduction in both systolic and diastolic blood pressures by more than 20 mmHg when the patient stands up after lying down, but there is no acceleration of the heart rate.[140] This form of hyoptension may cause syncope. Various remedies have been tried for this condition, these include corticosteroids, beta-adrenergic blocking agents and monoamine-oxidase inhibitors. On the basis that inhibition of prostaglandins might reverse the vasodilatation, Kochar and Itskovitz[81] treated four patients with indomethacin (Indocid) with success.

Syncope also sometimes occurs initially following a thoracolumbar sympathectomy performed to alleviate malignant hypertension. In the benign forms it can sometimes be avoided by wearing a tight abdominal belt, elastic stockings and a less tight collar when this is a contributory cause. When the condition has been explained patients learn to rise more slowly and, if they feel faint or ataxic, sit down lowering their head as far as possible while contracting their abdominal muscles. Ephedrine can be given in doses of 25 mg three or four times every day and is sometimes a useful adjuvant to other measures. Amphetamine sulphate

5–10 mg is an alternative substance, but may cause anorexia in patients in whom it is undesirable and contribute to emotional disturbances. Atropine sulphate 0.4–0.6 mg three to four times daily is also effective, but produces an unpleasant dryness of the mouth.

Drug syncope

This is largely a cause of postural hypotension. The drugs that produce this are the ganglion blocking agents, notably:

pentolinium	(Ansolysen)
mecamylamine	(Inversine, Mevasine)
pempidine	(Perolysen, Tenormal)

and the sympathetic blocking agents which are still being used:

guanethidine	(Ismelin)
bretylium tosylate	(Bretylate)

This condition can sometimes be avoided by the wearing of elastic stockings and a tight abdominal belt. It is a characteristic of patients who are treated with these drugs that they have to keep moving from foot to foot, contracting their leg muscles (e.g. if they stand talking for any length of time). Characteristically, deep sighing breaths need to be taken from time to time.

Syncope arising from metabolic disorders

Syncope quite commonly occurs when there is a total body Na^+ depletion. This can develop in otherwise healthy people who have for psychogenic or other reasons severely restricted their salt intake until the pattern described on page 28 has been produced. It more readily occurs in patients who have taken large doses of amphetamine for psychotherapy, during which a sodium diuresis sometimes occurs and food and salt intake has been restricted because of the associated anorexia. It also occurs in symptomless hyponatraemia (see p. 30), in which a normal diet is taken and extraneous therapy is not a factor in the resetting of the osmotic activity of the body fluids at a lower level than normal.

Potassium depletion will also cause syncope (Guyer, 1964),[66] especially when it is associated with an abnormal endocrine secretion resulting, for example, from carcinoma. It commonly occurs in patients suffering from cirrhosis of the liver, patients with cardiac disease who have become K^+ depleted following chronic malnutrition and diuretic therapy, and ulcerative colitis, especially when the onset of a localized neoplastic focus has contributed to electrolyte imbalance.

Spontaneous hypoglycaemia is a further cause of syncope. Hypoglycaemic syncope also occurs in such conditions as liver disease, in which there is depletion of glycogen stores and hypersensitivity to insulin, in conditions of hyperinsulinism arising from a pancreatic islet-cell adenoma or carcinoma and other endocrine disorders, for example, pituitary anterior lobe deficiency (Simmond's disease and neoplasia), adrenocortical insufficiency, hypothyroidism and lesions of the midbrain. Hypoglycaemia occurs also during pregnancy and lactation, malabsorption syndrome and, quite commonly, from no known cause (idiopathic hypoglycaemia). Its onset often follows major physical activity and sometimes after large amounts of sugar have been ingested and the stimulus to secrete insulin is maintained. Syncope does not normally occur until the blood sugar has fallen below 2 mmol/l (40 mg%).

Anaemia

Continuous bleeding from any site giving rise to a normocytic iron deficiency-type of anaemia or a macrocytic anaemia produced by metabolic disorders, such as pernicious anaemia and steatorrhoea, may be associated with syncopal attacks. Sudden haemorrhage commonly causes fainting and, therefore, is an almost invariable accompaniment of a large haematemesis.

Severe anaemia is one of the causes of fainting in the supine position (e.g. in bed), but a haemoglobin concentration of less than 5 g% appears to be necessary for this to occur. Although pernicious anaemia occurs more commonly in the female, beware of the male with a megaloblastic anaemia.

Cough syncope

This normally follows a prolonged paroxysm of coughing, usually of a nonproductive nature and caused by irritation of the upper respiratory tract. It sometimes results from laryngeal spasm, but more commonly results from an increase in intrathoracic pressure, obstruction to the venous return and fall in cardiac output (Valsalva effect). The face becomes plethoric and cyanosed and the patient may suffer from a mild feeling of faintness, making it necessary to sit on a chair, or he may fall to the ground with complete loss of consciousness. Patients who suffer from chronic obstructive lung disease may increase their intrathoracic pressure to almost 300 mmHg during a paroxysm of violent coughing.[139] A further factor may be the rise in intracranial pressure, as it has been found that the pressure of the cerebrospinal fluid rose to the same level as that recorded within the thorax.

Cardiac syncope

Aortic stenosis

The first indication of this condition may be abrupt and sudden, syncope coming on without warning after a period of unaccustomed exercise. It has been known to occur, for example, after climbing stairs hurriedly when a lift has been out of action. Although it may cause sudden death, loss of consciousness is usually of short duration and is preceded by intense pallor. Because it is often associated with cardiac failure, syncope arising from this cause sometimes responds to digitalization. Aortic incompetence may also cause syncope.

Adams–Stokes attacks

These are characterized by syncope and convulsions. ECG recordings normally show ventricular asystole, but sometimes paroxysmal ventricular fibrillation may occur with spontaneous reversion (Gable, 1965).[52]

Ball-valve thrombus

This is a condition which is very rarely diagnosed in life. When a massive thrombus occupies the left atrium during mitral stenosis with atrial fibrillation, it may intermittently block the mitral valve orifice reducing the cardiac output to very nearly zero. It may be a cause of sudden death. Severe breathlessness precedes syncope. There is a loss of peripheral pulses and marked peripheral cyanosis, especially of the extremities, ear lobes, fingers and tip of the nose. Angina pectoris is commonly present.

Diagnosis may be made by the fact that the profound peripheral cyanosis is intermittent and that relief of the dyspnoea, angina pectoris and peripheral cyanosis may be obtained by adopting a prone knee–chest position with the forehead touching the floor, similar to that of a Mohammedan at prayer. The only treatment available is surgical, when splitting of the mitral valve is performed at the same time.

Myxoma of the atrium

This is a primary tumour arising from the interatrial septum, being attached to this structure by means of a pedicle and developing in either atrium.

It is associated with a high erythrocyte sedimentation rate (ESR), anaemia and pyrexia. Small pieces of the tumour may become detached, giving rise to pulmonary emboli from the right atrium and peripheral emboli from the left atrium. Syncope probably arises from a myxoma of the right atrium blocking the IVC or the tricuspid orifice. When it develops in the left atrium, syncope occurs in a similar manner to that resulting from a massive thrombus occupying the left atrium, intermittently blocking the mitral orifice as in mitral stenosis. Atrial fibrillation, however, is not a common feature of the condition, although it sometimes occurs. Myxoma of the atrium may give rise to paroxysmal nocturnal dyspnoea, pulmonary oedema, congestive cardiac failure and sudden death. Deterioration of the patient's condition occurs much more rapidly than when mitral stenosis is the primary disease process. X-ray appearances are similar to those found in mitral stenosis, but angiocardiography may reveal a filling defect of the atrium. At cardiac catheterization, pulmonary hypertension and raised left atrial pressure may be found. Syncope may be relieved by means of adopting the prone knee–chest position and treatment consists of surgical removal of the myxoma.

Congenital cyanotic heart disease
Syncope commonly occurs in infants, often after a period of restlessness and crying, who are suffering from Fallot's tetralogy, Eisenmenger syndrome, complete transposition of the great vessels, primary pulmonary stenosis or complete anomalous pulmonary venous drainage. It is associated with an increase in the degree of cyanosis and the infant may convulse during the period of unconsciousness. Frequent attacks are indicative of a poor prognosis. Some relief may be obtained by keeping the infant in an oxygen tent so that pulmonary hypertension is reduced, by digitalization 0.1 mg/lb (0.05 mg/kg) body weight and by giving morphine sulphate 1 mg/10lb (4.5 kg) body weight during an attack. When the attacks are frequent, corrective surgery should be performed as soon as possible.

The hemiblock
In the early 1960s it was recognized that people who had right bundle branch block and left axis deviation frequently suffered from syncopal attacks. It is now realized (see p. 343) that people who have conduction blocks in two of the three fascicles may also suffer from disease of the remaining fascicle, so that intermittently a complete block (all three fascicles) can develop. The syncopal attack, therefore, is an Adams–Stokes attack.

Syncope was investigated prospectively by Dhingra et al.[37] in 186 patients who had chronic bifascicular block. Syncope was found to occur in 21 of 124 patients who had right bundle branch block and left *anterior* hemiblock, in 3 of 24 patients with right bundle branch block and left *posterior* hemiblock, and 6 of 38 patients with left bundle branch block. The LBBB is a bifascicular block (see p. 344). They concluded that permanent cardiac pacing appeared to be indicated only in those patients who had experienced a serious bradyarrhythmia.

Cardiac arrhythmias
Virtually any cardiac arrhythmia can cause syncope. The most common atrial tachyarrhythmias include atrial fibrillation, atrial flutter, paroxysmal atrial tachycardia, Wolff–Parkinson–White syndrome and tachybradycardia (sick sinus syndrome). The ventricular tachyarrhythmias include ventricular tachycardia, ventricular fibrillation, failure of an artificial pacemaker, tricyclic antidepressant toxicity and those syndromes associated with a prolonged Q–T interval, such as Jervell and Lange–Nielson and Ramano–Ward syndromes. The bradyarrhythmias include complete heart block, sick sinus syndrome, myocardial ischaemia and artificial pacemaker failure.

All these arrhythmias may be associated with *exercise syncope*.

Subclavian steal syndrome
Severe atheroma in the aortic arch and its branches may produce unconsciousness, for example when vigorous exercise is performed with one or both arms.

In 1954, Eastcott et al.[46] demonstrated that it was possible to relieve intermittent attacks of hemiplegia by surgery to the internal carotid artery. In 1960, Contorni[31] described a syndrome that was characterized by diplopia, dizziness, tinnitus, loss of hearing, ataxia and syncope.

Retrograde flow occurring in the cerebral circulation giving rise to transitory cerebral ischaemia was also reported by Reivich et al.[120] Prodromal signs, such as transitory loss of vision (amaurosis fugax), paraesthesiae and transient cerebellar signs, have been found to occur, and these frequently accompany carotid artery stenosis.

The condition sometimes develops spontaneously, but is commonly precipitated by significant activity of the *left* arm. It results from the flow of blood being diverted from the vertebral artery and away from the brain into the subclavian artery as blood flow through the arm increases. The term 'subclavian steal syndrome' was created by the Editors of the *New England Journal of Medicine* in 1961 following the confirmation of the findings by a number of investigators.[112]

The condition is caused by occlusion of the subclavian artery at its source and it can be relieved by the artificial anastomosis of the internal carotid to the subclavian artery by means of a Dacron graft or the anastomosis of the *right* subclavian to the *left* subclavian, distal to the block. It has been found that any exercise, such as walking, even without undue activity of the arms, can lead to the onset of syncope in this condition.

Quinidine syncope

Syncope resulting from paroxysmal ventricular fibrillation has been reported after quinidine, sometimes following very small doses. Selzer and Wray[136] reported their findings in eight patients. It is well known that ventricular fibrillation may occur following the use of this drug, but spontaneous reversal to a normal rhythm has not been previously stressed. External cardiac massage and other resuscitative measures should be started at once.

Micturition syncope

This is most commonly seen in young to middle-aged men who rise to micturate after being asleep or recumbent for a long period of time.[67,116,135] The causes and pathogenesis of the condition have not been clearly identified, but include postural hypotension, vagal inhibition of heart beat, and the Valsalva effect.

Swallow syncope

Patients suffering from oesophageal spasm, achalasia and peptic-ulcer-induced strictures are subject to syncopal attacks.[3,90,91] Various cardiac arrhythmias have been observed. These include sinus and junctional (nodal) bradycardia, SA block, AV block, complete heart block and numerous premature ventricular ectopic beats and even asystole. When these are mediated by the vagus nerve, treatment with atropine can prevent a syncopal attack.

In the majority of people suffering from swallow syncope the lesion has been found to be benign, but Tomlinson and Fox[157] reported a case of carcinoma of the oesophagus associated with syncope. This patient underwent a severe sinus bradycardia, either following swallowing or during fibreoptic endoscopy performed under anaesthesia. As in other cases, the bradycardia causing the syncopal attack was relieved by atropine and, in the case of Tomlinson and Fox, by removal of the carcinoma by surgery.

Weightlifter's syncope

Loss of consciousness of a transitory nature is a relatively common occurrence in weightlifters. There is a marked rise in intrathoracic pressure during the period of lifting the heavy weight, so that a Valsalva effect is produced. In addition, it has been noted[30] that hyperventilation, and therefore a fall in PCO_2 which may cause vasoconsricttion in the central nervous system, frequently precedes the lifting manoeuvre. This form of syncope therefore may be related to hyperventilation syndrome.

Pulmonary embolus

Clinicians can be severely misled by pulmonary embolus. For example, a 32-year-old black male was seen in the emergency department having fainted 20 minutes earlier. A careful examination was performed and a chest radiograph was taken. The patient was not cyanosed, had no pleural pericordial or pleuropericordial friction rub. There was no shortness of breath, no haemoptysis, pleuritic pain or tachycardia. The ECG was normal, $S_1 Q_3$ pattern (S wave in lead 1 and Q wave in lead 3) was absent. His oral temperature was normal. There was no calf tenderness and Hamman's sign was absent. The blood pressure was normal and there was no postural hypotension when it was measured in the erect position.

The classic triad of pyrexia, tachycardia and tachypnoea, which may have been present initially, could not be elicited. The patient was anxious not to enter hospital as he had travelled from Africa on business. An arterial blood sample to elicit a fall in PO_2, which is not reflected in the appearance of the mucous membranes, was not obtained; nor was the lactate dehydrogenase (LDH) level (which is frequently elevated) measured. Three days later the author attended this patient's post-mortem examination during which very long emboli, approximately 1 cm in diameter, were found in both lungs.

When collapse occurs, external cardiac massage and general resuscitative measures should be taken, even when the diagnosis has not been made.

Coronary occlusion

Syncope, collapse and sudden shortness of breath were the first findings in only 12% of patients in the Oxford linkage study.[79] Nevertheless, syncope must alert the clinician to the necessity of investigating the cause, even in the absence of chest pain.

Pregnancy

Syncopal attacks may occur at any time during pregnancy, but are more common when there is associated anaemia, myocardial disease and frank myocardial failure. Orthostatic hypotension is, however, quite a common feature and may be in part caused by the gravid uterus pressing backwards upon the inferior vena cava and thus interfering with the venous return to the heart.

Pulmonary Embolus

This is an acute emergency, which may cause instantaneous death or acute cardiac failure. It is most commonly caused by peripheral thrombi arising from the deep calf veins of the legs or from the pelvic veins following surgery. It is more common in the obese subject, but can arise in the malnourished patient. Another cause of pulmonary embolus is atrial fibrillation when the emboli arise from the right atrium. It also arises during congestive cardiac failure and myocardial infarction and mitral stenosis. Air may be introduced during surgery and fat emboli may follow bone fractures.

Certain conditions predispose towards pulmonary embolism. These are age, prolonged bedrest, surgical intervention of any kind, lethargy and lack of movement and a low cardiac output. Another most important predisposing cause is dehydration, especially in the postoperative period as this produces haemoconcentration and an increase in blood viscosity. It occurs following multiple fractures even when treatment during the period which follows resuscitation is carefully planned in order to avoid it appearing. Very rarely pulmonary embolus occurs following childbirth.

While during the years preceding 1968 pulmonary embolism accounted for between 2000 and 3000 deaths each year in the UK alone, there is evidence that there has been a rise in the incidence of the condition associated with the use of oral contraceptives.* A greater degree of interest is being displayed in the treatment and prevention of this condition because diagnosis has been improved by means of pulmonary angiography, studies using radio-isotopes such as technetium, ultrasound and body scanning.

The high incidence of pulmonary embolism is reflected in the figures of Sevitt and Gallagher,[137] who found that, at post-mortem examination, approximately 20% of patients admitted to the Birmingham Accident Hospital had experienced a pulmonary embolus. Over 90% of the patients were aged 50 or more years. The incidence of pulmonary embolism varied with the condition and was present in 49–60% of patients who died following fracture of the femur or tibia. Patients who had died followng trauma to the abdomen, thorax or cerebrum demonstrated pulmonary embolism in only 5.5% of cases. Death occurred in the majority of cases in the first 1–2 hours. The most common cause of pulmonary embolism was deep venous thrombosis. Although diagnosis has been made easier, the main approach to this condition should be that of prevention. It is therefore evident that, in addition to correct hydration and early mobilization, treatment by administration of 'low-dose heparin' can be added, although this is not without its dangers and some controversy surrounds this method of prevention.

Clinical presentation

In a series of 23 patients in whom angiography had confirmed the presence of a large pulmonary embolism, the following presentation was found (Miller and Sutton, 1970).[104]

Sudden onset of dyspnoea	87%
Collapse	70%
Mid-sternal chest pain	22%
Pleuritic chest pain	22%
Haemoptysis	9%

Premonitory episodes of small, pulmonary embolic phenomena occurred in 48% of patients in this series (Miller and Sutton, 1970).[104] They were associated with pleuritic pain and haemoptysis; cardiac arrest occurred in only 3 out of 23 patients. However, a cardiac arrest occurred more commonly and had a higher incidence when

* There is also evidence of myocardial infarction being associated with oral contraceptives (Engel et al., 1977; Waxler, 1971).[47,169]

pulmonary embolus was investigated by Sutton et al.[152]

Faintness or syncopal attack and associated dyspnoea is almost certainly associated with a fall of cardiac output. The diagnosis of pulmonary embolism, however, is sometimes difficult to make because when pulmonary embolus occurs, the severe, central pain in the chest is similar to that of an acute myocardial infarction. Syncope is more likely to develop if the patient is upright. Because of the obstruction to blood flow through the pulmonary arteries, the right ventricle becomes distended and the venous pressure rises abruptly. It is not unusual for patients to prefer to lie flat following pulmonary embolism and, while inspiratory and expiratory rhonchi are often heard, they may be either absent or not a prominent feature.

The obstruction to the flow of blood produces a situation which is depicted in Fig. 51B (p. 119), when there is a sudden and immense increase in the physiological dead space of the lungs. Thus there is ventilation without perfusion. As a result of this, tachypnoea, hyperpnoea and tachycardia develop. A readily recognizable massive increase in respiratory effort occurs. This is associated with marked cyanosis. The arterial oxygen tension is reduced and, because of the gas exchange occurring in unobstructed parts of the lung, the PCO_2 falls. The arterial blood is desaturated. Although the high venous pressure is present, the intense respiratory effort may, on occasions in the obese individual, make the detection of the raised jugular venous pressure (JVP) difficult. There is peripheral vasoconstriction and cyanosis and the blood pressure is low. The apex of the heart is frequently bounding in character.

The ESR is often raised and a leucocytosis follows 24 hours after the episode. On auscultation there is pulmonary consolidation, and within a few hours of it occurring a pleural effusion which may be bloodstained is commonly present. A friction rub is sometimes heard, especially when there is the pleuritic type of pain. Quite commonly, therefore, pulmonary embolism of this mild type is misdiagnosed as being pneumonia of acute onset.

On auscultation of the heart, in addition to the tachycardia, the heart sounds may be faint and distant. The pulmonary second sound in severe pulmonary embolus is frequently absent because the ventricular end-diastolic pressure rises to equal the pulmonary artery diastolic pressure. Hyperventilation may make auscultation of the heart sounds difficult to hear, especially when both inspiratory and expiratory rhonchi are present.

The physical signs encountered in pulmonary embolism have been well documented by a number of investigators Miller and Sutton (1970).[104]

Sinus tachycardia	97%
Gallop rhythm (S_3 or S_4)	83%
Raised JVP	80%
Cyanosis	74%
Hypotension, systolic pressure less than 80 mmHg	37%

Associated with these findings are those attributable to a low cardiac output such as a cold clammy skin associated with sweating, cold extremities and the pallor that is generalized throughout the body. When a pulmonary embolism occurs (e.g. postoperatively), and a urinary catheter is in situ, urinary output either ceases or falls abruptly immediately following pulmonary embolism. The gallop rhythm may be either presystolic S4 or protodiastolic S3. In the presence of a sinus tachycardia, these sounds produce a summation gallop. Occasionally, pulses paradoxus may be present (Küssmaul, 1873).[22,86]

Chest X-ray

The plain chest X-ray may have no changes visible, especially as right ventricular enlargement is commonly difficult to identify. The lung vascular markings, however, may be decreased and, if the embolus is predominantly in one artery, the decreased vascular markings on one side may be counterbalanced by a plethora of lung markings on the other. Fluid may accumulate in a fissure on the affected side. Increase in size of the pulmonary conus is sometimes seen.

Pulmonary angiography

When facilities are available for pulmonary angiography to be performed at short notice, this should be achieved by exposing an antecubital vein and passing a catheter into the main pulmonary artery. The degree of occlusion of the pulmonary vessels can be clearly demonstrated and the extent of the embolus defined. This procedure is not without its dangers as the replacement of blood by radio-opaque material in the alveolar capillaries may be sufficient to increase the physiological dead space, as described above, to such a degree that ventricular fibrillation is precipitated. This does not preclude survival of the patient if facilities for rapidly performing a Trendelenberg operation are available.

Pulmonary embolism and ECG

The changes in the ECG arise from the obstructive effects of the embolism on the heart. It has been known for quite large emboli to produce no effects in the ECG or to produce changes that mimic myocardial infarction that are either long-standing or even permanent. There can be transient supraventricular arrhythmias or a simple sinus tachycardia, which may develop later into junctional tachycardia, atrial fibrillation or atrial flutter.

Dilatation of the right atrium, in addition to causing the above, produces P pulmonale which implies tall P waves in leads II, III and AVF. The dilated right atrium should also produce a qR complex in the right chest leads (V_{3R}, VI).[146] Transient right bundle branch block, first, second and third degree block may also occur and are considered to be the result of dilatation of the right ventricle.

Inverted T waves and deviation of the S–T segment occurs in the right chest leads and are considered to be the result of not only the increased work load of the right ventricle but also acute coronary insufficiency.

The axis of the heart in the frontal plane rotates to the right, producing right axis deviation with a marked clockwise rotation of the heart in the horizontal plane. When this occurs to a marked degree, deep S waves are seen in the standard limb leads. It has been emphasized by McGinn and White (1935),[102] Solokow and Lyon (1949),[148] and Katz (1946)[77] that pulmonary embolus gives rise to an S wave in lead I and a Q wave in lead III ($S_I Q_3$ pattern) and that there is S–T elevation with 'staircase ascent'. A full review of the changes are given by Lipman et al. (1972).[92]

Massive pulmonary embolus

This always presents an acute emergency and in a number of cases death is instantaneous or follows within a few minutes. The patient is suddenly seized with severe agonizing breathlessness and has a feeling of impending death. A severe pain in the chest, similar to that of cardiac infarction and radiating through to the back, accompanies the onset of the episode. Occasionally, the patient loses consciousness completely or has transitory episodes of syncope. There is marked pallor, widespread cyanosis, the hands and feet are cold and there is profuse sweating. The pulse is rapid and of very poor volume and the blood pressure is low. This usually differs from the early onset of acute pulmonary oedema, which may, however, sometimes accompany the condition. There is an immediate rise in the jugular venous pressure (JVP), and the pulmonary second sound is generally accentuated and a gallop rhythm is commonly present. Reflex narrowing of the bronchial tree often occurs so that there are inspiratory and expiratory rhonchi.

Treatment

The main pattern of treatment is to combat shock, relieve the strain on the right ventricle, and dilate the vessels that have been reflexly made to contract so that cardiac output is increased and perhaps in order to allow the emboli to move to a more distant and therefore safer vessel. It is also essential to relieve pain, anxiety and discomfort of the patient. The patient must be given oxygen immediately and if necessary have assisted ventilation which should be continued until the acute episode has passed.

Morphine sulphate 10–15 mg i.m. or pethidine (demerol) 100 mg should be given to relieve the pain and anxiety. Theophylline-ethylenediamine (Aminophylline) 0.5–1 g should be given slowly intravenously. Atropine sulphate 0.6 mg is sometimes given to relieve the reflex contraction of the vessels and also the reflex contraction of the bronchi when it is present. Shock should be treated with the pressor drugs as described on page 231 in the manner that has been suggested for myocardial infarction. The intravenous injection of the papaverine is sometimes extremely effective. Although it is one of the opium alkaloids, it has no analgesic action and very little action on the central nervous system. It has a quinidine-like action in the sense that it depresses conductivity and prolongs the refractory period of heart muscle. The smooth muscle of all arteries, including that of the coronary vessels, is relaxed by this substance and the reflex contraction of the vessels in the pulmonary tree is reversed by it. Its action is transitory however, lasting from only a few seconds to a few minutes— 100 mg of the substance should be diluted and given over a period of 10 minutes intravenously and this dose should be repeated after a further 15 minutes. The infusion of streptokinase has been found to be of value.

Anticoagulation

This should be carried out in the same way as for cardiac infarction, but it is preferable that a dose of 10 000 units (100 mg) should be given intravenously as early as possible.

Prevention

We have seen how massive pulmonary embolus commonly arises in those patients who are confined to bed, usually in the postoperative period. Early ambulation is becoming less popular as a means of avoiding pulmonary embolus, although there is no doubt that prolonged bedrest is a contributory cause. However, so much is often lost and so little gained by the routine procedure of getting a patient to sit in a chair on the day following a major surgical intervention that it is far more important to maintain a state of adequate hydration, together with active ankle movements, than to force a sick and unwilling patient to sit in a chair where he remains even more immobile than in a bed. To increase the flow of blood along the veins of the calf, alternate plantar and dorsiflexion of the foot must occur. In no other way can the muscle pump be made to work, and although other movements at the thigh and knee may assist by increasing cardiac output and causing an increased flow of blood through the pelvic veins, these exercises will not increase the flow of blood through the muscles of the calf. Breathing exercises increase the venous return to the heart and transmit a negative pressure along the great veins and are therefore of value when performed correctly. The calves should be felt routinely by a medical attendant at least once a day and, if pain is found to be present, the patient should be placed on anticoagulants immediately and the foot exercises should be intensified. Anticoagulant therapy must be continued for at least 6 weeks and, if repeated emboli have occurred, it may have to be continued for 3–6 months. Withdrawal of the anticoagulant must proceed slowly, the dose being decreased by small amounts each time.

Low-dose heparin

The use of low-dose heparin for the prevention of venous thromboembolism was first suggested by Sharnoff et al.[138] in 1962. Since then, a Multi-Centre International Trial (1975)[111] has clearly demonstrated that small doses of heparin, given subcutaneously, can effectively reduce the incidence of postoperative deep vein thrombosis. The usual method of administration is the subcutaneous injection of 5000 units of calcium heparin 8-hourly.

Not only has low-dose heparin been found to be of value in the prevention of postoperative venous thromboembolism, but McCarthy et al.[100] have shown that it is of value in people suffering from acute strokes; at least 60% of patients suffering from stroke have associated deep vein thrombosis, and post-mortem studies have revealed that approximately 50% of the people admitted to hospital because of a stroke have evidence of pulmonary embolism.[35]

The use of low-dose heparin is, however, not without its critics. It has not been found of value in preventing thromboembolism in patients who have suffered a fractured neck of femur,[109] and the prophylactic effect of subcutaneous heparin following myocardial infarction has been found by some[167] but not by others.[68]

In relation to the prevention of postoperative thromboembolism, some workers have found it necessary to abandon the use of low-dose heparin,[19] because life-threatening postoperative bleeding, and also wound haematomata were found in some patients. Although the author has not performed a study in this field, low-dose heparin appears to be effective following, for example, thoracic surgery for aortocoronary bypass and other conditions.

It is, however, important to exclude, for example, the presence of a peptic ulcer as this can bleed profusely and neutralization of the heparin with protamine sulphate has to be instituted immediately. This is obviously important when bleeding is even suspected from any source.

Dissecting Aneurysm of the Aorta

This is an important but uncommon condition which may easily be mistaken for acute coronary occlusion because it is associated with severe pain, shock and syncope. A dissecting aneurysm occurs when there is a splitting of the media with or without rupture of the intimal lining of the vessel and blood is extravasated within the vessel wall. This originates either from the vasa vasorum or from the lumen of the aorta when there is splitting of the intima. Sometimes a re-entry point is made so that occlusion does not occur. If partial obliteration of the aortic lumen results from the dissection, the arterial pressures above the obstruction are increased and those below the obstruction are decreased. Quite commonly the dissection begins in the ascending aorta and sometimes spreads along its whole length into its branches. In these circumstances the blood pressures obtained in one arm may differ from those in the other arm. When the aneurysm dissects proximally it may enlarge the aortic ring so that aortic incompetence of either rapid or gradual onset may result, making the treatment of cardiac failure, possibly pulmonary oedema and, later, aortic valve replacement, necessary. If the dissection extends further, it may give rise to a haemopericardium and death from the acute onset of cardiac tamponade.

Dissection of the aorta commonly occurs in patients with connective tissue disorders, such as Marfan's syndrome. Coarctation of the aorta is also a predisposing cause, as is hypertension. Dissection of the aorta sometimes occurs during pregnancy and is known to be a rare complication of labour. It sometimes occurs in early life as an acute painful episode and is only detected when it gives rise later to cardiac failure resulting from aortic incompetence or when the pulses and blood pressure measurements are found to be widely different in different limbs. Calcification of the clotted blood in the wall of the false lumen is sometimes detected on X-ray. Arteriography by means of a catheter passed in a retrograde direction through one of the femoral vessels may also help in the diagnosis of the condition some years later, but difficulty may be experienced in passing the catheter further than the point of re-entry.

Signs and symptoms

An extremely severe pain which has a sudden onset and is stabbing in character is felt in the chest extending through to the back, down into the abdomen and radiating distally to the head and neck and to the lower limbs. In the early stages the blood pressure falls, there is peripheral cyanosis, pallor and sweating. After a short period the blood pressure in one or both arms may be raised. If the dissection involves vessels supplying the spinal cord, there may be associated neurological signs. The urine may contain casts, albumin and blood if the dissection involves one or more of the renal vessels. Either hypotension or vessel involvement may give rise to acute renal failure. Dyspnoea, resulting from cardiac failure, especially when there is involvement of the coronary vessels producing myocardial ischaemia from hypotension, is commonly present in the acute stage.

X-ray changes

There may be widening of the mediastinum, increase in the size of the heart shadow from cardiac failure or leakage of blood into the pericardium, and the shadow formed by the aorta is characteristically widened. Small pleural effusions may be present.

ECG changes

A characteristic pattern of myocardial infarction may be present and almost invariably occurs when the dissection involves the coronary vessels.

Treatment

Every effort should be made to resuscitate a patient with a dissecting aneurysm because of the increasing success of surgical intervention. Rob and Kenyon (1960)[122] suggested that the contraindications for surgical intervention were only those of fulminating dissections, severe cardiac tamponade, a progressive disease process or anuria. Experience has shown that it is possible that the contraindications might in some cases be revised, and the complication of anuria avoided by raising the plasma osmolality (Brooks, 1964).[20]

Immediate treatment

Pain must be relieved by means of injection of morphine sulphate 15 mg. Treatment of shock is by means of blood replacement and not by means of vasopressors which are, in general, contraindicated. Oxygen by mask or tent should be administered to relieve the dyspnoea. Hydrocortisone 100–300 mg should be administered intravenously to assist in the relief of the hypotension. In almost all cases it is wise for digitalization to be started so that myocardial failure may be prevented because it is an almost invariable accompaniment of dissection of the aorta in the elderly. Although it may be argued that anticoagulants may prevent thrombosis in some of the vessels, their use increases the difficulties associated with surgery and in practice appears to afford little benefit. Some surgeons believe that anticoagulants are contraindicated.

Cardiac Tamponade

This condition is a result of blood or fluid being contained within the pericardium so that it interferes with the beating of the heart. Occasionally, sterile effusions of large volumes are seen; these are of unknown aetiology. Others arise from tuberculosis, rheumatic carditis, myxoedema, anasarca, and malignant disease. Purulent effusions may arise from infective processes within the lungs or thoracic cavity, blood-spread infections, especially in those patients who have a low resistance arising from diabetes or chronic renal disease, trauma and surgical intervention. A haemopericardium occurs after open-heart surgery or penetrating wounds, leakage of blood from a dissecting aneurysm or an aneurysmal dilatation of a coronary vessel caused by periarteritis nodosa or rupture of the myocardial wall from cardiac infarction.

Clinical characteristics

When cardiac tamponade develops slowly over a period of hours the following signs and symptoms may be detected. As the effusion increases there is increasing dyspnoea, a tachycardia of increasing frequency and rise of the central venous pressure (CVP) reflected in engorgement of the external jugular veins and enlargement of the liver. The systemic arterial blood pressure falls. A weak pulse of poor volume is felt at the wrist and elsewhere, but its volume may be increased during expiration and decreased during inspiration; this phenomenon is referred to as pulsus paradoxus. During inspiration, tension within the pericardium is increased because of descent of the diaphragm so that further impairment of ventricular filling is produced. A fall in the venous pressure may be observed during systole as contraction of the ventricles reduces the tension and, therefore, less impedance is offered to the venous return. When the chest is percussed, dullness over the precordium extends outside its normal limits. On auscultation the heart sounds are faint and distant and a friction rub may be detected.

As the condition progresses the tachycardia becomes faster, the hypotension more severe and peripheral cyanosis more marked. Characteristically, when cardiac tamponade has been present for some hours there is a fall in the plasma $[Na^+]$ level and sometimes also a fall in the plasma $[K^+]$ level. A marked fall in the venous oxygen saturation occurs which, when it is below 30%, is an indication of impending cardiac arrest. The sinus tachycardia is insensitive to digitalis and, if cardiac tamponade is suspected, large doses should be avoided because they may lead to ventricular fibrillation.

Cardiac tamponade is probably most commonly seen after open-heart surgery and, unfortunately, the classical symptoms and signs are often obscured or absent. When the pericardium is closed or has become adherent to the posterior wall of the sternum it is not uncommon for cardiac tamponade to be produced by relatively small volumes of blood or fluid. In the early postoperative hours, therefore, cardiac tamponade may occur without any undue rise in heart rate or marked rise in venous pressure because of hypovolaemia. Hypotension does not respond to blood transfusion. A blood transfusion of small volume causes a marked rise in CVP without any change in the systemic arterial pressure. When hypotension results from both cardiac tamponade and hypovolaemia, damage to the kidneys is most likely. It is not an uncommon experience to observe an immediate rise in arterial blood pressure following surgical relief of the tamponade and the removal of only 200 ml of blood from an adult pericardium. The abrupt rise in arterial blood pressure, however, is followed very soon by an equally abrupt fall and is associated with a low CVP. Blood transfusion then has an immediate effect in producing a return of arterial blood pressure and CVP to normal limits. The explanation of the misleading absence of classical physical signs following open-heart surgery is obscure, but intrinsic impairment of myocardial function must play its part. When the condition frequently gives rise to marked hyponatraemia it is commonly associated with acute renal failure.

Chest X-rays, although of value in demonstrating the slow accumulation of fluid, are sometimes of relatively little value after open-heart surgery.

Treatment

If cardiac tamponade is produced by an effusion of fluid within the pericardium, paracentesis may be performed in order to relieve it. In the case of a haemopericardium, when there may be a large volume of clotted blood and paracentesis is therefore ineffective, an elective surgical procedure must be performed.

Paracentesis is performed by passing a needle to the left of the sternum through the fifth intercostal space, or by infiltrating the skin in the region of the epigastrium just to the left of the xiphoid process and passing a long needle at an approximately 30° angle to the skin to the anatomical left of the xiphisternum. When the needle has penetrated 1–2 inches (2.5–5.0 cm), according to the degrees of fatness of the patient, fluid may be withdrawn.

Heart Failure

The heart fails when the ventricles are unable to cope with demands made upon them and the output falls below its pre-existing level. Because the failing ventricles do not empty to the same degree, less blood is removed from the atria and, therefore, from the veins that drain into them.

Eventually the pressure within the ventricle during diastole is raised and this is transmitted to the atria and in turn to the veins.

In left ventricular failure the raised pulmonary venous pressure leads to congestion of the lungs. Pulmonary oedema occurs when the pressure within the capillaries rises above the osmotic pressure exerted by the plasma proteins. A rise of left atrial pressure above 25–30 mmHg therefore results in pulmonary oedema and lung damage.

In right ventricular failure, referred to as 'congestive cardiac failure', there is no congestion of the lungs, but the raised central and peripheral venous pressure gives rise to congestion of the liver and other organs and to peripheral oedema. The volume of blood within the great veins has to be increased by 10% before the venous pressure rises, and while this is developing the condition is one of incipient congestive cardiac failure.

Left ventricular failure results from aortic valve disease (incompetence or stenosis), hypertension, coronary artery disease, mitral incompetence, myopathies and systemic diseases (such as pernicious anaemia) which produce fatty degeneration of the heart.

Right ventricular failure develops as a consequence of:

1. left heart failure associated with pulmonary hypertension;
2. lung disease associated with increased pulmonary vascular resistance and pulmonary hypertension (including pulmonary embolus);
3. congenital lesions on the right side of the heart (e.g. pulmonary stenosis);
4. right ventricular infarction (see p. 287).

Right ventricular failure, occurring in isolation, is one of the conditions in which a central venous pressure (CVP) measurement or interpretation of the increased jugular venous pressure (JVP) may mislead the physician. A diuretic may be prescribed even when pulmonary oedema is not present. The resultant loss of water can lead to hypovolaemia and reduced perfusion of the tissues. We have to consider the heart to be functionally two separate pumps;[18,129] failure to do so can complicate the treatment of acute right heart failure.[54] The dramatic benefit that is sometimes seen following the infusion of glucose, insulin and K^+ solutions in cardiogenic shock could be due to the presence of some degree of right ventricular infarction and correction of the circulating blood volume.

When passing a Swan–Ganz catheter through the right atrium, the pressure measured from the midaxillary line may be found to be raised, but when the mean pulmonary capillary wedge pressure is measured it can be found to be low, the normal mean pressure being 8–12 mmHg.

As the pulmonary venous pressure rises as a result of left ventricular failure, the pulmonary arterioles constrict, the pulmonary resistance and pulmonary artery pressure rise and strain is placed upon the right ventricle. Both pulmonary and peripheral venous congestion can then occur together and some writers retain the term 'congestive cardiac failure' for this form of right heart failure.

Congestive Cardiac Failure

Congestive heart failure is a manifestation of underlying pathology of the myocardium or the lungs or both. It is a term used to describe a collection of signs and symptoms produced by a number of different conditions. Cardiac failure is caused by ischaemic changes of the myocardium, acute rheumatism, widespread respiratory disease producing pathological changes in the lung, hypertension of renal or other origin, thyrotoxicosis, arrhythmias, anaemia, especially of the megaloblastic type (see p. 366), congenital heart disease, arteriovenous aneurysm, Paget's disease of the bone, beri-beri, myxoedema, diphtheria, toxic myocarditis, infective myocarditis, collagen disease (polyarteritis nodosa, disseminated lupus erythematosus etc.), haemochromatosis, atrial myxoma or potassium depletion or excess.

As the heart fails and is unable to expel the blood it receives onwards around the systemic circulation, an increase in the pressure of the right atrium and the venous system occurs. This pressure is transmitted backwards along the venous system to the jugular veins, to the liver, and along the venules to the capillaries, thus Starling's equilibrium of fluid exchange into and out of the capillaries is upset, leading to the formation of oedema. Water is retained in the body because renal blood flow and the glomerular filtration rate (GFR) are reduced. As the central arterial pressure decreases the secretion of antidiuretic hormone (ADH) and aldosterone increases.

As cardiac failure develops there is a concomitant increase in left ventricular end-diastolic pressure and dilatation of the left ventricle. In a radiograph of the lungs taken in the upright position, diversion of blood to the upper lobes with consequent increased prominence and expansion of the upper lobe pulmonary veins can be observed.

The diversion or redistribution of blood to the upper lobes is due to the accumulation of fluid in the lower lobes under gravity (West et al., 1965).[173] The dilatation and engorgement of the pulmonary veins are due to increased pulmonary venous pressure leading to perivascular oedema.[87,105,121] The fluid collects largely in the interalveolar septal wall and the perivascular interstitial space. Before pulmonary oedema develops, blurring of the edges of the pulmonary vessels and short white lines can be seen perpendicular to and reaching the pleura, indicating the oedema-thickened inter-lobular septa which are not normally visible. These are Kerley's B lines (Fleming and Simon, 1958).[49]

Symptoms

The patient complains of a feeling of tiredness and lethargy and usually dyspnoea, especially on exercise, although this is less marked when the condition arises from right ventricular failure, as opposed to left ventricular failure. Sometimes the main complaint of the patient is swelling of the ankles. The raised venous pressure gives rise to congestion of the stomach which causes anorexia, nausea and vomiting. This leads to malnutrition and loss of weight and is one of the problems which affects long-term care. In a similar manner engorgement of the hepatic vessels gives rise to pain and discomfort under the right costal margin.

Although extreme lucidity is generally present, when untreated congestive cardiac failure has been present for some time, mental disorientation and bizarre behaviour often develop. The patient may become extremely childish, develop a puerile manner of talking, may continuously suck a finger or a lip or become aggressive and illustrate characteristics of paranoia.

Physical signs

Three classic physical signs of congestive cardiac failure are as follows.

1. Elevation of the central venous pressure (CVP).
2. Enlargement of the liver, associated with tenderness on palpation.
3. Oedema, which becomes manifest when the limb is held in a dependent position.

1. The raised central venous pressure (CVP) becomes apparent on examination of the jugular veins when the patient is placed in such a position that the thorax is at an angle of 45° to the horizontal. The jugular venous pulse, which decreases in height during deep inspiration and when the patient sits upright but increases when the pressure is applied over the liver (hepatojugular reflex), sometimes requires careful inspection and good illumination in order to be detected. When the venous pressure is extremely high, and especially if the patient is obese, venous pulsation may be detected only with difficulty and this can lead to an error in diagnosis and treatment.

2. Hepatic enlargement can be detected by laying the patient completely flat and feeling the edge of the liver below the costal margin as it moves up and down below the fingertips after the patient has been asked to breathe deeply in and out. There is also dullness to percussion over the liver area which extends down below the costal margin. In the presence of marked functional tricuspid incompetence, both enlargement and pulsation of the liver become prominent.

3. Oedema in congestive cardiac failure is characterized by pitting on pressure. Unfortunately, this is the least reliable of any of the physical signs, because it is produced by so many other factors such as renal disease, hypoproteinaemia, phlebothrombosis, allergic phenomena and capillary permeability produced by acute toxic infections. Other characteristics of congestive cardiac failure are as follows.

Breathlessness

Breathlessness, at first on exercise and later at rest, is a cardinal sign of left ventricular failure. It is therefore seen primarily in congestive cardiac failure when it is secondary to left ventricular failure. A history of nocturnal dyspnoea is usually indicative of left ventricular failure, although it can also occur when there is obstruction to the mitral valve orifice, at high altitudes and as a result of overhydration. Dyspnoea may be experienced by some patients with congestive failure in the absence of left ventricular failure when, for example, it is a feature of the primary lung disease. Breathing may become periodic when the cardiac failure is at an advanced stage. Cheyne[29] first described this form of respiration in 1818 and Stokes (1854) recognized that it was related to cardiac disease.[150] The rate and depth of respiration is irregular, the depth of respiration gradually increasing whereupon it ceases for 20–30 seconds, during which time the patient becomes cyanosed. It then begins again, at first slowly, then increasing both in rate and depth, whereupon the cyanosis disappears and then, after a period of hyper-ventilation, respiration ceases once again. This may be continued for minutes or for hours and in extreme cases, usually of a terminal nature, for days. It is well known that Cheyne–Stokes respiration occurs in conditions other than cardiac failure (e.g. lesions of the central nervous system such as meningitis, brain tumours, cerebral haemorrhage and thrombosis, narcotic poisoning with morphine or barbiturates etc., and in endocrine disorders such as myxoedema and Addisonian crisis).

Pleural effusions can develop and may be bilateral, contributing to the development of respiratory insufficiency. On auscultation, râles are frequently heard in the basal areas of the lungs.

Cyanosis

When the cardiac output falls, the amount of blood that is available for tissue perfusion is reduced, perhaps to the region of 1–1.5 litres/minute. The oxygen saturation of the blood in the arterial tree is normal, but because the amount of oxygen extracted by the tissues is greater, the venous oxygen saturation falls to approximately 45–50%. Contraction of the vessels in the periphery is a result of poor perfusion, and it is in these regions that cyanosis is most obvious. If gas exchange at alveolar levels is in any way impaired by pathological changes in the lungs, desaturation of the arterial blood is also present and the venous oxygen saturation falls still further. Increased tissue anoxia and the reduced oxygen tension in coronary blood then exacerbate the impairment of myocardial function.

Although marked peripheral cyanosis is produced by advanced mitral stenosis when the rise in left atrial pressure rises and pulmonary hypertension develops, the arterial oxygen saturation is normal. The peripheral cyanosis is a result of a markedly decreased cardiac output. When the left atrial pressure rises above 30 mmHg (i.e. above the oncotic pressure exerted by the plasma proteins) the onset of pulmonary oedema is an ever-present danger. The rise in pulmonary artery pressure is followed, after a period of time, by functional tricuspid incompetence and, when this has developed, dyspnoea becomes a less prominent feature of the condition.

Oliguria

A low cardiac output is always associated with retention of water. The reduced blood flow through the kidney leads to a reduced glomerular filtration rate (GFR) and the decreased filling of the arterial vascular tree causes an endocrine response similar to that of haemorrhagic shock. Secretion of anti-diuretic hormone (ADH) and aldosterone is increased. A urine of relatively high specific gravity which contains little sodium is therefore excreted. It invariably also contains traces of albumin, a few leucocytes and red cells and commonly granular and hyaline casts. The blood urea is frequently raised in congestive cardiac failure and in most cases does not rise above 13–20 mmol/l (80–120 mg%). In extremely severe cardiac failure, it may rise to the region of 58 mmol/l (350 mg%) or higher.

Jaundice

When there is a great increase in CVP and engorgement and enlargement of the liver is marked, jaundice develops. This is of the regurgitant or obstructive type and can be of a very severe degree, the plasma total bilirubin reaching 7 mg% or more. The urobilinogen content of the urine is increased and the urine darkens when allowed to stand exposed to the air. The tests for bile are positive and the froth, when the urine is shaken, is found to have a yellow tinge. Jaundice also results from the reabsorption of blood following pulmonary infarction and is, therefore, typical of a haemolytic jaundice rather than as a result of impaired hepatic excretion.

Pulmonary Oedema and Acute Left Ventricular Failure

Pulmonary oedema can arise from a number of different conditions. It is most commonly the result of left ventricular failure, but mitral valve obstruction (caused by mitral stenosis, a large left atrial thrombus, or a left atrial myxoma) will also produce the condition. This is because the pressure within the left atrium rises and is transmitted along the pulmonary veins so that the pressure with the lung capillaries exceeds the oncotic pressure of the plasma proteins.

Pulmonary oedema is produced following the rapid infusion of very hypertonic salt solutions, rapid blood transfusions, especially in the presence of primary myocardial insufficiency or a gross metabolic acidosis. It also occurs following exposure to irritant gases, at very high altitudes, and as a result of overhydration during the anuric phase of acute renal failure, and immediately following burns and trauma. This is particularly evident when there is present an added factor that lowers the blood pressure and misleads the clinician so that an excess of fluid is administered. An example of this (see p. 218) is a fractured skull causing neurogenic (normovolaemic) shock in the presence of earlier blood loss from other sites. A CVP measurement helps to avoid excessive infusion. Drowning (see p. 385) also gives rise to pulmonary oedema.

Pulmonary oedema is usually of dramatic, sudden onset, often appearing in an unpredictable manner, except for the fact that it quite commonly occurs in the early hours of the morning when the patient has been asleep for most of the night. It is often preceded by frequent attacks of nocturnal dyspnoea, orthopnoea and breathlessness on exertion. The patients are woken from sleep by extremely severe dyspnoea and feel as if they are about to die. Quite commonly coughing produces frothy sputum which may be tinged with blood. On auscultation, widespread coarse bubbling crepitations are heard all over the chest, and loud rhonchi are heard during inspiration and expiration. The expiratory rhonchi are the most marked and

give rise to the term 'cardiac asthma'. The blood pressure is commonly raised during an attack and in addition to the sounds of valvular disease a fourth sound (presystolic gallop rhythm) may be heard.

In those cases in which pulmonary oedema has not developed fully, the patient is severely dyspnoeic, sits up (i.e. on the edge of the bed), is peripherally cyanosed and greatly distressed but has few or no abnormal pulmonary sounds apart from a few scattered expiratory rhonchi. It is at this stage that misdiagnosis has been made because the condition has been ascribed either to bronchial asthma or to hysterical hyperventilation. When the attack has developed fully, cyanosis, as in bronchial asthma, is a major feature of the condition. Because the treatment of bronchial and cardiac asthma is so different, it is essential that a mistake should not be made in diagnosis and that, if there is any doubt whatsoever, a safe form of treatment applicable to both conditions should be used. Radiographs (Figs. 10.15–10.17) can assist in diagnosis. In bronchial asthma the blood pressure is not normally raised appreciably, signs

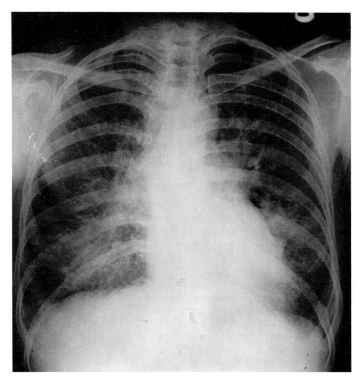

Fig. 10.15 Interstitial pulmonary oedema.

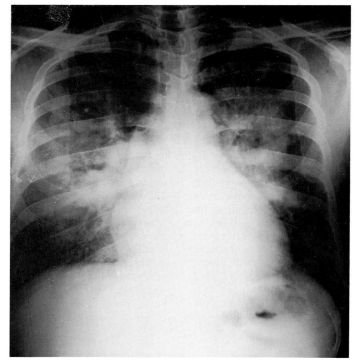

Fig. 10.16   Pulmonary oedema showing characteristic 'butterfly wing' pattern on X-ray of chest.

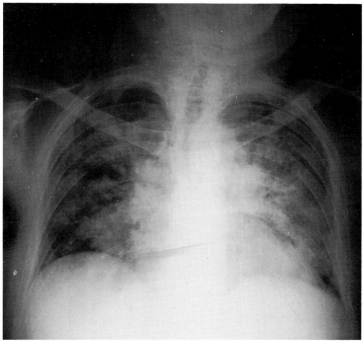

Fig. 10.17   Diffuse pulmonary oedema seen in a patient with left ventricular failure following coronary occlusion.

of myocardial pathology are usually completely absent and the loud bubbling crepitations which are dominant in cardiac asthma are not prominent on auscultation. The form of the breathlessness is also usually very different. The laboured breathing caused largely by obstruction during expiration is usually vastly different from the gross inspiratory and expiratory dyspnoea of cardiac asthma and, although descriptions of the two conditions may sound very much the same in practice, in most cases they are easily observed to be clinically separate entities. There is no doubt, however, that it is possible, especially at the onset of pulmonary oedema arising from myocardial insufficiency, that a misdiagnosis can be made. The greatest danger is that adrenaline (epinephrine) should be given when the correct diagnosis is cardiac asthma, since the irritability of the myocardium is increased, therefore increasing the chances of ventricular fibrillation and death. Whereas, in bronchial asthma, adrenaline (epinephrine) is often the treatment of choice.

Treatment of pulmonary oedema

The patient should be sat up in a chair or on the edge of the bed and be allowed to breathe in the position he finds most comfortable. Sometimes the patient prefers to stand rather than sit down so that blood tends to collect in the lower limbs. Morphine sulphate 15 mg should be injected immediately intramuscularly. Pethidine (meperidine, Demerol) 100 mg intramuscularly is an alternative treatment, but is usually not nearly as effective. Atropine sulphate 0.6 mg should be injected slowly intravenously. This immediate treatment relieves the anxiety and tension, depresses the respiratory centre so that active deep breathing can be maintained, while the anticholinergic drugs help to reduce the secretions of the bronchial mucosa and relieve the bronchial constriction. However, this degree of sedation can lead to severe respiratory depression and death. The clinician should be prepared to ventilate the patient artificially.

Oxygen should be administered by any means available as rapidly as possible with high flows of the gas through a mask or spectacles. Humidification of gas is unnecessary, and perhaps contraindicated, but it may be bubbled through with ethyl alcohol (Luisada, 1951)[94] as it is known that this agent prevents foaming and will help to dilate the bronchial tree and, although absorbed only in small quantities, may assist in sedation. If a rapid tachycardia is present and if there is any suggestion of myocardial insufficiency, atropine sulphate should be given intramuscularly. If the patient is capable of swallowing, sodium amytal 180 mg should be given by mouth, and if not by deep intramuscular injection. Theophylline-ethylenediamine 0.25–1 g should be given slowly intravenously and repeated after 20 minutes if no effect is discernible. This substance sometimes has a dramatically beneficial effect upon the dyspnoea.

When digitalization is indicated and the patient has not received digitalis preparations previously, it should in most cases be performed rapidly. The most rapid digitalization may be obtained with ouabain (Strophanthin-G) given intravenously in doses of 0.5 mg. Digoxin in a dosage of 0.5–1 mg is almost equally effective.

In most cases the patient's condition improves following administration of 100% O_2, by mask or endotracheal intubation, combined with diuretic therapy (see p. 367).[11]

It is important to reduce the volume of blood in pulmonary circulation. In addition to placing the patient in the semi-upright position, the 'bloodless venesection' can be tried in the first instance. This entails placing blood pressure cuffs around all four limbs and expanding the cuffs at a pressure which is midway between the systolic and diastolic pressures so that venous return is impeded. They are released in turn at intervals of 10–15 minutes for 2 or 3 minutes each time. When frequent recordings of blood pressure are being made, one cuff on each arm can be released alternately. If the patient does not respond to these measures, a unit of blood must be removed from the circulation. A large-bore needle is inserted into the vein in the antecubital fossa, the blood pressure cuff expanded so that it is midway between systolic and diastolic pressures, and blood is allowed to flow rapidly into a container so that its volume can be measured. In the adult between 500 and 800 ml can be removed with safety.

A rapidly acting diuretic, preferably ethacrynic acid 50–75 mg i.v. or frusemide (Lasix) 100–200 mg i.v. should be given. If these are not available, bumetanide (2 mg) should be given by deep intramuscular injection or i.v. and if necessary repeated after 20 min. It is important that mersalyl or any other diuretic should not be injected into an oedematous thigh where absorption is slow and its action delayed.

In the grossly hypertensive patient the blood pressure may be lowered by the subcutaneous or intramuscular injection of pentolinium (Ansolysen) 2–5 mg. An alternative method of treatment is hexamethonium bromide (Vegolysen) given intravenously in doses of 1 mg separated by at least

1 minute. Either substance enhances the pooling of blood in the lower limbs and therefore reduces the volume of blood in the pulmonary circulation.

Pressure and massage applied to the carotid sinus have been advocated in patients with hypertension or coronary artery disease and are said to relieve acute pulmonary oedema in about 80% of those patients who are suffering from these conditions (Lown and Levine, 1961).[93] The pressure and massage produce a bradycardia and hypotension.

The following case illustrates the ease with which even a small blood transfusion may produce pulmonary oedema when myocardial insufficiency is present.

Case history. A 30-year-old woman in her 32nd week of pregnancy had been attending an antenatal clinic for some weeks and was found to have a persistently low haemoglobin concentration which did not respond to oral treatment with iron compounds. She was admitted to hospital and given bed-rest, and because her haemoglobin was so dangerously low (29%), it was decided to transfuse her with whole blood. One unit (540 ml) was given over a period of 5 hours, after which a second unit was begun at the same rate. When only a small volume of this had been transfused it was observed that she had become dyspnoeic, which developed markedly over the next 5 minutes. A nurse considered this to be a transfusion reaction and fortunately stopped the drip immediately. When observed at this time the patient was cyanosed, restless, anxious and grossly dyspnoeic. She was put in the sitting position on the side of the bed and sphygmomanometer cuffs were applied to all four limbs and inflated midway between her systolic and diastolic pressures. Atropine 0.6 mg was given intravenously. Morphine sulphate 15 mg was also given—half intravenously and half intramuscularly. Theophylline-ethylenediamine (Aminophylline) 0.5 g was also given intravenously and repeated 5 minutes later when no obvious effect was produced.

After a few minutes it was apparent that these measures were ineffective and the condition was getting worse. The patient voiced the opinion that she was about to die. A widebore needle with tubing attached and a bowl were available for venesection. The needle was inserted into the medial basilic vein and the blood pressure cuff on the upper arm maintained just below the systolic pressure. A unit of blood was removed within a few minutes and improvement in respiration followed immediately. Within a very short space of time the adventitious sounds within the lungs disappeared, the tachycardia subsided and the jugular venous pressure (JVP) returned to normal. Although slow digitalization was begun, no diuretic was given.

This episode killed the fetus and spontaneous recovery from the macrocytic anaemia occurred, many primitive cells being found in the bloodstream 2 days later. The blood haemoglobin concentration rose rapidly and no further treatment was necessary.

It should be noted that at 32 weeks of pregnancy the cardiac output is raised to its maximum level and begins to decline after this period. Also the presence of a macrocytic anaemia gives rise to fatty infiltration of the heart ('tabby cat heart') so that myocardial failure can occur spontaneously. The dangers of blood transfusion in this condition when treatment with folic acid is inadequate are well illustrated. Although every precaution was taken to give the blood slowly, it would have been advisable to have transfused the blood together with a rapidly acting diuretic such as ethacrynic acid[88] or frusemide (Lasix) now that these preparations are available. Even if packed cells had been transfused, left ventricular failure may have developed. There seems little doubt that if prompt and active medical treatment had not been available immediately the patient would have died.

Treatment of cardiac failure

Because chronic cardiac failure produces such great alterations in fluid and electrolyte balance, this aspect of the condition is reviewed in Chapter 2.

Bed-rest and sedation

In the early stages of congestive cardiac failure complete bed-rest is essential, although this may be relaxed a little as treatment takes effect so that the patient may sit out of bed for an increasing length of time and later take moderate exercise. The measures outlined in 'long-term care' (see p. 436) must be maintained. Sedation is essential in order to relieve anxiety and, when dyspnoea is present, morphine sulphate 15 mg or heroin 10 mg should be given. A useful preparation for long-term sedation is hydroxyzine HCl (Atarax) in doses of 25 mg b.d., t.d.s. or q.d.s. and this may be combined with morphine if necessary. In the elderly, heroin is a safer drug to use or alternatively the dose of morphine sulphate should be reduced to 10 mg or pethidine 50 mg should be given intramuscularly.

Digitalis

Ouabain

The digitalizing dose is 0.25–0.75 mg. Ouabain is unsuitable for *maintaining* digitalization, but it acts more rapidly than other preparations when given intravenously.

Digoxin

The digitalizing dose is 0.75–1 mg, the maintenance dose is 0.25–0.75 mg daily. In most adults 0.25 mg b.d. is sufficient to maintain digitalization, but some patients will require 0.25 mg t.d.s. once or twice a week. By this means gross digitalis intoxication can be avoided and adequate quantities for therapeutic purposes administered.

When digitalizing infants, tablets containing 0.0625 mg per tablet and an elixir containing 0.05 mg/ml are available for intramuscular and intravenous route. The ampoules available for adult use are suitable for infants; it must be remembered, however, that intramuscular digoxin is painful and in the shocked adult as well as in the child rapid digitalization is performed in the kindest manner when it is given intravenously through a plastic tube inserted into the vein or a Gourd needle. The area for the site of insertion is infiltrated with 2% procaine, using a small 'diabetic' needle.

Infants are digitalized with digoxin 0.1 mg/lb (0.1 mg/500 g) body weight every 4–6 hours until digitalization is complete. The maintenance dosage is 0.01 mg/lb (0.01 mg/500 g) body weight daily in divided doses.

Digitoxin is almost completely absorbed from the gut, but is less rapid in its digitalizing effects when given intravenously. It tends to cause less vomiting in sensitive people and its maintenance dose is 0.05–0.2 mg per day. Lanatoside C (Cedilanid) is similarly of value when vomiting which is not the result of digitalis toxicity becomes a problem. The digitalizing dose of Cedilanid is 6–8 mg and the maintenance dose 0.5–2.5 mg.

Diuretics

There are a number of diuretics that work well and produce an almost immediate response even when the glomerular filtration rate (GFR) is low. The earliest of these diuretics were ethacrynic acid (Edecrin) and frusemide (Lasix) and these are still being used. Ethacrynic acid is particularly useful in children with fluid retention following open-heart surgery. For example, 25 mg given intravenously to a 10-year-old child who has interstitial pulmonary oedema and a low arterial PO_2 has a most dramatic effect upon the arterial PO_2 and the appearance of the chest X-ray. Ethacrynic acid can be given intravenously in doses of 25–75 mg and in obese patients weighing more than 75 kg it can be given in doses of 100 mg i.v.

Frusemide (Lasix) can be given in doses of 50–100 mg i.v., but when these doses are ineffective as much as 400 mg i.v. can be administered with safety. It can be used as a test for the presence of acute renal failure.

Bumetanide (Burinex) produces a diuresis within a few minutes following its administration. It is given in doses of 1–2 mg i.v., and these doses can be repeated after 20 minutes.

When an immediate response is not required, the diuretic can be given orally. Chlorothiazide was one of the early effective diuretics and is still being used in many parts of the world. It is given in doses of 0.5–1 g orally followed by a further dose of 0.5–1 g 4 hours later.

Hydrochlorothiazide is given in doses of 25–100 mg orally, according to the severity of the fluid retention. Bumetanide is given orally in doses of 1–5 mg/day.

An increase in urine $[K^+]$ occurs with chlorothiazide even in the presence of a normal plasma $[Na^+]$, so that K^+ depletion is more likely to occur with this group of drugs. It is, therefore, of the greatest importance that, in order to avoid digitalis intoxication, oral K^+ replacement in the form of KCl 4–6 g/day in divided doses should be given every day, whether a diuretic is administered or not. Indeed, it is preferable to administer KCl on those days on which the diuretic is not given because most, if not all, of the administered K^+ is lost when a diuretic is given at the same time.

Aldosterone antagonists such as spironolactone (Aldactone) 25–50 mg q.d.s., triamterene (Dytac) 50 mg t.d.s. or q.d.s. and amiloride (Midamor) 5 mg b.d. may be used in conjunction with diuretics. In patients resistant to diuretics the combination of, for example, spironolactone 25–50 mg and triamterene 50 mg can be given, but great care has to be taken that K^+ retention does not occur, even when only one of these diuretics is used. The dangers from hyperkalaemia and sudden death from this cause cannot be overstressed. Spironolactone particularly may give rise to painful nipples and gynaecomastia in the male and to gout. All diuretics can cause raised uric acid and glucose levels.

Prednisone (Deltacortone, Decortisyl, Di-Adreson) 5–30 mg/day and triamcinolone (Adcortyl, Aristocort, Ledercort) 4–16 mg/day have low salt-retaining properties and may assist diuretic therapy in producing an improved diuresis in resistant cases.

The diuretics of the 'thiazide group' alone may raise the blood uric acid level giving rise to gout, and may also cause a latent state of diabetes mellitus to become manifest or may exacerbate the condition when it already is established.

Vasodilator therapy

Vasodilator agents can be a useful adjunctive form of therapy in the management of both acute and chronic heart failure. The possible benefit of vasodilator therapy was recognized more than 30 years ago,[21,75,130] but since the 1960s studies have demonstrated a marked improvement in haemodynamic function and cardiac index with acute and chronic cardiac failure.[51,59,60,61,155] Vasodilator therapy was found to be of benefit in severe mitral regurgitation.[28]

A number of factors contribute to the benefits observed, but the therapy is based largely upon reduction of afterload that is commonly increased in the failing heart.

Substances that act as arteriolar dilators increase cardiac output by reducing peripheral vascular resistance. Such substances are hydralazine and minoxidil. Hydralazine (Apresoline) is given orally in doses of 25–50 mg or by slow intravenous injection of 20 mg. When given by infusion it is diluted in 0.9% saline or 5% sorbitol solution.

Minoxidil (Loniten) is given orally in doses of 2.5–5 mg. Severe hypotension can occur with both if given in excessive doses. Nifedipine (Adalat), salbutamol (Ventolin) and pirbuterol (Exirel) appear to have similar haemodynamic effects.

Nitrates, in addition to producing coronary, cerebral and other vascular dilatation, act mainly by redistributing the blood volume by venodilatation, producing a fall in the pulmonary venous pressure, a fall in pulmonary capillary wedge pressure and right atrial pressure. Nitrates may be given by tablet sublingually, topically using a cream containing, for example, 2% glyceryl trinitrate which is rubbed on the skin, or intravenously. An oral spray containing a metered dose of 0.4 mg of glyceryl trinitrate to be sprayed into the mouth is now available (Nitrolingual). A large oral dose of isosorbide trinitrate (100 mg) is reported to increase the cardiac output of patients suffering from severe cardiac failure.[114]

Vasodilators that produce both a fall in arteriolar constriction and an increase in venous pooling are captopril, nitroprusside, phentolamine, trimazosin and prazosin.

These substances, to a varying extent and for a varying period of time when given in a single dose, reduce the pulmonary artery, capillary wedge and right atrial pressures, while increasing cardiac output. The systemic arterial blood pressure tends to fall, sometimes precipitously, as the peripheral vascular resistance decreases.

Sodium nitroprusside is diluted 50 mg in 500 or 1000 ml of 5% dextrose and infused at a rate which produces the desired effect. This is usually in the region of 0.5–1.5 μg/kg body weight per minute. An infusion rate of 60–70 μg/minute is usually effective in the adult, although much faster rates, 700 or 800 μg/minute, are required when treating a hypertensive crisis and the lower dilution is then desirable.

Captopril is an angiotensin II antagonist and is probably the most promising of the vasodilator agents, especially for long-term use. The haemodynamic effects of a single oral dose of 25 mg last for 6–8 hours,[27] and only relatively small doses are required, little haemodynamic improvement from larger doses having been found.[2] Enalapril can also be used.

Prazosin HCl (Hypovase, Minipress) is a postsynaptic β-receptor blocking agent. It produces a significant increase in cardiac output and decreases pulmonary venous pressure, but may cause a precipitous fall in arterial blood pressure associated with the first dose.

There is, however, no indication that vasodilator therapy is superior to conventional treatment, either for acute or chronic cardiac failure. Many deaths occurring in the acute stage following vasodilator treatment alone are not reported, and conventional treatment might well have been better, but uncontrolled studies to date do not present a powerful indication for their general use. In individual cases, however, there is no doubt about the haemodynamic improvement that results from their administration, especially when conventional treatment alone has not resulted in a satisfactory degree of improvement.

Water intake and diet

Because water retention occurs in congestive cardiac failure it should be restricted, especially in the early stages, to the minimum required for metabolic purposes and comfort. When the patients become attuned to water restriction they are usually able to plan their daily water intake unconsciously so that they are unaware of doing so. This is usually a much kinder form of control than rigid salt restriction, which in itself has pathological consequences.

Although a restriction of sodium intake has its place in the treatment of cardiac failure in its early stages, it is inevitable that a patient placed on a low-salt diet and also given diuretics will become sodium depleted, and when this occurs the diuretics fail to act. It is by no means an uncommon picture to see a bedfast patient with gross oedema on a salt-restricted diet, a plasma sodium in the region of 125 mmol/l (mEq/l), and resistant to all forms of diuretic therapy. Only salt replacement and water restriction offer any hope for this type of patient, for if this state of affairs is not corrected, the prognosis is poor and operative mortality is high. Large doses of frusemide (e.g. 400 mg) or bumetanide may be used, when a large diuresis is considered to be advisable. Care must be taken to note that an abrupt depletion of sodium as well as potassium may follow in these circumstances. This is more likely to occur when a patient is on a sodium-restricted diet. Intravenous theophylline-ethylenediamine (aminophylline, Cardophylin, Ethophyllin) 0.5–1.0 g will enhance the effect of diuretics on occasions. Ethacrynic acid and frusemide commonly result in a diuresis when other diuretics have failed to act.

Venous engorgement of the stomach itself leads to anorexia and even the obese patient, in whom it is advisable that weight loss should take place, reverts to a state of chronic malnutrition and anaemia if recovery from congestive cardiac failure is prolonged. A salt-free diet contributes to this state of affairs and in the author's opinion, in many cases, shortens rather than extends the life of the majority of patients. The fact that in the grossly oedematous patient the total body sodium is raised above normal values when the plasma sodium is low, is only a further indication of the failure of existing forms of therapy. It means that a disproportion between total body water and extra-cellular $[Na^+]$ has been allowed to develop.

In the already anorexic patient specialized diets containing large quantities of protein, such as Casilan and Complan, are often not acceptable and it is essential that food should be made palatable by means of sauces etc. An easily available form of concentrated nourishment is in evaporated milk in which the fat is homogenized and, therefore, easily absorbed by the gut, and the protein concentration is high. When this is mixed with fruit juices or added liberally to canned fruit, both the calorie requirements and the essential fat and amino acid requirements are largely satisfied.

References

1. Adams, R. (1827). Cases of diseases of the heart, accompanied with pathological observations. *Dublin Hosp. Rep.*, **4**, 353.

2. Ader, R., Chatterjee, K., Ports, T., Brundage, B., Hiramatsu, B. and Parmley, W. (1980). Immediate and sustained hemodynamic and clinical improvement in chronic heart failure by an oral angiotensin converting enzyme inhibitor. *Circulation*, **61**, 931.

3. Alstrup, P. and Pederson, S. A. (1973). A case of syncope on swallowing secondary to diffuse oesophageal spasm. *Acta. med. Scand.*, **193**, 365.

4. Ashman, R. and Hull, E. (1937). *Essentials of electrocardiography for the student and practitioner of medicine.* New York: MacMillan.

5. Bayley, R. H., LaDue, J. S. and York, D. J. (1944). Electrocardiographic changes (local ventricular ischemia and injury) produced in the dog by temporary occlusion of a coronary artery, showing a new stage in the evolution of myocardial infarction. *Amer. Heart J.*, **27**, 164.

6. Befeler, B. (1975). The hemodynamic effects of Norpace. *Angiology*, **26 (part II)**, 99.

7. Befeler, B., Castellanos, A., Wells, D. E., Vagueiro, M. C. and Yeh, B. K. (1975). Electrophysiologic effects of the antiarrhythmic agent disopyramide phosphate. *Amer. J. Cardiol.*, **35**, 282.

8. Benfey, B. G. and Varma, D. R. (1966). Anti-sympathomimetic and sympathomimetic drugs. Propranolol and phentolamine on atrial refractory and contractility. *Brit. J. Pharm.*, **26**, 3.

9. Bett, I. H. N. (1968). Hypotension after oral propranolol. *Lancet*, **i**, 302.

10. Bexton, R. S. and Camm, A. J. (1982). Drugs with class III antiarrhythmic action. *Pharmacol. & Therapeutics*, **17**, 315.

11. Bhatia, M. L., Singh, I., Machanda, S. C., Khanna, P. K. and Ray, S. B. (1969). Effect of frusemide on pulmonary blood volume. *Brit. med. J.*, **2**, 551.

12. Bigger, J. T. Jr., Bassett, A. L. and Hoffman, B. F. (1968). Electrophysiological effects of diphenylhydantoin on canine Purkinje fibers. *Circ. Res.*, **22**, 221.

13. Bigger, J. T. Jr. and Jaffe, C. C. (1971). The effect of bretylium tosylate on the electrophysiologic properties of ventricular muscle and Purkinje fibers. *Amer. J.*

Cardiol., **27**, 82.

14. Bigger, J. T. Jr. and Mandel, W. J. (1970). Effect of lidocaine on the electrophysiological properties of the ventricular muscle and Purkinje fibers. *J. Clin. Invest.*, **49**, 63.

15. Boulos, G. and Brooks, D. K. (1986). In preparation.

16. Boura, A. L. A. and Green, A. F. (1959). The actions of bretylium: adrenergic neurone blocking and other effects, *Brit. J. Pharmacol.*, **14**, 536.

17. Boura, A. L. and Green, A. F. (1965). Adrenergic neurone blocking agents. *Ann. Rev. Pharmacol.*, **5**, 183.

18. Bradley, R. (1976). *Studies in Acute Heart Failure*, p. 1. London: Edward Arnold.

19. Britton, B. J., Finch, D. R. A., Gill, P. G., Kettlewell, M.G. W. and Morris, P. J. (1977). Low-dose heparin. *Lancet*, **ii**, 604.

20. Brooks, D. K. (1964). Osmolar, electrolyte and respiratory changes in hemorrhagic shock. *Amer. Heart J.*, **68**, 574.

21. Burch, G. E. (1956). Evidence for increased venous tone in chronic congestive heart failure. *Arch. Int. Med.*, **98**, 750.

22. Burdine, J. A. and Wallace, J. M. (1965). Pulsus paradoxus and Kussmaul's sign in massive pulmonary embolism. *Amer. J. Cardiol.*, **15**, 413.

23. Burrows, G. D., Vohra, J., Hunt, D., Sloman, J. C., Scoggins, B. A. and Davies B. (1976). Cardiac effects of different tricyclic antidepressant drugs. *Brit. J. Psychiatry.*, **129**, 335.

24. Butler, V. P. and Chen, J. P. (1967). Digoxin-specific antibodies. *Proc. Natl. Acad. Sci.*, **57**, 71.

25. Cardinal, R. and Sasyniuk, B. I. (1978). Electro-physiological effects of bretylium tosylate on subendo-cardial Purkinje fibers from infarcted canine hearts. *J. Pharmacol. Exp. Therap.*, **204**, 159.

26. Castellanos, A. and Lemberg, L. (1971). Diagnosis of isolated and combined blocks in the bundle branches and the divisions of the left branch. *Circulation*, **43**, 971.

27. Chatterjee, K. and Parmley, W. W. (1983). Vasodilator therapy for acute myocardial infarction and chronic congestive heart failure. *J. Amer. Col. Cardiol.*, **1**, 133.

28. Chatterjee, K., Parmley, W. W. and Swan, H. J. C. (1973). Beneficial effects of vasodilator agents in severe mitral regurgitation due to subvalvular apparatus. *Circulation*, **48**, 684.

29. Cheyne, J. (1818). A case of apoplexy in which the fleshy part of the heart was converted into fat. *Dublin Hosp. Rep.*, **2**, 216.

30. Compton, D., Hill, P. Mc. N. and Sinclair, J. D. (1973). Weight-lifter's blackout. *Lancet*, **ii**, 1234.

31. Contorni, L. (1960). Il circolo collaterale vertebro-vertebrale nella obliterazione dell arteria suclavia alla suaorigine. *Minerva Chir.*, **15**, 268.

32. Cooley, D. A. (1980). Private communication.

33. Coull, D. C., Crooks, J., Dingwall-Fordyce, I., Scott, A. M. and Weir, R. D. (1970). Amitriptyline and cardiac disease. *Lancet*, **ii**, 590.

34. Davis, L. D. and Temte, J. V. (1968). Effects of propranolol on the transmembrane potentials of ventricular muscle and Purkinje fibers of the dog. *Circ. Res.*, **22**, 661.

35. Denham, M. J., James, G. and Farran, M. (1973). The value of 125I fibrinogen in the diagnosis of deep vein thrombosis in hemiplegia. *Age & Ageing*, **2**, 207.

36. De Sanctis, R. W., Block, R. and Hutter, A. M. (1972). Tachyarrhythmias in myocardial infarction. *Circulation*, **45**, 682.

37. Dhingra, R. C., Denes, P., Wu, D., Chuquimia, R., Amat-y-Leon, F., Wyndham, C. and Rosen, K. M. (1974). Syncope in patients with chronic bifascicular block; significance, causative mechanisms and clinical implications. *Ann. Int. Med.*, **81**, 302.

38. Dhurandhar, R. W., Teasdale, S. J. and Mahon, W. A. (1971). Bretylium tosylate in the management of refractory ventricular fibrillation. *Canad. med. Assoc. J.*, **105**, 161.

39. Doherty, J. E., Perkins, W. N. and Flanigan, W. J. (1967). The distribution and concentration of tritiated digoxin in human tissue. *Amer. J. Int. Med.*, **66**, 116.

40. Dollery, C. T., Emslie-Smith, D. and McMichael, J. (1960). Bretylium tosylate in the treatment of hyper-tension. *Lancet*, **i**, 296.

41. Dollery, C. T., Emslie-Smith, D. and McMichael, J. (1960). Bretylium tosylate in the treatment of hyper-tension. *Lancet*, **ii**, 261.

42. Dreifus, L. S., Watanabe, Y., Haiat, R. and Kimbiris, D. (1971). Atrioventricular block. *Amer. J. Cardiol.*, **28**, 371.

43. Dreifus, L. S. (1975). Electrophysiology of Norpace. *Angiology*, **26**, 111.

44. Dreifus, L. S., Filip, Z., Sexton, L. and Watanabe, Y. (1973). Electrophysiological and clinical effects of a new antiarrhythmic agent: Disopyramide (Abst). *Amer. J. Cardiol.*, **31**, 129.

45. Dreifus, L. S., de Azevedo, I. M. and Watanabe, Y. (1974). Electrolyte and antiarrhythmic drug interaction. *Amer. Heart J.*, **88**, 95.

46. Eastcott, H. H. H. G., Pickering, G. W. and Robb, C. G. (1954). Reconstruction of internal carotid artery in patients with intermittent attacks of hemiplegia. *Lancet*, **ii**, 994.

47. Engel, H. J., Hundeshagen, H. and Lichtlen, P. (1977). Transmural myocardial infarction in young women taking oral contraceptives. Evidence of reduced regional coronary flow in spite of normal coronary arteries. *Brit. Heart J.*, **39**, 477.

48. First, S. R., Bayley, R. H. and Bedford, D. R. (1950). Peri-infarction block: electrocardiographic abnormality occasionally resembling bundle branch block and local ventricular block of other types. *Circulation*, **2**, 31.

49. Fleming, P. R. and Simon, M. (1958). The hemo-

dynamic significance of intrapulmonary septal lymphatic lines (Lines B of Kerley). *Fact. Radiol. J.*, **9**, 33.

50. Fogoros, R. N. (1984). Amiodarone-induced refractoriness to cardioversion. *Ann. Int. Med.*, **100**, 699.

51. Franciosa, J. B., Guiha, N. M., Limas, C. J., Rodriguera, E. and Cohn, J. N. (1972). Improved left ventricular function during nitroprusside infusion in acute myocardial infarction. *Lancet*, **i**, 650.

52. Gable, A. J. (1965). Paroxysmal ventricular fibrillation with spontaneous reversion to sinus rhythm. *Brit. Heart J.*, **27**, 62.

53. Gallagher, J. J., Pritchett, E. L. C., Benditt, D. G. and Wallace, A. G. (1977). High dose disopyramide phosphate: an effective treatment for refractory ventricular tachycardia (Abstr.). *Circulation*, **55, 56** (Suppl. III), 225.

54. George, R. J. D. and Bihari, D. (1982). Acute right heart failure complicated by hypovolaemia. *Brit. med. J.*, **284**, 1159.

55. Gilmore, J. P. and Siegel, J. H. (1962). Mechanism of the myocardial effects of bretylium. *Circ. Res.*, **10**, 347.

56. Gokhale, S. D. and Gulati, O. D. (1961). Potentiation of inhibitory and excitatory effects of catecholamines by bretylium. *Brit. J. Pharmacol.*, **16**, 327.

57. Gokhale, S. D., Gulati, O. D. and Kelkar, V. V. (1963). Mechanism of the initial adrenergic effects of bretylium and guanethidine. *Brit. J. Pharmacol.*, **20**, 362.

58. Goodman, D. J., Rosen, R. M., Cannon, D. S., Rider, A. K. and Harrison, D. C. (1975). Effect of digoxin on atrioventricular conduction: studies in patients with and without autonomic innervation. *Circulation*, **51**, 251.

59. Gould, L., Zahir, M. and Ettinger, S. (1969). Phentolamine and cardiovascular performance. *Brit. Heart J.*, **31**, 154.

60. Gould, L., Zahir, M., Shariff, M. and Giuliani, N. (1970). Phentolamine: use in congestive heart failure. *Jpn. Heart J.*, **11**, 17.

61. Gould, L., Zahir, M., Shariff, M. and Giuliani, N. (1970). Phentolamine: use in pulmonary edema. *Jpn. Heart J.*, **11**, 141.

62. Grant, R. P. (1956). Left axis deviation: an electrocardiographic-pathologic correlation study. *Circulation*, **14**, 233.

63. Grant, R. P. (1958). Left axis deviation. *Mod. Concepts. Cardiovasc. Dis.*, **27**, 437.

64. Grant, R. P. (1959). Peri-infarction block. *Prog. Cardiovasc. Dis.*, **2**, 237.

65. Greenspan, K., Steinberg, M., Holland, D. and Freeman, A. R. (1974). Electrophysiologic alterations in cardiac dysrhythmias: antiarrhythmic effects of aprinidine. *Amer. J. Cardiol.*, **33**, 140.

66. Guyer, P. B. (1964). Stokes–Adams attacks precipitated by hypokalaemia. *Brit. med. J.*, **2**, 427.

67. Haldane, J. H. (1969). Micturition syncope: two case reports and a review of the literature. *Canad. med. Assoc. J.*, **101**, 712.

68. Handley, A. J. (1972). Low-dose heparin after myocardial infarction. *Lancet*, **ii**, 623.

69. Hoffman, B. F. (1958). Action of quinidine and procainamide on single fibers of dog ventricle and specialized conducting system. *An. Acad. Bras. Cienc.*, **29**, 365.

70. Hoffman, B. F. and Bigger, J. T. (1971). Antiarrhythmic drugs. In *Drills Pharmacology in Medicine*, 4th edn. p. 824. Edited by J. R. DiPalma. New York: McGraw-Hill.

71. Hulting, J. and Jansson, B. (1977). Antiarrhythmic and electrocardiographic effects of single oral doses of disopyramide. *Eur. J. Clin. Pharmacol.*, **ii**, 91.

72. Hulting, J. and Rosenhamer, G. (1976). Antiarrhythmic and hemodynamic effects of intravenous and oral disopyramide in patients with ventricular arrhythmia. *J. Int. Med. Res.*, **4** (Suppl. 1), 90.

73. Hurst, J. W., Paulk, E. A., Proctor, H. D. and Schlant, R. C. (1964). Management of patients with atrial fibrillation. *Amer. J. Med.*, **37**, 728.

74. Josephson, M. E., Caracta, A. R., Lau, S. H., Gallagher, J. J. and Damato, A. N. (1973). Electrophysiological evaluation of disopyramide in man. *Amer. Heart J.*, **86**, 771.

75. Judson, W. E., Hollander, W. and Wilkins, R. W. (1956). The effects of intravenous Apresoline (hydralazine) and cardiovascular and renal function in patients with and without congestive heart failure. *Circulation*, **13**, 664.

76. Karim, A. (1975). The pharmacokinetics of Norpace. *Angiology*, **26** (Suppl. 1), 8.

77. Katz, L. N. (1946). *Electrocardiography*, 2nd edn. Philadelphia: Lea and Febiger.

78. King, R. M., Zipes, D. P., deNicoll, B. and Linderman, J. (1974). Suppression of ouabain-induced ventricular ectopy with verapamil and reversal with calcium. *Amer. J. Cardiol.*, **33**, 166.

79. Kinlen, L. J. (1973). Incidence and presentation of myocardial infarction in an English community. *Brit. Heart J.*, **35**, 616.

80. Kirpekar, S. M. and Furchgott, R. F. (1964). The sympathomimetic action of bretylium on isolated atria and aortic smooth muscle. *J. Pharmacol. Exp. Therap.*, **143**, 64.

81. Kochar, M. S. and Itskovitz, H. D. (1978). Treatment of idiopathic orthostatic hypotension (Shy-Drager Syndrome) with indomethacin. *Lancet*, **i**, 1011.

82. Kounis, N. G. (1979). Iatrogenic 'torsade de pointes' ventricular tachycardia. *Postgrad. med. J.*, **55**, 832.

83. Krikler, D. M. and Curry, P. V. L. (1976). Torsade de pointes, an atypical ventricular tachycardia. *Brit. Heart J.*, **38**, 117.

84. Kubasik, W. P., Brody, B. B. and Barold, J. J. (1975). Problems of measurement of serum digoxin by commercially available radioimmunoassay kits. *Amer. J. Cardiol.*, **36**, 975.

85. Kus, T. and Sasyniuk, B. I. (1975). Electrophysiological actions of disopyramide phosphate on canine ventricular muscle and Purkinje fibers. *Circ. Res.*, **37**, 844.

86. Küssmaul, A. (1873). Über schwielige Mediastino-Pericarditis und den paradoxen Puls. *Berl. Klin. Wchnschr*, **10**, 433, 445, 461.

87. Lavender, J. P. and Doppman, J. (1962). The hilum in pulmonary venous hypertension. *Brit. J. Radiol.*, **35**, 303.

88. Ledingham, J. G. (1964). Ethacrynic acid parenterally in the treatment and prevention of pulmonary oedema. *Lancet*, **i**, 952.

89. Leveque, P. E. (1965). Antiarrhythmic action of bretylium. *Nature*, **207**, 203.

90. Levin, B. and Posner, J. B. (1972). Swallow syncope. Report of a case and review of the literature. *Neurology*, **22**, 1086.

91. Lichstein, E. and Chadda, K. D. (1972). Atrioventricular block produced by swallowing, with documentation by His bundle recordings. *Amer. J. Cardiol.*, **29**, 561.

92. Lipman, B. S., Massie, E. and Kleiger, R. E. (1972). *Clinical Scalar Electrocardiography*, 6th edn. Chicago: Year Book Medical Publisher.

93. Lown, B. and Levine, S. A. (1961). The carotid sinus. Clinical value of its stimulation. *Circulation*, **23**, 766.

94. Luisada, A. A. (1951). The mechanism and treatment of pulmonary edema. *Illinois Med. J.*, **100**, 254.

95. Luomanmake, K., Heikkila, J. and Hartel, G. (1975). Bretylium tosylate. Adverse effects in acute myocardial infarction. *Arch. Int. Med.*, **135**, 515.

96. Manolas, E. G., Hunt, D., Dowling, J. T., Luxton, M., Vohra, J. K. and Sloman, G. (1979). Collapse after oral disopyramide. *Brit. med. J.*, **2**, 1553.

97. Marchlinski, F. E., Gansler, T. S., Waxman, H. L. and Josephson, M. E. (1982). Amiodarone pulmonary toxicity. *Ann. Int. Med.*, **97**, 839.

98. Marcus, F. I., Fontaine, G. H., Frank, R. and Grosgogeat, Y. (1981). Clinical pharmacology and therapeutic applications of the antiarrhythmic agent, amiodarone. *Amer. Heart J.*, **101**, 480.

99. Marrott, P. K., Ruttley, M. S. T., Winterbottam, J. T. and Muir, J. R. (1976). A study of the acute electrophysiological cardiovascular action of disopyramide in man. *Eur. J. Cardiol.*, **4**, 303.

100. McCarthy, S. T., Robertson, D., Turner, J. J. and Hawkey, C. J. (1977). Low-dose heparin as a prophylaxis against deep-vein thrombosis after acute stroke. *Lancet*, **ii**, 800.

101. McComb, J. M., Logan, K. R., Khan, M. M., Geddes, J. S. and Adgey, A. A. J. (1980). Amiodarone-induced ventricular fibrillation. *Eur. J. Cardiol.*, **11**, 381.

102. McGinn, S. and White, P. D. (1935). Acute cor pulmonale resulting from pulmonary embolism. *J. Amer. med. Assoc.*, **104**, 1473.

103. Millar, J. S. and Vaughan Williams, E. M. (1981). Anion antagonism—a fifth class of antiarrhythmic action? *Lancet*, **i**, 1291.

104. Miller, G. A. and Sutton, G. C. (1970). Acute massive pulmonary embolism. Clinical and haemodynamic findings in 23 patients studied by cardiac catheterization and pulmonary arteriography. *Brit. Heart. J.*, **32**, 518.

105. Milne, E. N. C. (1973). Correlation of physiologic findings with chest roentgenology. *Radiol. Clin. N. Am.*, **11**, 17.

106. Mobitz, W. (1924). Über die unvollständige Störung der Erregungsuberleitung wischen Vorhof und Kammer des menschlichen Herzens. *Z. Ges. Exp. Med.*, **41**, 180.

107. Moir, D. C., Crooks, J., Cornwell, W. B., O'Malley, K., Dingwall-Fordyce, I. and Turnbull, M. J. (1972). Cardiotoxicity of amitriptyline. *Lancet*, **ii**, 561.

108. Moll, A. and Lutterotti, M. (1951). Die beurteilung des 'diskrepaztypus der R-Zacke' (rt. SII, SIII-Bild des Ekg). *Z. Kreislaufforsch*, **40**, 737.

109. Morris, G. K. and Mitchell, J. R. A. (1976). Warfarin sodium in prevention of deep venous thrombosis and pulmonary embolism in patients with fractured neck of femur. *Lancet*, **ii**, 869.

110. Moysey, J. O., Jaggarao, N. S. V., Grundy, E. W. and Chamberlain, D. A. (1981). Amiodarone increases plasma digoxin concentrations. *Brit. med. J.*, **282**, 272.

111. Multi-Centre International Study (1975). Improvement in prognosis of myocardial infarction by long term beta-adrenoreceptor blockade using practolol. *Brit. med. J.*, **III**, 735.

112. New England Journal of Medicine (1961). A new vascular syndrome 'the subclavian steal'. *N. Engl. J. of Med.*, **265**, 912.

113. New York Heart Association (1969). *Diseases of the Heart and Blood Vessels: Nomenclature and Criteria for Diagnosis*. New York: Little, Brown & Co.

114. Packer, M., Meller, J., Medina, N., Gorlin, R. and Herman, N. (1979). Equivalent hemodynamic effects of intravenous nitroprusside and high oral doses of oral isosorbide dinitrate in severe heart failure. *Circulation*, **59,60** (Suppl. II), 182.

115. Pamintuan, J. C., Dreifus, L. S. and Watanabe, Y. (1970). Comparative mechanisms of antiarrhythmic agents. *Amer. J. Cardiol.*, **26**, 512.

116. Proudfit, W. L. and Forteza, M. E. (1959). Micturition syncope. *N. Engl. J. of Med.*, **260**, 328.

117. Pryor, R. and Blount, S. G. (1966). The clinical significance of true left axis deviation. Left intraventricular blocks. *Amer. Heart J.*, **72**, 391.

118. Rango, R. E., Warnica, W., Ogilvie, R. I., Kreeft, J. and Bridger, E. (1976). Correlation of disopyramide pharmacokinetics with efficacy in ventricular tachyarrhythmia. *J. Int. Med. Res.*, **4**, (Suppl. 1), 54.

119. Ranney, R. E., Dean, R. R., Karim, A. and Radzialowski, F. M. (1975). Disopyramide phosphate: pharmacokinetic and pharmacologic relationships of a new antiarrhythmic agent. *Arch. Int. Pharmacodyn.*

Ter., **191**, 162.

120. Reivich, M., Holling, H. E., Roberts, B. and Toole, J. F. (1961). Reversal of blood flow through the vertebral artery and its effects on cerebral circulation. *N. Engl. J. of Med.*, **265**, 878.

121. Rigler, L. G. and Surprenant, E. E. (1967). Pulmonary edema. *Seminars on Roentgenol.*, **2**, 1.

122. Rob, C. and Kenyon, J. R. (1960). Dissecting aneurysms. *Brit. med. J.*, **1**, 1384.

123. Rosen, K. M. (1973). Junctional tachycardia. Mechanisms, differential diagnosis and management. *Circulation*, **47**, 654.

124. Rosenbaum, M. B. (1968). Types of right bundle branch block and their clinical significance. *J. Electrocardiology*, **1**, 221.

125. Rosenbaum, M. B. (1969). Intraventricular trifascicular blocks. Review of literature and classification. *Amer. Heart J.*, **78**, 450.

126. Rothfeld, E. L. and Voorman, D. M. (1975). The ailing A–V junction. *Heart and Lung*, **4**, 909.

127. Rowlands, D. J., Howitt, G. and Markman, P. (1965). Propranolol (Inderal) in disturbances of cardiac rhythm. *Brit. med. J.*, **1**, 891.

128. Ryan, M. J., Temtw, J. and Lown, B. (1974). Evaluation of a new antiarrhythmic agent, disopyramide phosphate. (Abst). *Circulation*, **49, 50** (Suppl. 1), 79.

129. Sarnoff, S. J. and Berglund, E. (1954). Starling's law of the heart studied by means of simultaneous right and left ventricular function curves in the dog. *Circulation*, **9**, 706.

130. Sarnoff, S. J. and Farr, H. W. (1944). Spinal anesthesia in the therapy of pulmonary edema: a preliminary report. *Anesthesiology*, **5**, 1.

131. Sbarbaro, J. A., Rawling, D. A. and Fozzard, H. A. (1979). Suppression of ventricular arrhythmias with intravenous disopyramide and lidocaine: efficacy comparison in a randomized trial. *Amer. J. Cardiol.*, **44**, 513.

132. Schamroth, L. (1980). *The Disorders of Cardiac Rhythm*. Vol. 1. p. 107. London: Blackwell Scientific Publications.

133. Schamroth, L., Kriker, D. M. and Garrett, C. (1972). Immediate effects of intravenous verapamil in cardiac arrhythmias. *Brit. med. J.*, **224**, 73.

134. Schneider, J. F., Tomas, H. E., Kreger, B. E., McNamara, P. M. and Kannel, W. B. (1979). Newly acquired left bundle-branch block: The Framingham Study. *Ann. Int. Med.*, **90**, 303.

135. Schoenberg, B. S., Kuglitch, J. F. and Karnes, W. E. (1974). Micturition syncope—not a single entity. *J. Amer. med. Assoc.*, **229**, 1631.

136. Selzer, A. and Wray, H. W. (1964). Quinidine syncope. Paroxysmal ventricular fibrillation occurring during treatment of chronic atrial arrhythmias. *Circulation*, **30**, 17.

137. Sevitt, S. and Gallagher, N. G. (1959). Prevention of venous thrombosis and pulmonary embolism in injured patients. *Lancet*, **ii**, 981.

138. Sharnoff, J. G., Kass, H. H. and Mistica, B. A. (1962). A plan of heparinization of the surgical patient to prevent postoperative thromboembolism. *Surg. Gynecol. Obstet.*, **115**, 75.

139. Sharpey-Schafer, E. P. (1953). The mechanism of syncope after coughing. *Brit. Heart J.*, **2**, 860.

140. Shy, G. M. and Drager, G. A. (1960). A neurological syndrome associated with orthostatic hypotension: a clinico-pathologic study. *Arch. Neurol.*, **2**, 511.

141. Singh, B. N. and Vaughan Williams, E. M. (1970). The effect of amiodarone, a new anti-anginal drug, on cardiac muscle. *Brit. J. Pharmacol.*, **39**, 657.

142. Smith, T. W., Butler, V. P. and Haber, E. (1969). Determination of therapeutic and toxic serum digoxin concentrations by radioimmunoassay. *N. Engl. J. of Med.*, **281**, 1212.

143. Smith, T. W. and Haber, E. (1970). Digoxin intoxication: the relationship of clinical presentation to serum digoxin concentration. *J. Clin. Invest.*, **49**, 2377.

144. Smith, T. W. and Haber, E. (1973). Clinical value of radioimmunoassay of the digitalis glycoside. *Pharmacol. Rev.*, **25**, 219.

145. Sodi-Pallares, D., Bisteni, A., Medrano, G. A. and Ayola, C. (1960). *Electrocardiography and vectorcardiography, clinical cardiopulmonary physiology*. New York: Grune & Stratton.

146. Sodi-Pallares, D., Medrano, G. A., Bisteni, A. and Ponce de leon, J. J. (1970). *Deductive and polyparametric electrocardiography*. Mexico: Instituto Nacional de Cardiologia de Mexico. (Translated by Carlos R. Macossay, MD, Houston, Texas and Marvin Dunn, MD, Kansas City, Kansas.)

147. Sodi-Pallares, D. and Rodriguez, M. I. (1952). Morphology of the unipolar leads recorded at the septal surfaces: its application to the diagnosis of left bundle branch block complicated by myocardial infarction. *Amer. Heart J.*, **43**, 27.

148. Solokow, M. and Lyon, T. P. (1949). The ventricular complex in right ventricular hypertrophy as obtained by unipolar precordial and limb leads. *Amer. Heart J.*, **38**, 273.

149. Stokes, W. (1846). Observations on some cases of permanently slow pulse. *Dublin Quart. J. Med. Sci.*, **2**, 73.

150. Stokes, W. (1854). *The Disease of the Heart and the Aorta*. p. 320. Dublin: Hodges and Smith.

151. Strasberg, B., Arditti, A., Sclarovsky, S., Lewin, R. F., Buimovici, B. and Agmon, J. (1985). Efficacy of intravenous amiodarone in the management of paroxysmal or new atrial fibrillation with fast ventricular response. *Int. J. Cardiol.*, **7**, 47.

152. Sutton, G. C., Honey, M. and Gibson, R. V. (1969). Clinical diagnosis of acute massive pulmonary embolism. *Lancet*, **i**, 271.

153. Tartini, R., Kappenberger, L., Steinbrunn, W. and

Meyer, U. A. (1982). Dangerous interaction between amiodarone and quinidine. *Lancet*, **i**, 1327.

154. Taylor, S. H., Saxton, C., Davies, P. S. and Stoker, J. B. (1970). Bretylium tosylate in prevention of cardiac dysrhythmias after myocardial infarction. *Brit. Heart J.*, **32**, 326.

155. Taylor, S. H., Sutherland, G. R., MacKenzie, G. J., Staunton, H. P. and Donald, K. W. (1965). The circulatory effects of intravenous phentolamine in man. *Circulation*, **31**, 741.

156. Thorstrand, C. (1974). Cardiovascular effects of poisoning with tricyclic antidepressants. *Acta. med. Scand.*, **195**, 505.

157. Tomlinson, I. W. and Fox, K. M. (1975). Carcinoma of the oesophagus with 'swallow syncope'. *Brit. med. J.*, **II**, 315.

158. Van Durme, J. P., Bogaert, M. G. and Rosseel, M. T. (1974). Effectiveness of aprindine, procainamide and quinidine in chronic ventricular dysrhythmias. *Circulation*, **50**, 111.

159. Vaughan Williams, E. M. (1970). Classification of antiarrhythmic drugs. In: Symposium on cardiac arrhythmias, p. 499. Edited by E. Sandøe, E. Flensted-Jensen and K. H. Olsen. Södertälje, Sweden, A. B.: Astra.

160. Vaughan Williams, E. M. (1980). *Antiarrhythmic Action*. London: Academic Press.

161. Vismara, L. A., DeMaria, A. M., Miller, R. R., Amsterdam, E. A. and Mason, D. T. (1975). Effects of intravenous disopyramide phosphate on cardiac function and peripheral circulation in ischemic heart disease *Clin. Res.*, **23**, (Abstr). 87A.

162. Vismara, L. A., Mason, D. T. and Amsterdam, E. A. (1974). Disopyramide phosphate: clinical efficacy of a new oral antiarrhythmic drug. *Clin. Pharmacol. Therap.*, **16**, 330.

163. Vismara, L. A., Vera, Z., Miller, R. R. and Mason, D. T. (1977). Efficacy of disopyramide phosphate in the treatment of refractory ventricular tachycardia. *Amer. J. Cardiol.*, **39**, 1027.

164. Ward, D. E., Camm, A. J. and Spurrell, R. A. J. (1980). Clinical antiarrhythmic effects of amiodarone in patients with resistant paroxysmal tachycardias. *Brit. Heart J.*, **44**, 91.

165. Ward, J. W. (1976). The pharmacokinetics of disopyramide following myocardial infarction with special reference to oral and intravenous dose regimens. *J. Int. Med. Res.*, **4**, (Suppl. 1), 49.

166. Warlow, C., Ogston, D. and Douglas, A. S. (1972). Venous thrombosis following strokes. *Lancet*, **i**, 1305.

167. Warlow, C., Terry, G., Kenmure, A. C. F., Beattie, A. G., Ogston, D. and Douglas, A. S. (1973). A double-blind trial of low doses of subcutaneous heparin in the prevention of deep-vein thrombosis after myocardial infarction. *Lancet*, **ii**, 934.

168. Watanabe, Y. and Dreifus, L. S. (1977). *Cardiac arrhythmias: Electrophysiologic basis for clinical interpretation*. p. 4. New York: Grune & Stratton.

169. Waxler, E. B. (1971). Myocardial infarction and oral contraceptive agents. *Amer. J. Cardiol.*, **28**, 96.

170. Waxman, M. B. and Wallace, A. G. (1972). Electrophysiologic effects of bretylium tosylate on the heart. *J. Pharmacol. Exp. Therap.*, **183**, 264.

171. Wellens, H. J. J., Lie, K. I., Bär, F. W., Wesdorp, J. C., Dohmen, H. J., Düren, D. R. and Durrer, D. (1976). Effect of amiodarone in the Wolff–Parkinson–White syndrome. *Amer. J. Cardiol.*, **38**, 189.

172. Wenckebach, K. F. (1899). Sur analyse des unregelmässigen pulses. *Z. Klin. Med.*, **37**, 475.

173. West, J. B., Dollery, C. T. and Heard, B. E. (1965). Increased pulmonary vascular resistance in the dependent zone of the isolated dog lung caused by perivascular edema. *Circ. Res.*, **17**, 191.

174. Winkle, R. A., Mason, J. W., Griffin, J. C. and Ross, D. (1981). Malignant ventricular tachyarrhythmias associated with the use of encainide. *Amer. Heart J.*, **102**, 857.

175. Wit, A. L. and Cranefield, P. F. (1974). Verapamil inhibition of the slow response: a mechanism for its effectiveness against reentrant AV nodal tachycardia. *Circulation*, **50**, 146.

176. Wit, A. L., Steiner, C. and Damato, A. N. (1970). Electrophysiologic effects of bretylium tosylate on single fibers of the canine specialized conducting system and ventricle. *J. Pharmacol. Exp. Therap.*, **173**, 344.

177. Yeh, B. K., Sung, P. and Scheriag, B. J. (1973). Effects of disopyramide on electrophysiological and mechanical properties of the heart. *J. Pharm. Sci.*, **62**, 1924.

178. Zipes, D. P., Nobel, R. J., Carmichael, R. T., Rowell, H. and Fasola, A. F. (1975). Relations between aprindine concentration (APR) heart rate, ischemia, and ventricular fibrillation (VF) in dogs. *Amer. J. Cardiol.*, **35**, 179.

Further Reading

For Further Reading see page 379.

BETA-BLOCKERS AND THE AUTONOMIC NERVOUS SYSTEM

The autonomic system controls the involuntary and autonomic functions of numerous circulatory, metabolic and physiological aspects of the body. It can be divided into:

(a) the sympathetic system or, more correctly, the sympathoadrenal system; and
(b) the parasympathetic nervous system.

Sympathetic System
(alpha- and beta-adrenoreceptors)

The concept of the sympathetic system with adrenoreceptors was originated by Langley (1905–1906)[18] when investigating the action of curare on skeletal muscle. In 1906 Dale[11] applied the concept to the understanding of the action of ergot on the 'sympathetic myoneural junction', which he said could be called 'the receptor mechanism for adrenaline'.

In his classic paper in 1948, Ahlquist[3] divided the receptors as follows.

1. *Alpha-adrenoreceptors* which are associated with most excitatory functions, vasoconstriction, stimulation of the uterus, the nictitating membrane in animals, the ureter and dilator pupillae, and one important non-excitatory function, intestinal relaxation.

2. *Beta-adrenoreceptors* which are associated with most inhibitory functions, vasodilatation, relaxation of uterine and bronchial musculature, and one important excitor function, that of myocardial contraction. Probably the most important influence on recent day-to-day medication has been the inhibition of beta-autonomic receptor stimulation of myocardial contraction, together with the control of cardiac rhythms, via the beta-receptor sites.

Alpha-receptor distribution

The alpha receptors tend to be located in readily definable localized areas and are found predominantly, but not exclusively, in blood vessels, mainly in the arterioles. The areas most heavily supplied with alpha-receptors are the kidneys, splanchnic area and the skin. Innervation is supplied from the postganglionic fibres of the sympathetic nervous system. They respond to the sympathetic stimulating substances such as adrenaline (epinephrine) and noradrenaline (norepinephrine) and give rise to vasoconstriction.

This is quite different from the *beta-receptors* which are widely distributed throughout the body and produce a large number of different physiological effects. It is clear, however, that inhibition of some beta-receptors will enhance the action of the alpha-receptors, as the latter are left free to act without opposition.

Also, although *all* the alpha-receptors are innervated, only some beta-adrenoreceptors are innervated. This is particularly true of the heart and this fact has proved to be of fundamental importance in therapy.

Beta-1- and beta-2-adrenoreceptors

The pharmacological action of some substances appears to be more pronounced on the receptor sites of certain tissues than on others. This led Lands *et al.* (1967)[17] to the concept that more than one type of beta-receptor was present, and this view was later reinforced by Collier and Dornhurst (1969).[8] Beta-receptors can therefore be divided into two groups:

beta-1-receptors—present in heart and adipose tissue;
beta-2-receptors—present in the smooth muscle of the bronchi, arterioles, intestine, kidney and liver.

These receptor sites of the sympathoadrenal system cannot be identified by histological means, but only by their response to pharmacological stimuli. The subdivision of adrenergic receptor sites has great merit, especially with regard to therapy and elucidating the pathophysiology of acute conditions. Practolol (Eraldin), for example (now withdrawn from routine use), appears to have beta-blocking activity which is virtually confined to adipose tissue and the heart.

Sympathetic stimulation of the heart

Sympathetic stimulation of the heart is therefore produced by two main pathways, 'direct' and 'indirect'.

1. *Direct.*

(a) Beta-receptors in the atria are stimulated by sympathetic postganglionic nerve fibres. These receptors mediate an increase of the heart rate and they are therefore called *chronotrophic* receptors.

(b) Beta-receptors in the ventricles mediate an increase of the speed and force of myocardial contraction and are called *inotropic* receptors.

2. *Indirect*. Preganglionic sympathetic nerves supplying the adrenal medulla cause the release of catecholamines which stimulate both the alpha- and beta-receptors whether innervated or not.

Drugs may have a positive or negative effect with regard to chronotropism or inotropism.

Circulatory responses to infused catecholamines

We can now look at the response of the body when catecholamines are infused intravenously. The chemical neurotransmitter at all postganglionic sympathetic nerve endings is noradrenaline.[25] When noradrenaline is infused, both *alpha*- and *beta*-receptors are stimulated. However, the alpha-receptors are predominantly affected and this results in an elevation of the blood pressure due to vasoconstriction and reflex slowing of the heart. Noradrenaline appears to have little effect on the non-innervated beta-receptors.

When adrenaline is infused, it is the beta-receptors that are largely stimulated. Both the heart rate and the force of ventricular contraction are increased, and the diastolic pressure is reduced due to the dilatation of the peripheral arterioles. The vasodilator activity of adrenaline predominates over its minor vasoconstrictor action on the alpha-receptors, although alpha-receptor activity can be demonstrated to be present if a beta-receptor blocking drug is given prior to the infusion of adrenaline. When the synthetic vasopressor isoprenaline (isoproterenol, Suscardia) is infused, it can be demonstrated that, quite uniquely, only the beta-receptors, whether innervated or not, are stimulated. The beta-agonistic effect of isoprenaline is shared with other substances.

Beta-adrenoreceptor antagonists (beta-blockers)

Those chemical substances that have the property of preventing or reducing the stimulation of the beta-adrenoreceptors by catecholamines are referred to as 'beta-blockers'. These substances do not appear to modify the release of catecholamines from either the adrenal medulla or the sympathetic nerve endings. They appear to act at the beta-receptor sites and only relatively small concentrations of the drug are required. Their action is dose related so that if an increase in catecholamine

excretion occurs, the action of the catecholamine predominates over the beta-blocking activity of the substance. In addition, the effect is reversible, and withdrawal of the drug rapidly leads to a reduction in beta-blocking activity.

In addition to their beta-blocking activity, this group of substances has additional pharmacological properties. These properties vary from one preparation to another and are related to the chemical structure of the drug. The drugs available for clinical use are increasing at a rapid rate and some of these are listed in Table 10.3.

Table 10.3   Beta-blockers

Generic (or approved) name	Trade name	Oral dose (mg)
Acebutolol	Sectral	100–400
Alprenolol	Aptin	40–320
Atenolol	Tenormin	50–400
Labetalol	Trandate	300–2400
Metoprolol	Lopressor	50–400
Oxprenolol	Trasicor	40–320
Orciprenaline	Alupent	20–80
Pindolol	Visken	5–30
Practolol	Eraldin	*
Propranolol	Inderal	40–320
Timolol	Blocadren	15–50

*The oral form of practolol has been withdrawn; this drug is only given intravenously.

Obstructive lung disease

Because of the effects of these drugs on the beta-2-receptors located in the bronchi, constriction of the bronchioles may occur in patients suffering from asthma and chronic obstructive lung disease. It would appear that the cardioselectivity of the beta-blocking preparations may be of little benefit with regard to the initiation of increased airway resistance in view of the fact that oxprenolol (Trasicor) has been demonstrated to produce a reduction in the forced expiratory volume following both oral[6] and intravenous[7] administration.

Disturbances of glucose metabolism

As we have seen, the metabolism of glucose and its initiation by the autonomic nervous system are complicated and, in health, the beta-receptor activity plays only a relatively small part. However, when the glucagon stores in the liver are reduced, as in patients suffering from diabetic ketosis and in juvenile diabetics, so that the mobilization of glucose from glycogen is limited, blocking of the beta-2-receptors may precipitate hypoglycaemia (Kotler, 1966).[16] Although in uncomplicated diabetes the use of substances such as propranolol (Inderal), which block beta-1- and beta-2-receptors, may not in practice affect the overall control of the patient,[4] there is accumulating evidence that it is preferable to use preparations which selectively block only the beta-1-receptors when treating cardiac conditions. All beta-receptor blocking agents, especially propranolol, should be used with caution in the labile diabetic who has frequent hypoglycaemic attacks, and it has been noted that because of the exacerbation of this condition, the patient may pass rapidly into coma without warning and without developing the adrenergic symptoms and signs which normally precede the onset of hypoglycaemia.[1] There is some evidence[12] that atenolol (Tenormin), which is selectively a beta-1-inhibitor, is preferred for use in diabetics.

Phaeochromocytoma

The only indication for a beta-blocking agent (e.g. propranolol) in this disease would be the presence of a cardiac arrhythmia to a marked degree. Propranolol causes vasoconstriction because it opposes the vasodilating effects of adrenaline. The degree of hypertension is therefore increased. The hypertensive effect of the beta-blocker is more marked when the tumour is primarily adrenaline (epinephrine) secreting. However, because beta-1-receptors of the heart are also blocked, it has a beneficial effect in reducing the tachyarrhythmia caused by the catecholamines secreted by the phaeochromocytoma. However, beta-blockers should never be used in this condition without concomitantly using an alpha-receptor blocking drug such as phentolamine (Rogitine).[10,21]

During surgery phentolamine has to be given in large doses because handling the gland before all the veins have been ligated causes severe hypertension. Repeated intravenous injections of 40–50 mg of phentolamine may be required even after preoperative treatment.

Labetalol (Trandate) induces beta- and alpha-adrenergic blockade with rapid onset. Theoretically, it is therefore an ideal agent for the pretreatment of phaeochromocytoma. There have been a number of reports of its use in this condition.[2,5,15,23] It is given intravenously in doses of 50 mg over a period of 1 minute.

Membrane-stabilizing activity

This is sometimes referred to as the quinidine effect when it applies to the heart. It has the ability of stabilizing phase 4 of the action potential (see p. 301). It also has the ability of slowing the rate of rise of the action potential and increases the refractory period of the myocardial muscle, after depolarization. It is this fact that formerly contributed to the finding by the Multicentre International Study reported in the *British Medical Journal* in 1975[19] which demonstrated that in 3038 patients there was a marked fall in the death rate due to myocardial infarction. This trial had to be abandoned because the investigators used practolol which was shown during the study to cause the serious oculocutaneous and peritoneal reactions that were noted during the period of study. The long-term prophylactic antiarrhythmic effects of beta-blockers in patients with angina pectoris and hypertension have also been reported.[9,13,14,22,24] Since that time an extensive study has been performed in Norway with timolol (Blocadren). This has demonstrated clearly the protective effects associated with a lowered mortality following myocardial infarction.

Selectivity

Because the beta-blocking activity has different effects at different beta-receptor sites, preparations are now available which have actions which are specifically beneficial in readily definable conditions. For example, because propranolol has an agonist effect on beta-2-receptors, it has to be used with caution when given to patients suffering from asthma.

Contraindications

It is a matter of clinical judgement whether to withhold beta-blockers under specific medical circumstances. For example, for a diabetic patient with generalized vascular disease who is having numerous cardiac arrhythmias following aorto-coronary bypass, when only propranolol is available, by keeping the dose to the minimum amount and stopping treatment as soon as possible success can be achieved. Care must be taken that the vasoconstrictor (beta-2) effect does not precipitate gangrene, for example in the feet.

Surgery

Because beta-blockers change the responses to stress in general, it may be necessary to withdraw the drug 24 hours before elective surgery is performed. However, when a dysrhythmia is seriously threatened, complete withdrawal of the drug may be impracticable, and a reduction in dose, for example by half, may then be indicated. Careful ECG monitoring should be maintained in the postoperative period.

During emergency surgery a severe bradycardia may develop and this is sometimes associated with bradycardic shock, especially when certain anaesthetic agents (e.g. cyclopropane and trichlorethylene) are used.

Reversal of the bradycardia can be achieved either by the infusion of isoprenaline (isoproterenol Isuprel, Saventrine) or the administration of atropine 1–2 mg intravenously.

Alcoholism

Because of the hypoglycaemic action of alcohol, the administration of beta-blocking agents to chronic alcoholics should be carried out cautiously, and intravenous injection of beta-blockers should be performed in a critical care area where intravenous glucose is readily available. This is important because hypoglycaemia may be produced in the non-alcoholic after taking alcohol in association with sugar-containing diluents.[20]

References

Beta-blockers

1. Abramson, E. A. and Arky, R. A. (1968). Role of beta-adrenergic receptors in counterregulation to insulin-induced hypoglycemia. *Diabetes*, **17**, 141.
2. Agabiti Rosei, E., Brown, J. J., Lever, A. F. and Robertson, A. S. (1976). Treatment of phaeochromocytoma and of clonidine withdrawal hypertension with labetalol. *Brit. J. clin. Pharmacol.*, **3**, Suppl. 3, 809.
3. Ahlquist, R. P. (1948). A study of adrenotropic receptors. *Amer. J. Physiol.*, **153**, 586.
4. Allison, S. P., Chamberlain, N. J., Miller, J. E., Ferguson, R., Gillett, A. P., Bemand, E. V. and Saunders, R. A. (1969). Effects of propranolol on blood sugar, insulin and free fatty acids. *Diabetologia*, **5**, 339.
5. Bailey, R. R. (1979). Labetalol in the treatment of a patient with phaeochromocytoma: a case report. *Brit. J. clin. Pharmacol.*, **8**, Suppl. 2, 141.
6. Beumer, H. M. and Hardonk, H. J. (1972). Effects of beta-adrenergic blocking drugs on ventilatory function in asthmatics. *Eur. J. clin. Pharmacol.*, **5**, 77.
7. Chatterjee, S. S., Perks, W. H., Decalmer, P., Sterling, G. M., Cruickshank, J. M., Croxson, R. S. and Benseon, M. K. (1976). Cardioselective and non-cardioselective beta-blockers in obstructive airways disease.
8. Collier, J. G. and Dornhurst, A. C. (1969). Beta-receptors—different for respiratory stimulation and bronchodilatation. *Nature*, **223**, 1283.
9. Coltart, D. J., Gibson, D. G. and Shand, D. G. (1971). Plasma propranolol levels associated with suppression of ventricular ectopic beats. *Brit. med. J.*, **1**, 490.
10. Cooperman, L. H., Engelman, K. and Mann, P. E. G. (1967). Anesthetic management of pheochromocytoma employing halothane and beta-adrenergic blockade. *Anesthesiology*, **28**, 575.
11. Dale, H. D. (1906). On some physiological actions of ergot. *J. Physiol.*, **34**, 163.
12. Deacon, S. P. and Barnett, D. (1976). Comparison of atenolol and propranolol during insulin-induced hypoglycaemia. *Brit. med. J.*, **II**, 272.
13. Fitzgerald, J. D. (1975). Beta blocking drugs as anti-arrhythmic agents. *Int. J. clin. Pharmacol.*, **II**, 235.
14. Jewitt, D. E. and Singh, B. N. (1974). The role of beta-adrenergic blockade in myocardial infarction. *Prog. cardiovasc. Dis.*, **16**, 421.
15. Kaufman, L. (1979). Use of labetalol during hypotensive anaesthesia and in the management of phaeochromocytoma. *Brit. J. clin. Pharmacol.*, **8**, Suppl. 2, 229.
16. Kotler, M. N., Berman, L. and Rubenstein, A. H. (1966). Hypoglycaemia precipitated by propranolol. *Lancet*, **ii**, 1389.
17. Lands, A. M., Arnold, A., McAnliff, J. P., Luduena, F. P. and Brown, J. G. (1967). Differentiation of receptor systems activated by sympathomimetic amines. *Nature*, **214**, 597.
18. Langley, J. N. (1906). Croonian Lecture, 1906. On nerve endings and on special excitable substances in cells. *Proc. Roy. Soc. Lond.*, **LXXVII**, 170.
19. Multicentre International Study. (1975). Improvement in prognosis of myocardial infarction by long-term beta-adrenoreceptor blockade using practolol. *Brit. med. J.*, **III**, 735.
20. O'Keefe, S. J. D. and Marks, V. (1977). Lunchtime gin and tonic: a cause of reactive hypoglycaemia. *Lancet*, **i**, 1286.
21. Ross, E. J., Pritchard, B. N. C., Kaufman, L.,

Robertson, A. I. G. and Harries, B. J. (1967). Preoperative and operative management of patients with phaeochromocytoma. *Brit. med. J.*, **I**, 191.

22. Schamroth, L. (1966). Immediate effects of intravenous propranolol on various cardiac arrhythmias. *Amer. J. Cardiol.*, **18**, 438.

23. Stewart, P. A. (1982). Adrenal phaeochromocytoma in familial neurofibromatosis with initial control of hypertension by labetalol. *J. Roy. Soc. Med.*, **75**, 276.

24. Stock, J. P. P. (1966). Beta-adrenergic blocking drugs in the clinical management of cardiac arrhythmias. *Amer. J. Cardiol.*, **18**, 444.

25. Von Eular, U. S. (1947). Investigation on nature of substance liberated during stimulation of sympathetic nervous system. *Nordisk Medicin.*, **33**, 629.

Further Reading

Anonymous. (1986). Recurrent ventricular tachycardia: adverse drug reaction. *Brit. med. J.*, **292**, 50.

Bigger, J. T. (Editor) (1984). Symposium on flecainide acetate. *Amer. J. Cardiol.*, **53**, No. 5.

Braunwald, E. (Editor) (1984). *Heart Disease. A Textbook of Cardiovascular Medicine.* 2nd edition. Philadelphia, W. B. Saunders.

Caron, F. J., Libersa, C. C., Kher, A. R., Kacet, S., Wanszelbaum, H., Dupuis, B. A., Poirier, J-M. and Lekieffre, J. P. (1985). Comparative study of ecainide and disopyramide in chronic ventricular arrhythmias. A double-blind placebo-controlled crossover study. *J. of Amer. Coll. of Cardiol.*, **5**, 1457.

Escoubet, B., Coumel, P., Poirier, J. M., Maison-Blanche, P., Jaillon, P., Leclercq, J. F., Menasche, P., Cheymol, G., Piwnica, A., Lagier, G. and Slama, R. (1985). Suppression of arrhythmias within hours after a single oral dose of amiodarone and relation to plasma and myocardial concentrations. *Amer. J. Cardiol.*, **55**, 696.

Gray, R. I., Bateman, T. M., Czer, L. S. C., Conklin, C. M. and Matloff, J. M. (1985). Esmolol: A new ultrashort-acting beta adrenergic blocking agent for rapid control of heart rate in postoperative supraventricular tachyarrythmias. *J. of Amer. Coll. of Cardiol.*, **5**, 1451.

Hampton, J. R. (Editor) (1985). *Cardiovascular Disease.* London: William Heinemann.

Krikler, D. M. (1985). The Foxglove, 'The Old Woman from Shropshire' and William Withering. *J. Amer. Coll. Cardiol.*, **5**, no. 5, 3A.

McKenna, W. J., Oakley, C. M., Krikler, D. M. and Goodwin, J. F. (1985). Improved survival with amiodarone in patients with hypertrophic cardiomyopathy and ventricular tachycardia. *Br. Heart J.*, **53**, 412.

Chapter 11
Ventricular Fibrillation and Cardiac Arrest

Sudden Death

When ventricular fibrillation occurs the contractions of the myocardium are ineffective. There is no co-ordinated movement between one part of the myocardium and another. In appearance the heart is blue, flaccid and flattened. Superficially, it has fine or coarse serpiginous, writhing or twitching movements superimposed upon a fine fibrillar tremor. The heart is no more effective functionally than when there is no contraction of the myocardium at all and is said to be asystolic. The term 'cardiac arrest' is applied to it because the normal pumping action of the organ is absent, but some authors prefer to retain this term for asystole. It is possible, however, to obtain a normal electrocardiogram (ECG) from an asystolic heart and this has been observed frequently after open-heart surgery, both in man and animals. During ventricular fibrillation the output of the heart (and therefore the blood pressure) falls virtually to zero and the pulses become impalpable. The subject has the appearance of death, the pupils dilate and the skin has a greyish-yellow colour.

The electrocardiogram (ECG) reveals an uncoordinated series of irregular waves. These may be rapid or slow and may vary in voltage (Fig. 11.1). An electroencephalogram (EEG) tracing shows a straight line (an isoelectric trace). This occurs on all occasions when the flow of blood to the brain is stopped, for example it is produced when 'inflow occlusion' is applied to the right ventricle by means of tapes placed around the superior and inferior venae cavae for the purpose of operating upon the pulmonary valve. Reducing the body temperature does not alter the production of an isoelectric EEG tracing.

The moment ventricular fibrillation occurs respiration also ceases and may not start again when a normal rhythm has been restored. Anoxia, therefore, becomes apparent immediately and a normal cardiac action cannot be established unless the lungs are artificially ventilated.

Causes of ventricular fibrillation

Anoxia
The normal rate of oxygen consumption for the whole body of the adult is in the region of 250–300 ml/minute but if the rest of the body consumed

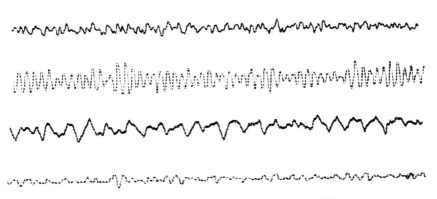

Fig. 11.1 Different patterns of ventricular fibrillation seen on the electrocardiogram (ECG).

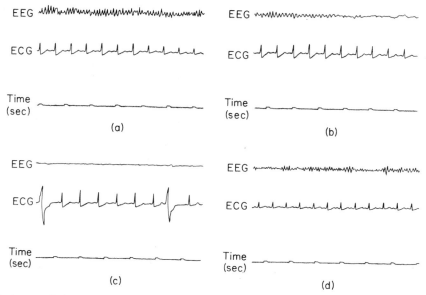

Fig. 11.2   An electroencephalogram (EEG) and electrocardiogram (ECG) recorded during inflow occlusion of the right ventricle for the purpose of relieving pulmonary valve stenosis. The patient, aged 6 years, was cooled to 29°C in the oesophagus (a) just before occluding the venae cavae, (b) at the time of applying occlusion, (c) during occlusion while surgery to the valve was being performed, and (d) 90 seconds after relief of occlusion. The EEG is returning to normal. The period of inflow occlusion lasted for 3.5 minutes.

oxygen at the same rate as the myocardium, 9 litres/minute would be required.[54] It is not surprising, therefore, that anoxia has such a profound effect upon this organ (Fig. 11.2). Unlike the brain, however, which also requires an adequate oxygen supply, the myocardium is able to use its stores of adenosine triphosphate (ATP) for a short period of time and continue metabolism until they are exhausted. Also unlike the brain,[64] the myocardium is not permanently damaged by a few minutes of anoxia.

Anoxia is a common cause of ventricular fibrillation and is most likely to be seen when patients who appear to have recovered from the anaesthetic are left unattended after an operation. It has also been reported after the use of the antibiotic kana-mycin (see p. 147). If respiratory inadequacy leads to desaturation of the arterial blood, the myocardium is unable to beat effectively. When a relatively moderate degree of hypoxia is present (i.e. an arterial oxygen saturation of 70%–80%) marked hypertension, together with a tachycardia, is commonly observed. Hypertension and tachycardia give place to bizarre complexes on the ECG which are followed by a bradycardia (Fig. 11.3) and profound hypotension. If these are observed during an anaesthetic, for example because of obstruction to the flow of gas, the situation can usually be corrected in time. For this reason continuous monitoring of the ECG during some operations is advisable, and for less important procedures the Keating blood pressure pulse

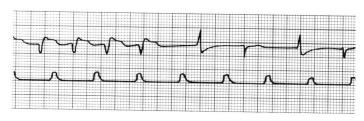

Fig. 11.3   Bradycardia and bizarre electrocardiogram (ECG) caused by anoxia during an anaesthetic. The lower trace denotes time in seconds. (See also p. 383.)

monitor,[36] which is easily applied to the pulp of the finger, is of great value.

The sequence of changes with regard to the blood pressure and heart rate in response to acute anoxia is reproduced in the varying circumstances of acute obstruction to the respiratory tract by a foreign body, infection or trauma, the failure of an artificial ventilator, or the sudden failure to breathe following an anaesthetic. However, the rise in blood pressure and heart rate does not occur when postoperative failure to breathe is caused by a metabolic acidosis (see p. 142).

It is of value to follow the sequence of events leading to ventricular fibrillation through in its classic form from the moment acute obstruction (for example) begins. These events can be conveniently divided into stages.

1. The heart rate and blood pressure increase.
2. The heart rate increases even further and the blood pressure rises to very high values.
3. The heart rate increases to an extremely fast rate, 300 beats/minute or more, and the blood pressure falls.
4. The heart rate slows so that there is a severe bradycardia. Even if by definition a bradycardia (less than 60 beats/minute) is not present (Fig. 11.4), many of the contractions of the myocardium are ineffective so that there is no transmission to the radial pulse.

Case history. A 23-year-old woman suffered a flail chest as a consequence of her chest hitting the steering wheel of her car in a road traffic accident. The ribs on both sides of the sternum were fractured. She was placed in the intensive care ward and, following an initial tracheal intubation, a tracheotomy was performed and controlled artificial ventilation of the lungs was instituted. The bow of the tape, attached to the cuffed tracheostomy tube to keep it in place, was tied behind the neck, but it loosened and allowed the tracheostomy tube to move forward when she moved. The right-angled tube changed its position so that the lower open end was occluded as it impinged against the posterior wall of the trachea. The inflated cuff, freed from the pressure of the tracheal walls, expanded so that it completely occluded the lumen of the trachea and made removal of the tracheostomy tube difficult until it was deflated.

With the changes in heart rate (R–R interval), the ECG was automatically recorded at the central monitoring area. The rise in blood pressure, which was monitored using a catheter placed in the femoral artery and connected to a transducer, was noted to pass through the stages described above.

Following a severe tachycardia, the bradycardia seen in Fig. 11.4 appeared. Removal of the tracheostomy tube and allowing the minimal spontaneous ventilation possible to occur with an O_2 catheter placed in the tracheostomy, resulted in improvement in the ECG.

Further anoxic changes occurred when the tracheostomy tube was re-inserted. With the restoration of artificial ventilation of the lungs, the tachycardia returned and persisted for over 10 minutes.

It cannot be stressed more strongly than one breath of air, when given immediately, can return a patient from the point of death to recovery.

Although the bradycardia of anoxia was reported in the first edition of this book (Brooks, 1967),[13] nurses are still not being taught its significance. Recently, a patient died in the recovery room of a hospital following relatively minor surgery; a bradycardia of 44 beats/minute was recorded by the nurse 10 minutes before death, but no action was taken because the nurse was unaware of its significance.

Diseases of the valves and myocardium

Ventricular fibrillation is sometimes precipitated by sudden exertion in the presence of valvular disease such as aortic stenosis or incompetence and mitral stenosis or incompetence. Adams-Stokes attacks, paroxysmal ventricular tachycardia and other arrhythmias may also develop into ventricular fibrillation. Further causes are myocardial ischaemia, fatty infiltration of the heart arising from macrocytic anaemia, diphtheritic carditis and toxic myocarditis caused by an overwhelming infection.

Myocardial infarction (coronary occlusion)

Ventricular fibrillation may occur at any time following myocardial infarction. It has been observed within a few minutes of the onset of pain or after many hours when the condition appears to have become quiescent. Although pain of increasing severity and electrocardiographic evidence of advancing myocardial infarction indicate the probability of ventricular fibrillation, the absence of these factors does not preclude its occurrence. Neither is the size of the area of infarction necessarily the deciding factor in the production of ventricular fibrillation, especially in the early stages, although it is well known from experiments on dogs that the larger the area of ischaemia caused by occluding the coronary vessels the more

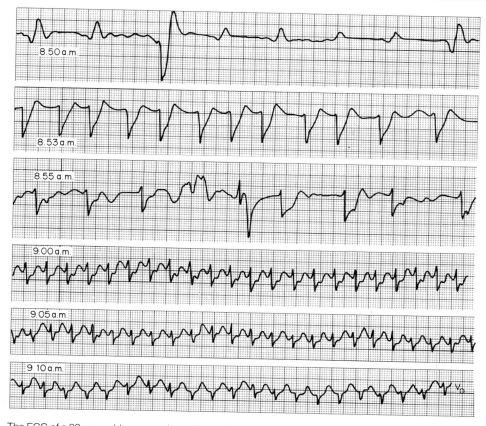

Fig. 11.4   The ECG of a 23-year-old woman who suffered a flail chest as a result of a road traffic accident. The ECG was being recorded automatically at the central nursing station when the R-R interval changed as a result of anoxia when the tracheostomy tube became misplaced and the balloon occluded the trachea.

The 8.50 a.m. trace is that of an anoxic heart. Most of the ventricular complexes would not be transmitted to the pulse and would appear as a severe bradycardia on palpation.

The 8.53 a.m. trace was recorded when the cuff of the tracheostomy tube was deflated and the tube removed, and a little, but inadequate, spontaneous respiration was possible and oxygen was administered into the trachea via a catheter.

The 8.55 a.m. trace was recorded during the short period required for re-inserting the tracheostomy tube. Serious anoxic changes and bradycardia are present.

The subsequent traces, taken at 9.00 a.m., 9.05 a.m. and 9.10 a.m., are those of a sinus tachycardia that was present when ventilation of the lungs using 100% oxygen had been re-established. Note that the tachycardia persisted for more than 10 minutes after the event.

readily it can be made to occur. It would seem, however, that in man when there is already an abnormal blood supply to the heart muscle, an imbalance in electrical activity is often the major factor causing ventricular fibrillation.

Diabetes mellitus
Sudden death occurring in patients suffering from diabetes is reviewed on page 293.

Cardiac catheterization and angiocardiography
Whenever these procedures are performed, the equipment for dealing with a sudden cardiac arrest should always be readily available. The incidence of cardiac arrest during these procedures is, however, low, except in Ebstein's disease,[70] where there is displacement and malformation of the tricuspid valve. Hypersensitivity to iodine during angiocardiography, cholecystography, urography and arteriography has been implicated. However, in many of the cases recorded other factors such as respiratory failure, anaesthesia, myocardial ischaemia or the presence of cyanotic heart disease may have played an important part.

Drugs

Sudden death can be caused by the intravenous injection of digitalis, quinidine sulphate, adrenaline (epinephrine), isoprenaline and calcium and potassium salts.

Preparations of digitalis are normally extremely safe to use and have none of the dangers, when given intravenously for the first time, that are associated with the other substances mentioned below. They are sometimes dangerous when given after previous therapy with digitalis of high dosage in patients who have a low plasma $[K^+]$, and very rarely in the presence of congenital cardiac defects. Ventricular fibrillation tends to occur only when digitalis toxicity is already established.

Now that ethacrynic acid (Edecrin), frusemide (Lasix) and bumetanide (Burinex) are available, they can be infused intravenously with safety when, in an emergency, a rapid diuresis is required. Pulmonary oedema and the acute onset of congestive cardiac failure, for example following coronary occlusion, are two of the conditions in which it may be necessary to administer an intravenous diuretic.

Adrenaline can cause ventricular fibrillation when accidentally injected into a vessel or when injected into the heart in which asystole has been produced by other means (e.g. hypothermia). It is, however, of value during cardiac massage in that it may convert a fine fibrillation into a coarse one so that electrical defibrillation can be performed more easily. It also assists in producing an adequate perfusion pressure.

Quinidine in very small doses may produce ventricular fibrillation in the hypersensitive patient. This may be manifested by repeated attacks of syncope (see p. 353) or sudden death. There is no way of predicting hypersensitivity in the individual patient and a single tablet may cause a fatal arrhythmia. This aspect is dealt with further on page 326.

Potassium salts may produce ventricular fibrillation or asystole followed by ventricular fibrillation, when injected rapidly into a vein. The effect is transient and is most readily reversed if active steps are taken to maintain ventilation, to apply external or internal cardiac massage and to administer Ca^{++} salts and $NaHCO_3$ solution intravenously or directly into the heart. Early electrical defibrillation can then be achieved. If safety is to be ensured, potassium chloride should not be given intravenously at a rate faster than 20 mmol/hour (mEq/hour). Care should be taken to ensure that there is an adequate urine excretion because gradual rise of plasma potassium concentration following acute renal failure will also lead to ventricular fibrillation.

Psychotropic agents

The tricyclic antidepressants, amitriptyline, nortriptyline and orphenadrine, can give rise to serious arrhythmias which lead to ventricular fibrillation. When these drugs are taken as an overdose, ventricular fibrillation may occur frequently during a convulsion. Treatment is described on page 328. A metabolic acidosis is virtually always present and its correction can alone return the patient to a sinus rhythm or assist in the relief of the arrhythmia and convulsions. The convulsions can be treated successfully with paraldehyde 10 ml i.m. given in divided doses (e.g. 5 ml into each thigh muscle).

While sudden death during exercise has become recognized with increasing frequency, especially in joggers suffering from coronary artery disease, the association of anabolic steroids taken during training by athletes has been questioned as being a cause (Harries, 1985).[30]

Calcium salts may produce asystole or ventricular fibrillation in patients who are already suffering from arrhythmias resulting from digitalis intoxication; calcium chloride ($CaCl_2$) has a greater degree of ionization than calcium gluconate and is more likely to produce this. Calcium gluconate should therefore be used routinely or when there is any doubt as to the possible ill-effects of the administration of calcium salts.

Hypothermia

During the elective cooling of the body to low temperatures for the purpose of occluding major vessels or performing open-heart surgery, ventricular fibrillation frequently occurs when the temperature in the oesophagus falls below 28°C. In some centres the body has been cooled electively by surface cooling to much lower oesophageal temperatures (e.g. to 17°C). Ether anaesthesia has been used in these special circumstances. Accidental exposure to as low as 18°C with survival has been recorded. In the majority of cases reduction of body temperature by surface cooling is limited by the hazard of ventricular fibrillation. An account of the physiology and biochemistry of cooling is given in Chapter 7.

Electrocution and lightning

In all civilized societies deaths from electrocution are increasingly common, and as electronic apparatus is more widely used in hospitals for recording and monitoring body functions and for clinical measurement, the dangers from this source become greater.[43] On average, approximately 140 people are killed each year in the UK from electrocution. Only very small currents are required to produce ventricular fibrillation and a direct current is generally more dangerous than an alternating current. Every year between 2 and 12 (average seven) people are killed by lightning in this country. The measures to be taken are those described under cardiac arrest.

Even though the patient may appear to be dead, it is important that steps are taken immediately to perform expired air ventilation and the general measures of cardiopulmonary resuscitation described below.

The importance of resuscitation was emphasized by Critcheley in 1934[21] when reporting the effects of electrocution from a high-tension cable and lightning. In 1951 the results of lightning striking a church in East Africa were described by Marriott.[48] The congregation numbered approximately 300 and the lightning strike rendered more than 100 unconscious, most of whom made a spontaneous recovery. Only six people were killed. Transfusions of plasma were recommended for the burns and prolonged artificial respiration, for several hours if necessary, was advocated.

Spontaneous recovery with or without injury has been well documented. The report by Silverman[61] is an illustration. A woman was working in her kitchen when lightning struck. It blew a hole in the roof, ripped off the door and destroyed a nearby chicken house. The woman was rendered unconscious for 5 minutes. Her left shoe was completely destroyed. She suffered superficial burns across her entire chest, abdomen and left calf, which were 5 cm wide, zig-zag in shape, extended down to her left foot. Her ear bled profusely, her left cheek became swollen and her eyebrow and eyelashes were singed. She was rendered permanently deaf, although her burns healed well.

An inability to move following spontaneous recovery is described in many accounts.[60,65] For example, a tea stall at the Ascot races in England was struck by lightning during a severe thunderstorm.[2] One woman was killed instantly, many people were rendered unconscious and many more were thrown to the ground and were dazed. When they tried to stand, they found they were unable to use their limbs, and this effect lasted for variable periods of time. Forty-five people were taken to hospital; 2 of these died (1 from a skull fracture), and 12 were unconscious for more than 5 minutes. One person had a perforation of the eardrum and altogether five people suffered hearing loss. The burns in all cases were superficial.

Few attempts have been made to resuscitate those who have been killed by lightning, either by people who were close by and survived, or by those who witnessed the event. Schallock[59] reported that a row of football players was rendered unconscious when struck by lightning, but no attempts were made to resuscitate the one who was killed, although all the others stood up uninjured after being thrown to the ground. There are, however, heroic exceptions, including that reported by Taussig[65] and Ravitch et al.[56] A 10-year-old boy was struck by lightning when riding a bicycle. He was carried unconscious to a nearby school where back press/arm lift artificial respiration was applied. He arrived at hospital, apparently dead, 22 minutes after being struck, having been given artificial respiration for 7 minutes. He was pulseless, he had not breathed, his pupils were dilated and he was cyanotic. He was given mouth-to-mouth ventilation. The chest was opened and no bleeding occurred. There was no heart beat. Adrenaline (epinephrine) was injected into the left ventricle and internal cardiac massage was begun. Five minutes after admission to hospital, the heart began to beat and ineffective respiratory efforts began. The patient was placed on an artificial ventilator for 3 days. He remained comatose or unconscious for 6 days, but was eventually discharged with no impairment of his IQ.

Haemorrhage

A sudden massive haemorrhage may produce cardiac arrest in two ways. Firstly, although major blood loss of relatively slow onset causes hyperventilation, a sudden rapid loss of blood (e.g. following the loosening of a suture around a major vessel after surgery) leads to complete cessation of respiratory effort. Anoxia then either causes or contributes to producing ventricular fibrillation. Secondly, a sudden fall of arterial pressure reduces the flow of blood to the coronary vessels and leads to acute myocardial ischaemia, which together with anoxia invariably causes the heart to fibrillate.

Drowning

Between 1500 and 2000 people are drowned in Great Britain every year, the majority in rivers, about 200–300 are drowned in the sea.

The prime cause of cardiac arrest in drowning is anoxia, and steps must be taken to correct this as rapidly as possible.

It can never be hoped that artificial means of cardiac massage and ventilation of the lungs during cardiac arrest will equal normal function. As the seconds pass, the possibilities of successful resuscitation become less and the probability of residual neurological damage becomes greater. There is no time for careful investigations or lengthy procedures, such as bronchoscopy to clear airways, because one breath of expired air from a medical attendant causing the patient's lungs to inflate directly after cessation of respiration is more valuable than 100 inflations with pure oxygen given 3 or 4 minutes later.

As Miles (1962) has pointed out, the rescuer, if possible, should begin mouth-to-mouth ventilation while still in the water, supporting the unconscious victim with one arm while occluding the nostrils with the free hand.[49] So little water can be removed from the lungs once it has entered that valuable time is lost by attempting to do so. Once on land, the presence of an effective heart beat must be confirmed and, if this is absent, external cardiac massage should be begun immediately. If the attendant is working alone, only intermittent inflation of the lungs can be performed. There is therefore no time to make good the oxygen debt which has already accrued. In a similar manner the cardiac output of the artificially massaged heart is therefore less than that of the heart that is beating spontaneously so that the tissue oxygen debt from this source must inevitably increase. Because of these factors it is essential that the reaction of the attendants must be immediate, determined and decisive.

Some people who drown lose consciousness without the inhalation of any water into the lungs, and death from anoxia is caused by breath-holding and 'glottic spasm'. When a small quantity of water is inhaled during consciousness an intense burning pain is felt in the chest and this itself may prevent the further inhalation of water. When water has entered the lungs, pulmonary oedema develops and positive pressure ventilation with oxygen is then required.

Case history. A 41-year-old European woman with a long psychiatric history took a moderately large dose of barbiturates and jumped into a canal. She was pulled out of the water by men who were fishing. She was transported to the accident and emergency department rapidly by ambulance; during this time she had received expired air resuscitation by means of a Brook airway. She was admitted in an unconscious state, and soon afterwards an endotracheal tube was passed and ventilation with 100% O_2 was begun. During intubation she was found to have a gross bradycardia, which was almost certainly due to anoxia (see p. 383), for which 10 ml of 10% calcium gluconate was given, and she passed immediately into ventricular fibrillation.

Conversion to a sinus rhythm was obtained with a single DC shock of 200 J (watt/seconds). A severe sinus bradycardia was present following cardioversion which responded to atropine 0.4 mg i.v. The bradycardia at this stage was therefore not due to anoxia. Shortly after admission the patient's rectal temperature was 35.2°C. The results of blood gas analysis at that time (Table 11.1) revealed a raised PCO_2 (110 mmHg) and a low PO_2 (64 mmHg), in spite of the fact that the patient was being ventilated manually at a fast rate with 100% O_2 supplied from a Boyle's anaesthetic apparatus at 12 litres/minute.

Although the blood gas levels were being measured, an infusion of 200 ml of 8.4% $NaHCO_3$ (200 mmol/l, mEq/l) was begun. Pink-stained frothy fluid of pulmonary oedema was sucked from the endotracheal tube im-

Table 11.1 A case of attempted drowning. Various parameters measured in a 41-year-old woman who jumped into a canal after taking a large dose of barbiturates. Note the low PO_2 in spite of being ventilated with 100% oxygen, and the high PCO_2 when blood was taken following admission. Note also the low haemoglobin as a result of haemolysis following inhalation of fresh water; this is apparent in the low haemoglobin concentration the day following admission

	pH	PCO_2	PO_2	[HCO_3^-]	Base excess	Hb	PCV	[Na^+]	[K^+]
Following admission 100% O_2 NaHCO$_3$ begun	6.90	110	64	21	−12			138	3.7
After 200 mmol (mEq) NaHCO$_3$ and 100% O_2	7.34	52	44	28	+1	16.0	48.0	130	3.4
Day following admission	7.38	48	54	28	+2	12.3	36.4	148	4.1
Third day extubated breathing O_2 by mask	7.43	38	66	25	+2	10.2	33.0	135	4.1
Fourth day	7.45	42	98	28	+5	9.3	32.0	144	4.7
Fifth day						10.4	32.0	137	4.1
Ninth day						12.3	38.0		

pH at 37°C; PCO_2, blood CO_2 tension in mmHg; PO_2, blood O_2 tension in mmHg; [HCO_3^-], blood bicarbonate concentration calculated from PCO_2 and pH; PCV, packed cell volume (%); [Na^+], plasma sodium concentration (mmol/l, mEq/l); [K^+], plasma potassium concentration (mmol/l, mEq/l).

mediately following its insertion and this did not disappear completely for 24 hours. A chest X-ray confirmed the presence of pulmonary oedema affecting both lungs uniformly. A catheter passed into the bladder demonstrated the urine to be uniformly blood-stained, indicating the early onset of haemolysis.

Ventilation with 100% O_2 was continued, although some voluntary respiratory effort occurred soon after cardioversion. However, the arterial blood PO_2 was low (44 mmHg). The percentage of inhaled O_2 was not reduced to 50% until the day following admission.

The blood pressure fell and urine output decreased approximately 1 hour after admission of the patient to the emergency department. Dopamine infused at the rate of 10 μg/kg per minute was begun; this raised the blood pressure to just above 80 mmHg systolic. Urine output fell below 30 ml/hour and no increase in output was obtained following 50 mg frusemide (Lasix) given intravenously. However, a good response was obtained following the infusion of 250 ml of 20% mannitol given over a few minutes, and a second infusion was given more slowly over 2 hours.

The following day the patient was jaundiced, the heart rate was 100 beats/minute in sinus rhythm, the blood pressure was 110/70 mmHg when dopamine was infused. Moist sounds were heard in both lungs. A radiograph, which revealed that bilateral alveolar opacities typical of patchy pulmonary oedema were still present, nevertheless demonstrated a marked improvement as clearing of the alveolar oedema had progressed. There was, however, little improvement in blood gases and ventilation of the lungs was continued using 50% O_2 and air, at a tidal volume of 700 ml, and ventilation rate of 18/minute. The PCO_2 was slightly raised (48 mmHg), the PO_2 was low (54 mmHg) and the acid–base state was normal.

Improvement in the patient's condition gradually continued and towards the evening of the second day urine output was satisfactory, the degree of oxygenation was greatly improved and no difficulty was experienced in maintaining a satisfactory blood pressure with dopamine infusions. The limbs and peripheries were warm to the touch. The patient was not hyperpyrexial, and the vasodilator action of dopamine was probably a contributory factor.

On the third day after admission, although haemolysis was still progressing and the haemoglobin concentration was still falling, and at this stage was 9 g%, the urine was not pigmented. Oxygenation of the arterial blood was satisfactory; the minute and tidal volume increased when the patient breathed spontaneously, so that the endotracheal tube was removed.

Progressive improvement in the chest X-ray occurred and haemolysis ceased by the fifth day. Ampicillin and gentamicin were given from the first day, and gentamicin levels were monitored. Although the blood urea and creatinine rose, no significant degree of renal impairment occurred.

The patient made a complete recovery. No impairment of intelligence developed, even though severe anoxia and ventricular fibrillation had occurred when there was no significant fall in body temperature. Renal failure did not develop and severe hypo-osmolality of the plasma was not observed because of the infusion of hypertonic sodium bicarbonate. Nevertheless, the plasma [Na^+] fell to 130 mmol/l (mEq/l), although 200 mmol of $NaHCO_3$ had been infused. However, there is no doubt that a large volume of water had entered the circulation via the lungs because of the fall in plasma [Na^+], the pulmonary oedema, haemolysis and haemoglobinuria. The haemolysis may have been confined to the lungs, the red cell envelope being damaged by the canal water present in the alveoli. The use of 100% O_2 did not in any way exacerbate the patient's respiratory problems and was essential in the early stages to maintain even minimal oxygenation.

Much emphasis has been placed on the differentiation between fresh-water and sea-water drowning. If water is not inhaled, as in the majority of cases, the resuscitative procedures are those that apply to any form of acute anoxia. Even when water is inhaled, the basic procedures are identical, and Rivers et al.[57] have emphasized that early treatment is an important factor in survival and that differentiation between the two forms of fresh-water and sea-water drowning should not delay its institution. When they reviewed the published data, in addition to assessing the significance of their own findings, they observed that biochemical and haematological investigations were unlikely to assist in diagnosis and could be misleading if blood analysis was allowed to influence treatment. This was in keeping with the views of Miles.[50]

Rivers et al. also stressed the importance of secondary drowning where, after an initial successful treatment of the acute anoxia, a protein-rich fluid is exuded into the alveoli during the following 24 hours. Secondary drowning caused by sea water is more severe and is associated with a much higher mortality than that due to fresh water.

Because of the degree of anoxia and loss of lung compliance, it is unlikely that when it occurs expired air resuscitation will be sufficient to maintain life for very long. Routine admission to hospital following apparent successful initial resuscitation was advocated by Miles[50] and Rivers et al.[57]

Varying degrees of haemolysis have been reported[26,52] associated with fresh-water drowning. A severe bleeding diathesis, which required transfusion, was reported by Culpepper.[23] It responded to fresh frozen plasma (FFP), but severe hypovolaemia developed with a central venous pressure (CVP) of 2 cmH$_2$O and the patient succumbed. Correction of the blood volume may be an important factor in drowning.

Immersion in sea water

Although death can occur from hypothermia, death from immersion at sea has been reported by a number of non-medical sources before significant cooling could have taken place. In 1981, Harries et al.[31] reported two cases of ventricular fibrillation occurring when only a moderate degree of hypothermia had developed.

The Diagnosis of Cardiac Arrest

When cardiac arrest occurs at normal body temperature, permanent brain damage can only be avoided with certainty if action is taken within 3 minutes. When ventricular fibrillation follows coronary occlusion, the onset is frequently quite sudden and all premonitory warning signs are absent. The author has treated a number of non-surgical patients who were successfully resuscitated when ventricular fibrillation occurred during the recording of an ECG. Frequently, however, especially in postoperative cases, cardiac arrest is often preceded by hypotension. If there is prolonged anoxia, hypertension occurs initially, followed later by hypotension and a bradycardia (see p. 383).

Respiratory failure

Therefore, as the clinician approaches the patient, apart from the developing yellow-tinged wax-like appearance of death, the first thing that should be noticed is the absence of respiration or slow agonal respiration with jaw tug. This is probably the most important of all the physical signs at the very beginning, because it so frequently precedes cardiac arrest that it is sometimes possible to prevent ventricular fibrillation by artificial ventilation if seconds are not lost in debate and the painfully slow accumulation of the perfect positive pressure equipment. One breath of expired air or one partial inflation of the lungs from an incompletely filled rebreathing bag through an ill-fitting mask is far more valuable than unlimited oxygen supply through a correctly placed endotracheal tube 1 minute later. Absence of breathing is, therefore, the first sign that any clinician should note. Agonal respiration may, however, be present for a short period after the onset of ventricular fibrillation.

If cardiac arrest occurs during a surgical procedure, absence of spontaneous respiration will nowadays not usually be of any significance as in almost all cases respiration is controlled by the anaesthetist. Cyanosis, however, is a clear indication that cardiac arrest is imminent or has occurred. Continuous pulse and blood pressure monitoring as a routine has been discussed on page 381.

Dilatation of the pupils

The most important physical sign next to spontaneous ventilation is that the pupils dilate widely immediately following cessation of the heart beat. They are readily observed after raising the eyelids and are a very good indication of the effectiveness of the cardiac massage. Unless there is a significant reduction in the size of the pupils when cardiac massage is performed, it almost always indicates that an inadequate supply of oxygenated blood to the body is being maintained. It is quite common to observe pupils that are dilated shortly after the onset of ventricular fibrillation, constrict and become small as soon as cardiac massage is performed. They remain small as long as massage is continued properly, but when the medical attendant begins to tire and the pulse becomes less easily palpable, then the pupils become dilated once again. They constrict once more either when renewed efforts are made or when cardiac massage is taken over by another person. During anaesthesia the pupils may become dilated with atropine, halothane and ganglion-blocking agents. Morphine sulphate and its derivatives produce constriction of the pupils and the author has seen this in an alcoholic who had died after a road accident. Hypothermia also causes the pupils to dilate, but the pupils return to normal size as rewarming proceeds.

General appearance

The general appearance is one of death. As soon as arrest of the circulation occurs the mucous membranes become greyish-white and the skin develops a translucent yellowish appearance.

The pulses

During shock the radial and sometimes the brachial pulses are not palpable. Quite commonly these pulses disappear when vasopressor agents have been given, but the carotid and femoral pulses are usually palpable. In extremely obese people the femoral pulse may be difficult to palpate unless pressure is applied to disperse the fluid fat lying below the skin.

During cardiac arrest none of the pulses is palpable. The absence of a pulse is an absolute sign of inadequate perfusion of tissues. It is sometimes the only physical sign that is of value in the anaesthetized patient. Although an absent pulse may also be the sign of excessive blood loss or septic shock, the procedure for cardiac arrest must be instituted immediately. External cardiac massage, which gives time for other factors to be assessed and investigated, reduces the danger of an emergency thoracotomy being performed unnecessarily.

Bleeding

It is sometimes suggested that if there is any doubt as to whether cardiac arrest has occurred, a vessel should be cut. A proviso is placed in many wills that a vein should be cut in order to make certain that death has occurred. This is, however, frequently a misleading sign. Bleeding can occur from the veins through an incision in the skin even after cardiac arrest. It is unnecessary to incise an artery as its pulsation alone is sufficient to determine whether it is being perfused under pressure. Absence of bleeding from the skin surface is present when there is gross dehydration or accidental hypothermia and cardiac arrest has not occurred. When searching for veins in order to set up intravenous drips in grossly dehydrated patients, who were hypotensive from this cause, bleeding has been frequently completely absent from the numerous small incisions made in the arms or legs. These incisions, when left open until the patient has been resuscitated with intravenous fluids, begin to bleed after a litre or more of fluid has been infused rapidly.

Electrocardiogram and electroencephalogram

Although sometimes, especially during surgery, an electrocardiogram (ECG) and electroencephalogram (EEG) have been recorded at the time of cardiac arrest, in the majority of cases these and similar aids are absent. Ventricular fibrillation will be readily apparent from the ECG. We have already seen how the EEG becomes isoelectric as soon as the circulation to the brain stops. Some indication of impending disaster may be given when desaturation of the arterial blood precedes cardiac arrest. A bradycardia is noted on the ECG and abnormal 3 and 4 cycle/second waves make their appearance on the EEG. These are very similar to the 3 and 4 cycle/second waves appearing during haemorrhagic shock when desaturation of the arterial blood occurs.

Absence of heart sounds

Searching for heart sounds in the patient with cardiac arrest is to be condemned, as is bronchoscopy before attempting to inflate the lungs. Every second counts and there is an appalling lack of appreciation of the situation when external cardiac massage is delayed so that numerous people may listen and confirm the findings. If, as sometimes happens, it is necessary to allow many people to listen in turn because the situation is so highly charged with controversy as to diagnosis and method of treatment, the person who is to listen to the heart should be ready with the stethoscope firmly placed in the ears with the bell on the left chest at the apex of the heart, ready to listen as soon as external cardiac massage is stopped for a moment. This may be permitted at repeated intervals. The person performing external cardiac compression should take no notice of those around him, apart from the anaesthetist or other attendant who is performing positive pressure ventilation.

External (closed chest) cardiac massage

Although it had been known for some time that an effective circulation could be produced and had been demonstrated in animals,[6] it was not until the experiments of Kouwenhoven et al.[42] when it was shown that external cardiac massage in conjunction with external electrical defibrillation would make resuscitation possible, that this method became widely used. It has now been performed so successfully all over the world and has either saved or helped to save so many lives that it should always be the first step taken after cardiac arrest.

Technique of external cardiac massage

The technique involves compressing the heart between the sternum and the vertebral bodies and raising the intrathoracic pressure. Although apparatus is available for this in various forms,[3] it can be performed successfully using the hands alone.

The sternum consists of a manubrium, a body which during development was composed of four sternabrae and a xyphoid process. The junction of the manubrium with the first sternabra is demarcated by the angle of Louis, which is the site of articulation of the second costal cartilage (Fig. 11.5). The space between the body of the sternum and the bodies of the thoracic vertebrae at the level of the third and fourth sternabrae is occupied in the main by the heart (Fig. 11.6). It is, therefore, at this point that external compression is most likely to be effective. The patient should be placed supine on a hard rigid surface, such as the floor or a table, which supports the entire length of the body. An operating table is, of course, ideal because it can be tilted; an ordinary bed can be placed on blocks. If the patient is lying on the ground, cushions or books should be placed under the buttocks or sacrum so that the level of this part of the body is raised. Whenever possible the legs should be elevated 30°–40° to facilitate the venous return to the heart while allowing adequate perfusion of the limbs. Wooden boards should be kept in all wards so that when a patient is in bed they can be placed below the mattress without interrupting the closed chest compression for very long. When the attendant is alone the fact that the patient is in bed and not on a rigid surface should not delay external cardiac massage, but when a sufficient number of people are present and the patient can be transferred with ease to the floor or other rigid surface, this should be performed as rapidly as possible so that pressure can be applied more effectively.

The palm of one hand is placed at the lower end of the body of the sternum, that is to say that part which is formed from the lower two sternabrae (Figs. 11.5 and 11.7), in such a way that pressure is transmitted directly along the radius and the ulna. The other hand is placed upon the back of the first hand so that the combined pressure transmitted along both arms is available for moving the sternum (Fig. 11.7). The person performing the massage should be positioned in such a way that maximum force can be applied at as fast a rate as possible. If the patient is on the ground, the attendant can either stand or kneel. In treating the large obese patient with a rigid thorax it may be necessary to stand in order to use all the available weight and force of the attendant. When the patient is lying in bed it is almost always essential to stand in order to perform effective external cardiac massage, and when cardiac arrest occurs on the operating table, then it is almost impossible to achieve an effective cardiac output without standing upon a chair or stool so that the feet are just below the level of the table. In addition to adequate pressure it is necessary to apply external cardiac massage at an adequate rate. The minimum rate acceptable in the adult is 60/minute because it must be remembered that when cardiac output is reduced the rate should be increased. The rate of 80/minute is probably the maximum that can be maintained by the normal, fit healthy person for any length of time, although speeds in excess of this can be performed for short periods. It is for this reason that mechanical means of performing external cardiac massage have been advocated and designed. Adequate pressure applied at a rate which is too slow is always insufficient and almost invariably precludes recovery, even if the slow rate is maintained for only a few minutes. An arterial blood pressure of 70–100 mmHg can be achieved by external cardiac massage, and when massage is performed correctly patients may become conscious in the presence of continued ventricular fibrillation recorded on the ECG. They then may talk and groan, although there is complete amnesia of the events afterwards.

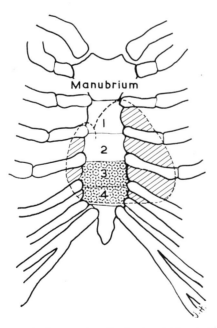

Fig. 11.5 A diagram showing the heart lying behind the sternum and rib cage. The darkly shaded area of the lower two sternabrae marks the area over which pressure should be applied for external cardiac massage.

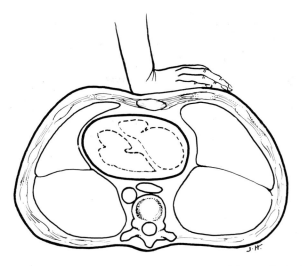

Fig. 11.6 This shows how the space between the lower end of the sternum and the vertebral column is largely occupied by the heart.

Compression of the lower end of the sternum does not produce an adequate ventilation of the lungs, although air may flow in and out of the upper respiratory tract giving the impression that adequate ventilation of the lungs is being achieved.

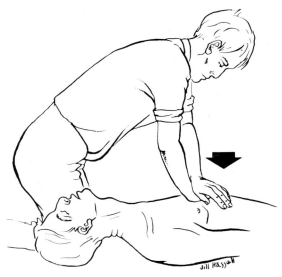

Fig. 11.7 The technique of external cardiac massage. It can also be performed in a similar manner when kneeling beside the abdomen.

Measurements of tidal volume have been made that show that this does not occur. Some improvement in ventilation may be obtained by periodically transferring the pressure applied by the palms of the hands to each side of the sternum so that they lie more laterally and towards the axillary aspects of the thoracic cage. When pressure is applied simultaneously through both palms there is an increase in tidal volume, but it is still very small and does not compensate for positive pressure ventilation.

The simplest method of inflating the lungs is by expired air ventilation ('mouth-to-mouth or mouth-to-nose breathing').

Ventilation of the lungs and the 'new' cardiopulmonary resuscitation (CPR)

It has been advocated that when the attendant is working alone and has to perform both tasks, there should be six compressions of the chest and then a breath. There should be four compressions of the chest followed by a breath when one attendant is performing the chest compression and another is ventilating the lungs. This method has worked very well, and when an endotracheal tube has been passed and 100% oxygen is being administered, as many as ten compressions of the chest have been performed repeatedly before a breath has been given, with success. The ability to do this depends upon the elasticity of the chest wall, and therefore the age of the patient, and the speed at which external cardiac massage is performed.

It has been demonstrated, however, that an improved cardiac output can be obtained by raising the intrathoracic pressure by intermittently ventilating the lungs at the *same time* that compression to the chest wall is applied.[19] This has also been the author's impression during many resuscitations, and if the pressure of gas in the inflating anaesthetic or resuscitator bag is not allowed to rise to excessive levels, the lungs are not damaged. However, if the release valve on the apparatus does become ineffective and a high pressure is transmitted down the endotracheal tube, damage can occur, and compression of the chest wall can exacerbate this circumstance. The reservations with regard to applying too high an inflation pressure still remain.

However, to obtain a satisfactory cardiac output, the pressure within the thorax should rise to 80 mmHg. If damage to the thoracic cage, liver, etc., is to be avoided, this pressure can be reached only by inflating the lungs at the same time as compression of the sternum.

Expired air resuscitation (mouth-to-mouth, mouth-to-nose breathing)

Expired air resuscitation is performed by pinching the patient's nostrils, taking a deep breath and placing one's own mouth over that of the unconscious victim so that a firm seal is made, while exhaling forcibly (Fig. 11.8). In this way air is forced into the lungs. If positioning of the head is so difficult that it is impossible to have one hand free, then it is sometimes possible to occlude the nostrils with one's own cheek.

The jaw of the unconscious person who is lying in the supine position falls backwards (downwards towards the ground), taking the tongue with it. This effectively blocks the air-pathway to the larynx while not usually completely occluding the oronasopharyngeal passage. The tongue presses against the bodies of the cervical vertebrae from which it is separated by the soft tissue of the posterior wall of the pharynx, producing typical ball-valve obstruction (Fig. 11.9). If one takes a deep breath and breathes out very forcibly, this can usually be overcome without any special manoeuvres, but the air-pathway which offers the least resistance is obtained when the head is hyperextended at the atlantooccipital joint and the jaw tilted forwards (upwards) (Fig. 11.10). Because of the large cross-sectional area (Fig. 11.11) that is available for the free flow of air both inwards and outwards, much larger tidal volumes can be obtained at lower pressures than by any other manoeuvre, including the insertion of a Guedel airway.

In practice, however, it is very difficult and tiring to maintain the position of hyperextension of the head in the unconscious patient and efforts to do so can sometimes impair the whole process of mouth-to-mouth respiration. An almost equally effective opening of the airway can be obtained in the unconscious patient by pushing the jaw forward (upwards) as far as the movement at the temperomandibular joint will allow[28] (Figs. 11.12 and 11.13). If obstruction by the tongue is allowed to occur and forceful expiration is used in an attempt to inflate the lungs, a greater quantity of air will pass into the stomach. This is partly because the obstruction persists as passive deflation of the lungs takes place and air enters the stomach during

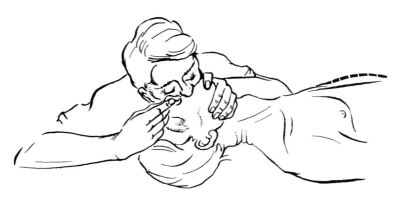

Fig. 11.8 Expired air resuscitation; mouth-to-mouth breathing. Note the elevation of the jaw, extension of the neck and squeezing the nostrils.

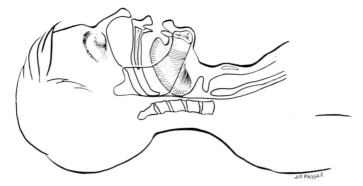

Fig. 11.9   A diagram showing the 'ball valve' produced by the tongue, as the jaw to which it is attached falls backwards in the unconscious patient. The airway is then occluded.

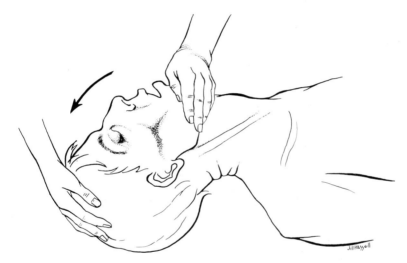

Fig. 11.10   Extension of the neck and lifting the jaw forwards and upwards produces a clear airway.

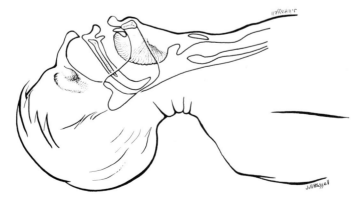

Fig. 11.11   The large open airway produced by the manoeuvre shown in Fig. 11.10.

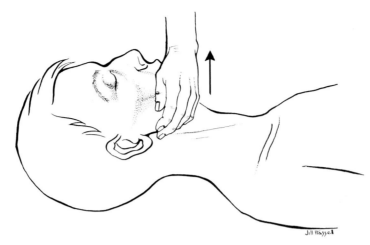

Fig. 11.12   Lifting the jaw forwards and upwards will also produce an open airway and this may be more easily performed when working alone.

both phases of the respiratory cycle. Although expired air resuscitation has been known from the earliest times and is mentioned in the Bible (see p. 1) it went 'out of fashion' with the advent of the 'germ theory' and the work of Pasteur. This aspect of mouth-to-mouth breathing and the real dangers associated with it in patients with respiratory diseases such as tuberculosis or when the patient has vomited, should never be taken too lightly, especially when teaching people who have had no medical training.[32]

The simplest method of overcoming the aesthetic aspects of mouth-to-mouth ventilation is to tear a small hole in a pocket handkerchief and, having placed the torn edges of the slit behind (below) the teeth of the patient, to breathe through the hole. It is more simple but less effective to fold the handkerchief and place it around the mouth. This, however, tends to move and a less efficient seal is obtained.

Numerous forms of simple apparatus have been designed in order to make mouth-to-mouth resuscitation easier and to provide an airway. Probably the best of these is the Brook airway. This simple device has an oral airway, a mouth guard which acts as an efficient seal when placed over the lips, and a non-return valve. In the words of Brook *et al.* it will 'improve airway patency, remove the repugnancy and protect the user against the danger of communicable disease'.[7,8,9]

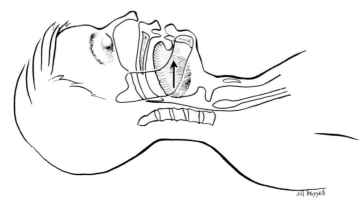

Fig. 11.13   The smaller but adequate airway produced by lifting the mandible.

Positive pressure ventilation can be applied by means of various forms of equipment specially designed for use in an emergency. As we have already seen (p. 3) in the very early times, use was made of the ordinary fire bellows. Today numerous designs are available[22] that are so constructed that they may be pressed with either the hand or foot or motivated by means of a cylinder of oxygen.

The simplest piece of apparatus which a practitioner should keep with him for use in an emergency is the self-inflating bag, such as the Ambu, the Ruben or the Dräger bag. All these require a non-return valve of the Ruben type and a face mask. An inexpensive model, the Laerdal bag, in a compact case designed expressly for this purpose is supplied by the British Oxygen Company.

The best airway is provided by a cuffed endotracheal tube, but this is difficult to pass successfully without a laryngoscope. As Whitby pointed out, however, it has long been known that if the head and chest are raised so that the patient is in the sitting-up position with the neck extended and the mouth facing upwards, a number eleven cuffed tube may be dropped into the larynx with very little difficulty when the vocal cords are relaxed. Smaller tubes pass even more easily.[68] The author can confirm the ease with which this can be performed. In addition to the fact that the endotracheal tube is ready to be attached to an anaesthetic apparatus or artificial ventilator, it is also available for expired air respiration.

It is essential to note as described above that, if forceful positive pressure ventilation is performed at the same time as forceful external cardiac massage, the pressure within the thoracic cavity rises and it is now considered to be the most important factor in achieving an adequate cardiac output. It is advocated that inflation of the lungs should be performed at the *same* time as chest compression.

Internal cardiac massage

Indications
Although internal cardiac massage is not used very often, except after open-heart surgery, when it is obvious that external cardiac massage is ineffective in maintaining an adequate circulation (i.e. when a pulse cannot be felt over the carotid or femoral vessels and the pupils remain dilated), the chest should be opened and internal cardiac massage should be performed. In the presence of cardiac tamponade from, for example, bleeding following trauma or open-heart surgery, it is virtually impossible to obtain an adequate perfusion of the tissues by external compression of the chest wall. Even when ventricular fibrillation follows coronary occlusion, factors may be present which allow only inadequate tissue perfusion. The time taken to open the chest wall is time that is irretrievably lost so that a decision must be made and the emergency thoracotomy must be performed as rapidly as possible, care being taken only to avoid damaging the lungs and the heart itself.

Thoracotomy
Any doctor is capable of performing a thoracotomy. It is performed in an emergency in a completely unwashed, unsterile manner and probably because antibiotics are used routinely the incidence of infection is extremely low.[1] All that is required is a scalpel blade, and the author can recall one patient who is alive today only because an extremely keen house surgeon kept a large scalpel blade attached to the inside cover of his medical diary with sticking plaster. The incision is made from just to the left of the body of the sternum to the axilla, preferably along the fourth left intercostal space. The fifth and sixth spaces will do equally well and in the female the lower level of the breast should be chosen. The incision should be as long as possible, but in the first instance an opening sufficient to admit one hand will permit compression of the heart against the posterior aspect of the sternum. When this has been performed several times the size of the incision should be increased so that the ribs may be parted and both hands may enter the thoracic cavity in order to perform bimanual cardiac compression. Enlargement of the incision can be interrupted so that compression of the heart against the sternum with one hand can be repeated at intervals. Once external compression of the chest has ceased, ventilation of the lungs should be continued at as fast a rate as possible to ensure maximum gas exchange and the greatest oxygen saturation of the arterial blood, when the circulation is once again restored by manual compression of the heart. Hyperventilation is not contraindicated at this stage as accumulation of CO_2 must have occurred.

Effective cardiac massage producing maximum possible output cannot be achieved while the pericardium is intact. After the heart has been squeezed a number of times and the incision made large enough to expose it within its coverings, the pericardium should be opened with scissors and the heart uncovered.

When cardiac massage is performed on a small child or infant, adequate cardiac output, blood pressure and perfusion of tissues can be achieved with one hand alone. One hand can also be used for cardiac massage in the adult by continuing to squeeze the heart against the sternum, but generally this is inefficient. In the adult, the greatest output is obtained when the heart is squeezed between both hands. Figures 11.14 and 11.15 are photographs taken when a man was successfully resuscitated after cardiac arrest in the operating theatre. The patient was a 75-year-old man who had been in intractable cardiac failure for many months and who had been anaesthetized for only a few minutes for a minor operation. He had been adequately ventilated from the very beginning and throughout the period of ventricular fibrillation was hyperventilated with 100% oxygen and infused with sodium bicarbonate solution. External cardiac massage was ineffective and the chest was opened within 2 minutes. After 2 or 3 minutes of bimanual massage the heart was successfully defibrillated. Figure 11.14 shows the left hand being placed behind the heart and the right hand about to squeeze the heart from infront. Figure 11.15 shows the hands just relaxing after having compressed the heart. The photographs were taken just after defibrillation when the heart was still flaccid and contracting poorly and when its output was being augmented by manual compression.

Massage of the fibrillating heart should be continued for a minimum of 2–3 hours, and when a team of medical attendants is present successful resuscitation can still be achieved after many hours as long as the basic biochemical and physiological changes are kept in mind and any abnormality is, when possible, corrected.

Disadvantages of External Cardiac Massage

It is important to note the disadvantages, even though in the majority of circumstances this is the method of choice.

Inadequate blood flow

External cardiac massage is a life-saving procedure, but sometimes compression of the heart by means of pressure exerted on the lower part of the body of the sternum is insufficient to maintain

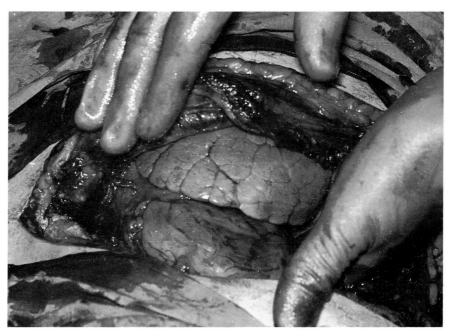

Fig. 11.14   Internal cardiac massage. The chest has been opened and the left hand is passing behind the heart. The heart can then be squeezed between the two hands.

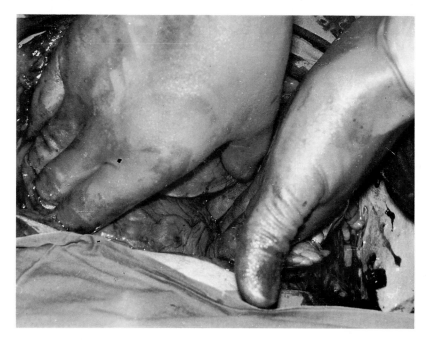

Fig. 11.15   The hands are just relaxing having squeezed the heart.

an adequate cardiac output. It is sometimes said that when closed chest resuscitation fails to maintain a satisfactory perfusion it is because it is performed badly. This is by no means true; closed chest resuscitation may be unsuccessful even when performed by experienced people.

The most common causes of inadequate output of oxygenated blood are too high an inflation pressure of the lungs and an inadequate venous return, but even the correction of these factors does not always result in an adequate pulse pressure which allows the carotid and femoral vessels to be palpated and cause the pupils to constrict. Although cardiac tamponade is an obvious condition in which external chest compression is ineffective, there are many cases in which it is impossible to find any real cause. It so happens that many of these patients in the less advanced age-groups (e.g. 40–50 years), are suffering from coronary infarction. Some of the patients under the age of 40 years appear to be suffering from active syphilis, and a Wassermann reaction and Kahn test should be performed routinely.

People who take an active part in resuscitation are never surprised when closed chest massage fails to work satisfactorily and this must be expected in some patients. It is important that internal cardiac massage should not be delayed when it is apparent that the blood supply to the brain is insufficient, as reflected by an absent carotid pulse, or one of poor volume, and dilatation of the pupils.

Fracture of ribs

When effective cardiac massage is performed it almost inevitably results in the fracture of some of the ribs forming the thoracic cage. This may result in complications which impair respiration after resuscitation, which is made worse by pneumothorax resulting from penetration of the lung, haemothorax and surgical emphysema. When the ribs are brittle and many are fractured on both sides, the elastic recoil of the sternum is lost and this impairs both the usefulness of cardiac compression and ventilation. This may result in a flail chest which requires positive pressure ventilation for a prolonged period.

Lung damage

In addition to penetration of the lungs by a rib, the combination of positive pressure ventilation and closed chest cardiac massage can result in parenchymal lung, haemorrhage and pneumothorax. In its mildest form haemoptysis results and in its worst form the lung damage is so widespread that recovery is impossible. People who suffer from emphysema are at a disadvantage in two ways. In the first place they are difficult to ventilate and, in the second, the presence of bullae makes rupture of the lung and pneumothorax more probable. This danger is reduced when care is taken to ventilate the lungs in such a way that the intra-thoracic pressure is not unduly raised.

Bruising and laceration of the liver

Laceration of the liver is most likely to occur when pressure is applied to the sternum at too low a level, so that much force is transmitted through the xiphisternum. Fatal intraperitoneal haemorrhage can occur.[4,35,53] Even when great care is taken to apply pressure over the area formed by the lower two sternabrae, bruising of the viscus is not uncommon. It is, therefore, of some importance to be aware of the danger of a too forceful compression of the chest and upper abdominal wall.

Damage to the heart

Quite commonly at *post mortem* it is possible to discern bruising of the heart muscle, and rupture of the heart has been reported in association with fracture of the sternum. It is also possible to tear the great veins at their point of entry into the heart. Rupture of the heart is most likely to occur when cardiac arrest takes place a few days after a myocardial infarction, and a large area of softening caused by necrosis is present.

Fracture of the sternum

This is a relatively uncommon complication of closed chest massage and is probably due to excessive force being used. When it has occurred, emboli of bone marrow have been found in the pulmonary arteries at autopsy.[35,39]

Pericardial effusion

Trauma to the internal aspect of the pericardium may give rise to a sterile non-haemorrhagic pericardial effusion. If the patient has been treated with anticoagulants prior to cardiac arrest, the effusion may be haemorrhagic. This effusion may give rise to cardiac tamponade some days later and because it is usually of relatively slow onset it demonstrates the classical signs of this condition which are: a raised central venous pressure (CVP), faint and distant heart sounds, tachycardia, low systolic blood pressure, enlargement of the liver and increased heart size shown by percussion and X-ray.

Advantages of Internal Cardiac Massage

Even when external cardiac massage is ineffective, compression of the heart between both hands in the adult, or by one hand in the child, almost always produces a satisfactory rise in output. The only exceptions to this are when the heart is dilated, blue and flaccid and when it fails to fill with blood as compression is released. Even when the heart fails to fill, cardiac output may be improved by massaging the abdominal contents upwards towards the diaphragm, by raising the feet and legs (e.g. by placing them on a chair), and by tilting the body, when this is possible, so that the head is dependent. Improvement in myocardial tone may also be produced by an injection of adrenaline (epinephrine). There is no doubt that the major advantage in internal cardiac massage is the fact that a constantly high output can be maintained when pressure is applied correctly. It has the disadvantage that when a thoracotomy is performed in an emergency, under non-sterile conditions, there is a danger of infection, although the incidence is extremely low.

When internal cardiac massage and ventilation of the lungs are performed properly, the cardiac output is sufficient with ventricular fibrillation present to allow the patient to regain consciousness while the chest is open and the patient sedated with pethidine (Demerol) or N_2O. The patient reported by Stewart et al. (1962).[63] was able to put out his tongue when requested to do so.

Respiration

Once the chest is opened the dangers associated with positive pressure inflation largely disappear, although it must be remembered in the presence of emphysematous bullae, too vigorous an inflation may still produce a pneumothorax. Opening the chest overcomes the dangers associated with a markedly raised intrathoracic pressure produced by combined pressure on the lower end of the sternum and vigorous lung inflation. Expansion of the lung is made remarkably easier, even in patients suffering from chronic lung disease.

It does mean, however, that once the chest is opened positive pressure ventilation has to be continued until it is closed surgically, with underwater drainage if necessary. When patients become conscious they are almost always irrational and their movements are too powerful to control. They may in fact tear at their own lung with their fingers and, although they are unable to breathe and expand their lungs, they do not tolerate positive pressure ventilation when it is applied by mouth-to-mouth breathing (expired air resuscitation) or by face masks, with or without a Guedal airway. Every breath that is inadequate for the oxygen requirements of the patient makes the return of ventricular fibrillation a greater possibility. When this degree of restlessness occurs in the powerful adult, it may be essential to produce muscle relaxation by the intravenous injection of *d*-tubocurarine 15–30 mg. Large doses should be avoided because of the association of this drug with hypotension. A normal anaesthetic is then necessary in order to close the chest.

Administration of intracardiac drugs

Giving drugs through the closed chest is largely a waste of time unless performed correctly. The time lost in starting external cardiac massage and ventilation of the lungs very often offsets any benefit that may be derived from the drug itself. Injection of material into the heart is by no means simple. Time is frequently lost in debating the distance of the point chosen from the sternal edge which should be not greater than 1 cm to the left of the sternum. In practice a needle 6–8 cm long is passed through the fourth or fifth intercostal space at the left sternal edge, in the antero-posterior direction (vertically downwards). The heart can also be injected through the diaphragm as in paracentesis (see p. 359).

Defibrillation

Electrical defibrillation of the heart may be performed with greater ease when the electrodes are applied directly to the myocardium, but internal defibrillation has the disadvantage that burning may damage the heart. It should be noted that external defibrillation can still be performed even after a thoracotomy.

Biochemical changes during cardiac arrest

The biochemical changes manifest during and after cardiac arrest are the result of tissue anoxia and the absence of a transport mechanism which removes the products of metabolism to an organ where they are incorporated into the normal biochemical pathway.

Blood oxygen tension

When the arterial blood is analysed it is found to be well saturated with oxygen (e.g. 96%) during external cardiac massage and expired air resuscitation. This degree of arterial blood oxygen saturation is maintained as long as expansion of the lungs with air is continued. Desaturation of arterial blood follows as soon as ventilation is stopped. The fact that fully oxygenated blood is usually obtained from arteries during skilled resuscitation has led one author to suggest that anoxia cannot be the cause of some of the biochemical changes, such as the metabolic acidosis. However, it must be borne in mind that because the flow of fully oxygenated blood is so small, complete extraction of oxygen occurs as blood perfuses the tissues, and samples of both peripheral and central venous blood show complete desaturation (Table 11.2). There is, consequently, during both external and internal cardiac massage, a maximum arteriovenous oxygen difference.

Table 11.2 Blood pH, 'standard bicarbonate', PCO_2 and oxygen saturation in a patient undergoing external cardiac massage because of ventricular fibrillation

	pH	St. bic.	PCO_2	O_2 sat.	PO_2
Arterial	7.07	16.5	75	92	96
Venous	6.99	15.7	92	40	21

pH = Blood pH at 38°C
St. bic. = Standard bicarbonate mmol/l (mEq/l)
PCO_2 = Partial pressure of CO_2 mmHg
O_2 sat. = Oxygen saturation %
PO_2 = Partial pressure of O_2 mmHg
The venous sample was taken from the femoral vein 1 minute before the arterial sample was taken from the femoral artery. The patient was being ventilated with 100% oxygen through an endotracheal tube by means of a rebreathing bag. The cardiac massage was so effective that the patient was 'awake' during the sampling. Successful defibrillation was achieved after treatment with procainamide and infusions of 2.74% $NaHCO_3$. These figures are similar to those found in numerous other cases and can be compared with those seen in haemorrhagic shock.

It is important to note the following points. Cardiac output must be kept at as high a level as possible and during external cardiac massage a number of people, preferably those who have had some training, are required. Arterial desaturation indicates inadequate alveolar ventilation. Furthermore, at any given ventilation rate, the smaller the cardiac output the less probability there is of the arterial blood oxygen tension falling to low levels. This is because the slower the rate of blood flow through the lungs the greater the time there is for gas exchange to take place in the alveolar capillaries.

Movement of water and electrolytes

As a result of an inadequate supply of oxygen to the tissues, certain intrinsic alterations in cellular integrity occur. Water and sodium pass into the intracellular fluid (ICF) from the extracellular fluid (ECF). A rise in the packed cell volume (PCV) and plasma protein content follows as the volume of the ECF is reduced. This phenomenon of haemoconcentration always appears when there is a marked increase in arteriovenous difference of oxygen content and appears to be a function of the venous oxygen content. It also occurs when the heart begins to fail during surface cooling to low temperatures. A decrease in the volume of ECF in the presence of haemorrhagic shock (see p. 185) has been observed. The movements of fluid with changes in body metabolism, including anoxia, have been reviewed by Robinson.[58]

The infusion of relatively dilute (2.74%) $NaHCO_3$ solution tends to reduce haemoconcentration by providing fluid, and therefore reducing blood viscosity and increasing tissue perfusion.

Another aspect of anoxia is the loss of K^+ from the cells and a subsequent rise in plasma concentration. Within a few minutes of the onset of ventricular fibrillation the plasma $[K^+]$ may have reached 7 mmol/l (mEq/l), and rises further as time passes. This does not prevent the re-establishment of a heart beat when calcium salts and sodium bicarbonate are injected either into the heart or intravenously. A rapid fall in the plasma potassium concentration follows when an adequate cardiac output and normal systolic blood pressure have been restored.

A fall in the plasma $[Na^+]$ is frequently observed during the days following cardiac arrest, even when a large volume of $NaHCO_3$ solution has been infused during the arrest period and moderate water restriction has been enforced during the recovery period.

Blood pH

Because of insufficient oxygen, there is a rise in the lactic acid content and a fall in the bicarbonate ion concentration of the ECF. As a result of an inadequate circulation, CO_2 is slowly eliminated so that there is a large arteriovenous difference of CO_2 tension (PCO_2). These factors produce an extremely low blood pH which is often in the region of 6.8 or 6.9. The low pH and low bicarbonate levels in the blood have a profound effect upon myocardial function under many circumstances. This observation is still surrounded by much controversy.

During experiments into profound hypothermia (Kenyon et al., 1959)[37] it was found that after rewarming, the blood pressure would not rise above very low values, the dogs made no spontaneous respiratory effort, there were no reflexes present and all the animals appeared to be decerebrate. When it was noted that at this time the plasma $[HCO_3^-]$ was extremely low (less than 4 mmol/l), steps were taken to correct this base deficit. Isotonic, 1.4% $NaHCO_3$ was infused in an empirical manner until normal plasma concentrations of HCO_3^- were obtained. A remarkable change in the physiological condition of the dogs took place: the dogs were by no means 'decerebrate' when the acid–base state had been corrected. The conjunctival 'eyelash' reflex returned and was present even after sedation with pethidine (Demerol) and during light anaesthesia. The blood pressure rose, there was an excellent cardiac output and a low central venous pressure (CVP). When bicarbonate was infused from the beginning of the operation, no problems in coagulation of the blood occurred and the animals survived with no apparent neurological damage after circulatory arrest for 45 minutes at 9°C in the porta hepatis.

The most significant change, apart from improvements to the neurological status and respiration of the animals, was that which occurred in the myocardium. Vasopressors, such as noradrenaline (norepinephrine), which had previously been ineffective were able to raise the blood pressure without difficulty, though they were not required. Calcium salts, which had also been ineffective, had a powerful inotropic and chronotropic effect when the plasma $[HCO_3^-]$ was normal. Furthermore, cardiac arrhythmias did not occur.

At that time vascular surgery was developing (see p. 13) and it was observed that following replacement of the abdominal aorta, made necessary by an aneurism, a similar condition to that seen in the dogs sometimes developed in man at normal body temperature when the clamps on the aorta and femoral vessels were released. This is sometimes called 'washout acidosis', but at that time, although both isotonic sodium bicarbonate and calcium chloride were given with improvement in the patients' condition, no careful study was made. A similarity was also observed between the dogs at the end of the hypothermia experiments and the patients who underwent vascular surgery, and cardiac arrest in man.

The condition was investigated by Brooks and Feldman[14,15] and a syndrome which was similar to that previously called 'neostigmine-resistant curarization' was described. A recommendation, based on the results reported which demonstrated the presence of a severe metabolic acidosis and many other measurements that had been made, was that bicarbonate solution should be infused *routinely* during cardiac arrest. The solution chosen was 2.74% $NaHCO_3$ which had twice the osmolality of plasma.

The *Lancet*, in an editorial in 1962, noting that the presence of a metabolic acidosis had been reported by other workers, accepted the earlier recommendation by Brooks and Feldman (1962)[14] that bicarbonate solutions should be infused routinely.[44] In the same journal Stewart *et al.*[63] confirmed the presence of a metabolic acidosis during cardiac arrest and also advocated the infusion of bicarbonate solutions.

If resuscitative measures are taken immediately after the onset of cardiac arrest, the development of a major metabolic acidosis is avoided and the fall in $[HCO_3^-]$ may never reach significant levels, although it always develops when the restoration of the heart beat is at all delayed. Immediate measures for the treatment of cardiac arrest are usually taken when it occurs in the operating theatre or fortuitously in hospital, for example in the casualty department or during a ward round. It is under these circumstances that successful resuscitation is most probable. Because there has been insufficient time for a metabolic acidosis to develop, special measures for its correction are frequently unnecessary. Sometimes, however, especially when acute cardiac failure and subsequent fall in systemic blood pressure have preceded ventricular fibrillation, a plasma $[HCO_3^-]$ as low as 8 or 9 mmol/l (mEq/l) can be detected after 1 or 2 minutes.

The restoration of an adequate cardiac output produces some improvement in the degree of metabolic acidosis and this is specially so when the period of circulatory arrest has been short. The low level of plasma HCO_3^- usually lasts 5–6 hours, although 48 hours is quite common and in some patients it may persist for many days. The presence of a metabolic acidosis tends to increase the irritability of the myocardium and can contribute to the recurrence of ventricular fibrillation after a normal rhythm has been obtained. This has been observed even when cardiac arrest has occurred in the casualty department of the hospital and resuscitative measures have not been delayed very long. Electrical defibrillation of the heart, both externally and internally in the presence of the metabolic acidosis, has been found to be impossible. Even when, initially, electrical defibrillation has been successful, effective beating of the heart has not been maintained for longer than a few minutes.

When the metabolic acidosis has been corrected by infusions of hypertonic sodium bicarbonate solution, defibrillation of the heart has been achieved with little difficulty and there has been no tendency for the heart to revert to the abnormal rhythm.

The other aspect of acid–base balance, the retention of CO_2, also requires attention. External cardiac massage may be associated with the fracture of some ribs, so that spontaneous ventilation is impaired. Expansion of the lungs may also be hindered by cardiac failure and pulmonary oedema. For these reasons artificial ventilation may be necessary in the early post-arrest period. When retention of CO_2 develops it is 'uncompensated' because it has occurred acutely and the pH is low. This is a further reason for advocating the routine infusion of sodium bicarbonate in all cases of cardiac arrest (Brooks and Feldman, 1962).[14,15] Sodium lactate was not recommended because the infusion of this substance is not followed by a rise in blood pH or $[HCO_3^-]$ for many hours and, because of the already raised lactate concentration, it may initially contribute to the metabolic acidosis. A report of a case later that same year[63] confirmed that electrical defibrillation of the heart was not possible until the infusion of sodium lactate was replaced with hypertonic sodium bicarbonate.

Because of the decrease in the ECF volume that follows tissue anoxia, a solution of sodium bicarbonate which has twice the osmolality of plasma is probably preferable. In this way expansion of the ECF can take place while the volume of fluid that must be infused in order to correct the metabolic acidosis is kept within convenient limits and an adequate plasma $[Na^+]$ is obtained. Although the use of much stronger solutions has been advocated by other workers who have used them successfully in the process of resuscitation, the 2.74% solution appears in practice to be the safest and most universally applicable. Approximately 500 ml to 1 litre may be required to correct the acidosis that occurs in the adult. Even when electrical defibrillation has been successful in the absence of an infusion of alkali, 500 ml of the 2.74% solution may be required daily for the first 2 or 3 days following arrest, in order to maintain a normal acid–base state. It has been shown by Clowes[20] and Brooks[12] that an abnormal acid–base state may have a profound effect on cardiac output. If excess alkali is infused, it is rapidly excreted in the urine. We have noticed that even after a prolonged period of ventricular fibrillation and periods of gross hypotension, no impairment in renal function has resulted when hypertonic sodium bicarbonate solution has been infused soon after the onset of cardiac arrest. It is possible that the maintenance of a hyperosmolar plasma has contributed to the protection of the kidneys.[11,16,17]

Some protection to the brain may also be given by the early infusion of alkali.[14,37,45]

Tris hydroxymethyl amino-methane (THAM)

This substance, introduced by Nahas for the correction of acid–base deficits in man (see p. 97) is a highly effective buffer. Its effect in assisting defibrillation of the heart in the presence of a gross metabolic acidosis cannot be doubted. Because of its ability to enter the cells it is capable of buffering accumulations of fixed acids in the ICF. It has, however, certain disadvantages that may make it less satisfactory than sodium bicarbonate. It lowers the blood sugar, an effect which may be contraindicated, and it in no way compensates for the movement of Na^+ into the cells. It does, however, effectively lower the K^+ concentration in the plasma. Because sodium bicarbonate is so effective in assisting the resuscitation of even the most severely ill patient and because it is a natural substance which is already present in the body fluids and is available in an immediately administrable form, the author has continued to prefer it to THAM.

Calcium

The effect of Ca^{++} upon the myocardium is antagonistic to that of K^+. For these reasons it is necessary to inject solutions containing freely ionizable calcium either intravenously or directly into the ventricle. An improved heart action is often seen following an injection of calcium gluconate or calcium chloride into the right ventricle. Sudden improvement has been observed after a 'final injection' of calcium salts into the heart has been given, and it seemed that the heart was never going to beat effectively again and that resuscitation was impossible. Calcium chloride is more highly ionized than calcium gluconate and is, therefore, in some ways preferable—10 ml of 10% solution injected into the right ventricle so that it passes through the relatively small volume of blood in the pulmonary circulation and then into the left side of the heart may give rise to spontaneous defibrillation.

However, it must also be recognized that Ca^{++} may itself cause ventricular fibrillation, especially when there is pre-existing digitalis intoxication of a marked degree. When the plasma $[K^+]$ rises as a result of anoxia during circulatory arrest, the factor of digitalis intoxication is neutralized and the injection of calcium salts becomes an essential part of therapy. One must also be aware of the reduced effectiveness of calcium salts in the presence of a marked metabolic acidosis and it may be necessary to correct this aspect of biochemical change before a response to Ca^{++} is observed.

Blood sugar

A rise in the blood sugar concentration is a common association of cardiac arrest as well as of haemorrhagic shock. Values in the region of 15–20 mmol/l (300 to 400 mg%) are quite common in blood taken for analysis after the restoration of an adequate circulation. The blood sugar may be raised for many days following resuscitation and no treatment is required. This may be the result of a process similar to that occurring during gross haemorrhage. It may assist the metabolism of the brain when a normal circulation is re-established and also helps to maintain the osmolality of the body fluids. This was especially noticeable in dogs after cardiac arrest at low temperatures and has since been found to apply to man.

Restoration of the Heart Beat

We have seen how marked biochemical changes are associated with circulatory insufficiency and even when resuscitative measures can be applied at the onset of ventricular fibrillation, immediate steps should be taken towards correcting them. When external cardiac massage is used it may be impossible to inject substances intravenously unless it so happens that an intravenous infusion has been previously established. It is possible to 'cut down' and expose a vein through a small skin incision if the insertion of a cannula through a needle is found to be too difficult.

Electrical defibrillation

Electrical defibrillation of the heart in man was first reported by Beck et al.,[5] although it had been previously demonstrated in dogs in 1899 by Prévost and Battelli[55] who used a high-voltage alternating current of 24 000 to 48 000 volts when the electrodes were placed in the mouth and rectum of the animal and 220 volts when an electrode was placed on the surface of the heart. The use of high-voltage currents for external defibrillation has also been investigated by others,[25,34] but because of the dangers associated with alternating currents of high potential Wiggers[69] recommended that thoracotomy should be performed, because lower voltages were required when the electrodes were applied directly to the heart. He advocated repeated electrical shocks at intervals of 1–1.5 seconds, a method which he referred to as 'serial defibrillation'. In 1939 Gourvich and Juniev described the use of external defibrillation in dogs after 8 minutes of ventricular fibrillation, rhythmical compression of the chest having been performed.[27] The electric shock was supplied by the discharge of a single condenser.[29] In 1956 Zoll et al. described the use of external defibrillation using an alternating current of 180–720 volts when one electrode was placed at the upper end of the sternum and the other just below the left nipple.[71] In 1951 Kouwenhoven described an apparatus[41] which delivered a current of 5 amps at 60 cycles/minute at a potential of 480 volts for 0.25 seconds and in 1961 reported 15 patients who were successfully defibrillated after external cardiac massage.[40]

Many forms of apparatus are now readily available for external defibrillation. Since the work of Lown (1963), who showed that when the electrical impulse was synchronized so that the current was applied at a time that did not coincide with the downstroke of the T wave on the ECG fibrillation was not induced, direct current defibrillators delivering high peak potentials of very short duration have been used with safety.[47] The positioning of the electrodes usually advocated is one at the upper end of the sternum and the other just to the left at the lower end of the sternum. Defibrillation can also be achieved successfully by placing the electrodes on each side of the chest. This method has to be used when the chest is re-opened, after a midsternal incision has been performed for cardiac surgery. The negative electrode is placed near the apex of the heart.

It is usual in the adult to begin with a charge of 200 J (watt/seconds) and to increase the charge by 50-J increments to 400 J (watt/seconds) if the lower charge is unsuccessful.

In the infant the regimen advocated by Harvey and Marcovitch[32] should be used. The charge required is between 20 J and 50 J.

The consequences of cardioversion

Evidence has been presented that repeated electrical cardioversion can produce cardiac necrosis.[24,66,67] The Italian patient quoted below, however, developed no problems following repeated cardioversion, although there was a significant rise in creatinine phosphokinase (CPK) activity. Cann and Corke[18] have reported cardioversion repeated 125 times with no evidence of necrosis. The patient had taken 200 tablets of the tricyclic antidepressant dothiepin HCl (Prothiaden) (each tablet contained 25 mg), and the patient developed ventricular fibrillation which responded to cardioversion of 150 J (watt/seconds). Positive pressure ventilation using 40% oxygen was administered, and over the subsequent 18 hours ventricular fibrillation recurred more than 125 times. On each occasion sinus rhythm was obtained after a shock of 50–150 J. In this particular case, the authors state that the rate of occurrence of ventricular fibrillation was not influenced by the administration of lignocaine, mexiletine, disopyramide, procainamide, magnesium sulphate and phenytoin.

Case history. A 32-year-old Italian woman underwent tricuspid valve replacement which was made necessary by severe rheumatic carditis. She recovered from the operation after a lengthy stay in the intensive care ward. She was about to leave hospital, having been under the care of her own cardiologist when she suddenly collapsed in her room. She was defibrillated immediately and was transferred back to the intensive care ward; she developed ventricular fibrillation a second time, before she could be placed in her bed. During the next 24 hours it was necessary to defibrillate her more than 68 times, and it was found that her plasma $[K^+]$ was 2.8 mmol/l (mEq/l). Her plasma $[Mg^{++}]$ was normal but it was not until 2 g of $MgSO_4$ had been given intravenously that recurrent ventricular fibrillation ceased, although KCl had been infused at a rate of 20 mmol/l per hour and her plasma $[K^+]$ had returned to 4.0 mmol/l (mEq/l). All the cardiac enzymes were raised above normal limits, but there was no impairment of cardiac function. The defibrillator that was used was a very early model which had to be discharged by an attendant after the electrodes had been correctly positioned on the chest wall and held in place by the clinician. The terminology used to instruct the nurse to discharge the defibrillator was 'hit her'. When the patient had recovered and had been placed on a non-effervescent form of oral K^+ replacement containing KCl, she asked "why was it necessary to hit me so often?" Because she was defibrillated on a number of occasions immediately after ventricular fibrillation appeared on the cathode ray oscilloscope, there had been time for her to hear and retain the instruction. She returned to Italy to the publishing firm where she worked with no mental impairment.

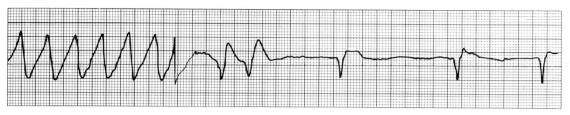

Fig. 11.16　Ventricular escape rhythm following cardioversion. The recording was switched off at the time of the cardioversion. The rhythm prior to cardioversion was a ventricular tachycardia.

Arrhythmias following Cardioversion

Four main abnormal rhythms can be observed following attempted or partially successful defibrillation.

1. A bradycardia is commonly observed which is either a ventricular escape rhythm (Fig. 11.16) or a junctional escape rhythm. Occasionally, as in Fig. 11.17, they may be seen together. Both rhythms may be associated with atrioventricular block. When the junctional beat is conducted aberrantly or when hypoxia is present, the QRS complex may be wide and the differentiation of these two beats may be difficult. The presence of a marked metabolic acidosis may also contribute both to the arrhythmias and to the degree of aberrancy.

It is essential therefore that one should do the following.

(a) Confirm that the lungs are being adequately ventilated, preferably with as high a concentration of O_2 as possible.

(b) Increase the infusion of $NaHCO_3$ and make certain that 100 mmol is given intravenously as rapidly as possible.

(c) Give atropine 0.6 mg i.v. This may be repeated four times at 5-minute intervals. Although we are well aware that atropine will relieve sino-atrial block when P waves are visible on the ECG, it is also effective when they are absent (undetectable). Atropine can restore sinus rhythm even when there appears to be no SA node activity at all and no P waves can be seen in the leads that are being monitored until after it has been given. The total dose of atropine administered should not exceed 2.5 mg.

(d) An intravenous injection of 5–10 ml of 1 : 10 000 adrenaline (epinephrine) may be given and this is often effective, and does not appear to increase the risk of initiating a return of ventricular fibrillation. However, it is sometimes ineffective, in which case an infusion of isoprenaline (isoproterenol) should be begun, 5 mg in 1 litre of 0.9% saline, given at a rate of 10–20 drops/minute, or at a rate that allows the frequency of the heart beat to be maintained above 60 beats/minute in the presence of a systolic blood pressure that is greater than 80 mmHg.

2. A supraventricular rhythm which has a normal or rapid ventricular rate. Although this is often a sinus tachycardia, it is frequently atrial fibrillation. The latter rhythm has been seen to accord a favourable prognosis.[46] This rhythm does not usually occur in the presence of hypoxia or a metabolic acidosis, but when these rhythms are present a satisfactory blood pressure can usually

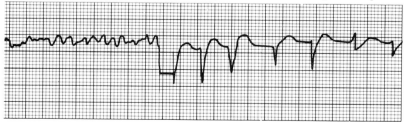

Fig. 11.17　Electrocardiogram (ECG) showing the conversion of ventricular fibrillation into a normally beating heart producing a systolic blood pressure of 120 mmHg. The bizarre, initially ventricular then junctional pattern rapidly gave way to a normal sinus rhythm trace. The ECG was switched off at the time of electrical defibrillation.

be recorded. Correction of atrial fibrillation can usually be obtained by synchronized DC cardioversion. It is safe to give lignocaine, 100–200 mg i.v., in the presence of the supraventricular arrhythmias in order to prevent the recurrence of ventricular fibrillation. A continuous infusion of lignocaine at a rate of 2–4 mg/minute is advisable following restoration of the heart beat.

3. Ventricular asystole. This can be caused by four main factors: hypoxia, a metabolic acidosis, hyperkalaemia, or severe damage to the myocardial muscle. It is necessary to assume in the initial stages that the myocardium has not been damaged, and indeed its presence may never be established except with special staining methods performed *post mortem*.

Therefore it is necessary to do the following.

(a) Confirm that adequate ventilation (preferably with oxygen) is being maintained, and that an endotracheal tube is not misplaced, (e.g. in the oesophagus), or located in a bronchus, so that only one lung is being ventilated. When expired air resuscitation is being performed it should be established that the neck is extended, the tongue is not occluding the airway and that expansion of the lungs is being achieved.

(b) Infuse a further 100 mmol of $NaHCO_3$.

(c) Inject into the heart, through the 4th or 5th intercostal space (see p. 399), 3 ml of 1:10 000 adrenaline (epinephrine) or give 1 ml of 1 : 1000 or 10 ml of 1 : 10 000 adrenaline intravenously. Note that external cardiac massage should be continued throughout the injection, except when the intracardiac injection is being performed. Both the intracardiac and intravenous injections can be repeated at 5-minute intervals.

(d) Calcium chloride 5 ml into the heart or 10 ml intravenously can also be given before the injection of adrenaline (epinephrine) is repeated. The calcium solution can be added to the syringe containing 1–3 ml of 1 : 10 000 adrenaline.

(e) When asystole is due to a high plasma $[K^+]$ it is almost always in clinical practice iatrogenic and results from the infusion of KCl at a rate that is greater than 20 mmol (mEq/hour). On many occasions it is because 40 mmol of KCl have been added to the burette of a giving-set used in the recovery room or intensive care ward, and the rate of administration has inadvertently been increased. It is necessary to perform external cardiac massage and ventilation until the high plasma $[K^+]$ has been dispersed, to give calcium salts (e.g. $CaCl_2$ 10 ml i.v.) to correct the metabolic acidosis and, if necessary, to administer adrenaline (epinephrine) or isoprenaline as described above.

4. Recurrent ventricular fibrillation. Recurrent or persistent ventricular fibrillation is a common problem. Initially, it has to be assumed that it can be corrected by adequate ventilation and oxygenation, by correcting the metabolic acidosis, raising the voltage of the electrical activity of the fibrillating heart by means of 1–3 ml of 1 : 10 000 adrenaline into the heart together with 5–10 ml of calcium gluconate 10% or $CaCl_2$ 10%. This should be tried before repeating a DC shock of 300–400 J in the adult. A bolus injection of 200–300 mg lignocaine (lidocaine) can be given intravenously. Propranolol 1 mg i.v. may also be effective, as may procainamide 300 mg i.v. Bretylium tosylate 300–400 mg i.v. can assist in achieving conversion from ventricular fibrillation, sometimes without repeating the DC cardioversion.

Internal defibrillation

When the chest has been opened one electrode is placed behind the heart and the other in front and a single electric shock of between 10 and 20 J (watt/seconds) is given. Greater current values are unnecessary and expose the heart to a greater risk of damage.[38] If defibrillation is not successful, the voltage is increased by degrees from the lower to the higher figure and the duration of the shock gradually made longer. If this is ineffective, then a number of single shocks may be given at rapid intervals as advocated by Wiggers.[69]

Immediately following the electric shock the heart goes into a period of asystole and after a short space of time bizarre QRS complexes appear on the ECG which gradually transform into a normal pattern (Fig. 11.17). Initially, there may be complete dissociation of the atrial and ventricular impulses, but as time passes a sinus rhythm is normally resumed.

Adrenaline (epinephrine)
When the patient is first seen the heart may be still and asystolic or the rate of fibrillation may be so slow that the heart appears to be in asystole, even when the chest has been opened, for example after open-heart surgery. Such a heart is difficult to defibrillate. Asystole and slow ventricular fibrillation may be converted into rapid ventricular fibrillation by injecting 0.5–2.0 ml 1 : 10 000 solution of adrenaline (epinephrine) into the right ventricle. Even when ventricular defibrillation is possible, the heart frequently returns to its previous state of ventricular fibrillation within a very short space of time. Further treatment should then be applied.

Injections into the heart through the chest wall

Injections into the heart are made through the 4th and 5th intercostal spaces. It is well recognized from ultrasound echograms that during life the only area that does not have lung anterior to, and therefore covering, the heart is approximately 2.5 cm (1 inch) wide, lateral to the left sternal border. This applies to most people, although in some the area free from lung may be a little narrower or a little wider.

Injection through the chest wall in the adult is best performed 1 cm (or one finger's breadth) lateral to the left sternal border in the 4th or 5th intercostal space, at right angles to the chest wall (the cardiac needle should pass immediately antero-posteriorly). The plunger should be withdrawn *gently* until blood is seen to enter the syringe. The solution in the syringe is then injected into the right ventricle. External cardiac massage is continued up to the time of performing the injection and recommenced immediately following the injection.

Injection of the heart may also be performed by passing the cardiac needle into the heart from below the diaphragm. The needle is passed through the skin of the upper abdominal wall and directed upwards (cephalad) 1 cm to the left of the sternum and through the combined layers of the diaphragm and parietal pericardium. The left ventricle is entered and blood can be withdrawn into the syringe before the injection is made.

Correction of acid–base changes

We have already discussed how the early correction of the deficit of base that accrues during hypoxia and circulatory insufficiency may be essential to the well-being of the patient (see p. 400). The effect of infusions of sodium bicarbonate in allowing easy low-voltage electrical defibrillation to take place is often quite dramatic. It has frequently been observed that the cardiac output, after defibrillation, is markedly increased when the metabolic acidosis is corrected. Often a slow fibrillation may be converted into a rapid, coarse fibrillation by means of sodium bicarbonate infusions alone and spontaneous defibrillation can then sometimes occur. The metabolic acidosis should always be corrected because of these factors and because the myocardial function is improved and the tendency to fibrillate again, after the heart beat has been re-established, is reduced.

Although there are many schemes for assessing the amount of alkali required from plasma bicarbonate concentrations, they are in practice of very little value because of the poor perfusion rates that are present during and after circulatory arrest. These do not allow the blood to reflect tissue acid–base characteristics accurately. The degree of metabolic acidosis depends upon the following.

1. The metabolic state and cardiac output of the patient before cardiac arrest.
2. The time that elapses between cardiac arrest and the provision of cardiac massage and ventilation.
3. The effectiveness of the cardiac massage, whether internal or external, and the ventilation of the lungs.
4. The length of time that elapses from the onset of cardiac massage.

A sample taken shortly after the onset of cardiac arrest may show a relatively normal $[HCO_3^-]$ in the plasma, but after a few minutes of external cardiac massage when some degree of tissue perfusion will have taken place a second plasma sample will reveal a very low plasma bicarbonate concentration (Table 11.3). Treatment therefore can only be given satisfactorily by infusing volumes of sodium bicarbonate solution that are safe, effective and of a suitable tonicity. For reasons that we have already discussed, the most suitable solution to use is one that contains 2.74% $NaHCO_3$, with twice the osmolality of plasma. The 60-kg adult can safely be infused with 200 ml (67 mmol, mEq) of this solution in 10–15 minutes; 500 ml (166 mmol, mEq) may be required before any effect is observed and this volume can be infused with safety over a period of 20–30 minutes; 3–3.5 ml/kg body weight should be infused in the first instance. In the large adult greater quantities may be required and in the very young both the initial and final quantities have to be reduced proportionally; when possible, frequent readings of pH and assessments of PCO_2 and plasma bicarbonate should be taken so that there is some indication of the quantitative acid–base change that is taking place. It must be borne in mind, however, that the distribution of the infused solution throughout the fluid spaces of the body is relatively slow and raised concentrations of HCO_3^- are rapidly reduced as partitioning between the compartments takes place. Because of this, and also because excessive bicarbonate levels are corrected by means of renal excretion, a moderately raised blood pH and $[HCO_3^-]$ following a rapid infusion of alkali should not be considered to indicate that too great a volume of $NaHCO_3$ has been infused. Between 100 and 350 mmol (mEq) of $NaHCO_3$ will be required by the average adult.

Table 11.3 Blood pH, 'standard bicarbonate', PCO_2 and oxygen saturation in a patient undergoing external cardiac massage because of ventricular fibrillation

	pH	St. bic.	PCO_2	O_2 sat.	PCV
1	7.22	18.4	56	97	43
2	6.95	11.8	76	94	46

pH = Blood pH at 38°C
St. bic. = Standard bicarbonate mmol/l (mEq/l)
PCO_2 = Partial pressure of CO_2 mmHg
O_2 sat. = Oxygen saturation %
PCV = Packed cell volume %
Sample 1 was taken from the femoral artery at the beginning of external cardiac massage, the patient's lungs being inflated with oxygen. Sample 2 was taken 5 minutes later from the femoral artery before an infusion of sodium bicarbonate solution had been begun. Note the rise in packed cell volume.

The solution may be injected directly into the right ventricle, but when this is done it must be borne in mind that, unlike protein, electrolytes can diffuse across the alveolar capillary membrane and, therefore, produce pulmonary oedema. This is a greater hazard when the rate of infusion is rapid and the concentration of the solution is high. For this reason greater caution should be observed when this method of administration is used and the 8.4% solution containing 1 mmol/ml should never be given into the right ventricle. Solutions of $NaHCO_3$ in concentrations greater than 2.74% should always be given intravenously.

Calcium salts
A slow fibrillation is quite commonly converted into a rapid coarse form when calcium salts are administered, so that large quantities repeated at frequent intervals may be necessary. In the adult 5 ml of 10% solution of calcium gluconate may be injected into the right ventricle in the first instance and if this is ineffective repeated doses of 10 ml of the 10% solution may be given. In some cases it is necessary to use calcium chloride and doses of up to 10 ml of the 10% solution can be given at intervals. Spontaneous defibrillation has been observed following the use of calcium salts and they very often improve the heart action after electrical defibrillation, so that there is a marked rise in arterial blood pressure and an associated fall in central venous pressure (CVP).

Procaine and lignocaine
Lignocaine is used in order to facilitate defibrillation. It should be given intravenously in doses of 200 mg (10 ml of a 2% solution). Lignocaine can also be given in divided doses of 5 ml (100 mg) down the endotracheal tube as it is rapidly absorbed

from the lungs. It will also help in humidification.

Procaine HCl, procainamide (Pronestyl) and lignocaine (lidocaine, Xylocaine) slow down the rate at which the heart is fibrillating and may cause spontaneous defibrillation to occur.[51] On numerous occasions these substances have been found to facilitate electrical defibrillation. They may, however, depress the myocardium so that only weak, slow fibrillations occur. It is then impossible to revert the heart to a normal rhythm. The action of these substances is very largely reversed by adrenaline (epinephrine) or by one of the vasopressors acting primarily upon the heart, such as methylamphetamine, and these should be used if too slow a rate is observed to be present.

Procaine HCl and procainamide should be given intravenously in doses of 100–200 mg which should be repeated until the desired effect is observed, either by direct observation of the heart during internal cardiac massage or on the ECG.

Bretylium tosylate (Bretylate)
This substance was introduced as a hypotensive agent. It acts in this way by adrenergic neuron blockade. Although it is probably not suitable for routine use as an anti-arrhythmic agent, there are a number of reports (see p. 333) of it causing spontaneous defibrillation during cardiac arrest. It is given in doses of 5 mg/kg body weight or 350 mg i.v. to a 70-kg man. Its mode of action in causing spontaneous defibrillation is unknown, but its effectiveness in this respect can be confirmed by the author. Hypotension following restoration of the heart beat can be corrected using a vasopressor that has a vasoconstrictive action, such as metaraminol or *l*-noradrenaline.

Adrenaline (epinephrine)
The injection of adrenaline (epinephrine) intravenously 2 ml of 1 : 1000 solution may help in the restoration of the heart beat, but its main benefit is in improving the cardiac output during combined ventilation and external cardiac massage. An improved perfusion of the tissues is obtained but the pupils may dilate.

Isoprenaline sulphate (isoproterenol)
This sympathomimetic drug, which acts almost exclusively on the beta-receptors (see p. 291), is a potent cardiac stimulant and is given intravenously. It has both a positive inotropic and positive chronotropic effect. It may give rise to ventricular fibrillation after producing a rapid tachycardia, but during the past decade its widespread use intravenously has indicated that it is

not as dangerous a preparation as was previously thought. When used on selected cases it is considered by many clinicians to have *anti*-arrhythmic properties. It is the author's experience that when the cardiac output is improved, and consequently coronary blood flow is increased, there is quite definitely an anti-arrhythmic action. This has been noted by other clinicians who have treated cardiogenic shock occurring in a wide variety of conditions, such as post-myocardial infarction, toxic shock and drug toxicity (e.g. tricyclic antidepressant re-entry arrhythmias). It produces vasodilatation and bronchial relaxation.

If the cardiac rate is slow and the force of contraction of the myocardium is weak, following cardiac arrest, so that the blood pressure is inadequate, 2 mg of isoprenaline (isopropyl-noradrenaline, isoproterenol) may be added to 500 ml of isotonic saline and infused at 5–10 drops (2–4 µg) per minute or at a rate which is just sufficient to maintain an adequate blood pressure.

It may be necessary to continue this infusion for 48 hours or more and while there may be an increased tendency for ventricular fibrillation to recur in some patients, isoprenaline can be a valuable form of therapy, maintaining a normal heart rate and blood pressure in these special circumstances.

Beta-blockers

The action of beta-adrenergic blocking agents has been discussed in relation to other cardiac arrhythmias. These are sometimes of value in restoring a heart that is difficult to defibrillate when the acidosis has been corrected and other forms of treatment, such as procainamide, have been given.

The preparation propranolol (Inderal) has been shown to be of value[62] in preventing a recurrence of ventricular fibrillation. It should be given intravenously in doses of 1 mg. Practolol in doses of 5 mg i.v. is also of value.

Failure of external chest compression

The following case illustrates the steps to be taken when external defibrillation or external cardiac massage is unsuccessful.

Case history. A 40-year-old patient was sent to the casualty department because of pain in the chest. His blood pressure was 130/70 mmHg. The pain, which was typical of coronary occlusion, became increasingly severe so that he was given 15 mg of morphine, but within 5 minutes, while an ECG was being arranged, ventricular fibrillation occurred. External cardiac massage and positive pressure ventilation with a mask were begun immediately. An endotracheal tube was inserted a few minutes later. External defibrillation was attempted, but was unsuccessful. External chest compression over the lower end of the sternum failed to produce a palpable pulse.

The chest was opened and internal cardiac massage performed and defibrillation attempted. The internal bimanual cardiac massage produced palpable carotid and femoral pulses and the pupils remained small. 200 mg of procainamide were given intravenously and electrical defibrillation attempted. This was again unsuccessful. Defibrillation was achieved following a second injection of 200 mg of procainamide, but it was not maintained for more than a few seconds. Calcium chloride and procainamide were given repeatedly until 1200 mg of the latter had been administered, but a normal rhythm was not maintained for very long and not all the attempts at electrical defibrillation were effective. A blood sample taken at that time demonstrated a marked metabolic acidosis (Table 11.4). An infusion of 2.74% $NaHCO_3$ was given, 500 ml being infused over a period of 20 minutes, and electrical defibrillation was then successfully performed and the blood pressure rose almost immediately to 120/20 mmHg.

Table 11.4   Arterial blood pH, 'standard bicarbonate', PCO_2 and PCV in the patient resuscitated after cardiac arrest

	pH	St. bic.	PCO_2	PCV
1	6.91	10.5	70.0	49
2	7.25	15.3	33.5	44
3	7.46	25.5	37.0	37

pH = Blood pH at 38°C
St. bic. = Standard bicarbonate mmol/l (mEq/l)
PCO_2 = Partial pressure of CO_2 mmHg
PCV = Packed cell volume %
Sample 1 was taken before the infusion of $NaHCO_3$ when defibrillation was not possible. Sample 2 was taken 45 minutes after defibrillation, 500 ml of 2.74% $NaHCO_3$ having been infused. Sample 3 was taken 1 hour later when a further 400 ml of the same solution had been infused.

While the chest was being closed a blue infarcted area, 2.5 cm in diameter, was observed anteriorly on the left ventricle of the heart. Over 1 hour had elapsed from the onset of ventricular fibrillation. A further 540 ml of $NaHCO_3$ 2.74% was infused over 4 hours. The patient breathed spontaneously at the end of the anaesthetic and continued to maintain a blood pressure of 120/70 mmHg. He was not digitalized and no diuretic was necessary. The non-sterile thoracotomy did not become infected and no renal dysfunction developed.

This patient was very fortunate because many patients require assisted ventilation, digitalis or amrinone (see p. 289) has to be given because of cardiac failure and careful watch has to be maintained on water and electrolyte metabolism.

Resuscitation Trolley

Equipment and apparatus

Apparatus for positive pressure ventilation
Brook airway.

A self-inflating rebreathing bag (Ambu, Dräger, Ruben, BOC) correctly fitted to take face masks of various sizes.

Endotracheal tubes of all sizes with connections to rebreathing bag filled from an oxygen cylinder or the self-inflating bag.

Guedal airways.

Apparatus for tracheal intubation and toilet
Oxygen cylinder fitted with reducing valve, pressure gauge and flow meter.

Connections and tubing and anaesthetic bag for positive pressure ventilation through a mask.

Laryngoscope.

Catheters for suction.

Suction apparatus, either electrical or foot operated such as the Ambu suction apparatus.

Instruments for thoracotomy
Two scalpels (with one large blade (No. 24) and one small blade (No. 15)).

One easily assembled rib retractor, sufficiently powerful to allow access to the interior of the thorax when the incision made is too small.

One pair of dissecting (toothed) forceps.

One pair of medium-sized scissors for opening the pericardium.

Numerous sterile swabs, double wrapped in paper bags.

Four pairs of sterile surgical gloves.

Defibrillator
Apparatus for both external and internal defibrillation with electrodes of varying size. The electrodes used for internal defibrillation should be kept in easily opened sterile containers.

Medicines and pharmaceutical preparations
2.74% and 8.4% $NaHCO_3$ solution and drip sets for intravenous infusion.

Calcium chloride 10% solution.

Calcium gluconate 10% solution.

Lignocaine 1% or 2% solution.

Bretylium tosylate 100 mg in 2 ml.

Procainamide 100 mg/ml.

Procaine hydrochloride 1% solution.

Verapamil 5 mg in 2 ml.

Disopyramide.

Propranolol.

Practolol.

Adrenaline (epinephrine) 1 : 1000 for intravenous injection during arrest.

Adrenaline 1 : 10 000 solution for intracardiac injection.

Methylamphetamine ampoules containing 30 mg in 1.5 ml.

Mephenteramine 15 mg/ml.

l-noradrenaline.

d-tubocurarine.

Neostigmine.

Nalorphine 10 mg/ml.

Naloxone 0.02 mg/ml and 0.4 mg/ml.

Atropine 0.6 or 0.1 mg/ml.

Aminophylline 250 mg/10 ml.

Hydrocortisone for intravenous injection.

Methylprednisolone for intravenous injection.

Pentolinium tartrate for subcutaneous injection 5 mg/ml.

Isoprenaline 0.2 mg in 5 ml and isoprenaline 2 mg in 2 ml.

Frusemide 40 mg in 2 ml.

Ethacrynic acid for intravenous injection 50 mg.

Bumetanide 2 mg in 4 ml.

Dextrose 50%.

Summary of steps to be taken in emergency resuscitation

When alone
1. While maintaining an unobstructed airway, inflate the lungs as fully as possible once by means of expired air resuscitation, mouth-to-mouth (see Fig. 11.8) or mouth-to-nose ventilation, Brook airway or self-inflating bag and call for immediate assistance. Thump the lower end of sternum.

2. Apply external cardiac massage five or six times to the lower end of the sternum before inflating the lungs each time.

3. The patient, if in bed, should be placed upon a board or hard surface, if this is physically possible, and external cardiac massage continued at the rate of 60–80/minute.

4. The lungs should be inflated fully with one breath every five to eight compressions of the sternum.

5. Observe the pupils for size at the end of each period of external cardiac massage, so that its effectiveness can be assessed.

6. If assistance has not arrived and the external cardiac massage has not reduced the size of the pupils, an emergency thoracotomy can be performed, preferably through the fourth or fifth left intercostal space. It is then possible to continue internal cardiac massage and expired air resuscitation until help arrives, but in practice, except in the small child, this is extremely difficult.

7. If possible, attempt defibrillation with 300 J immediately.

When a resuscitation team is available

1. The patient should be placed on a hard surface preferably with the legs and feet raised; inflation of the lungs and external cardiac massage at 60–80/minute should be started immediately.

2. An endotracheal tube should be passed as soon as possible and the lungs inflated with oxygen. Positive pressure should be applied during a pause after every six to eight compressions of the lower end of the sternum. During other compressions of the thorax the lungs should be inflated *in unison* with the compression in order *to raise* the intrathoracic pressure.

3. An injection 2 ml of 1 : 1000 adrenaline should be given intravenously.

4. The carotid pulses should be felt and the size of the pupils observed. An ECG should be connected to the patient.

5. External defibrillation should be attempted as *early as possible*. It is important to note that external defibrillation can be used even after the chest wall has been opened and is used routinely after re-opening a midline split sternum incision.

6. An intravenous infusion of 2.74% sodium bicarbonate should be set up as soon after cardiac arrest as is feasible and a minimum of 200 ml (66 mmol, mEq) administered in the first 10 minutes and the drip continued until 500 ml (175 mmol, mEq/l) has been given over a period of 20–30 minutes. Another 500 ml may be required and can be given safely over the next period of 30 minutes. If the intravenous drip is running slowly, the bottle

of 2.74% $NaHCO_3$ should be replaced with one containing the 8.4% solution, (1 mmol/ml, mEq/ml), or the 4.2% solution.

7. If defibrillation by electrical means is difficult, it may be because of anoxia of the myocardium resulting from inadequate ventilation or external cardiac massage, or from inadequate correction of the metabolic acidosis. When these factors do not apply and the heart rate is rapid then calcium gluconate or calcium chloride (10 ml of 10% solution) or procainamide (Pronestyl) 100–200 mg of lignocaine (lidocaine, Xylocaine) 25 mg may be given intravenously. Propranolol (Inderal) 1–2 mg may also be given intravenously and, by its beta-adrenergic blocking action, may both facilitate defibrillation and assist in maintaining a normal rhythm. Bretylium tosylate 350–400 mg may, in addition to assisting defibrillation, induce spontaneous conversion to sinus rhythm.

8. If external cardiac massage is observed to be ineffective in maintaining an adequate perfusion as judged by absence of pulses and inability to make the pupils constrict, or if external electrical defibrillation is found to be impossible in some cases, the chest should be opened, through the 4th or 5th intercostal space.

9. When the heart is found to be flaccid and the fibrillations weak and slow then, if calcium chloride is found to be ineffective, 0.5–3.0 ml of 1 : 10 000 solution of adrenaline (epinephrine) can be injected into the right ventricle, and massage of the heart continued until an improvement in both tone and rate of fibrillation is obtained.

10. Once electrical defibrillation has been achieved, it is important that adequate ventilation with oxygen is continued, the metabolic acidosis corrected with alkali and the blood pressure maintained. If there has been a major haemorrhage, then blood transfusion should be given or plasma or dextran infused. If these measures and the continued injection of calcium salts are not effective, it may be necessary to give vasopressors.

11. In the post-arrest period care must be taken to treat cardiac failure with diuretics and, if necessary, with digitalis; to correct arrhythmias with oral propranolol, procainamide, disopyramide or tocainide, or if necessary intravenous lignocaine, verapamil and other anti-arrhythmic agents (see pp. 310 and 332); to observe any reduction in urine output and specific gravity;[10] to maintain correct fluid, electrolyte and acid–base balance; to treat cerebral anoxia with sedation, cooling and moderate dehydration; and to administer antibiotics, if necessary, intravenously.

References

1. Altemeier, W. A. and Todd, J. (1963). Studies on the incidence of infection following open chest cardiac massage for cardiac arrest. *Ann. Surg.*, **158**, 596.

2. Arden, G. P., Harrison, S. H., Lister, S. and Maudsley, R. H. (1956). Lightning accident at Ascot. *Brit. med. J.*, **1**, 1450.

3. Bailey, R. A. Browse, N. L. and Keating, V. J. (1964). Automatic external cardiac massage: a portable pneumatic external cardiac compression machine. *Brit. Heart J.*, **26**, 481.

4. Baringer, J. R., Salzman, E. W., Jones, W. A. and Friedlich, A. L. (1961). External cardiac massage. *New Engl. J. of Med.*, **265**, 62.

5. Beck, C. S., Pritchard, W. H. and Feil, H. S. (1947). Ventricular fibrillation of long duration abolished by electric shock. *J. Amer. med. Assoc.*, **135**, 985.

6. Boehm, R. (1877). Ueber Wiederbelebung nach Vergiftungen und Asphyxie. *Arch. exp. Path. Pharmak.*, **8**, 68.

7. Brook, M. H. (1960). Discussion on artificial respiration. *Proc. roy. Soc. Med.*, **53**, 311.

8. Brook, M. H. and Brook, J. (1960). Direct artificial respiration (D.A.R.): present-day teaching and group training requirements. *Canad. med. Assoc. J.*, **82**, 245.

9. Brook, M. H., Brook, J. and Wyant, G. M. (1962). Emergency resuscitation. *Brit. med. J.*, **2**, 1564.

10. Brooks, D. K. (1958). The modern treatment of anuria and oliguria. *Postgrad. med. J.*, **34**, 583.

11. Brooks, D. K. (1964). Osmolar, electrolyte and respiratory changes in hemorrhagic shock. *Amer. Heart J.*, **68**, 574.

12. Brooks, D. K. (1965). Physiological responses produced by changes in acid–base equilibrium following profound hypothermia. *Anaesthesia*, **20**, 173.

13. Brooks, D. K. (1967). *Resuscitation*, 1st edn, p. 254. London: Edward Arnold.

14. Brooks, D. K. and Feldman, S. A. (1962). Cardiac arrest and acidosis. *Lancet*, **i**, 1111.

15. Brooks, D. K. and Feldman, S. A. (1962). Metabolic acidosis: a new approach to 'neostigmine resistant curarisation'. *Anaesthesia*, **17**, 161.

16. Brooks, D. K., Williams, W. G., Manley, R. W. and Whiteman, P. (1963). Osmolar and electrolyte changes in haemorrhagic shock: hypertonic solutions in the prevention of tissue damage. *Lancet*, **i**, 521.

17. Brooks, D. K., Williams, W. G., Manley, R. W. and Whiteman, P. (1963). Respiratory changes in haemorrhagic shock. *Anaesthesia*, **18**, 363.

18. Cann, P. A. and Corke, C. F. (1981). Cardioversion 125 times without necrosis. *Brit. med. J.*, **282**, 1835.

19. Chandra, N., Weisfeldt, M. L., Tsitlik, J., Vaghaiwalla, F., Snyder, L. D., Hoffecker, M. and Rudikoff, M. T. (1981). Augmentation of carotid flow during cardiopulmonary resuscitation by ventilation at high airway pressure simultaneous with chest compression. *Amer. J. Cardiol.*, **48**, 1053.

20. Clowes, G. H. A., Alichniewicz, A., Del Guercio, L. R. M. and Gillespie, D. (1960). The relationship of postoperative acidosis to pulmonary and cardiovascular function. *J. thorac. cardiovasc. Surg.*, **39**, 1.

21. Critcheley, M. (1934). Neurological effects of lightning and electricity. *Lancet*, **i**, 66.

22. Croton, L. M. (1960). Recent developments in techniques of artificial respiration. *J. Inst. Sci. Technol.*, **6** (No. 2), 5.

23. Culpepper, R. M. (1975). Bleeding diathesis in fresh water drowning. *Ann. Int. Med.*, **83**, 675.

24. Dahl, C. F., Ewy, G. A., Warner, E. D. and Thomas, E. D. (1974). Myocardial necrosis from direct current countershock. *Circulation*, **50**, 956.

25. Ferris, L. P., King, B. G., Spence, P. W. and Williams, H. B. (1936). The effect of electrical shock on the heart. *Elect. Engng.*, **55**, 498.

26. Fuller, R. H. (1963). The clinical pathology of human near-drowning. *Proc. roy. Soc. Med.*, **56**, 33.

27. Gourvitch, N. L. and Juniev, G. S. (1939). Sur l'arrêt des tremulations fibrillaires du coeur par une décharge électrique. *Byull. éksp. Biol. Med.*, **8**, 56.

28. Greene, D. G., Elam, J. O., Dobkin, A. B. and Studley, C. L. (1961). Cinefluorographic study of hyperextension of the neck and upper airway patency. *J. Amer. med. Assoc.*, **176**, 570.

29. Gurvich, N. L. and Yuniev, G. S. (1947). Restoration of heart rhythm during fibrillation by a condenser discharge. *Amer. Rev. sov. Med.*, **4**, 252.

30. Harries, M. (1985). Deaths of athletes. *Brit. med. J.*, **290**, 656.

31. Harries, M. G., Golden, F. St. C. and Fowler, M. (1981). Ventricular fibrillation as a complication of salt-water immersion. *Brit. med. J.*, **283**, 347.

32. Heilman, K. M. and Muschenheim, C. (1965). Primary cutaneous tuberculosis resulting from mouth-to-mouth respiration. Report of a case. *New Eng. J. of Med.*, **273**, 1035.

33. Harvey, D. and Marcovitch, H. (1983). Paediatric emergencies. In *Modern Emergency Department Practice*, p. 302. Edited by D. K. Brooks and A. J. Harrold. London: Edward Arnold.

34. Hooker, D. R., Kouwenhoven, W. B. and Langworthy, O. R. (1933). The effect of alternating electrical currents on the heart. *Amer. J. Physiol.*, **103**, 444.

35. Jude, J. R., Kouwenhoven, W. B. and Knickerbocker, G. G. (1961). Cardiac arrest. Report of application of external cardiac massage on 118 patients. *J. Amer. med. Ass.*, **178**, 1063.

36. Keating, V. J. (1952). A simple pulse indicator. *Brit. med. J.*, **1**, 1188.

37. Kenyon, J. R., Ludbrook, J., Downs, A. R., Tait, I. B., Brooks, D. K. and Pryczkowski, J. (1959).

Experimental deep hypothermia. *Lancet*, **ii**, 41.

38. Kerber, R. E., Carter, J. Klein, S., Grayzel, J. and Kennedy, J. (1980). Open chest defibrillation during cardiac surgery: energy and current requirements. *Amer. J. Cardiol.*, **46**, 393.

39. Klassen, G. A., Broadhurst, C., Peretz, D. I. and Johnson, A. L. (1963). Cardiac resuscitation in 126 medical patients using external cardiac massage. *Lancet*, **i**, 1290.

40. Kouwenhoven, W. B., Jude, J. R. and Knickerbocker, G. G. (1961). Heart activation in cardiac arrest. *Mod. Conc. cardiov. Dis.*, **30**, 639.

41. Kouwenhoven, W. B. and Kay, J. H. (1951). A simple electrical apparatus for the clinical treatment of ventricular fibrillation. *Surgery*, **30**, 781.

42. Kouwenhoven, W. B., Milnor, W. R., Knickerbocker, G. G. and Chesnut, W. R. (1957). Closed chest defibrillation of the heart. *Surgery*, **42**, 550.

43. Lancet (1960). Annotation: Fatal shock from a cardiac monitor. *Lancet*, **i**, 872.

44. Lancet (1962). Annotation. Acidosis in cardiac arrest. *Lancet*, **ii**, 976.

45. Ledingham, I. McA. and Norman, J. N. (1962). Acid-base studies in experimental circulatory arrest. *Lancet* **ii**, 967.

46. Liberthson, R. R., Nagel, E. L., Hirschman, J. C. and Nussenfeld, J. D. (1974). Prehospital ventricular defibrillation. Prognosis and follow-up course. *New Engl. J. of Med.*, **291**, 317.

47. Lown, B., Kaid Bey, S., Perlroth, M. G. and Abe, T. (1963). Comparative studies of ventricular vulnerability to fibrillation. *J. clin. Invest.*, **42**, 953.

48. Marriott, H. L. (1951). Lightning effects. In *Medical Treatment—Principles and Their Application*, p. 300. Edited by G. Evans. London: Butterworth.

49. Miles, S. (1962). *Underwater medicine*. London: Staple Press.

50. Miles, S. (1968). Drowning. *Brit. med. J.*, **3**, 597.

51. Milstein, B. B. and Brock, R. (1954). Ventricular fibrillation during cardiac surgery. *Guy's Hosp. Rep.*, **103**, 213.

52. Modell, J. H. (1968). The pathophysiology and treatment of drowning. *Acta. Anaesth. Scand.*, **29** (Suppl.), 263.

53. Morgan, R. R. (1961). Laceration of the liver from closed-chest cardiac massage. *New Engl. J. of Med.*, **265**, 82.

54. Neil, E. (1965). Biochemical disturbances as a cause of cardiac arrest. In *Resuscitation and cardiac pacing*, p. 41. Edited by G. Shaw, G. Smith and T. J. Thompson. London: Cassell.

55. Prévost, J. L. and Battelli, F. (1900). Sur quelques effets des décharges électriques sur le coeur des mammifères. *J. Physiol. Path. gén.*, **2**, 40.

56. Ravitch, M. M., Lane, R., Safar, P., Steichen, F. M. and Knowles, R. (1961). Lightning stroke. Report of a case with recovery after cardiac massage and prolonged artificial respiration. *New Eng. J. of Med.*, **264**, 36.

57. Rivers, J. F., Orr, G. and Lee, H. A. (1970). Drowning. Its clinical sequelae and management. *Brit. med. J.*, **2**, 157.

58. Robinson, J. R. (1960). Metabolism of intracellular water. *Physiol. Rev.*, **40**, 112.

59. Schallock, G. (1957). Uber Eine ungewohnliche Form von Blitzschlagfolgen. *Zbl. Allg. Path.*, **88**, 245.

60. Schmidt, W., Grützner, A. and Schoen, H. R. (1957). Beobachlagfolgen bie Blitzschlagverletzungen unt er Berucksichtigung von Ekg. and Eef. *Deutsch. Arch. Klin. Med.*, **204**, 307.

61. Silverman, N. M. (1936). Unilateral deafness as a sequel to non-fatal lightning trauma. *J. Indiana Med. Ass.*, **29**, 530.

62. Sloman, G., Robinson, J. S. and McLean, K. (1965). Propranolol (Inderal) in persistent ventricular fibrillation. *Brit. med. J.*, **1**, 895.

63. Stewart, J. S. S., Stewart, W. K. and Gillies, H. G. (1962). Cardiac arrest and acidosis. *Lancet*, **ii**, 964.

64. Swann, H. G. and Brucer, M. (1951). The sequence of circulatory, respiratory and cerebral failure during the process of death; its relation to resuscitability. *Tex. Rep. Biol. Med.*, **9**, 180.

65. Taussig, H. B. (1968). "Death" from lightning—and the possibility of living again. *Ann. Int. Med.*, **68**, 1345.

66. Van Vleet, J. F., Thacker, W. A., Jr., Geddes, L. A. and Ferrans, V. J. (1977). Acute cardiac damage in dogs given multiple transthoracic shocks with a trapezoid wave generator. *Am. J. Vet. Res.*, **38**, 617.

67. Warner, E. D., Dahl, C. and Ewy, G. A. (1975). Myocardial injury from transthoracic defibrillator countershock. *Arch. Path.*, **99**, 55.

68. Whitby, J. D. (1962). Some early manuals of resuscitation. *Anaesthesia*, **17**, 365.

69. Wiggers, C. J. (1936). Cardiac massage followed by countershock in revival of mammalian ventricles from fibrillation due to coronary occlusion. *Amer. J. Physiol.*, **116**, 161.

70. Wood, P. (1956). *Diseases of the heart and circulation*, 2nd ed., p. 356. London: Eyre & Spottiswoode.

71. Zoll, P. M., Paul, M. H., Linenthal, A. J., Norman, L. R. and Gibson, W. (1956). The effects of external electric currents on the heart. Control of cardiac rhythm and induction and termination of cardiac arrhythmias. *Circulation*, **14**, 745.

Further Reading

Hanning, C. D. (1985). Editorial. "He looks a little blue down this end". Monitoring oxygenation during anaesthesia. *Brit. J. Anaesth.*, **57**, 359.

Chapter 12
Resuscitation from Coma and Long-Term Care

Diabetic Coma

Diabetic coma is a medical emergency of the highest order requiring constant attention to detail, a clear knowledge of the pathophysiology of the condition, determination to continue treatment until all danger has passed, and teamwork between the doctor, nursing staff and laboratory services. In order to be able to treat it properly we must follow the disease process from the beginning.

History

Thomas Willis described the sweetness of the urine of diabetes in the seventeenth century when the only sweetening agent was honey, and he therefore called it diabetes mellitus. He associated the disease with mental abnormality and thought it was caused by 'a long sorrow'.[102]

Progress towards understanding the disease was slow. By the middle of the nineteenth century it was realized that patients suffering from diabetes mellitus developed deterioration in the level of consciousness and frequently became comatose, and that the condition was commonly associated with deep breathing suggestive of 'air hunger' prior to death as described in 1874 by Kussmaul.[51]

Ketone bodies were first identified in the urine of patients with diabetes mellitus by Peters (1857)[71] and Gerhardt (1865).[37] They both described the production of a purple coloration when ferric chloride was added to the urine of patients suffering from diabetes. Von Jaksch (1885) showed that this colour reaction was due to the presence of acetoacetic acid.[91] Stadelmann (1883)[81] described the presence of a substance which he called 'crotonic acid', but Minkowski (1884)[62] and Kulz (1884)[49] identified this substance as 3-hydroxybutyrate.

During the early part of this century the cause of diabetic coma became a matter of some controversy. Opinions were divided between those who considered the coma to be the result of the toxic action of the ketone bodies[61,91] and those who considered it to be caused by the metabolic acidosis

that had been identified as present. A number of workers in the field were able to demonstrate that the toxicity of the ketone bodies was very low.[23,28,93,95] It was possible, by means of pH-sensitive dyes and blood bicarbonate measurements, to demonstrate that: (a) the relative acidity of the venous blood was increased, (b) the bicarbonate content of the blood was lowered, and (c) the urine contained large amounts of organic acids.

Even in these relatively early days when biochemical analysis was still being developed, patients who appeared to have developed diabetic coma, had a low venous blood pH and bicarbonate, were reported to have no ketone bodies in their urine.[26,81,90] Although, as has been shown (see p. 17), intravenous fluid was given as early as 1831 with good effect in certain conditions, its first recorded use in the treatment of diabetic acidosis was in 1874 by Hilton-Fagge,[42] who used a solution containing sodium phosphate and sodium chloride. Young (1903),[104] Williamson (1898),[101] Dickinson (1898)[24] and Von Noorden (1895)[92] used intravenous salt solutions. Because their patients improved (as with present knowledge we would expect from the increase in blood volume) and the solution used was not alkaline in character, further controversy was added with regard to the acidic nature of the coma. We now know that restoration of the fluid volume would be expected not only to produce clinical improvement, but also to reduce the degree of acidosis if this was partly caused by lactic acid. Although the discovery and identification of insulin by Banting and Best in 1922,[9] has made the treatment of diabetes possible, it has not prevented the development of diabetic ketosis in some patients.

The development of diabetic ketosis

The classical accounts of diabetes describe the effects of diabetic ketosis with dehydration and progressively increasing metabolic acidosis; as indicated in the first edition of this book,[14] the process, however, is not simple and is complicated by the movement of body water from the intracellular fluid (ICF) compartment to the extracellular fluid (ECF) compartment. We can follow these changes in three distinct phases, although one phase merges imperceptibly into the other. The period of time taken over each phase varies, it may be very short in one patient and relatively long in another.

Phase 1.   Before glucose can enter the cell, it has to be converted into glucose-6-phosphate under the hexokinase reaction which is controlled by insulin. In the absence of insulin, relatively little glucose can enter the cell and it therefore accumulates in the ECF. In the early stages of the development of diabetic coma, the extracellular concentration of glucose rises and this is reflected in a raised blood glucose concentration and dilution of the components of the vascular space, caused by the movement of water from the ICF to the ECF.

If in the hospital accident and emergency department one sees a patient presenting for the first time with diabetes in the very early stages of the condition, one finds that there is an expansion of the ECF (interstitial and vascular) at the expense of the fluid content in the ICF. The expansion of the ECF leads to dilution and this is seen when the [Na$^+$] of the plasma is measured and is found to be low, for example 130 mmol/l (mEq/l) or less. At this stage the [K$^+$] is usually within normal limits or only slightly raised, and the plasma protein concentration is diluted to a relatively small degree (Fig. 12.1). The plasma [HCO$_3^-$] is also reduced by only a minor degree.

It must be remembered that this stage of *relative* expansion of the ECF persists throughout the whole period of diabetic ketosis and is not reversed until sufficient insulin has been given to allow the excess glucose to pass back into the cells (Fig. 12.1a and b).

Phase 2.   With the rise in the extracellular glucose concentration, which is reflected in the high plasma glucose levels, glycosuria and an osmotic diuresis develop. This leads gradually to a reduction in total body water but, as the extracellular glucose concentration rises, the relative disparity in water content between the ICF and ECF increases. Dehydration therefore is *superimposed* upon the already *contracted* ICF and the *expanded* ECF (Fig. 12.1c). As dehydration proceeds, the plasma [Na$^+$] rises and returns to normal or near-normal values. The measured plasma [Na$^+$] can be misleadingly normal, for example 138 mmol/l

(mEq/l), unless the effect of the high concentration of glucose is borne in mind.* The calculation for obtaining the corrected plasma [Na$^+$] is given on page 422.

In addition to progressive dehydration, there is, during phase 2, a progressive increase in extracellular glucose concentration so that it frequently rises to above 50 mmol/l (1000 mg%). The plasma [K$^+$] rises, except in a small number of K$^+$-depleted patients. Although the ECF was initially expanded by the influx of water from the ICF (Fig. 12.1b), dehydration causes a contraction of the ECF as a whole so that it is smaller than it was before the onset of diabetic ketosis and severe hyperglycaemia. This includes a reduction in *blood volume*. Indeed, the most important factor maintaining the blood volume at this time is the raised plasma (ECF) glucose concentration. The expansion, even in phase 2, may be insufficient to maintain the blood pressure. Furthermore, the abnormal metabolism of the patient may lead to hypothermia and many patients suffering from severe diabetic ketosis have a low body temperature, when measured, for example, rectally with a low-reading thermometer. It should be noted at this time that there are three reasons why the plasma [HCO$_3^-$] is low: ketosis, hypovolaemia and hypothermia.

The reduced blood volume, hypothermia and abnormal metabolic state all contribute to a fall in blood pressure, and a self-potentiating condition then exists.

Phase 3.   In phase 3 of diabetic ketosis, markedly severe dehydration occurs so that there is an even more severe fall in blood pressure, sometimes associated with marked hypothermia and a gross metabolic acidosis. The plasma sodium concentration may rise (Fig 12.1d) so that hypernatraemia may be present, and values as high as 170 mmol/l (mEq/l) of Na$^+$ can be recorded. As demonstrated above, the shift of water from the ICF to the ECF persists and the disproportionate accumulation of water in the ECF increases as the blood glucose concentration rises, the diabetic state becomes more severe and dehydration and loss of total body water by osmotic diuresis, progress.

In phase 3, however, even the hyperosmolality of the plasma and ECF is insufficient to maintain the blood volume, so that there is a reduction in

---

* Even when water is lost from the body because of the osmotic diuresis and the plasma [Na$^+$] rises to 'normal' or greater than normal values, relative dilution of the ECF is still present (see p. 415).

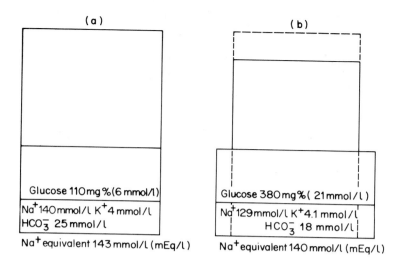

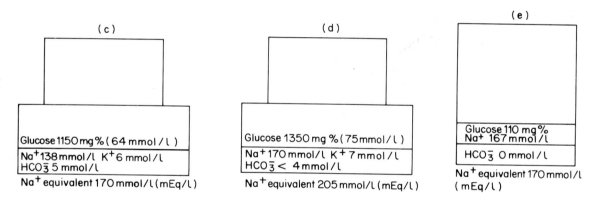

Fig. 12.1 (a) This shows the resting state of a diabetic patient with regard to the three main fluid compartments (see p. 19), demonstrating near normal values of glucose, [Na⁺], [K⁺], and [HCO₃⁻]. (b) This illustrates the changes that occur in the early stages of diabetic ketosis (phase 1) in which there is a shift of fluid from the intracellular fluid (ICF) into the extracellular fluid (ECF) resulting in dilution of [Na⁺]. Ketosis is beginning to appear so that there is a moderate fall in [HCO₃⁻]. The [K⁺] is beginning to rise. (c) The condition has progressed much further without treatment and dehydration has been superimposed upon the abnormal relative expansion of the ECF. The concentration of glucose in the ECF has risen to a marked degree and the patient is already beginning to be severely ill. A severe fall in [HCO₃⁻] has occurred due to both ketosis and lactacidosis. The plasma [K⁺] has increased significantly. This may be looked at as phase 3 which can progress to a more severe degree of dehydration. (d) Phase 3 has progressed so that there is a much greater degree of dehydration so that the plasma [Na⁺] has increased to 170 mmol/l (mEq/l). The patient at this stage is usually moribund. Virtually no HCO₃⁻ can be found in the plasma and the plasma [K⁺] has increased to 7 mmol/l (mEq/l) or more. Severe hypothermia is usually present at this stage. (e) This demonstrates the severe fall in blood volume that would occur if a patient in phase 2 or 3 is given insulin without first correcting the water (blood volume) deficit. It represents what might be seen if a patient illustrated in (c) were given intravenous insulin and only a minimal volume of fluid. In the presence of insulin, glucose would pass into the cell, expand the ICF, and the ECF would contract. But this results in a further reduction in blood volume with subsequent haemodynamic and circulatory effects.

It should be noted that although these stages can be seen if patients are carefully investigated in the emergency department, occasionally patients are seen late in Phase 3, with low plasma [Na⁺]. It would appear that a low cardiac output due to low blood volume, profound metabolic acidosis and hypothermia has reduced the glomerular filtration rate (GFR). These patients are hypotensive and usually have a poor prognosis.

Note: 18 mg% of plasma glucose = 1 mmol/l = 1 mosmol/l.

cardiac output and tissue perfusion. This causes a rise in the lactic acid concentration which is exacerbated by the hypothermia that is almost always present. Lactic acidosis is then superimposed upon the ketoacidosis.

We should now consider the sequence of events that would occur if, in either phase 2 or 3, insulin is given to the patient *before* the fluid deficit is corrected. The pathophysiological changes are clear. In the presence of insulin, glucose-6-phosphate can be formed and this will pass readily into the cells. When glucose-6-phosphate enters the cells as an osmotically active substance, water will leave the extracellular compartment, including the vascular compartment. When this occurs, the already depleted blood volume will decrease even further, leading to a further reduction in cardiac output and decreased tissue perfusion. This further decrease in tissue perfusion may lead to death. It can be said that the *only* factor maintaining the blood volume in the patient suffering from phase 2 and 3 of diabetic ketosis is the raised plasma glucose concentration.* It is important, therefore, that rehydration of the patient should be achieved and the blood volume expanded *before* insulin has had time to act.

Blood ketones

There is commonly some difficulty in interpreting blood ketone body concentrations. Although Nabarro in 1962[66] demonstrated that in most patients there was good correlation between the concentration of acetoacetate in the blood and the severity of diabetes, it has also been shown by Marliss et al.[59] that the ketoacidosis present in some patients may be due almost entirely to the beta-hydroxybutyric acid. Plasma acetone concentrations are also markedly elevated and, although significant variations occur in individual patients, the plasma acetone concentration may be four times that of the concentration of acetoacetate.[85] The plasma acetone concentration may remain elevated for 40 hours or more after the onset of diabetic ketosis, long after the blood glucose and beta-hydroxybutyric acid and acetoacetate concentrations have returned to normal. This must be one of the explanations for the ketonuria being present in some patients for several days following successful treatment.[16]

It has been shown that following insulin therapy, the concentration of beta-hydroxybutyrate de-

creases rapidly, while that of acetoacetic acid remains unchanged for a considerable period and may even rise slightly.[83]

Blood lactate

The contribution of lactic acid to the severity of the metabolic acidosis seen in diabetic ketosis has been the subject of much debate. If a standard is set in which lactic acidosis is assumed to be present when the concentration of lactate in the blood is 2 mmol/l (mEq/l) or greater, then the work of Oliva[70] would indicate that it is present in 29–55% of patients with diabetic ketosis.[70,84,97,103,106] Other workers[86] chose a concentration of 7 mmol/l (mEq/l) as the significant concentration of blood lactate. The frequency of lactic acidosis in this condition is then reduced. However, as the normal blood lactate concentration is very low, it must be accepted that any rise above normal is of clinical significance, and the concentration reflects the degree of hypovolaemia present or the severity of the reduction of tissue perfusion.

Alberti and Hockaday[1] studied 56 patients who had developed ketoacidosis. They arbitrarily divided them into two groups: (a) those with a blood lactate concentration below 2.5 mmol/l (mEq/l), and (b) those with a lactate concentration greater than 2.5 mmol/l (mEq/l). The patients in group (b), in which the concentration of lactate was in excess of 2.5 mmol/l (mEq/l), had a higher concentration of blood glucose, a lower [HCO_3^-] and a greater degree of hypovolaemia than the patients in group (a). The concentration of lactate in group (b) decreased with the use of fluids and insulin. The patients in group (a), in which the plasma lactate was less than 2.5 mmol/l (mEq/l), had other metabolic changes that were also less marked.

It is apparent, however, that as lactate production can be the result of a number of factors, such as hypovolaemia, reduced cardiac output and hypothermia which are present to a varying degree in different patients, a constant correlation between the degree of lactic acidosis and the severity of the hyperglycaemia cannot be found.

The syndrome of diabetes mellitus

This syndrome is characterized by a raised blood glucose level (hyperglycaemia) and glucose in the urine (glycosuria). It is associated with abnormal protein and fat metabolism and results from inadequate or completely absent secretion of insulin from the islets of Langerhans of the pancreas. It is seen in its purest form in children when the clinical

---

* The high concentration of glucose in the blood is, in short, keeping the patient alive by maintaining the circulation.

picture is not clouded by pathology that is either completely unrelated to the condition or a result of the disease process itself. Although hyperglycaemia and glycosuria may also be noted in the presence of abnormalities of the pituitary and suprarenal glands, as in Cushing's syndrome, the mechanism is different.

Physical signs

The physical signs of diabetes mellitus in both children and adults are very much the same. The most outstanding signs are loss of weight, even in the presence of an increased food intake, polyuria and polydipsia. The major difference between the child and the adult is the rate of onset of coma. Sometimes the child may present as a failure to thrive, or with polyuria and bedwetting following previous training. Not infrequently, however, children present as an acute emergency in a comatose or stuporous state. The adult may also present in this condition, though less commonly.

Pre-coma

In the pre-comatose state a hot dry skin is seen, the cheeks are flushed and acetone may be smelt in the breath. Hyperventilation is usually present, sometimes even at an early stage approximating in degree to the 'air hunger' of the fully developed condition. Nausea and vomiting may occur and are sometimes associated with marked abdominal pain. Quite commonly a child will complain, before the onset of the pre-comatose state, of vague muscle aches and discomfort.

Coma

In the fully developed condition of diabetic coma, the patient is unrousable, is breathing stertorously, inhaling a large volume of air at each breath. This is the 'air hunger' of Kussmaul and when seen is easily recognizable.[51] The signs of dehydration are present, the eyeball tension is low and the pulse is rapid and of poor volume. When the condition has developed to a dangerous degree the arterial blood pressure falls and peripheral cyanosis can be observed. Unless great care is taken in treatment, the state of shock persists and death results.

Pathophysiology of diabetes mellitus

The primary defect in diabetes is the inability to metabolize glucose, but this has a pronounced secondary effect on the metabolism of fat and protein. The severity of the disease is influenced by adrenocortical activity and diabetogenic hormones of the neurohypophysis.

Glucose is lost into the urine, the carbohydrate stores within the body are diminished, and the glycogen content of the liver becomes reduced as a result of glucogenesis. Protein is metabolized in an attempt to repair the body glucose content, this process being referred to as gluconeogenesis. In addition more fat is metabolized. The consequences of increased protein metabolism are wasting and potassium depletion, while increased fat metabolism leads to the accumulation of keto-acids (β-hydroxybutyric acid and acetoacetic acid) and hypercholosterolaemia. Because they are not metabolized, the ketone bodies, in the presence of incomplete glucose metabolism, are excreted in the urine and they add to the osmolar load of the glomerular filtrate which already contains an abnormally high glucose concentration. There is therefore an increase in the osmolar load presented to the renal apparatus so that a marked osmotic diuresis is induced and the body becomes depleted of water. The symptoms and signs of dehydration appear.

In addition to the increased solute excretion, other factors may lead to a disproportionate water loss. In the early stages of pre-coma, vomiting often occurs and is sometimes associated with diarrhoea. Also, the generalized metabolic disturbance leads to impairment of the concentrating ability of the renal apparatus.

Therefore, while loss of Na^+ and K^+ occurs to a marked degree, the relative loss of water is very much greater. When this water is replaced by isotonic saline only, hypernatraemia follows and less water is made available for rehydration of the cells where the need is greatest. This must be kept in mind when choosing intravenous therapy for resuscitation, as cellular rehydration can only be achieved by the infusion of a solution of fructose, glucose or hypotonic saline solutions. Hypernatraemia can also occur spontaneously, before giving intravenous infusions because of the disproportionate water loss.

Four basic factors may lead to reduced cardiac output and shock.

1. Reduced blood volume.
2. Gross metabolic acidosis.
3. Hypothermia.
4. Inadequate adrenocortical secretion.

As dehydration progresses the blood volume is reduced and this becomes one of the major factors in the production of peripheral circulatory failure or shock. With the onset of peripheral circulatory failure and the resultant decrease in tissue perfusion, the blood lactic acid concentration rises, the degree of metabolic acidosis becomes more marked and is reflected in further reduction of the bicarbonate ion concentration of the plasma, which has already fallen as a result of the accumulation of ketoacids in the ECF.

In the early stages of the development of diabetic acidosis the increased concentration of glucose in the ECF, which may eventually reach 65 mmol/l (1300 mg%) or more, causes a withdrawal of fluid from the ICF into the ECF with consequent dilution of the plasma electrolytes and protein. The continued disproportionate water loss, however, eventually leads to an increased sodium concentration in the plasma. When this occurs, severe dehydration is present and is almost always associated with hypotension and peripheral circulatory failure.

Physiological consequences of diabetic ketosis

We have seen how the osmotic load to the kidneys of glucose and ketoacids leads to water depletion. There is, in addition, a marked reduction of base so that a metabolic acidosis of marked proportions may develop (i.e. the plasma may contain only 6 mmol/l(mEq/l) of bicarbonate ion). There are also abnormal $[Na^+]$ and $[K^+]$ both within the plasma and within the body as a whole. These alterations in biochemistry lead to an altered function of organs not directly involved in the disease. These organs are the central nervous system, resulting in coma and marked hyperventilation, the myocardium, producing a reduction in cardiac output, and the suprarenal gland, increasing the adrenocortical secretions. In addition, as dehydration progresses and the blood volume is reduced, the general metabolism becomes more abnormal; the amount of adrenocortical hormone secreted may become inadequate. This can contribute to the development of hypotension. At this stage, therefore, we must look at one important aspect which has a great bearing on treatment and is not always stressed in descriptions of this condition. Although we know that in the presence of a high blood sugar more glucose enters some cells, the gradient between the ECF and the ICF is still marked. When the blood sugar concentration is raised, the effective osmolality exerted by this substance is also increased. When, therefore, a diabetic patient presents in coma, a major part of the force that is maintaining the blood volume is the osmotic pressure of the abnormally high glucose concentration within the plasma. This force may be greater than 40 mosmol/l.

Let us now consider what might happen if we treated a patient with a very high blood sugar level with insulin alone. Under its influence glucose would be metabolized and the concentration within the ECF would fall. The effective osmotic force of the ECF would be reduced so that water would then have to pass into the intracellular compartment in order to maintain osmotic uniformity. The volume of the ECF as a whole and therefore the plasma volume, already reduced by the processes of dehydration, would be further contracted. Peripheral circulatory failure, if already present, would be made worse and, if absent, might be precipitated. The importance of repairing the fluid deficit in the patient suffering from diabetic coma is thus made clear; it is apparent that treatment in this respect must be instituted *before* insulin, given therapeutically, has had time to act.

Another aspect we must consider is that of the gross metabolic acidosis. Diabetic ketosis is one of the conditions in which correction of the acidosis with sodium bicarbonate may have a dramatic effect on cardiac output and blood pressure. The attendant rise in blood pressure following the infusion of isotonic solution (1.4% $NaHCO_3$) occurs very shortly after the infusion of an adequate volume. It is interesting to note that it does not always have any effect upon ventilation unless infused in large volumes and the reason for this is possibly explained on page 93. It is sometimes said that because the ketoacids and, in the presence of shock, lactic acid, will be converted on recovery into bicarbonate ion (HCO_3^-), the infusion of sodium bicarbonate is unnecessary. It is also quite commonly stated that the infusion of sodium chloride helps to correct the metabolic acidosis, although accounts of *unsuccessful* treatment with isotonic saline demonstrate high plasma sodium levels in the presence of a bicarbonate ion concentration of 4 mmol/l (mEq/l). These recommendations should be ignored because, unless adequate tissue perfusion is re-established early in the process of resuscitation, accumulation of lactic acid and ketoacids continues and the stage at which active metabolism of organic acids occurs is never reached. It is true that a raised plasma bicarbonate level will be found in the recovery period, but this is rapidly corrected by renal excretion and the urine is then made alkaline.

Even when adequate fluid therapy is being instituted and the metabolic acidosis is corrected, the blood pressure may remain low and the peripheral circulation inadequate. Because some patients respond to large doses of intravenous hydrocortisone, it can be assumed that impairment of adrenocortical function has occurred and, although stabilization of the patient with insulin may be made more difficult during the 2 or 3 days following its use, this is a small price to pay for a live patient.

When patients present with relatively advanced diabetic ketosis, for example the later stages of phase 2 and the earlier stages of phase 3, it is found that they are often hypotensive, sometimes with an unrecordable blood pressure, that the $[HCO_3^-]$ is low, usually below 10 mmol/l (mEq/l), and that the plasma $[Na^+]$ ranges between 147 and 127 mmol/l (mEq/l) and the plasma $[K^+]$ is almost invariably raised. Jones et al.,[45] in a series of 12 patients who presented in the accident and emergency department, observed that the plasma $[K^+]$ could be as high as 7.0 mmol/l (mEq/l) (when the $[Na^+]$ was only 130 mmol/l (mEq/l)), and that only one patient who was cachectic and suffering from hepatic disease and renal disease had a low-normal $[K^+]$ of 3.6 mmol/l (mEq/l) (Table 12.1). It therefore follows that in the majority of patients the plasma potassium is raised, although in some, who are already suffering from a depletion of K^+, low values may be found. Thus the observation that infusions of sodium bicarbonate in the early stages of treatment of diabetic ketosis will cause cardiac arrest, because of the induction of hypokalaemia, is largely incorrect, but early values for plasma $[K^+]$ must be obtained.

A fall in rectal temperature occurred in most patients with diabetic ketosis.

The following case history illustrates the difficulty encountered in the management of the severely sick patient.

Case history. A 58-year-old woman who was a known diabetic was admitted to the accident and emergency department in a semiconscious condition. Her blood pressure was initially unrecordable when taken using the sphygmomanometer cuff, and palpation of the radial pulse. The rectal temperature was 33.2°C (91.76°F). Her respirations, although deep and slightly increased in rate, were not typically Kussmaul in character. Arterial blood analysis revealed that the pH was 6.8, $[HCO_3^-]$ was 5 mmol/l and the PCO_2 was 19 mmHg. A cannula was inserted and a venous blood sample was taken for analysis before an intravenous infusion of 0.9% NaCl was begun.

The $[Na^+]$ was 127 mmol/l (mEq/l), $[K^+]$ was 6.8 mmol/l (mEq/l), urea was 168 mg%, and blood sugar was 64 mmol/l (1152 mg%). A central venous pressure (CVP) cannula was also inserted and the CVP was found to be 13 cmH$_2$O after the infusion of 1 litre of fluid. A total of 200 mmol (mEq) of sodium bicarbonate was administered over a period of 20 minutes. When only 25% of this volume had been given, the blood pressure began to rise, and when approximately 50% had been infused the blood pressure rose to 110/60 mmHg. Following this infusion, blood gas analysis revealed pH 7.12, PCO_2 28 mmHg, $[HCO_3^-]$ 8 mmol/l (mEq/l), and base excess −21 mmol/l. Because of the raised blood sugar, a 10-unit dose of insulin was given intramuscularly and repeated every hour. Although the patient's physical condition had improved following the infusion of NaHCO$_3$ and she was warm peripherally, it was found that the $[HCO_3^-]$ had risen to only 8 mmol/l (mEq/l). The arterial blood PO_2 was 111 mmHg. A further 200 mmol (mEq) of 8.4% NaHCO$_3$ was begun and isotonic (0.9%) saline infusion continued, but because the CVP was +13 cmH$_2$O, both were given slowly. Improvement of the clinical condition continued and the CVP fell so that 5 hours after admission it measured +4 cmH$_2$O. It was noted at this time that the plasma $[Na^+]$ had increased to 145 mmol/l (mEq/l) and the plasma $[K^+]$ had fallen to 2.6 mmol/l (mEq/l). The blood glucose had fallen to 50 mmol/l (900 mg%).

It was therefore apparent that although a marked degree of metabolic acidosis was still present, a fall in $[K^+]$ had occurred. These figures indicate two factors: (a) the metabolism of 14 mmol of glucose per litre had caused a movement of fluid from the extracellular to the intracellular compartment; and (b) the plasma $[K^+]$ had fallen in association with the uptake of glucose by the tissues. An infusion of KCl at a rate of 20 mmol/hour (mEq/hour) was begun. Three and a half hours later a further blood sample showed that the $[Na^+]$ had increased to 149 mmol/l (mEq/l) and the $[K^+]$ was still only 2.6 mmol/l (mEq/l). The $[HCO_3^-]$ was 21 mmol/l (mEq/l) and the blood sugar was 37.8 mmol/l (680 mg%). An infusion of KCl was continued and no further bicarbonate was given. After a further 4 hours, the plasma $[Na^+]$ was 147 mmol/l (mEq/l) and the $[K^+]$ was 4.4 mmol/l (mEq/l). The blood glucose was 31.5 mmol/l (567 mg%). Fourteen hours after admission the blood glucose was 12.2 mmol/l (220 mg%) and no further insulin was given. The CVP remained at 4–5 cmH$_2$O and there was no evidence of any mental impairment or cerebral oedema. A transient rise in serum amylase occurred after this event and was associated with abdominal pain.

The gross acidosis that this patient developed was the result of both plasma ketosis and lactacidosis. The low plasma $[K^+]$ that developed

Table 12.1 The analysis of blood from 10 consecutive patients. Blood samples for analysis were taken shortly after arrival of these patients at the accident and emergency department

Patient's number	Age (years)	Glucose (mmol/l, mg%)	[Na+] (mmol/l, mEq/l)	[K+] (mmol/l, mEq/l)	Urea (mmol/l)	pH	PCO_2 (mmHg)	$[HCO_3^-]$ (mmol/l, mEq/l)	PO_2* (mmHg)	Hb (g%)	PCV (%)	Respiratory rate (breaths/minute)	Temperature (°C)	Blood pressure (mmHg)	Heart rate (beats/minute)
1	65	39.0 (702)	136	6.5	7.5	7.03	11	3	(130)	12.5		7		100/70	100
2	19	27.6 (497)	134	5.1	7.2	7.02	19	4	(130)	14.4	45	24	36.2	110/70	120
3	70	24.3 (437)	132	5.4	6.0	7.29	27	13	62	13.5	40	26	37.0	120/80	112
4	24	43.0 (774)	129	4.5	7.5	7.28	33	10	88	15.0	41	24	37.5	120/70	120
5	41	24.6 (443)	128	5.5	7.8	7.06	19	5	(139)	14.7	44	20	36.6	130/50	128
6	23	36.8 (662)	130	7.0		7.14	15	10	(117)	16.4	49	28	36.2	110/60	112
7	53	26.0 (468)	137	4.8		7.12	22	7	104	15.8	49	20	35.5	190/100	100
8	63	51.0 (918)	147	4.7	16.9	7.34	29	15	90	17.5			36.7	120/85	
9	35	41.0 (738)	126	4.9		7.15	13	9	100		48	32	36.4	115/80	
10	58	64.0 (1152)	127	6.8		6.81	19	5	(116)				33.2	Not recorded	147

*PO_2 values given in parentheses indicate values obtained from patients breathing O_2 by mask.

appeared to be unrelated to the acid–base state. Hypotension and hypothermia contributed to the metabolic acidosis. It is of interest that the patient's rectal temperature began to rise almost immediately following the infusion of bicarbonate and this, no doubt, assisted in her recovery. The more dilute solutions and 5% fructose were unavailable.

The day following treatment a raised plasma $[Na^+]$ of 150 mmol/l (mEq/l) or more is sometimes seen. This can be treated with infusions of half normal saline (0.45% NaCl) which increase the rate with which the abnormality is corrected. It is to be noted that in spite of the prolonged hypotension observed in these patients, it is rare for acute renal failure to develop. This is in keeping with the observations of Brooks et al. (1963)[17] that when a raised plasma osmolality is present, acute renal failure tends not to develop following profound hypotension.

Management of diabetic ketosis

Recovery from diabetic coma is directly related to its severity and duration and, therefore, also the quantitative aspects of treatment. If treatment is begun in the early stages of the condition, before consciousness is lost completely and the patient is said to be in 'pre-coma', relatively small doses of insulin given intramuscularly, combined with oral fluids assisted by the intravenous infusion of perhaps only a litre of normal saline will suffice. Nevertheless, it must be stressed that in severe cases inadequate treatment is common. With this in mind and because we are now familiar with the pathophysiology and abnormal biochemical findings of the condition, we can approach the stages of treatment in logical sequence related to their importance.

1. Monitor blood pressure, respiratory rate and electrocardiogram.
2. If patient is unconscious, aspirate the stomach to prevent the contents being inhaled.
3. Prepare for endotracheal intubation. Even when the patient is hyperventilating (Kussmaul respiration), respiratory arrest may occur, especially in the presence of a very severe metabolic acidosis and hypothermia.
4. Examine the urine for glucose and ketone bodies.
5. Take a blood sample and fill a haematocrit tube at the bedside. Send a sample to the laboratory for blood sugar estimations. Examine the rest of the blood for $[Na^+]$, $[K^+]$ and $[HCO_3^-]$. Ideally, an intravenous infusion should be set up at the same time as the blood sample is taken. Blood gases should be measured in an arterial blood sample. A full blood count should be obtained.

Choice of solution for infusion

Approximately 2 litres of fluid should be infused in the first hour; if control of blood sugar is slow and the osmotic diuresis persists, 10–12 litres of fluid may be required during the first 24 hours of treatment. The initial choice of solution will depend upon the severity of the condition; rapid infusion will be necessary if shock is present before the analysis of the serum electrolytes and bicarbonate concentration is known.

If severe peripheral circulatory failure has developed, it is beneficial to infuse 500 ml of isotonic sodium bicarbonate solution over a period of 20 minutes or less. Sodium lactate may produce some benefit by increasing the volume of the ECF but it will not change either the blood pH or its $[HCO_3^-]$ until further general improvement in the circulation occurs. Sodium lactate in this respect is very little better than sodium chloride, but neither of these should be withheld if they are the only solutions available.

It must be realized that if it is intended to infuse NaCl there can be no objection and every indication for the infusion of $NaHCO_3$, as the Na^+ content will not be appreciably different. If only hypertonic $NaHCO_3$, for example 8.4% (1 mmol/ml), is available, this can be used with success, as demonstrated in the case history on page 419.

We have seen how water is lost in disproportionately greater amounts relative to sodium loss so that hypovolaemia and cellular hydropenia may develop, either spontaneously or following fluid replacement with isotonic electrolyte solutions of either sodium chloride or sodium bicarbonate. In severe dehydration in the presence of hypernatraemia when water must be made available for cellular metabolism, 'half-strength' NaCl, or glucose or fructose should be administered.* Alternatively, isotonic glucose or fructose can be given. This form of therapy has been criticized because it may lead to water intoxication if given in excessive quantities in the presence of marked Na^+ depletion. In the absence of laboratory assistance, the infusion of 500 ml of isotonic electrolyte solution alternated with 500 ml of 5% or 2.5% glucose or fructose solution may be a safer form of treatment in the majority of patients, but in the very severely water-depleted case as

* Because it is unstable, $NaHCO_3$ solution cannot be administered safely in solutions more dilute than isotonic (1.4%).

described, the early infusion of half-strength solutions is indicated. Fructose is removed from the plasma of the diabetic and from the plasma of the normal man at the same rate. Although the anti-ketogenic activity of fructose in the absence of insulin is in doubt, fructose can be infused without giving rise to excessive mellituria. If available, therefore, half-strength saline or fructose is to be preferred for correcting a very large true water deficit that is causing hypernatraemia.

In the presence of high blood sugar concentrations, an assessment of the body water deficit cannot be made from estimates based on the plasma Na$^+$ concentration as on page 31. This is because the abnormal concentration of glucose has such a powerful osmotic action. For example, 6 mmol/l (180 mg%) of glucose in the plasma has the same effective osmolality as 5 mmol/l (mEq/l) of Na$^+$. In order to calculate the water deficit it is therefore necessary to correct the effective osmotic activity of the plasma glucose to equivalent concentrations of cation. This is illustrated by the following case.

Case history. A patient in diabetic coma weighing 52 kg had a serum [Na$^+$] of 158 mmol/l (mEq/l) and a plasma glucose concentration of 50 mmol/l (900 mg%).

18 mg% of glucose = 1 mosmol/l (mmol/l)

Therefore the effective osmolality of plasma glucose was 50 mosmol/l. This is equal to 25 mmol/l (mEq/l) of Na$^+$ because glucose, unlike NaCl, does not ionize in solution to produce two osmotically active particles.

The deficit of water in this case had to be assessed on an apparent plasma [Na$^+$] of 183 mmol/l (mEq/l).

158 + 25 = 183 mmol/l (mEq/l) of Na$^+$

The patient weighed 52 kg and would therefore have been expected to have approximately 31.2 litres of body water.

52 × 0.6 = 31.2 litres of body H$_2$O

Because the plasma [Na$^+$] was inversely proportional to the body water content, at the time of the investigation, her total body water was in the region of 23.8 litres.

$$\frac{\text{Normal [Na}^+]}{\text{Abnormal [Na}^+]} \times 31.2 = \frac{140}{183} \times 31.2 = 23.8$$

As her normal body water content was 31.2 litres, her fluid deficit was 31.2 − 23.8 = 7.4 litres. Because of some degree of sodium depletion, this figure would tend to under-estimate her fluid requirements and in fact

more than 8 litres of fluid were infused.

It is as well to note that the total osmolality of the plasma in this case was 374 mosmol/l, the plasma [K$^+$] being 4 mmol/l (mEq/l).

Treatment of potassium deficiency

Although, as we have seen, a total body deficit of potassium can exist in diabetic coma, it may not be apparent from plasma values because hyper-kalaemia is usually present, and frequently rises to 7 mmol/l (mEq/l) or more (Table 12.1).

A major potassium deficiency may give rise to muscle weakness, myocardial insufficiency and respiratory failure, sometimes leading to cardiac arrest. Steps should therefore be taken towards its correction as soon as possible. Preferably, KCl should be given orally in the liquid form. Because rapid absorption is required, the enteric-coated tablet is unsuitable in this case. A gram of KCl given in water or in milk is well tolerated and can be repeated at intervals.

During the treatment of diabetic ketosis it is well recognized that the plasma [K$^+$] falls, and this appears to be mainly a function associated with glucose metabolism and glycogen storage. As illustrated in the case history (see p. 000), a fall in plasma [K$^+$] occurs even in the presence of a metabolic acidosis so that the fall in plasma [K$^+$] appears to be independent of the acid–base state. Although it is well recognized that the infusion of Na$^+$ salts, especially NaHCO$_3$, increases the rate at which plasma [K$^+$] is reduced, it may be essential to infuse sodium bicarbonate during the initial stages of treatment. When the plasma [K$^+$] falls to 3 mmol/l (mEq/l), cardiac arrhythmias and muscle weakness can develop. When a low serum K$^+$ has been demonstrated and vomiting precludes the administration of K$^+$ by mouth, it is necessary to give the cation intravenously. It may be added to any solution that is being infused. The rate of infusion should not be faster than 20 mmol/hour (mEq/hour) if cardiac arrhythmias are to be avoided with certainty. Slower rates of infusion are necessary in children.

The degree of hydration can be checked by means of serial haematocrit readings. Plasma protein concentrations or plasma specific gravity may also be of assistance. As the packed cell volume (PCV) approaches a normal value and hyperventilation becomes less marked and blood glucose levels begin to fall, the rate of infusion of fluid may be slowed. It is at this time that a careful biochemical assessment of the parameters involved is of greatest value.

Cerebral oedema

Cerebral oedema is an unfortunate complication, commonly occurring in the apparently well-treated case of diabetic ketosis, which has been recognized for some time.[33,41,105] The aetiology of this complication is still unknown, but must result from the large changes that occur in the relative hydration of the fluid compartments and from the fact that the cerebrospinal fluid (CSF) content changes relatively slowly. Osmotic gradients can therefore readily occur.

It has also been suggested that treatment with hypertonic solutions of bicarbonate have instigated cerebral oedema when it has developed.[63] In addition it was considered that the development of cerebral oedema distinguished patients with fatal diabetic ketosis from those dying from hyperosmotic non-ketotic diabetic coma. Maccario and Messis,[57] however, reported a case of cerebral oedema occurring in a patient who developed hyperosmotic non-ketotic diabetic coma, and who was not treated with bicarbonate solutions. They reported that the patient resembled cases that they had previously studied.[56,58] They observed that excessive sodium administration appeared to play no part, but on admission the patient had a normal CSF pressure with a normal glucose content, and when cerebral oedema developed during treatment and a rapid fall in blood glucose concentration occurred, there was a concomitant rise in CSF pressure and CSF glucose concentration. The patient was treated with methylprednisolone 40 mg, 6-hourly for 4 days, and improvement was evident following the first day of treatment. Fluid intake was not restricted and an adequate urine output was maintained throughout. Successful recovery has also been reported by Frier and McConnell[34] following treatment with dexamethasone (Decadron), 10 mg i.m., followed by diazepam (Valium), 4 mg 6-hourly.

Cerebral oedema has also been reported in a diabetic patient receiving haemodialysis which resulted in a marked hyperglycaemia.[30] This patient also developed increased CSF pressure and papilloedema, having become deeply comatose. A relatively convincing explanation for the development of cerebral oedema—the accumulation of fructose and sorbitol in the CSF—has been postulated by Clements et al.[20] who found this occurred in hyperglycaemic dogs. Both fructose and sorbitol are osmotically active, do not diffuse readily through tissues and are not readily metabolized. There is, however, some evidence that the incidence of cerebral oedema is reduced by the regimen of 'small-dose' insulin described below, although severe overhydration should, where possible, be avoided.

Insulin

We have dealt with fluid and electrolytes first because these are the factors that are essential to the successful resuscitation of the patient who presents in coma. When the condition has developed in the latter stages of phase 2 and during the whole of phase 3, the patient is in danger (before treatment has begun) because of factors other than the plasma glucose concentration; these are, of course, cellular and total body dehydration, the low plasma bicarbonate concentration and the high plasma [K^+]. All these factors produce their own physiological effects as described above. As we have seen, the high blood glucose concentration is the *only* factor maintaining the blood volume. Insulin should therefore be administered slowly. The short-acting soluble or crystalline insulin should be given hourly in doses of 5–10 units i.m. The first dose can be given intravenously. The adult of average size (e.g. 75 kg body weight) requires 7 units of soluble insulin every hour. The slow administration of insulin given intramuscularly or intravenously, preferably by a constant infusion pump until the patient's blood sugar has fallen to 12 mmol/l (250 mg%), prevents sudden shifts of H_2O into the intracellular compartment and assists in preventing the onset of cerebral oedema. Insulin is then given according to the requirements of the patient.

Summary of treatment of the severely dehydrated patient

1. Take blood for investigation through the needle used for giving an intravenous infusion. If shock is present, the solution of choice is isotonic 1.4% sodium bicarbonate. Alternative solutions are 2.74%, 4.2% and 8.4% $NaHCO_3$ and isotonic sodium chloride. Isotonic fructose (5%) if available can also be used.

2. A total of 2 litres of fluid is infused during the first hour. A total of 1.5 litres should be infused during the second hour. Solutions may be alternated in volumes of 500 ml, for example:

first hour:

Insulin 7 units i.v.
500 ml sodium bicarbonate 1.8%, 15 minutes
500 ml sodium chloride 0.45%, 15 minutes
500 ml sodium chloride 0.9%, 15 minutes

500 ml fructose 5% or sodium chloride 0.45%, 15 minutes

second hour:

Insulin 7 units i.m.
500 ml sodium bicarbonate 1.4%, 15 minutes
500 ml sodium chloride 0.9%, 15 minutes
500 ml sodium chloride 0.45%, or fructose 5%, 15 minutes

3. Take a second blood sample for determination of blood sugar level, plasma [K+], [Na+] and [HCO$_3$], and PCV. Determine the effectiveness of treatment upon blood sugar level and rehydration. Begin repair of potassium depletion by infusing 20 mmol (mEq) of KCl in 0.9% NaCl by means of a *separate* infusion so that the rate of administration is independent of the infusion being used for repairing the blood volume and total body fluid deficit.

4. Continue to administer insulin to the adult in doses of 5–10 units/hour and continue infusions of fluid: 3–6 litres are given in the first 6 hours according to the severity of the condition. It may be necessary to repeat infusions of NaHCO$_3$ if there has been little improvement in the metabolic acidosis; and at this stage it is preferable to use the less dilute solutions (eg. 2.74% or 4.8% solution).

5. Continue estimations and treatment for as long as necessary. When some improvement has occurred, an intragastric tube can be passed and fluids containing KCl, sodium chloride or sodium bicarbonate given by this pathway. Stop intramuscular or intravenous insulin when blood sugar falls to 15 mmol/l (300 mg%).

6. If a low blood pressure persists or if peripheral circulatory failure is of a marked degree at the onset of treatment, intravenous hydrocortisone should be given in doses of 100–300 mg and repeated at intervals. When the patient has recovered consciousness, small frequent feeding of nutritious liquid foods should be given in order to repair deficiencies not accounted for, such as magnesium. Obtain an estimation of serum PO$_4$.

7. When the patient has recovered from coma and is being stabilized with insulin in the normal way, careful check must be maintained on cardiovascular function, water and electrolyte balance and infective processes. Bed-rest should be imposed for at least 3 days and intravenous vitamins should be given to prevent the onset of diabetic neuritis, which may be precipitated by the coma. Vitamin B$_{12}$ should be given intramuscularly.

Non-ketotic Hyperglycaemia (hyperosmolar non-ketotic diabetic coma)

As demonstrated above, even during the nineteenth century it was recognized that not all patients who develop diabetic coma had ketonuria as a concomitant finding. For example, in the 1880s Von Frerichs[90] and Dreschfeld[26] were able to demonstrate a type of diabetes that was characterized by hyperglycaemia typically accompanied by weakness, cold extremities, drowsiness, a pulse of poor volume and Kussmaul respiration. These patients either 'collapsed' or developed cardiac failure, but no acetone could be detected either in the expired air or in the urine. Death occurred within 10 to 20 hours of the onset of the condition. Similar cases were described by Rosenbloom in 1915[78] and Joslin in 1917.[46]

In 1914 Sellards[80] reported patients who had no ketonaemia but whose blood bicarbonate concentration was lowered and who responded well when treated with large amounts of alkali. In the same year Marriott[60] reported a very carefully performed quantitative study of the acidosis, and observed that there was no correlation between the blood and urinary concentrations of ketone bodies and the blood bicarbonate concentration.

Rosenbloom[78] realized, both from his review of the published papers available at that time and from his own patients, that a reappraisal of the aetiology of diabetes mellitus was necessary in view of the fact that acidosis could be present in the absence of ketonuria.

In 1925 Warburg,[96] reviewing the history of diabetic coma, reported four patients suffering from the condition, none of whom had acetonuria to a significant degree. All these patients suffered from renal disease. Warburg, without investigating this parameter, assumed that ketonaemia was present and that the renal disease prevented the excretion of the ketone bodies. In three of these patients this could be a possible explanation as increased urinary excretion of ammonia was observed.

In at least one of Warburg's patients this conclusion could not be met. The 57-year-old patient had previously been in good health and was admitted to hospital deeply comatosed, with a blood sugar concentration of 37.2 mmol/l (670 mg%). The patient was dehydrated, but the expired air did not smell of acetone and no acetone was present in the urine. Excretion of ammonia was not increased. This patient was treated with insulin and infusions of salt solutions; his condition improved rapidly, and he was discharged from hospital. Following this improvement no insulin was given initially, but further treatment with insulin was necessary at a later date.

Two major advances had been made which allowed the elucidation of the condition to be achieved more readily. One was the accurate and relatively simple measurement of bicarbonate in the body fluids by Van Slyke and Neil (1924)[88] and the other was the discovery of insulin by Banting and Best in 1922 and the subsequent investigations.[7,8,9] In addition Van Slyke and Palmer[89] reported a method of measuring organic acids in urine in 1920 following the earlier report of Van Slyke (1917)[87] giving the determination of beta-hydroxybutyric acid, acetoacetic acid and acetone in urine.

Following the therapeutic use of insulin, reports rapidly appeared stating that although ketonuria decreased shortly after insulin administration, acidosis frequently persisted.[12,18] In 1924 Starr and Fitz[82] reported two patients in whom unidentified organic acids were found in the urine and in whom the concentration of ketoacids in the blood could not account quantitatively for the degree of acidosis that was present. This is what they wrote in 1924 of a 53-year-old diabetic woman with polyuria and polydipsia.

> The history was not typical of diabetic coma. However, physical examination gave no evidence of any cerebral lesion; lumbar puncture was normal; there were no signs of uremia, and the patient had acidosis, acetonemia, glycosuria, acetonuria and a blood sugar concentration at entry of 0.53 per cent . . .
>
> The striking feature in this case was the marked degree of acidosis present in the first blood sample without a corresponding blood acetone body concentration, and the presence in the urine throughout of a large proportion of unidentified organic acid. We believe therefore that in this case, also, other acids than the acetone bodies were in part responsible for the acidosis present. The patient was given insulin and sodium bicarbonate at entry with an almost immediate improvement. After consciousness was regained a few hours later, the subsequent course in the hospital was uneventful.

Feinblatt, also in 1924,[29] reported a case of fatal hyperglycaemic coma associated with a low plasma [HCO$_3^-$] in whom the plasma gave no reaction for ketones and no acetoacetate was present in the urine. Other reports of this type of patient were published including Allen and Wishart (1923),[2] Sellards (1914)[80] and Marriott (1914).[60]

As we have seen, there were a number of reports and case histories that were almost certainly those of non-ketotic hyperglycaemia. The acidosis that was found to be present was later established to be due to lactate (lactic acidosis) caused by hypovolaemia. The incidence of the condition has become greater with the increasing use of steroids. In 1957 Sament and Schwartz[79] drew attention to the condition by reporting severe diabetic stupor which was not associated with ketosis, and in the same year De Graef and Lips[22] reported the occurrence of hypernatraemia in non-ketotic hyperglycaemia. The mortality rate from this condition is very high.[3,4,11,21,27,31,38,54,74]

Mental confusion is a common occurrence and may be associated with a bizarre dietary behaviour as thirst and mental confusion develop. One patient is reported to have consumed 9 quarts of skimmed milk in a single day; another patient, whose clinician did not recognize the condition, was found at home surrounded by the containers of carbohydrate-rich carbonated drinks. When untreated and the severity of the condition increases, grand mal seizures occur or positive Babinski reflexes and nystagmus, muscle tremor and fasciculations can be observed. The patient becomes dysphasic or aphasic and hyperthermic. Conversely, especially in the unconscious patient, hypothermia can occur. In spite of the absence of ketosis, Kussmaul ventilation can be observed.

The blood glucose levels can rise in this condition to very high values, for example a blood glucose concentration of 287 mmol/l (4800 mg%) was reported by Knowles.[48] The degree of dehydration that can develop is illustrated by the fact that Jackson and Forman[44] reported two patients who had PCVs of 90%.

Nevertheless, the potential danger and the gravity of the condition are often not recognized, and hyperglycaemia is often not established sufficiently early. This may account for the high mortality. The absence of Kussmaul breathing is sometimes blamed for the delay, even though it is not always present in diabetic ketosis and can be readily observed in the non-ketotic form of hyperglycaemia.

The degree of impairment of consciousness has a good correlation with the degree of hyperosmolality, in both diabetic ketosis[36] and non-ketotic hyperglycaemia.[4,35]

Causes of the non-ketotic hyperglycaemic crisis

A number of stressful conditions give rise to hyperglycaemia. These include haemorrhagic shock, hypothermia, cardiogenic shock, extra-corporeal circulation,[15] pulmonary embolism and burns.[77] They do not, however, normally lead to such high levels of blood glucose that an osmotic diuresis follows.

Peritoneal dialysis may give rise to the condition.[13,40,99] Treatment with steroids can lead to a severe non-ketotic hyperglycaemic crisis, for example during the early postoperative period following cardiac transplantation when the doses of steroids given are high, or during the continued treatment of respiratory failure caused by fat emboli. It can be precipitated by an acute respiratory infection in the bilaterally adrenalectomized patient receiving 'maintenance' doses of cortisone acetate (Brooks, 1972).[15] It should always be remembered that a significant section of the population are latent diabetics and this is made apparent following corticosteroid therapy.

It would appear, however, that in some diabetic patients, although there is insufficient circulating insulin to prevent severe hyperglycaemia, there is sufficient insulin to metabolize the fatty acids so that ketoacidosis is prevented.

Treatment of the non-ketotic hyperglycaemic crisis

The degree of hyperglycaemia is frequently much higher than that seen in diabetic ketosis so that patients present in phase 2, when dehydration or disproportionate H_2O loss is already beginning, or in phase 3, when dehydration and hypernatraemia are already established.

Treatment of the condition is therefore based on a similar pattern to that of diabetic ketosis, except that infusions of bicarbonate are not required unless lactic acidosis is so marked because of hypovolaemia and hypothermia that it gives rise to pathophysiological changes.

The rate at which fluid is infused is dictated by the degree of dehydration (plasma [Na^+] and PCV) that is present when treatment is begun.

1. Infuse 2 litres of 0.9% saline in 1 hour. Inject 10–15 units of soluble (crystalline) insulin intramuscularly every hour.
2. Infuse 1 litre of 0.45% saline during the following 2 hours. Inject 5–10 units of soluble (crystalline) insulin intramuscularly or intravenously every hour.
3. Take blood hourly (as in diabetic ketosis) for measurement of PCV, blood glucose, plasma [Na^+], [K^+] and [HCO_3^-].
4. Begin to repair plasma [K^+] by infusion of

KCl at a rate of 20 mmol/hour, using a separate intravenous infusion.
5. If the patient is unconscious, aspirate the stomach and catheterize the bladder. Establish that urine output is 30 ml/hour or more when infusing KCl.
6. Alternate isotonic (0.9%) NaCl with 0.45% NaCl every hour.
7. Stop 1-hourly insulin when the blood glucose level falls to 12 mmol/l (250 mg%) or 14 mmol/l (300 mg%) and give according to requirements.
8. Give intravenous vitamins, B_{12} and Mg^{++} ($MgSO_4$ 2 g i.v.) during subsequent 24–48 hours.

Hepatic Coma

The symptoms and signs of hepatic encephalopathy in patients with liver disease are readily recognizable when they develop slowly. Coma may, however, develop so rapidly that it is mistaken for cerebral thrombosis or other disease of the central nervous system. This is most likely to occur when it is accompanied by focal neurological signs such as a positive Babinski reflex or unequal pupils.

Signs and symptoms

As hepatic toxicity begins to develop, the intelligence becomes impaired and this is followed by bizarre behaviour and conversation. As the encephalopathy worsens muscular tremors appear in the hands and feet. This is sometimes called a 'flapping' or 'seagull' tremor, and it may become extremely severe. Hyperventilation is usually apparent clinically at this stage, but increased alveolar ventilation produced by an increased tidal volume without any rise in the respiratory rate usually occurs at the beginning of hepatic toxicity. Gradually, consciousness is lost, the eyes cease to focus, unilateral loss of muscle tone may develop, the Babinski reflex may become positive bilaterally or unilaterally and tendon reflexes may be unequal.

The picture, therefore, of a deeply unconscious patient insensitive to pain and unresponsive to commands, markedly hyperventilating with neurological signs is not unlike that seen when brain damage has occurred as a result of either thrombosis or coma.

There may, however, be jaundice and erythema of the palms, spider angiomata, ascites, oedema, caput medusae and hepatomegaly. Apart from hepatomegaly the other physical signs are all too often absent. Biochemical tests, however, are indicative of liver disease.

Biochemical changes

The patient with chronic hepatic disease tends to retain sodium and to lose potassium so that in the absence of water intoxication, the serum $[Na^+]$ tends to be high and serum $[K^+]$ to be low. The plasma $[HCO_3^-]$ is almost always raised except in the presence of liver necrosis (see p. 92) when it may be low. Because of hyperventilation the PCO_2 falls. The combined metabolic and respiratory alkalosis causes the blood pH to be high.

The importance of ammonia or ammonia-producing compounds, such as urea and protein, in the development of hepatic encephalopathy was first suggested by Phillips *et al.* (1952).[73] Urea is converted by *Eschericia coli* into ammonium and carbon dioxide so that the gut is a constant source of this compound. Ammonia is derived mainly from the large intestine and the administration of antibiotics inhibits the growth of the bacterial flora[25,32,72] and, therefore, of the incidence of hepatic encephalopathy.

The total protein in liver disease usually falls, but the most marked change is the fall in serum albumin and a rise in serum globulin. This causes a marked reduction in effective osmotic activity even when the total protein has a normal value.

Flocculation tests

The zinc sulphate[50] (normal 4–8 units), the thymol turbidity[55] (normal 0–4 units), and the thymol flocculation[67] (normal 0–4), and the cephalin cholesterol flocculation (0–4 +) tests are indicative of liver disease and increased concentrations of gamma globulin in the plasma.

Enzyme tests

Changes in the serum enzyme activity are also indicative of hepatic disease. The alkaline phosphatase (normal 3–13 King–Armstrong units, 1.5–4 Bodansky units) and the transaminases are raised. The serum glutamic oxaloacetic transaminase (SGOT), normal value 5–17 units/100 ml, and the serum glutamic-pyruvic transaminase (SGPT), normal value 4–13 units/100 ml, and the serum lactic dehydrogenase (SLDH), normal values being up to 500 units/100 ml, are not specific indications of hepatic disease, because raised values are also found in widely differing conditions, such as myocardial infarction, carcinoma, infectious mononucleosis. Isocitric dehydrogenase (ICD), normal values 3–10 units, is considered to

be the most specific enzyme reaction for parenchymatous liver damage.[10] Gamma glutamyl transferase (γ GT) level is also raised in a variety of primary and secondary liver disorders.[100]

Causes of hepatic coma

The biochemical cause or causes of hepatic coma are still largely unknown with certainty, because so many factors appear to contribute when it occurs. It is, however, known to be associated with high blood ammonium levels, although other products derived from the bacterial action upon protein in gut may also be important.

When liver disease is present hepatic encephalopathy and coma may be precipitated by:

(*a*) high-protein diet,
(*b*) haemorrhage from oesophageal varices so that blood enters the lumen of the gut,
(*c*) administration of ammonium compounds orally or intravenously, or of urea orally,
(*d*) administration of thiazide diuretics without potassium supplements;
(*e*) portacaval anastomosis,
(*f*) paracentesis abdominis for ascites,
(*g*) hyponatraemia.

Anastomosis of the portal and superior mesenteric vein to the inferior vena cava may precipitate hepatic encephalopathy when no primary liver disease is present and anastomosis is performed during resection of carcinoma of the pancreas.[43,53,76] Hemicolectomy prevented the recurrence of the encephalopathy. In the case reported, the operation was effective in a manner similar to that observed in the patient who underwent total colectomy with ileorectal anastomosis, reported by Atkinson and Goligher,[5] in whom recurrent attacks of coma were prevented even when an increased protein intake was allowed.

Treatment of hepatic coma and encephalopathy

One of the common causes of hepatic coma is bleeding either from oesophageal varices or from an associated gastric ulcer. In a sense it can be looked upon as the rapid ingestion of a large quantity of protein. The longer the protein stays in the gut the more severe and prolonged is coma. Purgation with magnesium sulphate and enemata assists in removing the cause unless further bleeding occurs.

When coma is precipitated by a high-protein diet, a high-glucose protein-free diet will often reverse the process during the pre-coma stage.

Oral antibiotics, especially neomycin, 6 g/day in divided doses, reduce the bacterial flora and therefore the concentration of toxic products absorbed from the large bowel. When coma has developed fully it is best treated by an intragastric tube down which is dripped continuously a daily intake of at least 100 g of glucose in a 10% or 20% solution, together with an adequate intake of water. Antibiotics are also administered down the tube. A careful fluid balance measurement must be maintained and if more than 1 litre of urine is being excreted, 4–6 g of KCl are given daily. If the urine output is reduced and excretion impaired, K^+ should be omitted or given with great caution. Hyponatraemia, which can follow paracentesis abdominis and also appears to contribute to the precipitation of hepatic coma, should be treated with hypertonic saline solutions, infused slowly as in water intoxication (see p. 31).

Glucose can be given intravenously in high concentration in large veins (the SVC or IVC) but, because the patient with cirrhosis of the liver is hypersensitive to insulin, the doses recommended during acute renal failure should not be used, otherwise hypoglycaemia will be produced. Insulin may be omitted from the drip or given in much smaller quantities. Frequent blood sugar estimations should be made initially. Cirrhotics are also sensitive to the synthetic hypoglycaemic agents such as tolbutamide. Resistance to infection is reduced so that great care must be taken to maintain sterility during insertion of the catheter and when changing infusion bottles.

We have seen that in patients with cirrhosis of the liver the acid–base state of blood is one of alkalosis, in both the metabolic and respiratory components during coma. A 'normal' plasma $[HCO_3^-]$ may therefore be regarded as a deficit of base, and when plasma levels only a little below normal are found, correction of this factor with infusions of $NaHCO_3$ can be made with clinical benefit. Some improvement in the degree of encephalopathy may be obtained with oral zinc supplements (Reding et al., 1984).[75]

Barbiturate Coma

In the first instance, as in all cases of coma, the prime concern of the clinician when treating a patient with barbiturate poisoning must be directed towards confirming whether the lungs are being adequately ventilated. Depression of respiration and anoxia[68] is the most common cause of death in this condition.

The patient may present in a hypoxic state at the very point of death. If, while the patient is in hospital, cardiac arrest occurs because of respiratory depression, reversion to a normal rhythm by electrical defibrillation, after either internal or external cardiac massage and positive pressure ventilation, is relatively easy. The author treated three patients who developed ventricular fibrillation in hospital; all survived. Resuscitative measures were taken immediately and electrical defibrillation was no problem once the desaturation of the arterial blood and the metabolic acidosis had been corrected. Barbiturates reduce metabolism at a cellular level so that the effects of hypoxia may not be as important in this condition as in others.

The patient may remain in coma for many days and require artificial ventilation for 5 days or more. Patients have been maintained first on controlled ventilation and later on patient-triggered pressure-cycled ventilation for 6 days using a plastic endotracheal tube. In this way tracheostomy has been avoided. No ill-effects followed this period of endotracheal intubation. The minute volume and tidal volume should be measured at frequent intervals, every 30 minutes in the early stages and later every hour. The same regimen as that for a cuffed endotracheal tube should be followed (see p. 167), the pressure within the cuff being released periodically and secretions in the lungs removed by suction. If ventilation is performed with dry (unhumidified) gases, 2 ml of 0.45% NaCl should be administered down the endotracheal tube every 30 minutes to 1 hour.

Gastric lavage

If the patient,has a cough reflex when first seen, gastric lavage can be performed immediately. This will remove tablets that are still within the stomach. The patient must be tilted in the head-down position so that inhalation of fluid into the lungs is avoided and care must be taken that the patient does not lapse into respiratory depression during the procedure. A slightly acid solution (e.g. a dilute solution of vinegar) should be used. If no cough reflex is present, tracheal intubation must be performed before gastric lavage.

Removal of absorbed barbiturates

Although patients can be maintained satisfactorily in barbiturate coma for many days when properly ventilated and kept in correct water and electrolyte balance, the assisted removal of the barbiturate, especially the long-acting preparations, may be necessary. In order to reduce the period of positive pressure ventilation or to avoid it becoming necessary, methods that increase renal excretions have been recommended for routine use.

Barbiturates are weak organic acids and are excreted by the proximal tubule as well as passing into the glomerular filtrate.[98] While passing through the rest of the nephron, barbiturate can be reabsorbed from the renal tubular fluid in a manner similar to the reabsorption of urea. This is most marked when the volume of urine is small and acid in reaction.[94] The converse, a rapid flow of alkaline urine, can be expected to increase barbiturate excretion, although only the excretion of phenobarbitone is known, without doubt, to be increased by a high urinary pH. Forms of treatment that achieve this state have been devised.

Myschetzky and Lassen have advocated the use of two solutions:[65,64]

(a) 50% urea in physiological saline;
(b) a solution containing sodium lactate, potassium chloride, sodium chloride and glucose.

Solution (a) causes a rapid diuresis and solution (b) is intended to make the urine alkaline while maintaining electrolyte balance. Hypernatraemia and hypokalaemia may develop, but they can be corrected by supplementing the intake of water and potassium salts. They advocated that 80 ml of urea solution (a) and 300 ml of the electrolyte solution (b) should be given every hour for 4 hours. If anuria has not developed, indicating peritoneal or haemodialysis, a brisk urine flow of 6 ml/minute should occur. Myschetzky and Lassen found that an average urine output of 12.1 litres/24 hours was obtained. This volume will cause marked dehydration if additional water is not given.

The organic buffer, tris hydroxymethyl aminomethane (THAM),[6] diuretics with physiological[69] saline and intravenous mannitol,[19] have also been tried. In many cases more than one barbiturate will have been taken, either intentionally or because they were combined in a single pill.

Peritoneal dialysis

Some workers in this field prefer peritoneal dialysis to a forced diuresis for the removal of barbiturate. After some experience it is easily performed and is probably justified when very high blood barbiturate levels are found.

Cerebral stimulants

In most centres the use of cerebral stimulants has been discarded completely and reliance has been placed solely upon maintaining adequate artificial ventilation, correct metabolic control and increasing the rate of excretion and removal of the barbiturate.

Cardiovascular system

In severe barbiturate poisoning accidental hypothermia may be produced and this, together with the intrinsic depression of myocardial activity, may cause severe hypotension. This is more marked when artificial ventilation is necessary and high inflation pressures are used to expand the lungs. Improvement in the patient's condition can be obtained by applying external heat, using if possible, a patient-triggered ventilator and injecting hydrocortisone in doses of 100–300 mg i.v. Following a period of cerebral anoxia resulting from respiratory depression, a raised body temperature may be found and cooling by exposure and cold wet towels may be necessary. Conversely, if the patient is exposed to a low ambient temperature, accidental hypothermia develops and death can occur from this cause when the dose of barbiturate taken is alone insufficient to kill.

Cardiac arrest due to barbiturate overdose

Case history. A 52-year-old patient with barbiturate poisoning was admitted to hospital on the point of death. Her pulse had been noted to be very weak. Cardiac arrest occurred while she was being transferred from the ambulance. External cardiac massage was begun immediately, an endotracheal tube was inserted and the lungs were ventilated with oxygen. An intravenous drip of 2.74% $NaHCO_3$ was set up. External cardiac massage produced a pulsation in the carotid arteries that was palpable only with difficulty, and the pupils remained dilated. A non-sterile thoracotomy was performed and the heart was electrically defibrillated at the first attempt when 350 ml of the bicarbonate solution had been infused over 15 minutes. The systolic blood pressure remained in the region of 70 mmHg while the chest was closed. Ventilation of the lungs was continued with a mechanical ventilator and the systolic blood pressure fell to 60 mmHg. The temperature of the patient was found to be 32.1°C (89.8°F). An arterial blood sample was taken when 750 ml of the bicarbonate solution had been infused and this revealed a marked metabolic and respiratory alkalosis (Table 12.2a). The ventilation was changed so as to conform with the Radford nomogram (see p. 134) and a rise in the blood pressure followed. A further rise in blood pressure to 100/50 mmHg followed the intravenous administration of 200 mg of hydrocortisone. The patient's temperature rose until it reached 38.88°C (102°F).

Sample (*a*) was taken during artificial ventilation; 2 days later positive pressure ventilation was stopped and the endotracheal tube was removed. Full return to consciousness had not been reached, but moderate hyperventilation continued. The patient's arterial blood continued to show a respiratory and metabolic alkalosis (Table 12.2 b) which was still present when she had returned to a normal level of consciousness after a further 2 days (Table 12.2c).

Table 12.2 Acid–base data taken at intervals of 2 days from a patient who suffered cardiac arrest as a result of barbiturate poisoning

	pH	Standard bicarbonate (mmol/l, mEq/l)	PCO_2 (mmHg)
(a)	7.83	30.2	12.0
(b)	7.53	28.0	32.5
(c)	7.51	26.2	30.0

pH = arterial blood pH at 38°C.

It is of interest to note that no infection resulted from the non-sterile thoracotomy and there was no impairment of renal function. The importance of avoiding a gross respiratory alkalosis in the hypothermic patient has been stressed (see p. 258).

Summary of treatment

1. Maintain adequate ventilation.
2. Perform gastric lavage with acidulated water.
3. Maintain cardiovascular system by means of warmth and hydrocortisone given intravenously.
4. Administer positive pressure ventilation when the tidal volume falls to 300 ml *before* respiratory arrest occurs. Remember the patient who accepts an endotracheal tube *needs* an endotracheal tube.
5. Administer alkali intravenously (e.g. $NaHCO_3$ 2.74%) in order to increase the rate of excretion of barbiturates. A forced diuresis with hyperosmolar solutions or diuretics may be indicated.
6. In very severe barbiturate poisoning peritoneal dialysis may be necessary.

7. Maintain correct water and electrolyte balance and adequate nutrition throughout.

Coma from Salicylate Intoxication

Aspirin poisoning may appear as an overdose given therapeutically, especially in infants when instructions to parents have been misunderstood. This occurs now less commonly because of the availability of pleasantly tasting aspirin tablets which contain only 100 mg. Aspirin poisoning also occurs accidentally in children when they take the adult tablets in mistake for sweets, and in adults who have attempted suicide. Salicylates may be detected in the urine by the addition of ferric chloride 10% drop by drop. At first the urine in a test tube may give a precipitate of phosphates, but on further addition of the ferric chloride the typical reddish-purple colour is obtained which, unlike ketone bodies, does not disappear on boiling.

Salicylates have a profound effect upon the metabolism of the body. Marked and obvious hyperventilation occurs by direct stimulation of the respiratory centre. Aspirin also sensitizes the respiratory centre to CO_2 so that it is sometimes given in acute respiratory failure. In the early stages increased alveolar ventilation occurs which is not clinically detectable (see p. 118) because there is no increase in respiratory rate, but only in tidal volume. Measurement of blood gases, however, show a fall in the arterial PCO_2. At a later stage marked and obvious hyperventilation occurs (respiratory rate and depth increase) and a marked reduction in arterial PCO_2 follows. When a concentration of salicylate in the blood reaches lethal levels, respiratory depression follows, bradycardia occurs and this is followed by ventricular fibrillation. The PCO_2 at this stage may be found to be raised in the presence of a marked metabolic acidosis and arterial blood oxygen desaturation.

Although salicylates are normally used as antipyretics, in toxic doses they raise the body temperature. When near-lethal intoxication in reached, hyperthermia gives place to hypothermia unless cardiac arrest occurs before this stage.

The salicylates themselves also produce a metabolic acidosis of large proportions and in addition sometimes give rise to the presence of ketone bodies. Impairment of cardiac output by the toxic action upon the myocardium may also cause a raised blood lactate and pyruvate concentration.[68] These changes in the body metabolism are readily reflected in measurements of the acid–base state of the blood.

Acid–base changes in salicylate poisoning

Initially, hyperventilation, which causes a fall in the PCO_2, produces a raised blood pH with little change in the metabolic component. Figures from Case A (Table 12.3) are taken from a patient who was being treated with large doses of aspirin for rheumatoid arthritis. The respiratory rate was not noticeably increased.

Table 12.3 Acid–base findings in patients with salicylate overdosage

		pH	Standard bicarbonate (mmol/l, mEq/l)	PCO_2 (mmHg)
Case A		7.47	23.4	30.0
Case B	(i)	7.56	23.1	23.5
	(ii)	7.57	28.3	28.0

pH = blood pH at 38°C.

The results for Case A are the findings in a man placed on high aspirin dosage for rheumatoid arthritis for 5 days. There was no dyspnoea, but a lowered PCO_2 is apparent.

The results for Case B are those described in the case history. B (i) was taken 1 hour after completion of a transfusion of 2 units of ACD (acid–citrate–dextrose) blood and an infusion of 300 ml (100 mmol) of $NaHCO_3$ (2.74% solution) and 50 mg of ethacrynic acid. Note how an isolated pH measurement alone would be misleading because the bicarbonate is still 1 mmol/l (mEq/l) below normal values.

Sample B (ii) was taken 24 hours later, and it will be seen that alveolar hyperventilation is still present, giving rise to a respiratory alkalosis, although the salicylate had been largely eliminated and a metabolic alkalosis was present.

When there has been attempted suicide and the patient is in coma, hyperventilation, which is readily detectable by clinical observation, soon occurs. The PCO_2 is lowered to such levels that a blood pH which is abnormally alkaline is always detected (e.g. 7.55 or more). This is so even in the presence of a major metabolic acidosis.* It can therefore be seen that this is one clinical condition in which a measurement of plasma bicarbonate or total carbon dioxide (TCO_2) is of little value, because it is reduced by both the respiratory and the metabolic component of acid–base balance. It is when the metabolic component, which may fall to below 10 mmol/l, is reduced that respiratory depression in this condition appears to occur,

although the actual level of bicarbonate concentration at which cessation of respiration appears varies between individual patients. Although, therefore, it is sometimes said that because hyperventilation tends to compensate for the fall in bicarbonate ion concentration alkali therapy is unnecessary, the infusion of $NaHCO_3$ is an essential part of therapy in some cases. The infusion of alkali in no way depresses the ventilation, it increases cardiac output and aids the secretion of salicylate in the urine.

Treatment of salicylate poisoning

In the first instance salicylates may give rise to polyuria, but this may become depressed if there is a toxic action upon the myocardium. It is essential, however, to increase urine output to the maximum, and fluids should therefore be infused as rapidly as is possible, bearing in mind the possibility of precipitating cardiac failure. A diuretic which does not give rise to a metabolic acidosis, such as ethacrynic acid or frusemide (Lasix), may also be given intravenously. In this way fluids may be given with greater safety. The use of the diuretic acetazolamide has sometimes been advocated because it tends to increase the blood pH. It has, however, been found to increase the mortality of animals receiving toxic amounts of salicylates.[47]

Very often the cause of suicide is another underlying disease process which is undiagnosed but will respond to treatment. The changes that occur in salicylate poisoning are readily illustrated below.

Case history. A 60-year-old woman was admitted to hospital in undiagnosed coma although it later transpired that she had taken 100 325-mg aspirin tablets some time during the night. While she was being examined she became grossly hypotensive so that her blood pressure and pulse were unrecordable, respiration ceased and after a period of bradycardia the heart beat became undetectable. External cardiac massage was begun and mephentermine (Mephine) 15 mg was given intravenously. Digoxin, 0.5 mg, was also given because it had been noticed on inspection that there was a raised jugular venous presse (JVP). After very few minutes spontaneous ventilation returned and the blood pressure rose to 110/50 mmHg. Hyperventilation was apparent. It was noticed that in addition to hyperventilation and raised neck veins, the patient's mucous membranes were extremely pale. A rapid cross-matching of blood was performed and 2 units were infused with the addition of 25 mg of ethacrynic acid to each unit.[52] When the blood had been given,

* An *alkalaemia* is present associated with the metabolic acidosis.

a haemoglobin estimation performed at that time gave a value of 30%. A blood film demonstrated a macrocytic megaloblastic anaemia. An estimation of plasma TCO_2 showed it to be 14 mmol/l. Arterial blood gases performed 1 hour later confirmed the hyperventilation and the base deficit. It was, therefore, decided to infuse sodium bicarbonate solution and 300 ml of 2.74% solution was given over a period of 25 minutes. Improvement continued and consciousness returned 5 hours later. The ethacrynic acid produced a large diuresis of 1.5 litres in the first hour and more than 3 litres in the 12 hours following its administration. Correction of a low haemoglobin concentration by giving a blood transfusion and intravenous vitamin B_{12} was continued. The patient's condition the following day was markedly improved and, although the respiratory rate had returned to 19 breaths/minute, increased alveolar ventilation was detectable on examination of the blood gases (Table 12.3).

Hyperventilation is a characteristic of large salicylate dosages because the effect on the respiratory centre persists for a considerable time after its administration. It is achieved by an increased depth of breathing and may not be clinically detectable on examination of the patient at this stage, any more than it is detectable in the early stages of salicylate poisoning. In addition to illustrating the importance of maintaining a good urine flow, of correcting the metabolic acidosis and maintaining hydration, this patient also shows that suicidal attempts are sometimes the result of organic disease processes and that one form of treatment in isolation may be insufficient to achieve success.

Coma from Addison's Disease

The adrenal glands lie at the upper poles of the two kidneys. One is cone shaped, the other is shaped like a half-moon. Anatomically, functionally and embryologically, both glands consist of two separate parts.

The cortex is of mesodermal origin and is laid down before the medulla, which is formed from ectoderm. The cortex of the gland is divided histologically into three separate layers or zones: the zona glomerulosa, the zona fasciculata and the zona reticularis. Each zone is considered to have its own special function. The zona glomerulosa, for example, is believed to be the site of aldosterone production, the zona reticularis is associated with the production of sex hormones and corticosteroids, and the zona fasciculata is associated with the precursors of steroids.

The adrenal medulla, which consists of chromaffin* tissue and sympathetic ganglion cells, forms adrenaline (epinephrine) and noradrenaline (norepinephrine) and, unlike the adrenal cortex, is not essential to life. This is because the substances it produces are also elaborated in chromaffin tissues scattered throughout the body and in sympathetic ganglion cells.

If both suprarenal glands are removed, however, death occurs within 15 days because of the loss of cortical secretions.

The adrenal cortex is stimulated by adreno-cortico-trophic hormone (ACTH) elaborated by the pituitary gland. It is suppressed by cortisone and cortisol (hydrocortisone). Various investigations have shown that ACTH does not stimulate the production or release of *all* cortical hormones. Aldosterone, for example, appears to be very largely removed from its control.

The adrenocortical steroids are usually divided into three main groups according to their predominant action upon body metabolism. This division is also very largely related to their chemical structure.

Mineralocorticoids

These are the salt-retaining steroids, aldosterone (which predominates), deoxycorticosterone, corticosterone and cortisol. Apart from aldosterone and deoxycorticosterone, the salt-retaining properties of these hormones is so weak that they are relatively ineffective in maintaining a positive salt balance after adrenalectomy. For therapeutic purposes a synthetic steroid, 9-α-fluorohydrocortisone (Fludrocortisone), is used because its metabolic effects are very nearly the same as those of the naturally produced hormone, aldosterone. The mineralocorticoids, in addition to promoting the retention of Na^+, cause an increased excretion of K^+ by the renal tubules.

Glucocorticoids

These steroids are cortisol, cortisone and corticosterone. Their main function within the body is largely concerned with carbohydrate, protein and fat metabolism, the response of the body to trauma and changes in water content. For example, these steroids must be present in order that the body can

---

* Chromaffin is the term used for denoting cells which have an affinity for stain.

react to a water load by excretion of a dilute urine. When given in excessive doses they produce water retention,† oedema and therefore sometimes cardiac failure and the symptoms and signs of Cushing's syndrome. Because of their effect on carbohydrate metabolism they produce hyperglycaemia and glycosuria. When absent they conversely produce hypoglycaemia and depletion of glycogen both in the liver and muscles.

By their action upon protein the glucocorticoids cause an increase in protein breakdown and thus promote gluconeogenesis.

Sex hormones

These substances may also have an effect upon water excretion and electrolyte metabolism. Androgens, oestrogens and progesterone are all formed in the adrenal cortex in both sexes.

Suprarenal insufficiency

When the suprarenal glands are destroyed or partially destroyed by tuberculosis, auto immune disease, acquired immunodeficiency syndrome (AIDS)[39] or by other circumstances such as spontaneous atrophy, the symptoms of adrenocortical insufficiency appear. The characteristic clinical features of the disease are lethargy, tiredness of great severity, hypotension, subnormal body temperature, pigmentation of the skin and mucous membranes seen on the roof of the mouth and buccal mucosa, and disturbances of water and electrolyte metabolism. Dehydration is produced, Na^+ is lost from the body and K^+ is retained. The blood sugar concentration is also reduced.

In the early stages lethargy and tiredness sometimes associated with polyuria and abdominal pains are often the only symptoms. As the disease progresses tiredness gives place to muscle weakness and medical advice is usually requested. Sometimes, however, especially if an unrelated infection, such as pneumonia, occurs, the patient may pass directly into a state of Addisonian crisis.

Although the temperature is usually subnormal, even in the presence of infective processes, hyperpyrexia has been noted in the absence of infection. Pigmentation is not always present. The blood pressure is low and may be recorded only with difficulty. In the preterminal stages ventilation is depressed and at a slow rate, giving rise to desaturation of the arterial blood. The patient cannot be roused. Examination of the skin reveals

dehydration and this is associated with a raised packed cell volume (PCV).

Blood analysis shows a low sodium concentration and a raised potassium concentration. The blood urea is high (e.g. 25 mmol/l, 150 mg%), and the blood sugar is low. Urgent replacement of salt and water is essential at this stage and must be accompanied by the injection intravenously of corticosteroids. The treatment is illustrated by the following case.

Case history. A 45-year-old man was admitted to hospital in a comatose state. His temperature was subnormal and his respiratory rate was 13/minute. Blood pressure was 65/35 mmHg. No pigmentation of the skin was visible. The patient was clearly dehydrated because of loss of skin elasticity. His packed cell volume (PCV) was 56%. Gentle inflation of the lungs with oxygen was performed and blood was taken for analysis. The following results were obtained: Na^+ 126 mmol/l (mEq/l), K^+ 7.1 mmol/l (mEq/l) and urea 24.9 mmol/l (150 mg%).

Analysis of a catheter specimen of urine demonstrated that it contained 120 mmol/l (mEq/l) of sodium and 40 mmol/l (mEq/l) of potassium. During the next 12 hours the patient was infused with 9 litres of normal saline i.v. and given 1500 mg of hydrocortisone i.v. When, after 6 hours, his blood pressure had risen to 110/70 mmHg and he was able to swallow, he was given 9-α-fluorohydrocortisone 0.5 mg p.o. Within 24 hours he had fully recovered and was able to converse normally. The following day his blood urea had fallen to 5.8 mmol/l (35 mg%) and he volunteered that he felt very much stronger than for many weeks previously. He was later maintained on oral cortisone and 9-α-fluorohydrocortisone.

Cerebral Embolus

Cerebral embolus today occurs commonly during an extracorporeal circulation. Air is frequently seen to lie within the coronary vessels following open-heart surgery. However, this does not always produce a cerebral embolus, although it is obvious that when air enters the left side of the heart it can be directed into the carotid vessels and thence into the brain. Therefore, the earliest signs of brain damage arising from emboli may be seen during the latter part of an open-heart operation using an extracorporeal circulation; these are hypertension and hyperpyrexia.

Cerebral emboli also occur as a result of valve prosthesis.

† A high plasma Na^+ is usually not seen because of the concomitant retention of H_2O.

Hypertension

When blood is infused from an extracorporeal apparatus into the patient only a small volume is required to produce an excessive rise in blood pressure. Pressures of above 200 mmHg may be obtained under these conditions. This, under extreme circumstances, may give rise to bleeding from the orifices such as the nose, and careful regulation of the circulating blood volume is therefore necessary. It is sometimes argued that the hypertension precedes brain damage and this may well be so, especially during an extracorporeal circulation involving hypothermia of a moderate degree or to such low temperatures that the procedure is referred to as profound hypothermia. During cooling and rewarming temperature gradients of not greater than 10°C (50°F) between the blood leaving the heat exchanger and the temperature of the nasopharynx of the patient should be maintained throughout the procedure. When brain damage occurs from any cause, numerous signs of central nervous system damage appear either early during the extracorporeal circulation or later.

Hyperpyrexia

If a heat exchanger has not been incorporated into the extracorporeal circulation, the onset of the very high temperature may occur towards the end of the period of extracorporeal circulation. If hypothermia has been used, rewarming of the patient may occur slowly, and will be followed by a marked rise of temperature when the operation has been completed. The normal afterdrop of temperature when the circulation of warm blood is stopped may still occur, but this is followed by the continuous rise of body temperature if measured at a central point such as the oesophagus or the rectum.

Focal neurological signs

Almost all anaesthetized patients will have received relaxants so that no reflexes will be elicited during anaesthesia, The only sign which will indicate brain damage is that of unequal pupils, but this is unreliable.

Postoperative physical signs

When cerebral embolus has occurred, the patient fails to regain consciousness at the end of the anaesthetic. The pupils may be of unequal size and the position of the eyes may be abnormal. When the effects of the anaesthetic have completely disappeared, the patient still fails to respond to painful stimuli. The breathing may be noisy and stertorous, and respiratory depression is not usually a major feature in this syndrome. Focal neurological signs then begin to appear. There may be, for example, a hemiplegia, a positive Babinski reflex or absent tendon reflexes and it is at this stage that the pupils become of unequal size. By this time the body temperature has often risen steeply and special measures have to be taken in order to reduce it. Fits of a predominantly Jacksonian type then make their appearance and these often increase in intensity as time progresses. A further rise in body temperature often occurs in the period immediately following a fit. Active voluntary movements by the patient may now be present, although the patient lies completely still and only moves just before a fit takes place. At times the patient may appear to be just returning to consciousness and even sometimes to be looking at the medical attendants and to be doing so in response to requests or commands. This, however, is misleading and it is important that no relaxation of treatment should take place as it is well known that the return to consciousness may take 6 weeks or more and that this will only be achieved by long, patient and accurate medical and nursing care. The management of the patient therefore has two aspects; first, the treatment that is necessary immediately following the embolus, and second, when the acute effects of the cerebral embolus have ended, it is necessary to maintain the essential vital functions in an unconscious, immovable and incontinent patient for a long period of time.

Aspects of treatment immediately following a cerebral embolus

Control of body temperature

The higher the body temperature rises the more frequent fitting appears to be. The violent muscular movements that take place during the fit contribute to a sharp rise in body temperature. It is, therefore, necessary to break this potentially lethal circle of events.

External cooling

The patient is covered with towels which have been dipped into cold or iced water and a fan is placed nearby so that a draught of cold air is blown across the body. In this way active cooling will begin. However, it is necessary continually to record the rectal temperature as a marked gradient of temperature can occur between the skin and other parts of the body. For example, a thermometer placed in the axilla or in the groin may read 35°C (95°F) while a thermometer placed in the rectum or the oesophagus at the same time may read 40.6°C (105°F) or more. It is sometimes recommended that chlorpromazine (Largactil) should be given by deep intramuscular injection in order to help to reduce the body temperature. In the author's opinion, however, there are few indications for this drug because large doses are often necessary before any effect can be seen and sometimes a profound fall in blood pressure results; on one occasion this has given rise to acute renal failure. If under certain circumstances it is found necessary to resort to the use of chlorpromazine (Largactil), individual doses of no greater than 100 mg should be given and these repeated with great caution. If a marked fall in blood pressure results, this will respond to the intravenous injection of adequate doses (e.g. 200 or 500 mg) of hydrocortisone.

Control of convulsions

By far the most effective treatment is the intramuscular injection of paraldehyde. This can be given in doses of 10 ml for an adult and repeated hourly until the fits cease. This is a safe form of therapy and no abnormal changes in the cardiovascular and respiratory system are seen. The effects of barbiturate drugs are disappointing in this condition, and barbiturates will rarely control fitting when used alone. However, they may be used to augment the effect of paraldehyde. Sodium phenobarbitone can be given intramuscularly in doses of 200 mg to an adult; the dose has to be reduced for children and infants. A child of 25 kg may safely be given 5 ml of paraldehyde intramuscularly and this dose repeated hourly in the same way as in the adult until fitting stops. A child of 25 kg would require 60 mg of sodium phenobarbitone. Diazepam (Valium) may also control the convulsions. It is given in doses of 5–10 mg i.v.

Blood pressure

In the presence of a normal cardiac output the patient who has suffered a cerebral embolus is extremely sensitive to changes in blood volume. In most cases there is a tendency towards hypertension and this is usually most apparent when damage to the central nervous system has occurred during the processes of an extracorporeal circulation. In the postoperative period, however, overtransfusion produces a marked rise in systemic arterial blood pressure and care therefore has to be taken to control the rate of blood transfusion so

that an excessive rise of systemic arterial pressure is avoided. It is probably not advisable to follow the trend of blood replacement being mathematically equal to estimated blood loss, but a moderate degree of hypovolaemia may produce a marked fall in blood pressure. It is therefore essential to maintain very close observation of this very important clinical factor.

Dehydration therapy

Because anoxic brain tissue may become oedematous, it has been advocated that hypertonic urea–glucose mixtures should be infused. The osmotic activity of these substances causes the withdrawal of water from all tissues and produces an osmotic diuresis with subsequent total body dehydration. This is reflected in raised plasma [Na^+], protein concentration and blood PCV (see p. 33).

It is known that the oedematous appearance seen in brain cells that have been anoxic is not present before 18 hours have elapsed, by which time fluid restriction will have had a similar effect without the consequences of a grossly altered body metabolism. In the author's experience no reduction in the frequency of fitting or other beneficial effects of treatment have resulted from its use.

Patients with brain damage may remain unconscious for many weeks, and they can be successfully resuscitated to live a normal life following a long period of unconsciousness when care is taken to maintain body function and metabolism.

Long-term care

Cerebral embolus is very similar in many ways to the condition that can be seen when anoxic brain damage has been caused by cardiac arrest. In these circumstances the same kind of aftercare is necessary.

Feeding

A severely ill or unconscious patient is unable to take either fluid or solid food orally. A careful fluid balance and adequate calorie intake have to be maintained. Fluid balance is described in Chapter 2.

Intravenous glucose and vitamins may maintain a patient for some weeks, but after some operations and in some clinical circumstances it may be necessary to continue intravenous feeding for 3 months. Intravenous amino acid preparations can be used successfully, although it is possible that hypophosphataemia can develop (see p. 55).

Infusion of purified protein fraction also assists in replacing essential factors.

Whenever possible an intragastric tube should be passed, the length of which should be measured so that there is some indication of its position in the alimentary tract. There is never any necessity for a normal diet not to be taken by an unconscious patient as long as absorption from the alimentary canal continues and there is no vomiting. Modern methods of pulverizing (blending) food are readily available at a moderate cost. It is, therefore, possible to produce a normal diet or a normal meal for a patient and then reduce it to a liquid form by placing it in a suitable machine with an adequate quantity of water. In this way it is possible to feed and nourish any sick person so that the fluid balance and a normal vitamin and electrolyte intake are maintained. If intrinsic renal disease is present or renal function is impaired, for example because of pyrexia, toxicity, cardiac failure etc., feeding presents a much more difficult problem and must be dealt with as described in Chapter 2. In the majority of cases, however, the severely ill and unconscious patient is exposed over a period of time to the danger of the wrong administration of the wrong food materials in the wrong quantities. The simplest manner in which the nutrition of a patient may be maintained is therefore with a simple normal pulverized (blended) diet.

Fluid requirements will vary according to the patient's size in the presence of a pyrexia, the temperature of the environment and the solute load to which the renal apparatus is exposed, in the form of urea and electrolytes. The average quantity of fluid the patient might need is dealt with in Chapter 2, but some indication of the patient's requirements will be obtained by measuring the urine specific gravity. A rise in specific gravity above 1.022 will indicate, in the absence of a high osmotic load, the necessity to conserve water, and it may therefore be necessary to increase the water intake.

Prolonged bed-rest
Degenerative changes begin to appear almost immediately the first 24 hours of complete bed-rest has begun. In the unconscious patient a decubitus ulcer of enormous size can be produced in less than 3 hours and loss of skin is almost invariably seen, even in the young patient, after being left immobile for 5 hours. Complete immobility in bed is dangerous. In general, decubitus ulcers can be prevented by correct nursing and physiotherapy.

It is necessary to turn the patient every half-hour and to prevent one limb pressing against another. The patient must be lifted so that skin is not rubbed against the sheets during moving.

An alternating pressure point pad unit, such as that produced by Talley Surgical Instruments, London, UK, which rhythmically alters the areas where the body presses against the mattress by means of an air compressor, is an important aid to nursing. The incontinent patient has to be kept clean and dry and the skin treated with lanoline or silicone creams. If a bed sore is produced, it should be treated with antibiotic creams and kept well padded and covered. Ultraviolet light, which in effect produces a 'sunburn', does not appear to have any outstanding beneficial effect in promoting healing.

Care of the mouth
The unconscious patient who is unable to take fluids orally is liable to develop monilia infections of the mouth and oral pharynx. The oral cavity must be cleansed with bland antiseptic mouthwash at regular intervals.

Care of the eyes
If the eyes are left uncovered and open for long periods of time, corneal ulceration may develop. Rinsing with isotonic saline or isotonic sodium bicarbonate helps to prevent this occurring, and the use of antibiotics or sulphonamide drops is rarely necessary. The eyelids may be kept closed by means of strapping placed over gauze.

Physiotherapy
The movement of the limbs by a trained physiotherapist, performed at least three times a day, greatly assists in the eventual rehabilitation of the unconscious patient. Assisted breathing and coughing help to reduce chest complications.

Keeping a patient alive through a prolonged period of unconsciousness is always a great challenge and often very rewarding, especially, for example, in a young patient after a car accident in whom apparent neurological damage disappears 6 months to 1 year later. Every effort should always be made to maintain accurate control over fluid, electrolyte, metabolic, cardiac and respiratory function.

References

1. Alberti, K. G. M. M. and Hockaday, T. D. R. (1972). Blood lactic and pyruvic acids in diabetic coma. *Diabetes*, **21**, 350.

2. Allen, F. M. and Wishart, M. B. (1923). Experimental studies in diabetes. V: Acidosis. *J. Metab. Res.*, **4**, 223.

3. Arieff, A. I. (1975). Nonketotic hyperosmolar coma with hyperglycemia. In *Diabetes Mellitus*, 4th edn, p. 181. Edited by K. E. Sussman and R. J. S. Metz. New York: American Diabetes Association.

4. Arieff, A. I. and Carroll, H. J. (1974). Cerebral edema and depression of sensorium in nonketotic hyperosmolar coma. *Diabetes*, **23**, 525.

5. Atkinson, M. and Goligher, J. C. (1960). Recurrent hepatic coma treated by colectomy and ileorectal anastomosis. *Lancet*, **i**, 461.

6. Balagot, R. C., Tsuji, H. and Sadove, M. S. (1961). Use of an osmotic diuretic—THAM—in treatment of barbiturate poisoning: alkalinizing action of drug and its ability to increase elimination of electrolytes in urine appears to facilitate clearance of barbiturates. *J. Amer. med Assoc.*, **178**, 1000.

7. Banting, F. G. and Best, C. H. (1922). The internal secretion of the pancreas. *J. Lab. Clin. Med.*, **7**, 251.

8. Banting, F. G., Best, C. H. and Collip, J. B. (1922). The effects of insulin on experimental hyperglycemia in rabbits. *Amer. J. Physiol.*, **62**, 559.

9. Banting, F. G., Best, C. H., Collip, J. B., Campbell, W. R. and Fletcher, A. A. (1922). Pancreatic extracts in the treatment of diabetes mellitus. *Canad. med. Assoc. J.*, **12**, 141.

10. Bell, J. L., Shaldon, S. and Baron, D. N. (1962). Serum isocitrate dehydrogenase in liver disease and some other conditions. *Clin. Sci.*, **23**, 57.

11. Bendezu, R., Wieland, R. G., Furst, B. H., Mandel, M., Genuth, S. M. and Schumacher, P. (1978). Experience with low-dose insulin infusion in diabetic ketosis and diabetic hyperosmolarity. *Arch. Int. Med.*, **138**, 60.

12. Bock, A. V., Field, H. and Adair, J. S. (1923). The acid base equilibrium in diabetic coma, being a study of five cases treated with insulin. *J. Metab. Res.*, **4**, 27.

13. Boyer, J., Gill, G. N. and Epstein, F. H. (1967). Hyperglycemia and hyperosmolarity complicating peritoneal dialysis. *Ann. Int. Med.*, **67**, 568.

14. Brooks, D. K. (1967). *Resuscitation*, 1st edn. p.00. London: Edward Arnold.

15. Brooks, D. K. (1972). Organ failure following surgery. In *Advances in Surgery*, p. 289. Chicago: Year Book Medical Publishers

16. Brooks, D. K. Unpublished observations.

17. Brooks, D. K., Williams, W. G., Manley, R. and Whiteman, P. (1963). Osmolar and electrolyte changes in haemorrhagic shock: hypertonic solutions in the prevention of tissue damage. *Lancet*, **i**, 521.

18. Campbell, W. R. (1922). Ketosis, acidosis and coma treated by insulin. *J. Metab. Res.*, **2**, 605.

19. Cirksena, W. J., Bastian, R. C. and Barry, K. G. (1962). Use of mannitol in exogenous and endogenous intoxications. In *Symposium on clinical and experimental use of mannitol*, pp. 31–2. Washington. D. C.: Walter Reed Army Institute of Research.

20. Clements, R. S., Prockop, L. D. and Winegrad, A. L. (1968). Acute cerebral edema during treatment of hyperglycemia. *Lancet*, **ii**, 384.

21. Danowski, T. S. (1971). Nonketotic coma and diabetes mellitus. *Med. Clin. North America.*, **54**, 683.

22. De Graef, J. and Lips, J. B. (1957). Hypernatraemia in diabetes mellitus. *Acta. med. Scand.*, **157**, 71.

23. Desgrez, A. and Soggio, G. (1907). Sur la nocivite des composes acetoniques. *Compt. rend. Soc. Biol. (Paris)*, **63**, 288.

24. Dickinson, R. (1898). Quoted by: Williamson, R. T. (1898). In *Diabetes Mellitus and its Treatment*, p. 399. Edited by J. Young. Edinburgh and London: Pentland.

25. Dintzis, R. Z. and Hastings, A. B. (1953). The effect of antibiotics on urea breakdown in mice. *Proc. nat. Acad. Sci., (Wash.)*, **39**, 571.

26. Dreschfeld, J. (1886). Diabetic coma. *Brit. med. J.*, **2**, 358.

27. Ehrlich, R. M. and Bain, H. W. (1967). Hyperglycemia and hyperosmolarity in an eighteen-month-old child. *New Engl. J. of Med.*, **276**, 83.

28. Ehrmann, R. (1913). Ueber das coma diabeticum. *Berlin Klin. Wschr.*, **1**, 11.

29. Feinblatt, H. M. (1924). Report of a fatal case of juvenile diabetic coma with insignificant ketonuria, and with a large amount of acetone in the spinal fluid. *Arch. Int. Med.,* **23**, 509.

30. Fernandez, J. P., McGinn, J. T. and Hoffman, R. S. (1968). Cerebral edema from blood-brain glucose differences complicating peritoneal dialysis second membrane syndrome. *N. Y. St. J. Med.*, **68**, 677.

31. Fineberg, S. E. and Levin, R. M. (1977). Diabetic ketoacidosis and nonketotic hyperosmolar hyperglycemic coma. In *Medical Emergencies: Diagnostic and Management Procedures from Boston City Hospital*, p.163. Edited by A. S. Cohen, R. B. Freidin and M. A. Samuels. Boston: Little Brown.

32. Fisher, C. J. and Faloon, W. W. (1957). Blood ammonia levels in hepatic cirrhosis; their control by the oral administration of neomycin *N. Engl. J. of Med.*, **256**, 1030.

33. Fitzgerald, M. G., O'Sullivan, J. and Malins, J. M. (1961). Fatal diabetic ketosis. *Brit. med. J.*, **i**, 247.

34. Frier, B. M. and McConnell, J. B. (1975). Cerebral oedema in diabetic ketoacidosis. *Brit. med. J.*, **2**, 208.

35. Fulop, M., Rosenblatt, A., Kreitzer, S. M. and Gerstenhaber, B. (1975). Hyperosmolar nature of

diabetic coma. *Diabetes*, **24**, 594.

36. Fulop, M., Tannenbaum, H. and Drever, N. (1976). Ketotic hyperosmolar coma. *Lancet*, **ii**, 635.

37. Gerhardt, C. (1865). Diabetes mellitus und aceton. *Wien. Med. Presse*, **6**, 673.

38. Ginsburg-Fellner, F. and Primack, W. A. (1975). Recurrent hyperosmolar nonketotic episodes in a young diabetic. *Amer. J. Dis. Child*, **129**, 240.

39. Guenthner, E. E., Rabinowe, S. L., Vanniel, A., Naftilan, A. and Dluhy, R. G. (1984). Primary Addison's disease in a patient with the acquired immunodeficiency syndrome. *Ann. Int. Med.*, **100**, 847.

40. Handa, S. P. and Cushner, G. B. (1968). Hyperosmolar hyperglycemic nonketotic coma during peritoneal dialysis. *Southern Med. J.*, **61**, 700.

41. Hayes, T. M. and Woods, C. J. (1968). Hyperosmolar non-ketotic coma. Lancet, **i**, 209.

42. Hilton-Fagge, C. (1874). A case of diabetic coma treated with partial success by the injection of a saline solution into the blood. *Guy's Hospital Reports*, **19**, 173.

43. Hubbard, T. B. (1958). Carcinoma of the head of the pancreas: resection of the portal vein and portacaval shunt. *Ann. Surg.*, **147**, 935.

44. Jackson, W. P. U. and Forman, R. (1966). Hyperosmolar nonketotic diabetic coma. *Diabetes*, **15**, 714.

45. Jones, P. N. G., Mahood, J. M., Pye, J. K., Thacker, C. R. and Brooks, D. K. (1980). Biochemical findings in diabetic ketosis in the accident and emergency department. (unpublished).

46. Joslin, E. P. (1917). *The Treatment of Diabetes Mellitus*, 2nd edn, p.88. Philadelphia and New York: Lea and Febiger.

47. Kaplan, S. A. and Del Carmen, F. T. (1958). Experimental salicylate poisoning: observations on the effects of carbonic anhydrase inhibitor and bicarbonate. *Pediatrics*, **21**, 762.

48. Knowles, H. C. (1966). Syrupy blood (editorial). *Diabetes*, **15**, 760.

49. Kulz, E. (1884). Ueber eine neue links drehende Saure (Pseudooxy-buttersaure; ein Beitrag zur Kenntniss de Zuckherruhr. *Sschr. Biol.*, **20**, 221.

50. Kunkel, H. G. (1947). Estimation of alterations of serum gamma globulin by a turbidimetric technique. *Proc. Soc. exp. Biol. (N.Y.)*, **66**, 217.

51. Kussmaul, A. (1874). Zur lehre vom diabetes mellitus. *Dtsch. Arch. Klin. Med.*, **14**, 1.

52. Ledingham, J. G. (1964). Ethacrynic acid parenterally in the treatment and prevention of pulmonary oedema. *Lancet*, **i**, 952.

53. McDermott, W. V., Adams, R. D. and Riddell, A. G. (1954). Ammonia metabolism in man. *Ann. Surg.*, **140**, 539.

54. McGurdy, D. K. (1970). Hyperosmolar hyperglycemic nonketotic diabetic coma. *Med. Clin. North. Am.*, **54**, 683.

55. MacLagan, N. F. (1944). The thymol turbidity test as an indicator of liver dysfunction. *Brit. J. exp. Path.*, **25**, 234.

56. Maccario, M. (1968). Neurological dysfunction associated with non-ketotic hyperglycaemia. *Archs. Neurol., Chicago*, **19**, 525.

57. Maccario, M. and Messis, C. P. (1969). Cerebral oedema complicating treated non-ketotic hyperglycaemia. *Lancet*, **ii**, 352.

58. Maccario, M., Messis, C. P. and Vastola, E. F. (1965). Focal seizures as a manifestation of hyperglycemia without ketoacidosis. *Neurology, Minneap.*, **15**, 195.

59. Marliss, E. B., Ohman, J. L., Aoki, T. T. and Kozak, G. P. (1970). Altered redox state obscuring ketoacidosis in diabetic patients with lactic acidosis. *N. Engl. J. of Med.*, **283**, 978.

60. Marriott, W. McK. (1914). The blood in acidosis from the quantitative standpoint. *J. Biol. Chem.*, **18**, 507.

61. Marx, A. (1910). Ueber die wirkung des buttersauren natriums auf dem organismus junger hungernder hunde, nebst bemberkungen zur lehre vom coma diabeticum. *Zschr. f. klin. Med.*, **71**, 165.

62. Minkowski, O. (1884). Ueber das vorkommen von oxybuttersaure in harn bei diabetes, ein beitrag zur lehre von coma diabeticum. *Arch. f. exp. Pathol. u. Pharm.*, **18**, 35.

63. Moore, J. (1975). Cerebral oedema in diabetic ketoacidosis. *Brit. med. J.*, **iii**, 540.

64. Myschetzky, A. and Lassen, N. A. (1963). Osmotic diuresis and alkalinization of the urine in the treatment of severe acute barbiturate intoxication. *Dan. med. Bull.*, **10**, 104.

65. Myschetzky, A. and Lassen, N. A. (1963). Urea-induced, osmotic diuresis and alkalinisation of urine in acute barbiturate intoxication. *J. Amer. med. Assoc.*, **185**, 936.

66. Nabarro, J. D. N. (1962). Treatment of severe diabetic ketosis. *Disorders of Carbohydrate Metabolism*, Edited by D. A. Pyke. London: Pitman.

67. Neefe, J. R. (1946). Results of hepatic tests in chronic hepatitis without jaundice; correlation with the clinical course and liver biopsy findings. *Gastroenterology*, **7**, 1.

68. Neil, E. (1965). Biochemical disturbances as a cause of cardiac arrest. In *Resuscitation and cardiac pacing*, p. 41 Edited by G. Shaw, G. Smith and T. J. Thomson. London: Cassell.

69. Ohlsson, W. T. L. and Fristedt, B. I. (1962). Blood lavage in acute barbiturate poisoning: ten years' experience. *Lancet*, **ii**, 12.

70. Oliva, P. N. (1970). Lactic acidosis. *Amer. J. Med.*, **48**, 209.

71. Peters, H. (1857). Untersuchungen uber die honigharnruhr. *Prag. Vierteljahr*, **55**, 81.

72. Phear, E. A., Ruebner, B., Sherlock, S. and Summerskill, W. H. J. (1956). Methionine toxicity in liver disease and its prevention by chlortetracycline. *Clin. Sci.*, **15**, 93.

73. Phillips, G. B., Schwartz, R. Gabuzda, G. J. and Davidson, C. S. (1952). The syndrome of impending

hepatic coma in patients with cirrhosis of the liver given certain nitrogenous substances. *New Engl. J. of Med.*, **247**, 239.

74. Podolsky, S. and Pattavina, C. G. (1973). Hyperosmolar nonketotic diabetic coma. A complication of propranolol therapy. *Metabolism*, **22**, 685.

75. Reding, P., Duchateau, J. and Bataille, C. (1984). Oral zinc supplementation improves hepatic encephalopathy. Results of a randomised controlled trial. *Lancet*, **ii**, 493.

76. Reynolds, V. H. and Wilson, R. E. (1961). Absence of recurrent ammonia intoxication following right hemicolectomy with anastomosis of the superior mesenteric vein to the inferior vena cava. *Ann. Surg.*, **154**, 826.

77. Rosenberg, S. A., Brief, D. K., Kinney, J. M., Herrera, M. J., Wilson, R. E. and Moore, F. D. (1965). The syndrome of dehydration coma and severe hyperglycemia without ketosis in patients convalescing from burns. *N. Engl. J. of Med.*, **272**, 931.

78. Rosenbloom, J. (1915). A form of diabetic coma, not due to the acetone bodies. *N. Y. Med. J.*, **102**, 294.

79. Sament, S. and Schwartz, M. B. (1957). Severe diabetic stupor without ketosis. *S. Afr. Med. J.*, **31**, 893.

80. Sellards, A. W. (1914). A clinical method of studying titratable alkalinity of the blood and its application to acidosis. *Johns Hopkins Hosp. Bull.*, **25**, 101.

81. Stadelmann, E. (1883). Ueber die uraschen der pathologischen ammoniakausscheidung beim diabetes mellitus und des coma diabeticum. *Arch. f. exp. Pathol.*, **17**, 443.

82. Starr, P. and Fitz, R. (1924). The excretion of organic acids in the urine of patients with diabetes mellitus. *Arch. Int. Med.*, **33**, 177.

83. Stephens, J. M., Sulway, M. L. and Watkins, P. J. (1971). Relationship of blood acetoacetate and 3-hydroxy-butyrate in diabetes. *Diabetes*, **20**, 485.

84. Strangaard, S., Nielson, P. E. and Bitsch, V. (1971). Blood lactate and ketone bodies in diabetic ketoacidosis. *Acta. med. Scand.*, **190**, 17.

85. Sulway, M. J. and Malins, J. M. (1970). Acetone in diabetic ketoacidosis. *Lancet*, **ii**, 736.

86. Tranquada, R. E., Grant, W. J. and Peterson, C. R. (1966). Lactic acidosis. *Arch. Int. Med.*, **117**, 192.

87. Van Slyke, D. D. (1917) Studies of acidosis. II. A method for the determination of carbon dioxide and carbonates in solution. *J. Biol. Chem.*, **30**, 347.

88. Van Slyke, D. D. and Neil, J. M. (1924). The determination of gases in blood and other solutions by vacuum extraction and manometric measurement. I. *J. Biol. Chem.*, **61**, 523.

89. Van Slyke, D. D. and Palmer, W. W. (1920). Studies of acidosis. XVI. The titration of organic acids. *J. Biol. Chem.*, **41**, 567.

90. Von Frerichs, F. T. (1884). *Ueber den Diabetes*, p.113. Berlin: August Hirschwald.

91. Von Jaksch, W. (1885). *Ueber Acetonurie und Diaceturie.* Berlin: Hirschwald.

92. Von Noorden, C. (1895). Ueber die fruhdiagnose der zucerkrankheit. *Zschr. f. artztl. Lanpraxis*, **4**, 161.

93. Von Walter, F. (1877). Intersuchungen uber die wirkung der sauren auf den thierischen organismus. *Arch. f. exp. Path. u. Pharm.*, **7**, 148.

94. Waddell, W. J. and Butler, T. C. (1957). The distribution and excretion of phenobarbital. *J. clin. Invest.*, **36**, 1217.

95. Waldvogel, R. (1903). In *Die Acetonkorper*. Stuttgart: F. Enke.

96. Warburg, E. (1925). Some cases of diabetic coma complicated with uraemia and some remarks on the previous history of diabetic coma. *Acta. med. Scand.*, **61**, 301.

97. Watkins, P. J., Smith, J. S., Fitzgerald, M. G. and Malins, J. M. (1969). Lactic acidosis in diabetes. *Brit. med. J.*, **1**, 744.

98. Weiner, I. M., Washington, J. A. and Mudge, G. H. (1959). Studies on the renal excretion of salicylate in the dog. *Bull. Johns Hopk. Hosp.*, **105**, 284.

99. Whang, R. J. (1967). Hyperglycemic nonketotic coma induced by peritoneal dialysis. *Lancet*, **i**, 453.

100. Wilkinson, J. H. (1976). *The Principles and Practice of Diagnostic Enzymology*. London: Edward Arnold.

101. Williamson, R. T. (1898). *Diabetes Mellitus and its Treatment*, p.399. Edited by J. Young. Edinburgh and London: Pentland.

102. Willis, T. (1684). *Practice of Physick, Treatise II, Pharmaceutice Rationalis. 1st. pt*, p.74. London: Dring, Hayer and Leigh.

103. Wise, P. H., Chapman, M., Thomas, D. W., Clarkson, A. R., Harding, P. E. and Edwards, J. B. (1976). Phenformin and lactic acidosis. *Brit. med. J.*, **1**, 70.

104. Young, D. (1903). Diabetic coma treated by transfusion. *Brit. med. J.*, **1**, 544.

105. Young, E. and Bradléy, R. F. (1967). Cerebral edema with irreversible coma in severe diabetic ketoacidosis. *N. Engl. J. of Med.*, **276**, 665.

106. Zimmet, P. Z., Taft, P., Ennis, G. C. and Sheath, J. (1970). Acid production in diabetic ketoacidosis; a more rational approach to alkali replacement. *Brit. Med. J.*, **3**, 610.

Index

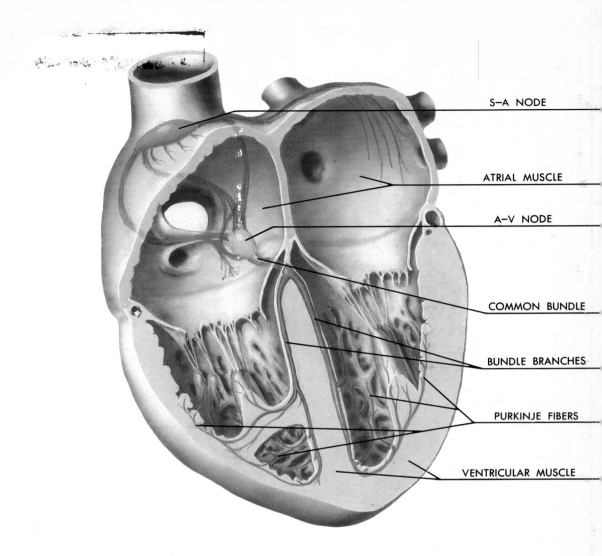

S-A NODE

ATRIAL MUSCLE

A-V NODE

COMMON BUNDLE

BUNDLE BRANCHES

PURKINJE FIBERS

VENTRICULAR MUSCLE

The heart uniquely combines three characteristics – automaticity, rhythmicity and contractility. This ability, which develops from a series of energy producing biochemical changes and the movement of at least three electrolytes, Na+, Ca++ and K+, through the cell wall, results in a series of action potentials that can be recorded at different sites within the heart.

This plate depicts the transmembrane potentials at different cardiac sites. It can be seen that these action potentials can be very different from that depicted on page 301 for ventricular muscle. For example, the action potential from the S-A node cell demonstrates two important differences: (1) the rate of rise of the upstroke of the action potential, phase 0, is low and is associated with the slow conduction of the impulse in the S-A node, and (2) a spontaneous, slow depolarization occurs so that there is no steady resting potential during phase 4. The slow spontaneous depolarization during phase 4, due to a shift in electrolyte through the membrane of the S-A node cell, is characteristic of automaticity in pacemaker cells.

Atrial muscle: The action potential recorded from an ordinary muscle fibre, demonstrates that the upstroke is rapid and the resting (phase 4) potential is steady and in this respect is similar to that of ventricular muscle.

Atrioventricular node: Action potentials recorded from fibres of the A-V node

demonstrate a low rate of rise. The extremely slow spread of the impulse through the A-V node results in the larger portion of the P-R interval. The depolarization in phase 4 results in automatic activity only in those fibres situated at the lower part of the node in close proximity to the common bundle.

His-Purkinje system (His bundles and Purkinje fibres): These action potentials recorded from the fibres of this part of the specialized conducting system have three important characteristics: (1) the rate of rise of the action potential is high and thus conduction is rapid; (2) the duration of the action potential is long and thus the refractory period is long; (3) under certain conditions this group of fibres may develop spontaneous phase 4 depolarization and become an automatic pacemaker (not shown), possibly due to pacemaker cells present within the fibres.

Ventricular muscle: The action potential which is described on page 301 illustrates the time of excitation and action potential duration for comparison with other records.

Sequence of excitation and the electrocardiogram: The seven tracings of transmembrane action potentials indicate the normal sequence of heart activation in relation to the schematic electrocardiogram shown below them. The colouring of the ECG trace suggests the temporal relationship of each